Carbon Ligands: From Fundamental Aspects to Applications

Carbon Ligands: From Fundamental Aspects to Applications

Editor

Yves Canac

MDPI • Basel • Beijing • Wuhan • Barcelona • Belgrade • Manchester • Tokyo • Cluj • Tianjin

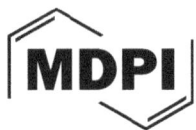

Editor
Yves Canac
LCC-CNRS
Université de Toulouse
Paul-Sabatier
Toulouse
France

Editorial Office
MDPI
St. Alban-Anlage 66
4052 Basel, Switzerland

This is a reprint of articles from the Special Issue published online in the open access journal *Molecules* (ISSN 1420-3049) (available at: www.mdpi.com/journal/molecules/special_issues/molecules_NovelElectronRichCarbonLigands).

For citation purposes, cite each article independently as indicated on the article page online and as indicated below:

LastName, A.A.; LastName, B.B.; LastName, C.C. Article Title. *Journal Name* **Year**, *Volume Number*, Page Range.

ISBN 978-3-0365-1350-8 (Hbk)
ISBN 978-3-0365-1349-2 (PDF)

© 2021 by the authors. Articles in this book are Open Access and distributed under the Creative Commons Attribution (CC BY) license, which allows users to download, copy and build upon published articles, as long as the author and publisher are properly credited, which ensures maximum dissemination and a wider impact of our publications.

The book as a whole is distributed by MDPI under the terms and conditions of the Creative Commons license CC BY-NC-ND.

Contents

Yves Canac
Carbon Ligands: From Fundamental Aspects to Applications
Reprinted from: *Molecules* 2021, 26, 2132, doi:10.3390/molecules26082132 1

Ronja Jordan and Doris Kunz
The Fascinating Flexibility and Coordination Modes of a Pentamethylene Connected Macrocyclic CNC Pincer Ligand
Reprinted from: *Molecules* 2021, 26, 1669, doi:10.3390/molecules26061669 5

Lakshmi Suresh, Ralte Lalrempuia, Jonas B. Ekeli, Francis Gillis-D'Hamers, Karl W. Törnroos, Vidar R. Jensen and Erwan Le Roux
Unsaturated and Benzannulated N-Heterocyclic Carbene Complexes of Titanium and Hafnium: Impact on Catalysts Structure and Performance in Copolymerization of Cyclohexene Oxide with CO_2
Reprinted from: *Molecules* 2020, 25, 4364, doi:10.3390/molecules25194364 17

Chandrakanta Dash, Animesh Das and H. V. Rasika Dias
Mercury(II) Complexes of Anionic N-Heterocyclic Carbene Ligands: Steric Effects of the Backbone Substituent
Reprinted from: *Molecules* 2020, 25, 3741, doi:10.3390/molecules25163741 39

Maura Pellei, Riccardo Vallesi, Luca Bagnarelli, H. V. Rasika Dias and Carlo Santini
Syntheses and Reactivity of New Zwitterionic Imidazolium Trihydridoborate and Triphenylborate Species
Reprinted from: *Molecules* 2020, 25, 3184, doi:10.3390/molecules25143184 49

Mathilde Bouché, Bruno Vincent, Thierry Achard and Stéphane Bellemin-Laponnaz
N-Heterocyclic Carbene Platinum(IV) as Metallodrug Candidates: Synthesis and ^{195}Pt NMR Chemical Shift Trend
Reprinted from: *Molecules* 2020, 25, 3148, doi:10.3390/molecules25143148 65

Manel Ouji, Guillaume Barnoin, Álvaro Fernández Álvarez, Jean-Michel Augereau, Catherine Hemmert, Françoise Benoit-Vical and Heinz Gornitzka
Hybrid Gold(I) NHC-Artemether Complexes to Target Falciparum Malaria Parasites
Reprinted from: *Molecules* 2020, 25, 2817, doi:10.3390/molecules25122817 75

Arnaud Peramo, Ibrahim Abdellah, Shannon Pecnard, Julie Mougin, Cyril Martini, Patrick Couvreur, Vincent Huc and Didier Desmaële
A Self-Assembling NHC-Pd-Loaded Calixarene as a Potent Catalyst for the Suzuki-Miyaura Cross-Coupling Reaction in Water
Reprinted from: *Molecules* 2020, 25, 1459, doi:10.3390/molecules25061459 95

Michał Pieczykolan, Justyna Czaban-Jóźwiak, Maura Malinska, Krzysztof Woźniak, Reto Dorta, Anna Rybicka, Anna Kajetanowicz and Karol Grela
The Influence of Various N-Heterocyclic Carbene Ligands on Activity of Nitro-Activated Olefin Metathesis Catalysts
Reprinted from: *Molecules* 2020, 25, 2282, doi:10.3390/molecules25102282 109

Rachid Taakili and Yves Canac
NHC Core Pincer Ligands Exhibiting Two Anionic Coordinating Extremities
Reprinted from: *Molecules* 2020, 25, 2231, doi:10.3390/molecules25092231 129

Henning Steinert, Christopher Schwarz, Alexander Kroll and Viktoria H. Gessner
Towards the Preparation of Stable Cyclic Amino(ylide)Carbenes
Reprinted from: *Molecules* **2020**, *25*, 796, doi:10.3390/molecules25040796 149

Ugo Authesserre, Sophie Hameury, Aymeric Dajnak, Nathalie Saffon-Merceron, Antoine Baceiredo, David Madec and Eddy Maerten
Complexes of Dichlorogermylene with Phosphine/Sulfoxide-Supported Carbone as Ligand
Reprinted from: *Molecules* **2021**, *26*, 2005, doi:10.3390/molecules26072005 161

Marius Klein, Nemrud Demirel, Alexander Schinabeck, Hartmut Yersin and Jörg Sundermeyer
Cu(I) Complexes of Multidentate *N,C,N*- and *P,C,P*-Carbodiphosphorane Ligands and Their Photoluminescence
Reprinted from: *Molecules* **2020**, *25*, 3990, doi:10.3390/molecules25173990 171

Lili Zhao, Chaoqun Chai, Wolfgang Petz and Gernot Frenking
Carbones and Carbon Atom as Ligands in Transition Metal Complexes
Reprinted from: *Molecules* **2020**, *25*, 4943, doi:10.3390/molecules25214943 187

Józef Drabowicz, Aneta Rzewnicka and Remigiusz Żurawiński
Selenonium Ylides: Syntheses, Structural Aspects, and Synthetic Applications
Reprinted from: *Molecules* **2020**, *25*, 2420, doi:10.3390/molecules25102420 235

Jan Bloch, Stefan Kradolfer, Thomas L. Gianetti, Detlev Ostendorf, Subal Dey, Victor Mougel and Hansjörg Grützmacher
Synthesis and Characterization of Ion Pairs between Alkaline Metal Ions and Anionic Anti-Aromatic and Aromatic Hydrocarbons with -Conjugated Central Seven- and Eight-Membered Rings
Reprinted from: *Molecules* **2020**, *25*, 4742, doi:10.3390/molecules25204742 281

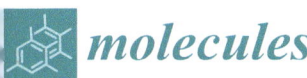

Editorial

Carbon Ligands: From Fundamental Aspects to Applications

Yves Canac

LCC–CNRS, Université de Toulouse, CNRS, UPS, CEDEX 4, 31077 Toulouse, France; yves.canac@lcc-toulouse.fr

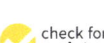

Citation: Canac, Y. Carbon Ligands: From Fundamental Aspects to Applications. *Molecules* **2021**, *26*, 2132. https://doi.org/10.3390/molecules26082132

Received: 1 April 2021
Accepted: 6 April 2021
Published: 8 April 2021

Publisher's Note: MDPI stays neutral with regard to jurisdictional claims in published maps and institutional affiliations.

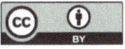

Copyright: © 2021 by the author. Licensee MDPI, Basel, Switzerland. This article is an open access article distributed under the terms and conditions of the Creative Commons Attribution (CC BY) license (https://creativecommons.org/licenses/by/4.0/).

Ligand design is at the forefront of many advances in various areas of chemistry such as organometallic chemistry, functional materials, and homogeneous catalysis. Faced with these challenges, the development of ligands has long been centered on elements of group 15 (N, P), and it is only more recently that carbon ligands have proven to be valuable alternatives. The predominance of N- and P-based ligands for many years was due to their high stability, as opposed to carbon ligands, which were supposed to be highly sensitive and reactive. The isolation of the first stable carbenes, namely, a phosphino(silyl)carbene by Bertrand et al. in 1988 [1], followed a few years later by the famous *N*-heterocyclic carbenes (NHCs) by Arduengo and co-workers [2] proved thus to be a trigger in the minds of chemists, leading very quickly to remarkable advances in both fundamental and applied fields of chemistry. However, if the advent of carbenes was a decisive factor, other carbon ligands demonstrated also their potential as Lewis bases in the activation of inert bonds, coordination chemistry, and homogeneous catalysis. Indeed, one must also mention the huge contribution of Schmidbaur in the chemistry of P-ylides which brought these carbon species to light [3]. Later on, different carbon ligands were developed based on a C-sp^2 coordinating carbon atom similar to NHCs or, alternatively, on a C-sp^3 coordinating carbon atom similar to phosphonium ylides. In the first category, we can mention the more recently reported cyclic alkylamino carbenes (CAACs) where one of the stabilizing N-atoms adjacent to the carbenic center is substituted by a quaternary carbon atom [4], and in the second category all other onium ylides in which the positively charged heteroatom is an N, As, S, or Se atom [5] without forgetting the N-heterocyclic olefins (NHOs) where the exocyclic ylidic carbon atom is stabilized by an imidazolium moiety [6]. Following Ramirez's pioneering report on carbodiphosphoranes [7], bis-ylide species also named carbones [8], which behave like strong σ- and π-donor carbon ligands due to the presence of two lone pairs at the central carbon atom, have also recently experienced a renewed interest in coordination chemistry with applications in catalysis [9]. While all the carbon ligands cited so far have the common feature of being globally neutral in their free state, anionic carbon ligands likewise play a fundamental role in modern chemistry. Both NHCs and ylides can be thus made anionic by deprotonation to form metalated dicarbenes and ylides which correspond to ditopic anionic NHCs [10] and yldiides [11], respectively. In these species, the introduction of a negative charge modifies the electronic properties resulting in an enhancement of the nucleophilicity with repercussions, in particular, in catalysis. Other anionic carbon ligands exhibiting alkyl, alkenyl, alkynyl, allyl, aryl, or cyclopentadienyl-based backbones differing in the hybridization state and the number of coordinating carbon atoms were also widely considered over the years from fundamental aspects to applications.

In this *Special Issue*, the majority of the different types of carbon ligands mentioned above have been gathered together. The NHCs which constitute the most developed family of neutral carbon ligands have been approached from two main directions by the different contributors, namely, from a synthetic point of view with the preparation of new carbenic structures, and for their applications either in catalysis or in biology. In the first direction, while Kunz et al. described the fascinating coordination chemistry of a strongly donor macrocyclic *C,N,C*-pincer ligand exhibiting pentamethylene tethered

NHC donor ends [12], Dias et al. were interested in the design of Hg(II) complexes bearing anionic maloNHC ligands [13], and Santini et al. in the chemistry of zwitterionic imidazolium borate species [14]. Regarding catalytic applications, Grela et al. reported the preparation of a family of nitro-activated Ru(II)-based olefin metathesis catalysts while evaluating the influence of the NHC ligand [15]. Huc et al. demonstrated that benzyloxycalix arene supported NHC-Pd(II) complexes were active for the Suzuki–Miyaura cross-coupling reaction in water [16], and Le Roux et al. focused on the preparation of Ti(IV) and Hf(IV) complexes containing tridentate bis-phenolate NHC core ligands for the copolymerization of cyclohexene oxide with CO_2 [17]. For biological purposes, Bellemin-Laponnaz et al. synthetized a series of Pt(IV) NHC complexes and studied their cytotoxicity against different cancer cell lines [18], and Gornitzka et al. prepared Au(I) NHC-artemether complexes to assess their antiplasmodial activity and cytotoxicity against mammalian cells [19]. Finally, in this category of sp^2-carbon ligands, the chemistry of NHC core pincer ligands bearing two anionic coordinating ends, especially phosphonium ylide moieties, was reviewed by us [20].

As a formal link between the two categories of neutral carbon ligands of interest, Gessner et al. reported a joint experimental and theoretical study on cyclic amino(ylide) carbenes based on pyrrole and trialkyl onium fragments where the carbenic center is expected to be stabilized by the strongly donating ylide substituent [21]. Bis-ylides were also considered, on the one hand by Sundermeyer et al. through the preparation of photoluminescent Cu(I) complexes of P,C,P-carbodiphosphorane-based ligands [22], and on the other hand by Maerten et al. with the coordinating behavior of phosphine-sulfoxide substituted carbones towards dichlorogermylene [23]. Those carbones, as well as carbido complexes featuring a naked carbon atom, were reviewed by Frenking et al. [24]. In the same family of carbon species characterized by the presence of a sp^3-carbon atom, selenonium ylides were described from synthetic and structural aspects to synthetic applications by Drabowicz et al. [25]. Anionic carbon ligands were also of primary interest in this issue, as illustrated with the report by Grützmacher et al. of alkaline metal salts based on trop (C_5H_{11}) and dbcot ($C_{16}H_{12}$) moieties and the characterization of a d^8-Rh(I) complex of the anionic trop ligand [26].

Funding: This research received no external funding.

Acknowledgments: The guest editor would like to thank all the authors that have contributed to this special issue and all the reviewers for the evaluation of the submitted articles.

Conflicts of Interest: The author declares no conflict of interest.

References

1. Igau, A.; Grutzmacher, H.; Baceiredo, A.; Bertrand, G. Analogous α, α′-bis-carbenoid triply bonded species: Synthesis of a stable $λ^3$-phosphinocarbene-$λ^5$-phosphaacetylene. *J. Am. Chem. Soc.* **1988**, *110*, 6463. [CrossRef]
2. Arduengo III, A.J.; Harlow, R.L.; Kline, M. A stable crystalline carbene. *J. Am. Chem. Soc.* **1991**, *113*, 361. [CrossRef]
3. Schmidbaur, H. Phosphorus ylides in the coordination sphere of transition metals: An inventory. *Angew. Chem. Int. Ed. Engl.* **1983**, *22*, 907. [CrossRef]
4. Lavallo, V.; Canac, Y.; Präsang, C.; Donnadieu, B.; Bertrand, G. Stable cyclic (alkyl)(amino)carbenes as rigid or flexible, bulky, electron-rich ligands for transition-metal catalysts: A quaternary carbon atom makes the difference. *Angew. Chem. Int. Ed. Engl.* **2005**, *44*, 5705. [CrossRef]
5. Urriolabeitia, E.P. Ylide ligands. In *Topics in Organometallic Chemistry*; Chauvin, R., Canac, Y., Eds.; Springer: Berlin/Heidelberg, Germany, 2010; Volume 30, p. 15.
6. Kuhn, N.; Bohnen, H.; Kreutzberg, J.; Bläser, D.; Boese, R. 1,3,4,5-tetramethyl-2-methyleneimidazoline—An ylidic olefin. *J. Chem. Soc. Chem. Com.* **1993**, *14*, 1136. [CrossRef]
7. Ramirez, F.; Desai, N.B.; Hansen, B.; McKelvie, N. Hexaphenylcarbodiphosphorane, $(C_6H_5)_3PCP(C_6H_5)_3$. *J. Am. Chem. Soc.* **1961**, *83*, 3539. [CrossRef]
8. Tonner, R.; Öxler, F.; Neumüller, B.; Petz, W.; Frenking, G. Carbodiphosphoranes: The chemistry of divalent carbon(0). *Angew. Chem. Int. Ed.* **2006**, *45*, 8038. [CrossRef] [PubMed]
9. Marcum, J.S.; Roberts, C.C.; Manan, R.S.; Cervarich, T.N.; Meek, S.J. Chiral pincer carbodicarbene ligands for enantioselective rhodium-catalyzed hydroarylation of terminal and internal 1,3-dienes with indoles. *J. Am. Chem. Soc.* **2017**, *139*, 15580. [CrossRef]

10. Wang, Y.; Xie, Y.; Abraham, M.Y.; Wei, P.; Schaefer III, H.F.; Schleyer, P.v.R.; Robinson, G.H. A viable anionic N-Heterocyclic dicarbene. *J. Am. Chem. Soc.* **2010**, *132*, 14370. [CrossRef] [PubMed]
11. Bestmann, H.J.; Schmidt, M. Synthesis of nitriles via the ylide anion of sodium cyanotriphenylphosphoranylidenemethanide. *Angew. Chem. Int. Ed. Engl.* **1987**, *26*, 79. [CrossRef]
12. Jordan, R.; Kunz, D. The fascinating flexibility and coordination modes of a pentamethylene connected macrocyclic CNC pincer ligand. *Molecules* **2021**, *26*, 1669. [CrossRef]
13. Dash, C.; Das, A.; Rasika Dias, H.V. Mercury(II) complexes of anionic N-heterocyclic carbene ligands: Steric effects on the backbone substituent. *Molecules* **2020**, *25*, 3741. [CrossRef] [PubMed]
14. Pellei, M.; Vallesi, R.; Bagnarelli, L.; Rasika Dias, H.V.; Santini, C. Syntheses and reactivity of new zwitterionic imidazolium trihydridoborate and triphenylborate species. *Molecules* **2020**, *25*, 3184. [CrossRef] [PubMed]
15. Pieczykolan, M.; Czaban-Jóźwiak, J.; Malinska, M.; Wozniak, K.; Dorta, R.; Rybicka, A.; Kajetanowicz, A.; Grela, K. The influence of various *N*-heteterocyclic carbene ligands on activity of nitro-activated olefin metathesis catalysts. *Molecules* **2020**, *25*, 2282. [CrossRef] [PubMed]
16. Peramo, A.; Abdellah, I.; Pecnard, S.; Mougin, J.; Martini, C.; Couvreur, P.; Huc, V.; Desmaële, D. A self-assembling NHC-Pd-loaded calixarene as a potent catalyst for the Suzuki-Miyaura cross-coupling reaction in water. *Molecules* **2020**, *25*, 1459. [CrossRef]
17. Suresh, L.; Lalrempuia, R.; Ekeli, J.B.; Gillis-D'Hamers, F.; Törnroos, K.W.; Jensen, V.R.; Le Roux, E. Unsaturated and benzannulated *N*-heterocyclic carbene complexes of titanium and hafnium: Impact on catalysts structure and performance in copolymerization of cyclohexene oxide with CO_2. *Molecules* **2020**, *25*, 4364. [CrossRef]
18. Bouché, M.; Vincent, B.; Achard, T.; Bellemin-Laponnaz, S. *N*-heterocyclic carbene platinum(IV) as metallodrug candidates: Synthesis and ^{195}Pt NMR chemical shift trend. *Molecules* **2020**, *25*, 3148. [CrossRef]
19. Ouji, M.; Barnouin, G.; Álvarez, A.F.; Augereau, J.M.; Hemmert, C.; Benoit-Vical, F.; Gornitzka, H. Hybrid gold(I) NHC-artemether complexes to target falciparum malaria parasites. *Molecules* **2020**, *25*, 2817. [CrossRef]
20. Taakili, R.; Canac, Y. NHC core pincer ligands exhibiting two anionic coordinating extremities. *Molecules* **2020**, *25*, 2231. [CrossRef]
21. Steinert, H.; Schwarz, C.; Kroll, A.; Gessner, V.H. Towards the preparation of stable cyclic amino(ylide)carbenes. *Molecules* **2020**, *25*, 796. [CrossRef]
22. Klein, M.; Demirel, N.; Schinabeck, A.; Yersin, H.; Sundermeyer, J. Cu(I) complexes of multidentate *N,C,N*- and *P,C,P*-carbodiphosphorane ligands and their photoluminescence. *Molecules* **2020**, *25*, 3990. [CrossRef]
23. Authesserre, U.; Hameury, S.; Dajnak, A.; Saffon-Merceron, N.; Baceiredo, A.; Madec, D.; Maerten, E. Complexes of dichlorogermylene with phosphine/sulfoxide-supported carbone as ligand. *Molecules* **2021**, *26*, 2005. [CrossRef]
24. Zhao, L.; Chai, C.; Petz, W.; Frenking, G. Carbones and carbon atom as ligands in transition metal complexes. *Molecules* **2020**, *25*, 4943. [CrossRef]
25. Drabowicz, J.; Rzewnicka, A.; Zurawinski, R. Selenonium ylides: Syntheses, structural aspects, and synthetic applications. *Molecules* **2020**, *25*, 2420. [CrossRef] [PubMed]
26. Bloch, J.; Kradolfer, S.; Gianetti, T.L.; Ostendorf, D.; Dey, S.; Mougel, V.; Grützmacher, H. Synthesis and characterization of ion pairs between alkaline metal ions and anionic anti-aromatic and aromatic hydrocarbons with π-conjugated central seven- and eight-membered rings. *Molecules* **2020**, *25*, 4742. [CrossRef] [PubMed]

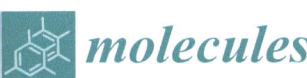 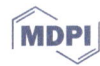

Article

The Fascinating Flexibility and Coordination Modes of a Pentamethylene Connected Macrocyclic CNC Pincer Ligand

Ronja Jordan and Doris Kunz *

Institut für Anorganische Chemie, Eberhard Karls Universität Tübingen, D-72076 Tübingen, Germany; Ronja.Jordan@uni-tuebingen.de
* Correspondence: Doris.Kunz@uni-tuebingen.de; Tel.: +49-7071-29-72063

Abstract: The coordination chemistry of an electron-rich macrocyclic CNC pincer-ligand consisting of two pentamethylene tethered N-heterocyclic carbene moieties on a carbazole backbone (bimca^{C5}) is investigated by mainly NMR spectroscopy and X-ray crystal structure analysis. A bridging coordination mode is found for the lithium complex. With the larger and softer potassium ion, the ligand adopts a facial coordination mode and a polymeric structure by intermolecular potassium nitrogen interactions. The facial coordination is also confirmed at a Cp*Ru fragment, while C-H activation under dehydrogenation at the alkyl chain is observed upon reaction with [Ru(PPh$_3$)$_3$Cl$_2$]. In contrast, Pd(OAc)$_2$ reacts under C-H activation at the central carbon atom of the pentamethylene tether to an alkyl-pincer macrocycle.

Keywords: pincer ligand; macrocycle; N-heterocyclic carbene; lithium; potassium; ruthenium; intramolecular C-H activation; dehydrogenation

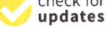

Citation: Jordan, R.; Kunz, D. The Fascinating Flexibility and Coordination Modes of a Pentamethylene Connected Macrocyclic CNC Pincer Ligand. *Molecules* **2021**, *26*, 1669. https://doi.org/10.3390/molecules26061669

Academic Editor: Yves Canac

Received: 26 February 2021
Accepted: 15 March 2021
Published: 17 March 2021

Publisher's Note: MDPI stays neutral with regard to jurisdictional claims in published maps and institutional affiliations.

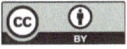

Copyright: © 2021 by the authors. Licensee MDPI, Basel, Switzerland. This article is an open access article distributed under the terms and conditions of the Creative Commons Attribution (CC BY) license (https://creativecommons.org/licenses/by/4.0/).

1. Introduction

Pincer-ligands, whose wingtips are tethered with simple or unfunctionalized hydrocarbon chains, are still very rare and an exception among phosphine pincer complexes [1,2]. For geometric reasons, bis(N-heterocyclic carbene) pincer ligands are more suitable for tethering. Notably, Chaplin and coworkers showed very interesting examples of macrocyclic CNC ligands that contain alkyl tethers between 8 and 16 C-atoms [3–5]. Their transition metal complexes showed particular properties depending on the ring size [6–8], but no reactivity at the tether itself.

Tethered CNC pincer complexes with smaller ring sizes are scarce [9], although potential ligand precursors are well known [10–14]. The interaction with the metal center should become stronger and influence its reactivity by steric restrictions.

When we reported on the improved synthesis of the so-called bimca ligand [15] (1,8-bis(imidazolin-2-ylidene)-3,8-di-*tert*-butylcarbazolide), a monoanionic CNC ligand, we also showed that a still relatively concentrated reaction mixture of 1,8-bis(imidazol-1-yl)-3,8-di-*tert*-butylcarbazol and 1,5-dibromopentane leads selectively to the bisimidazolium macrocycle **1a** (Hbimca^{C5})·2HBr [13]. However, until now, the coordination chemistry of this proligand remained unexplored. In the following, we will show that the tether leads not only to still unprecedented binding modes of the bimca ligand with alkali metals and to a suitable ligand for the facial coordination mode of the all sp^2-hybridized framework, but that the proximity of the pentamethylene chain can also induce intramolecular C-H activation resulting in either dehydrogenation to an olefinic or formation of a carbanionic donor site.

2. Results and Discussion

2.1. Alkali Metal bimca^{C5} Complexes

The first step of the synthesis of metal complexes is the generation of the monoanionic carbene ligand bimca^{C5} with 3 equiv. of a strong base, preferably an alkali metal base.

As the N-H moiety is more acidic than the two imidazolium moieties, the independent generation of only the carbene moieties is not possible.

After combining the proligand **1b** with 3.5 equiv. of Li(N(SiMe$_3$)$_2$) in tetrahydrofuran, the successful formation of the desired lithium-pincer complex **2** (Scheme 1) can be optically recognized by the yellow color of the solution that shows a blue fluorescence at λ = 460 nm under UV light (330 nm), as has been observed qualitatively for the [Li(bimca^{Me})] complex before [15]. In the ^{1}H NMR spectrum (THF-d$_8$), the absence of the N-H and imidazolium C-H signals indicates full deprotonation, and thus, generation of the carbene moieties. In the ^{13}C NMR spectrum, the carbene signal of the free NHC moiety would be expected at around 215 ppm. In our case, the signal at 204.5 ppm is characteristic for a coordination of the carbene moiety to lithium ions as it has been reported for other Li(bimca) complexes [13]. However, typically, the carbene signals of lithium complexes are shifted by about 20 ppm to higher field compared to the respective free carbenes. The carbene signal shows no direct ^{13}C-^{7}Li coupling, and in the ^{7}Li NMR spectrum, only one broad signal at 0.31 ppm is observed at room temperature, which indicates a fast exchange of the lithium ions between the complex and solvated Li$^+$ in solution on the NMR timescale. We had to cool the sample down to $-110\,^\circ$C to determine the coupling constant $^1J_{CLi}$ of about 24 Hz from the satellites of the Li signal at 2.06 ppm, which is separated at this temperature from the [Li(THF)$_n$]$^+$ signal at 0.65 ppm. At room temperature, the ^{1}H NMR spectrum shows 3 signals in a 2:2:1 ratio for the methylene protons, which indicates fast conformational interconversion of the axial and equatorial ring protons. At $-90\,^\circ$C, two separate signals for the axial and equatorial protons of the N-CH$_2$ moiety can be observed.

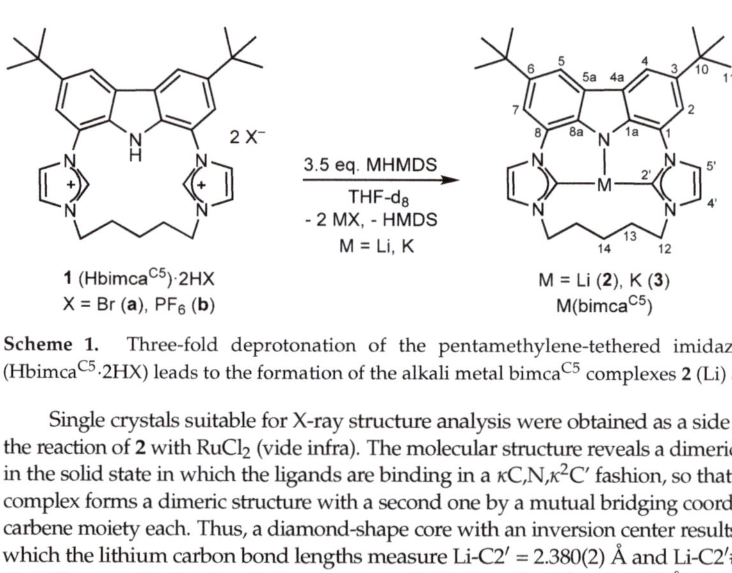

Scheme 1. Three-fold deprotonation of the pentamethylene-tethered imidazolium salts **1** (Hbimca^{C5}·2HX) leads to the formation of the alkali metal bimca^{C5} complexes **2** (Li) and **3** (K).

Single crystals suitable for X-ray structure analysis were obtained as a side product from the reaction of **2** with RuCl$_2$ (vide infra). The molecular structure reveals a dimeric arrangement in the solid state in which the ligands are binding in a κC,N,κ^2C' fashion, so that one Li-pincer complex forms a dimeric structure with a second one by a mutual bridging coordination of one carbene moiety each. Thus, a diamond-shape core with an inversion center results (Figure 1), in which the lithium carbon bond lengths measure Li-C2' = 2.380(2) Å and Li-C2'# = 2.257(4) Å. The other coordinating bonds are pronouncedly shorter (Li-C7' = 2.141(8) Å, Li-N = 1.965(5) Å). The formation of bridging Li(NHC) complexes with constrained geometry Cp-ligands has been recognized before [16].

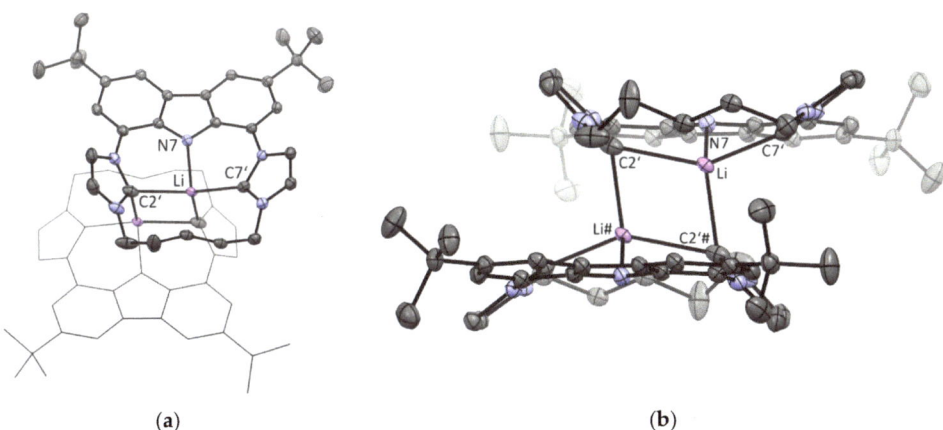

Figure 1. ORTEP-style plot of the molecular structure of [Li(bimca^{C5})] (**2**) in the solid state (anisotropic atomic displacement parameters at the 50% probability level). Hydrogen atoms are omitted for clarity. Multiple disordered solvent was removed applying the SQUEEZE routine. (**a**) Top view; the wireframe style of the symmetry equivalent lower part is used for clarity; (**b**) side view.

It can be excluded that this dimeric structure is the prevailing structure in a solution in tetrahydrofuran, as it has a lower symmetry and would give rise to eight signals in the aromatic region of the ^{1}H NMR spectrum, which is not observed.

Crystallographically characterized lithium complexes with NHC pincer or tripodal NHC complexes are very rare [17]. Due to the preferred tetrahedral coordination sphere as well as the small ion radius of the lithium ion, a symmetric T-shape pincer coordination seems not favorable. To probe whether larger alkali metal ions lead to the typical meridional coordination of the bimca ligand, we deprotonated the proligand **1** with 3 equiv. of KHMDS (potassium hexamethyldisilylamide) in THF-d_8. The blue fluorescence indicates full deprotonation, but vanishes upon darkening of the solution and precipitation of the complex **3**. Nevertheless, NMR spectra could be obtained from the diluted solution. The ^{1}H NMR spectrum shows the signal pattern of a symmetric complex and fast conformational changes in the alkyl chain. The four aromatic signals are upfield-shifted in comparison to lithium complex **2**, especially the signals of the imidazole backbone. This can be explained with the reduced Lewis-acidity of the potassium ion [18–21]. The reduced influence of the Lewis acid is also reflected in the upfield shift of the methylene signals H-12 and H-13 of the dangling alkyl tether, while the signal of H-14 is not affected. In the ^{13}C NMR spectrum, the carbene signal at 213.1 ppm lies very close to that of a comparable free carbene (~215 ppm) [19], which confirms the very weak binding of the potassium ion. From the filtrate we obtained small crystals that were subjected to X-ray structure analysis. The limited quality of the data due to multiple twinning and inclusion of powder in the crystal allows no discussion of bond lengths and angles, but the results confirm unambiguously the coordination mode of the ligand (Figure 2). The potassium is coordinated by five donor atoms. The bimca^{C5} ligand coordinates in a facial manner instead of the typical meridional pincer fashion. The nitrogen donor is not coordinating within the carbazole plane, but the potassium is oriented almost perpendicular to the plane. The carbazole nitrogen coordinates to the potassium center of the next complex monomer, which is oriented by a rotation of 180°, thus forming a polymeric structure along this two-fold axis with almost equidistant K-N bonds (3.0 Å) in a zig-zag fashion. The fifth coordination site is occupied by tetrahydrofuran.

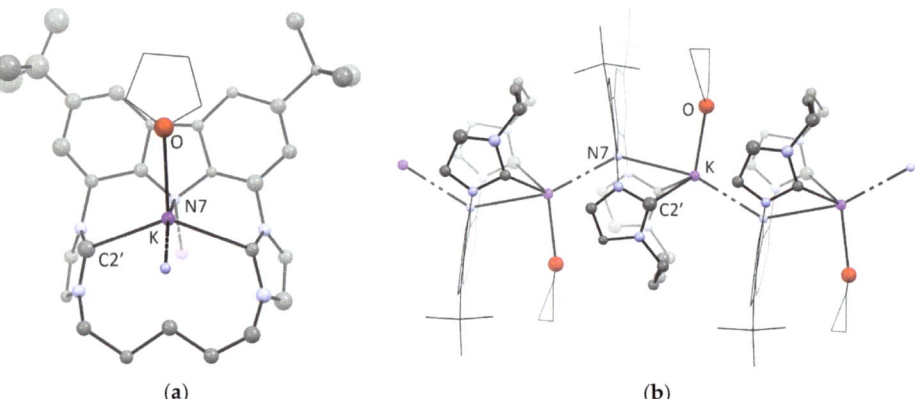

Figure 2. Two views of the isotropically refined structure of complex [K(bimca^{C5})] (**3**). For clarity, the wireframe style is used for the coordinated THF and the bimca framework where suitable. Co-crystallized solvent and hydrogen atoms have been omitted for clarity: (**a**) view along the two-fold axis polymer chain with one monomer depicted; (**b**) side view of the coordination polymer. The K(bimca^{C5})(THF) moieties are additionally coordinated by the carbazole nitrogen atom of the next complex that is rotated by 180° in a zig-zag fashion, thus forming a coordination polymer along a two-fold axis.

2.2. Ruthenium(II) bimca^{C5} Complexes

2.2.1. Facial Coordination of the bimca^{C5} Ligand

The facial coordination mode is untypical for fully sp^2 hybridized pincer ligands. An anionic CNP pincer ligand was reported to form a dimeric facially coordinated potassium complex in the solid state [22]. A dimeric K[Pd(bimca^{Me})] complex shows additional facial coordination to the potassium counterion [23].

We had shown earlier that the *N*-homoallyl substituted bimca ligand bimca^{Homo} is able to coordinate in a facial mode when the in situ-generated [Li(bimca^{Homo})] is reacted with [Ru (NCCH$_3$)$_3$Cp*]PF$_6$ [24]. The macrocyclic ligand bimca^{C5} should be even more suitable for this purpose due to the C5-tether. Therefore, we reacted [Li(bimca^{C5})] (**2**) with the ruthenium precursor and obtained the desired product complex **4** in 84% yield as a red solid (Scheme 2).

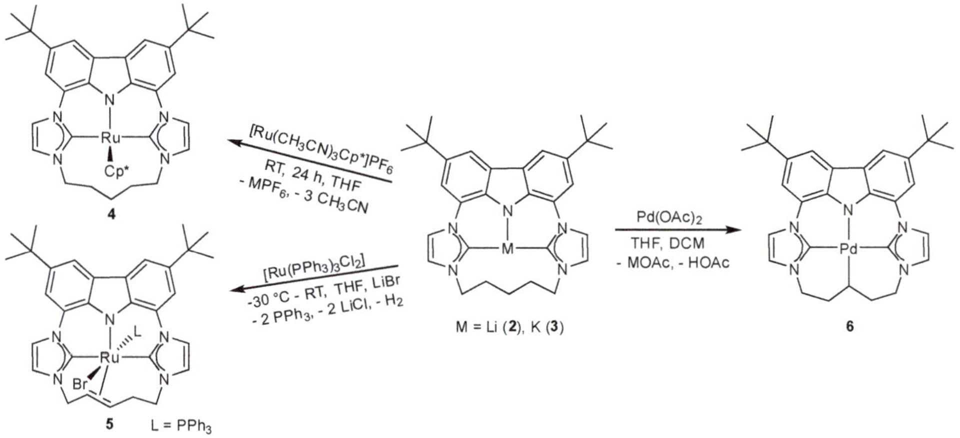

Scheme 2. Formation of Ru(II) and Pd(II) complexes with different coordination modes of the bimca^{C5} ligand from the in situ-generated alkali metal complexes **2** (Li) and **3** (K).

In the ^{1}H NMR spectrum, the four signals of the aromatic bimca protons indicate a C_s symmetry. With the help of 2D NMR spectra, including an NOE experiment as well as comparing the coupling constants with a DFT-optimized structure (which is almost identical to the molecular structure obtained by X-ray structure analysis (vide infra)), the six signals of the diastereotopic methylene protons can be assigned. The chemical shift difference between the signals of those protons pointing towards the metal center vs. those pointing away amounts to $\Delta\delta = 1.5$ ppm in case of the NCH$_2$ signals (H-12) and still $\Delta\delta = 1.0$ ppm for those of H-14 (Figure 3a). As anagostic interactions can be excluded due to the long H···Ru distances (>2.9 Å) [25], this can be explained with the magnetic effect of the metal.

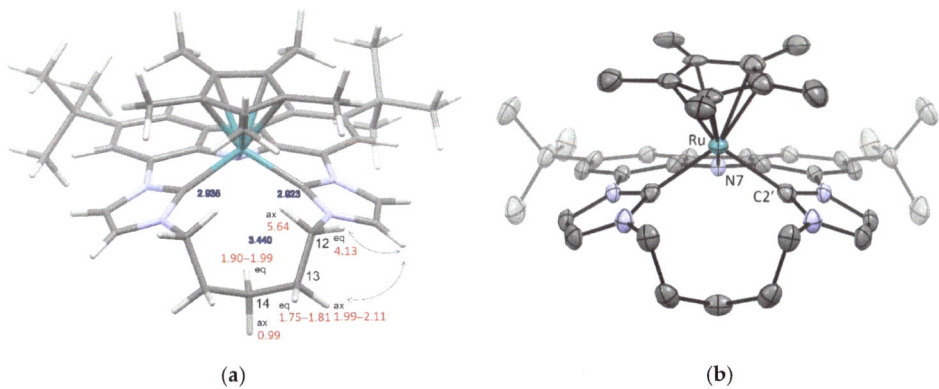

Figure 3. Molecular structure of complex **4**. (**a**) DFT-optimized structure showing the chemical shifts of the methylene signals (red) and important NOE cross peaks (black arrow) as well as the distance between the metal and close hydrogen atoms (blue); (**b**) ORTEP-style plot of the molecular structure of complex **4** (anisotropic atomic displacement parameters at the 50% probability level). Hydrogen atoms are omitted for clarity. The Cp* ligand is highly disordered.

From a concentrated solution of **4** in THF/diethylether at room temperature, red plates were obtained that were suitable for X-ray single crystal structure analysis. The facial binding mode of the bimca^{C5} ligand is confirmed (Figure 3b) and the overall geometry is similar to that reported for the bimca^{Homo} analogue [24]. The Ru atom is located 1.135 Å over the plane spanned by the donating carbene and carbazole nitrogen atoms.

The macrocyclic ligand should be ideal to avoid the formation of octahedral complexes with two meridionally coordinating pincer ligands, which is typically observed when reacting monoanionic pincer ligands with RuCl$_2$ or with FeCl$_2$ or IrCl(PPh$_3$)$_3$ under oxidation [26]. We also tried to obtain the ruthenocene analogue Ru(bimca^{C5})$_2$ with two facially coordinating bimca^{C5} ligands instead of one and one Cp* ligand, but reacting [Li(bimca^{C5})] with RuCl$_2$ did not result in a defined compound.

2.2.2. Complex Formation under Dehydrogenation of bimca^{C5}

When we reacted [Ru(PPh$_3$)$_3$Cl$_2$] with a freshly prepared solution of the potassium complex **3** in THF at −30 °C, red crystals formed after 24 h (Scheme 2). The product is only poorly soluble in THF, slightly soluble in dichloromethane, soluble in methanol and decomposes in DMSO. In the ^{1}H NMR spectrum the signal pattern indicates a mixture of at least two asymmetric complexes in a 1:0.4 ratio. The two multiplets at 5.20–5.27 (H-14) and 5.07–5.10 ppm (H-13) indicate the formation of a double bond, which is corroborated by the respective ^{13}C NMR signals at 81.6 (C13) and 88.4 (C14). All remaining signals in the alkyl region can be assigned to the six non-equivalent hydrogen atoms as well as the carbon signals by means of ^{1}H,^{13}C correlation spectroscopy and NOE experiments. Therefore, a dehydrogenation under C-H activation must have occurred so that complex **5** is the final reaction product. The formation of H$_2$ is not observed in the ^{1}H NMR spectrum; however, this might be the case due to its volatility. In methanol, a qualitative similar ^{1}H NMR spectrum is obtained. The peaks of the second isomer are partly covered by those of the main isomer. In the ^{31}P NMR spectrum two very close peaks at 64.3 and 67.8 ppm indicate the presence of two isomers of complex **5** with a similar constitution. The formation of a carbene complex by double C-H activation at the central carbon atom C14, as was observed with a pentenyldiphosphine ruthenium complex by Gusev in low amounts [27], was not observed in our case.

The red crystals were suitable for X-ray structure analysis. The molecular structure is depicted in Figure 4 and confirms the formation of a double bond that is coordinated to the Ru center at a distance of 2.208 (Ru-C13) and 2.284 Å (Ru-C14). A disorder in the alkyl chain prevents the discussion of C-C bond lengths. The Ru-Carbene bonds and the Ru-N bond are in a typical range. Due to the octahedral coordination mode and the non-symmetric dehydrogenated C5 chain, it becomes apparent that the other isomer could be the diastereomer obtained by inversion of the phosphine and bromido ligand.

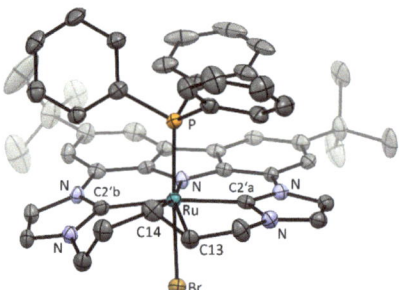

Figure 4. ORTEP-style plot of the molecular structure of complex [Ru(bimca^{C5H8})Br(PPh$_3$)] (**5**) (anisotropic atomic displacement parameters at the 50% probability level). Hydrogen atoms and two molecules of dichloromethane are omitted for clarity.

While C-H activation of arenes by Ru complexes is well established since its first mentioning by Chatt in 1962 [28,29] and the successive developments based on the Murai reaction [30–32], the inter- and intramolecular C-H activation of alkanes by Ru complexes is still rare [26,27]. The first observed cyclometallation was reported by Chatt from a Ru(0) intermediate in 1965 [29,33]. In the past few years, the dehydrogenation of alkanes by a Ru(0) catalyst was reported by Goldman [34] as well as its acceptorless variant with Ru(II) pincer catalysts by Roddick and Huang [35,36].

2.3. A macrocyclic Palladium(II) bimca^{C5} Complex by C-H Activation

To probe on a small scale whether Pd(II), which usually forms square planar complexes, is also suitable for an intramolecular C-H activation at room temperature, we reacted the freshly generated [Li(bimca^{C5})] in tetrahydrofuran with Pd(II) acetate (Scheme 2). The reaction mixture turned brownish and was left overnight at −30 °C. The solvent was removed in vacuo and the residue washed with pentane to obtain a light brown residue after drying.

The ^{1}H-NMR spectrum in dichloromethane-d$_2$ shows the symmetry reduced signal set with four aromatic signals and no typical signals of an olefin. The pentamethylene chain leads to five signals at 4.35 (12-H$_{eq}$), 4.22 ppm (12-H$_{ax}$), 2.30 (13-H$_{ax}$), 2.03 (14-H$_{ax}$) and 1.97 (13-H$_{eq}$) in a 2:2:2:1:2 ratio, which can be assigned based on the characteristic coupling pattern to the equatorial and axial protons (Figure 5). The diastereotopic signals also confirm the conformational stability of the pentamethylene chain that can be explained by a C-H activation at the C14 position under formation of a tetradentate macrocyclic ligand. In the ^{13}C NMR spectrum, the carbene signal is detected at 171.0 ppm and the Pd-C14 signal at 23.8 ppm. The latter is slightly shifted upfield compared to the signal of an NCN pincer ligand based on 1,5-bis(pyrazol-1-yl)pentane (δ = 2.54 (^{1}H)/28.4 (^{13}C)) [37].

In the HR-ESI mass spectrum, the molecule peak with its characteristic Pd isotope pattern is superimposed by the [M+H]$^+$ peak.

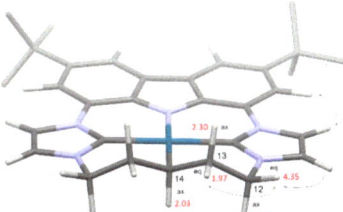

Figure 5. DFT (BP86/def2-TZVP)-optimized structure of [Pd(bimca^{C5H9})] (**6**), showing the chemical shifts of methylene and methine signals (red) and important NOE cross peaks (black arrow).

The C-H activation of an alkyl chain which is close to a Pd(II) center is well known from the formation of PCP or NCN pincer complexes from the reaction of Pd(II) acetate with 1,5-bis(phosphino)pentane in refluxing ethanol [38] or with 1,5-bis(N-heterocycle)pentane in refluxing acetic acid [37]. The ease of the C-H activation in our case can be rationalized with the proximity of the pentamethylene chain at the already-formed CNC pincer complex with an intramolecular deprotonation by the acetate ligand (concerted metalation deprotonation (CMD) mechanism) [39].

3. Materials and Methods

All reactions were carried out under argon atmosphere in dried and degassed solvents with Schlenk technique or in a glovebox (MBraun-Labmaster). Chemicals for synthesis were commercially available. Solvents were purchased from Sigma Aldrich and dried with an MBraun SPS-800 solvent purification system and degassed. Young NMR tubes from Deutero were used for measuring air- and water-sensitive products. NMR spectra were recorded using a Bruker AVANCE II+ 400 spectrometer or a Bruker AVANCE AVII+ 500. The chemical shifts (δ) are reported in [ppm] and the ^{1}H NMR spectra are referenced to the residual protonated solvent peak: δ_H (THF-d_7) = 1.72 and 3.57 ppm, δ_H (DMSO-d_5) = 2.50 ppm, δ_H (CDHCl$_2$) = 5.32 ppm and δ_H (CD$_2$HCN) = 1.94 ppm. ^{13}C{^{1}H} NMR spectra are referenced to the signal of the deuterated solvent: δ_C (THF-d_8) = 25.2 und 67.4 ppm, δ_C (CD$_2$Cl$_2$) = 53.8 ppm [40,41]. The following abbreviations were used: s = singlet, d = doublet, t = triplet, m = multiplet, p = pseudo and variations of them. Coupling constants (*J*) are expressed in [Hz]. 2D NMR correlation spectra were used for peak assignment. Mass spectra were measured on an APEX FT-ICR of Bruker und Daltonik Maxis 4G. UV/VIS spectra were collected using a Jasco V-770 UV-Visible/NIR spectrophotometer. Fluorescence spectra were recorded with a PTI Quantamaster QM4 spectrofluorometer equipped with a 75 W continuous xenon short arc lamp as an excitation source. The emission was monitored using a monochromator at 1200 grooves/mm and detected with a PTI P1.7R detector module (Hamamatsu PMT R5509-72 with a Hamamatsu C9525 power supply operated at 1500 V). Elemental analysis was carried out on a varioMICRO V1.9.2 of Elementar Analysensysteme GmbH. The measurements were recorded in the CHNS modus.

X-ray diffraction data were collected on a Bruker APEX Duo CCD with an Incoatec IμS microfocus sealed tube and QUAZAR optics for MoK$_\alpha$ radiation (λ = 0.71073 Å). Corrections for absorption effects were applied using SADABS or TWINABS. All structures were solved by direct methods using the ShelXle [42–44] software package for structure solution and refinement. In the case of structures **2** and **4** the SQEEZE routine was applied [45]. CCDC 2,064,676 (**3**), 2,064,677 (**4**), 2,064,678 (**5**) and 2,064,679 (**2**) contain the supplementary crystallographic data of this paper (Supplementary Materials). These data are provided free of charge by the joint Cambridge Crystallographic Data Centre and Fachinformationszentrum Karlsruhe Access Structures service, www.ccdc.cam.ac.uk/structures (accessed on 21 January 2021).

Calculations were performed based on density functional theory at the BP86/def2-TZVP [46–51] level implemented in Turbomole [52–61]. The RI-approximation [62–67] was used all over as well as the Grimme dispersion correction [68,69]. The cartesian coordinates of the geometry optimized structures are available as xyz-file in the Supporting Information.

3.1. Preparation of (Hbimca^{C5})·2HPF$_6$ (1b)

1 eq (Hbimca^{C5})·2HBr (1a) [13] was stirred in water for 20 min at 60 °C. Afterward, the suspension was filtered and 1 eq KPF$_6$ was added. Upon stirring for 2 h, the colorless product (Hbimca^{C5})·2HPF$_6$ (1b) precipitated and was filtered off, washed with water and n-hexane, and dried in vacuo. The yields were usually about 30%. The ^{1}H NMR-spectroscopic data are comparable to those of compound 1a [13]. Deviations in the chemical shifts of the signals of the acidic protons can be due to changes in hydrogen bonding of the different counterion as well as to variable concentrations of residual water from the deuterated solvent, which is a known phenomenon [13].

^{1}H NMR (400.11 MHz, DMSO-d$_6$): δ = 1.46 (s, 18H, H-11), 1.66–1.71 (m, 2H, H-14), 1.77–1.83 (m, 4H, H-13), 4.33–4.36 (m, 4H, H-12), 7.79 (d, $^4J_{HH}$ = 1.1 Hz, 2H, H-2/7), 8.05 (br s, 2H, H-4′), 8.27 (br s, 2H, H-5′), 8.60 (d, $^4J_{HH}$ = 1.1 Hz, 2H, H-4/5), 9.65 (s, 2H, H-2′), 11.18 (s, 1H, NH). ^{19}F NMR (376.48 MHz, DMSO-d$_6$): 70.2 (d, $^1J_{PF}$ = 711.4 Hz, PF$_6$).

3.2. General Procedure for the Generation of Alkali Metal bimca^{C5} Complexes

A suspension of proligand 1 (Hbimca^{C5})·2HX (X = Br (a), PF$_6$ (b)) and 3.5 equiv. of MHMDS (M = Li, K) were stirred in 0.5 mL THF-d$_8$ for 5 min.

Complex 2 (Li(bimca^{C5})): A yellow solution with a blue fluorescence under UV-light was obtained. ^{1}H NMR (400.11 MHz, THF-d$_8$): δ 1.50 (s, 18H, H-11), 1.85–1.90 (m, 2H, H-14), 2.07–2.13 (m, 4H, H-13), 4.11–4.13 (m, 4H, H-12), 7.05 (d, $^3J_{HH}$ = 1.7 Hz, 2H, H-4′), 7.35 (d, $^4J_{HH}$ = 1.7 Hz, 2H, H-2/7), 7.52 (d, $^3J_{HH}$ = 1.7 Hz, 2H, H-5′), 7.99 (d, $^4J_{HH}$ = 1.7 Hz, 2H, H-4/5). ^{13}C{^{1}H} NMR (100.61 MHz, THF-d$_8$): δ 23.9 (C14), 30.4 (C13), 33.0 [69] (C11), 35.3 (C10), 50.3 (C12), 111.4 (C2/7), 114.7 (C4/5), 119.9 (C4′ or C5′), 120.2 (C4′ or C5′), 127.7 (C4a/5a), 129.0 (C1/8), 135.5 (C3/6), 144.9 (C1a/8a), 204.4 (C2′). ^{7}Li NMR (194.37 MHz, THF-d$_8$): 2.06 (Li(bimca^{C5})), 0.65 (LiHMDS/LiX). UV/VIS (THF): λ_1 = 246 nm (ε = 8·10^3 L·mol^{-1}·cm^{-1}), λ_2 = 300 nm (ε = 5·10^3 L·mol^{-1}·cm^{-1}), λ_3 = 347 (ε = 2·10^3 L·mol^{-1}·cm^{-1}). Fluorescence (THF): λ = 460 nm (ex: 330 nm).

Complex 3 (K(bimca^{C5})): ^{1}H NMR (400.11 MHz, THF-d$_8$): δ 1.45 (s, 18H, H-11), 1.62–1.69 (m, 4H, H-13), 1.85–1.96 (m, 2H, H-14), 4.13 (pst, $^3J_{HH}$ = 4.7 Hz, 4H, H-12), 6.83 (s, br, 2H, H-4′), 6.96 (s, br, 2H, H-5′), 7.16 and 7.99 (each d, each $^4J_{HH}$ = 1.8 Hz, each 2H, H-4/5, H-2/7). ^{13}C{^{1}H} NMR (100.61 MHz): δ 32.9 (C11′), 33.5 (C13), 35.0 (C10), 52.3 (C12), 114.7 (C2/7 or C4/5), 115.0 (C2/7 or C4/5), 117.7 (C4′), 122.7 (C5′), 127.7 (C1/8), 130.7 (C4a/5a), 133.9 (C3/6), 148.1 (C1a/8a), 212.5 (C2′). The peak of C14 was not detected.

3.3. Synthesis of the Ru(II) Sandwich Complex 4 (Ru(bimca^{C5})Cp*)

A total of 40 mg (51.8 µmol, 1 eq.) of the proligand 1b (X = PF$_6$) and 33.1 mg (165 µmol, 3.2 equiv.) KHMDS were mixed in 1 mL tetrahydrofuran. After five minutes, the reaction was completed and the mixture cooled to −30 °C. The ruthenium precursor (24.0 mg, 51.6 µmol, 1 equiv.) [Ru(CH$_3$CN)$_3$Cp*]PF$_6$ was added to the solution under further cooling and stirring. Upon dissolving of the precursor, the solution was warmed to room temperature. After stirring for 24 h, the solvent was removed in vacuo and the remaining solid extracted with n-pentane. The extract was dried again in vacuo to obtain the product as a red solid in 28 mg (84%) yield. ^{1}H NMR (400.11 MHz, THF-d$_8$): δ 0.99 (ps dd, $^2J_{HH}$ = 14.3 Hz, $^3J_{HH}$ = 6.6 Hz, 1H, H-14$_{ax}$), 1.05 (s, 15H, Cp*), 1.47 (s, 18H, H-11), 1.75–1.81 (m, 2H, H-13$_{eq}$), 1.90–1.99 (m, 1H, H-14$_{eq}$), 1.99–2.11 (ps dt, 2H, $^{2,3}J_{HH}$ = 13.8 Hz, $^3J_{HH}$ = 6.6 Hz, H-13$_{ax}$), 4.13 (ps d, $^2J_{HH}$ = 13.3 Hz, 2H, H-12$_{eq}$), 5.64 (ps t, $^{2,3}J_{HH}$ = 13.2 Hz, 2H, H 12$_{ax}$), 7.24 (d, $^4J_{HH}$ = 0.8 Hz, 2H, H-2/7), 7.25 (d, $^3J_{HH}$ = 2.1 Hz, 2H, H-4′), 7.71 (d, $^4J_{HH}$ = 0.8 Hz, 2H, H-4/5), 7.91 (d, $^3J_{HH}$ = 2.2 Hz, 2H, H-5′). ^{13}C{^{1}H} NMR (100.61 MHz, THF-d$_8$): δ = 10.2 (Cp*-CH$_3$), 16.8 (C14) 33.0 (C11), 35.4 (C13), 35.6 (C10), 51.0 (C12), 83.4 (Cp*), 106.6 (C2/7),

114.2 (C4/5), 119.1 (C5′), 120.6 (C4′), 126.9 (C4a/5a), 129.2 (C1/8), 137.7 (C3/6), 143.4 (C1a/8a), 196.2 (C2′). MS (ESI$^+$, THF/CH$_3$CN, m/z) = 715.1 [C$_{41}$H$_{51}$N$_5$Ru+H]$^+$, 952.1 [C$_{41}$H$_{51}$N$_5$Ru+Ru+Cp*]$^+$. MS (HR-ESI$^+$, CH$_3$CN) calcd for [C$_{41}$H$_{51}$N$_5$Ru]$^+$ 715.31825; found 715.31911, relative mass deviation = 0.34 ppm.

3.4. Synthesis of the Macrocyclic Ru(II)(bimca^{C5}) Complex 5

A total of 20.3 mg (31.6 µmol, 1 eq.) (Hbimca^{C5})·2HBr (**1a**) and 20.4 mg (94.8 µmol, 3.3 eq) KHMDS were stirred in 2 mL tetrahydrofuran. The reaction was completed after five minutes and 30.0 mg (31.6 µmol, 1 eq.) [Ru(PPh$_3$)$_3$Cl$_2$] was added to the reaction mixture. After stirring for an additional five minutes, the mixture was stored for 24 h at −30 °C, whereupon the product precipitated as red crystals. They were filtered off and washed with n-pentane and diethyl ether 1 mL each. The NMR spectra show the formation of a mixture of two isomers in a 1:0.4 ratio.

Major isomer: ^{1}H NMR (400.11 MHz, dichloromethane-d$_2$): δ 1.45 (s, 18H, H-11), 1.93–2.03 (m, 1H, H-15), 3.29–3.34 (m, 1H, H-15), 4.09–4.13 (m, 1H, H-16), 4.43–4.55 (m, 2H, H-16, H-12), 4.75–4.81 (m, 1H, H-12), 5.07–5.10 (m, 1H, H-14), 5.20–5.27 (m, 1H, H-13), 7.29–7.35 (m, PPh$_3$), 7.38 (s, br, 1H, H-4′), 7.46–7.50 (m, PPh$_3$), 7.55–7.59 (m, PPh$_3$), 7.65 (s, br, 1H, H-2/7 or H-4/5), 7.63–7.70 (m, PPh$_3$), 7.76 (s, br, 1H, H-2/7 or H-4/5), 7.73 (s, br, 1H, H-4′), 7.98 (s, br, 1H, H-5′), 8.16 (s, 1H, H-2/7 or H-4/5), 8.17 (s, 1H, H-2/7 or H-4/5), 8.29 (s br, 1H, H-5′). Signal H-4′ is superimposed by the PPh$_3$ signal at 7.29–7.35 ppm. ^{13}C{^{1}H} NMR (100.61 MHz, dichloromethane-d$_2$): δ 31.3 (C15), 32.5 (C11), 32.5 (C11), 35.2 (C10), 35.3 (C10), 51.5 (C12 or C16), 52.1 (C12 or C16), 81.6 (C13), 88.4 (C14), 109.8 (C2/7), 111.4 (C2/7), 115.0 (C4/5), 115.1 (C4/5), 117.0 (C5′), 118.3 (C5′), 119.6 (C4′), 123.9 (C4′), 127.5 (C4a/5a), 127.8 (C4a/5a), 129.0 (CPPh$_3$), 129.1 (CPPh$_3$), 132.4–132.5 (CPPh$_3$), 134.1 (CPPh$_3$), 134.3 (CPPh$_3$), 135.8 (C1a/8a), 139.2 (C3/6), 139.5 (C-3/6). Signal C2′ was not detected and signal C1/8 is superimposed by the PPh$_3$ signal at 129.0–192.1 ppm.

Minor isomer: 1.55 (s, 18H, t-Bu), 2.64–2.73 (m, 1H, C$_5$H$_8$), 3.09–3.11 (m, 2H, C$_5$H$_8$), 3.53–3.58 (m, 1H, C$_5$H$_8$), 4.43–4.55 (m, 2H, C$_5$H$_8$), 4.98–5.04 (m, 1H, C$_5$H$_8$), 5.75–5.28 (m, 1H, C$_5$H$_8$), 7.29–7.33 (PPh$_3$), 7.40 (s br, 1H, ArH), 7.46–7.48 (PPh$_3$), 7.56–7.59 (PPh$_3$), 7.67–7.70 (m, PPh$_3$), 7.73 (s br, 1H, ArH), 8.06 (s br, 1H, ArH), 8.16–8.18 (2H, ArH), 8.25 (s br,1H, ArH). Two aromatic signals were not detected.^{31}P{^{1}H} NMR (MeOD-d$_4$, 161.97 MHz): δ = 67.8 (1P, PPh$_3$), 64.3 (0.4P, PPh$_3$, minor isomer). MS (ESI$^+$, MeOH, m/z) = 840.2 (100) [C$_{49}$H$_{49}$BrN$_5$PRu-Br]$^+$, 480.3 (10) [ligand]$^+$. CHN: (C$_{49}$H$_{49}$BrN$_5$PRu): Calcd C 63.98, H 5.37, N 7.61 found C 63.74, H 5.63, N 7.33.

3.5. Preparation of the Macrocyclic Pd(II) Complex 6

A total of 30.0 mg (46.8 µmol, 1 eq) (Hbimca^{C5})·2HBr (**1**) and 27.4 mg (164.4 µmol, 3.5 eq) LiHMDS were mixed and dissolved in 2 mL of tetrahydrofuran. Moreover, 10.5 mg (46.8 µmol, 1 eq) [Pd(OAc)$_2$] were added and the reaction mixture was kept at −30 °C for 24 h. After warming to room temperature, the solvent was removed in vacuo and the residue washed three times with 1 mL n-pentane. The product is a pale brown solid that is insoluble in tetrahydrofuran and soluble in dichloromethane.

^{1}H NMR (400.11 MHz, dichloromethane-d$_2$): δ 1.53 (s, 18H, H-11), 1.97 (d ps t, $^3J_{HH}$ ~ 2.6 Hz, $^{2/3}J_{HH}$~13.8 Hz, 2H, H-13$_{eq}$), 2.03 (tt, $^3J_{HH}$ = 2.6 Hz, $^3J_{HH}$ = 12.0 Hz, 1H, H-14$_{ax}$), 2.30 (ps qd, $^{2/3}J_{HH}$ ~ 12.9 Hz, $^3J_{HH}$ = 2.8 Hz, 2H, H-13$_{ax}$), 4.22 (pst d, $^{2/3}J_{HH}$ = 12.5 Hz, $^3J_{HH}$ = 1.7 Hz, 2H, H-12$_{ax}$), 4.35 (d ps t, $^2J_{HH}$ = 12.6 Hz, $^3J_{HH}$ = 3.3 Hz, 2H, H-12$_{eq}$), 7.13 (d, $^3J_{HH}$ = 1.9 Hz, 2H, H-4′), 7.69 (d, $^4J_{HH}$ = 1.4 Hz, 2H, H-2/7), 8.08 (d, $^3J_{HH}$ = 1.9 Hz, 2H, H-5′), 8.14 (d, $^4J_{HH}$ = 1.4 Hz, 2H, H-4/5). ^{13}C{^{1}H} NMR (100.61 MHz, dichloromethane-d$_2$): δ 23.8 (C14), 32.7 (C11), 35.4 (C10), 38.3 (C13), 53.4 (C12), 110.1 (C2/7), 114.8 (C4/5), 115.8 (C5′), 122.3 (C4′), 124.6 (C1/8), 126.7 (C4a/5a), 135.7 (C1a/8a), 138.6 (C3/C6), 171.0 (C2′). MS (HR-ESI$^+$, CH$_3$CN) calcd for [C$_{31}$H$_{35}$N$_5$Pd]$^+$ 583.19272; found 583.19679, relative mass deviation = 6.98 ppm; calcd for [C$_{31}$H$_{35}$N$_5$Pd+H]$^+$ 584.20001, found 584.19985, relative mass deviation = 2.27 ppm.

4. Conclusions

We have shown that the introduction of a pentamethylene tether into a CNC pincer ligand leads to a rich coordination chemistry and an increase of possible coordination modes. Due to the proximity of the alkyl tether at the metal center, C-H activation reactions were observed, which—depending on the nature of the metal and additional ligands—can lead to a dehydrogenation (Ru) or a deprotonation (Pd). Thus, the bimca^{C5} ligand can not only serve as a monoanionic pincer ligand, but also as a monoanionic (bimca^{C5H8}) as well as a dianionic (bimca^{C5H9}) tetradentate macrocyclic ligand. In addition, the hindered rotation of the carbene moieties in the tethered pincer ligand enhances a facial coordination mode (Ru, K). From this point of view, the formation of a dimeric lithium complex by a chelating and bridging coordination mode is rather unexpected and likely due to the small size of the lithium ion.

Especially the hapticity increase of the bimca^{C5} ligand leads to new options for the catalyst design as the ligand could play an active role in the activation of substrates or stabilize highly reactive intermediates. Studies on these aspects will be the topic of future research.

Supplementary Materials: The following are available online: SI containing the spectra of all new compounds, crystallographic information and the xyz-file of the calculated structures.

Author Contributions: Investigation, X-ray structure analyses and draft preparation R.J.; Supervision, DFT calculations, interpretation and writing—review and editing D.K. All authors have read and agreed to the published version of the manuscript.

Funding: This research received no external funding.

Data Availability Statement: The data is available in the Supplementary Material.

Acknowledgments: We thank Cäcilia Maichle-Mössmer and Fabio Mazzotta for help with the structure solution of the X-ray data, and Karl W. Törnroos for help with an earlier dataset of complex **5**. We also thank Wolfgang Leis for VT NMR measurements the MS facility for carrying out measurement and simulation of the MS spectra.

Conflicts of Interest: The authors declare no conflict of interest.

Sample Availability: Samples of the compounds might be available from the authors.

References

1. Hood, T.M.; Gyton, M.R.; Chaplin, A.B. Synthesis and rhodium complexes of macrocyclic PNP and PONOP pincer ligands. *Dalton Trans.* **2020**, *49*, 2077–2086. [CrossRef]
2. Leforestier, B.; Gyton, M.R.; Chaplin, A.B. Synthesis and group 9 complexes of macrocyclic PCP and POCOP pincer ligands. *Dalton Trans.* **2020**, *49*, 2087–2101. [CrossRef]
3. Andrew, R.E.; Chaplin, A.B. Synthesis, structure and dynamics of NHC-based palladium macrocycles. *Dalton Trans.* **2014**, *43*, 1413–1423. [CrossRef] [PubMed]
4. Andrew, R.E.; Chaplin, A.B. Synthesis and reactivity of NHC-based rhodium macrocycles. *Inorg. Chem.* **2015**, *54*, 312–322. [CrossRef] [PubMed]
5. Andrew, R.E.; Storey, C.M.; Chaplin, A.B. Well-defined coinage metal transfer agents for the synthesis of NHC-based nickel, rhodium and palladium macrocycles. *Dalton Trans.* **2016**, *45*, 8937–8944. [CrossRef] [PubMed]
6. Storey, C.M.; Gyton, M.R.; Andrew, R.E.; Chaplin, A.B. Terminal Alkyne Coupling Reactions through a Ring: Mechanistic Insights and Regiochemical Switching. *Angew. Chem. Int. Ed.* **2018**, *57*, 12003–12006. [CrossRef]
7. Leforestier, B.; Gyton, M.R.; Chaplin, A.B. Oxidative Addition of a Mechanically Entrapped C(sp)-C(sp) Bond to a Rhodium(I) Pincer Complex. *Angew. Chem.* **2020**, *59*, 23500–23504. [CrossRef]
8. Storey, C.M.; Gyton, M.R.; Andrew, R.E.; Chaplin, A.B. Terminal Alkyne Coupling Reactions Through a Ring: Effect of Ring Size on Rate and Regioselectivity. *Chem. Eur. J.* **2020**, *26*, 14715–14723. [CrossRef]
9. Biffis, A.; Cipani, M.; Bressan, E.; Tubaro, C.; Graiff, C.; Venzo, A. Group 10 Metal Complexes with Chelating Macrocyclic Dicarbene Ligands Bearing a 2,6-Lutidinyl Bridge: Synthesis, Reactivity, and Catalytic Activity. *Organometallics* **2014**, *33*, 2182–2188. [CrossRef]
10. Alcalde, E.; Ramos, S.; Perez-Garcia, L. Anion Template-Directed Synthesis of Dicationic [14]Imidazoliophanes. *Org. Lett.* **1999**, *1*, 1035–1038. [CrossRef]
11. Yuan, Y.; Gao, G.; Jiang, Z.-L.; You, J.-S.; Zhou, Z.-Y.; Yuan, D.-Q.; Xie, R.-G. Synthesis and selective anion recognition of imidazolium cyclophanes. *Tetrahedron* **2002**, *58*, 8993–8999. [CrossRef]

12. Radloff, C.; Gong, H.-Y.; Schulte to Brinke, C.; Pape, T.; Lynch, V.M.; Sessler, J.L.; Hahn, F.E. Metal-Dependent Coordination Modes Displayed by Macrocyclic Polycarbene Ligands. *Chem. Eur. J.* **2010**, *16*, 13077–13081. [CrossRef] [PubMed]
13. Jürgens, E.; Buys, K.N.; Schmidt, A.-T.; Furfari, S.K.; Cole, M.L.; Moser, M.; Rominger, F.; Kunz, D. Optimised synthesis of monoanionic bis(NHC)-pincer ligand precursors and their Li-complexes. *New J. Chem.* **2016**, *40*, 9160–9169. [CrossRef]
14. Lu, T.; Yang, C.-F.; Steren, C.A.; Fei, F.; Chen, X.-T.; Xue, Z.-L. Synthesis and characterization of Ag(I) and Au(I) complexes with macrocyclic hybrid amine N-heterocyclic carbene ligands. *New J. Chem.* **2018**, *42*, 4700–4713. [CrossRef]
15. Moser, M.; Wucher, B.; Kunz, D.; Rominger, F. 1,8-Bis(imidazolin-2-yliden-1-yl)carbazolide (bimca): A New CNC Pincer-Type Ligand with Strong Electron-Donating Properties. Facile Oxidative Addition of Methyl Iodide to Rh(bimca)(CO). *Organometallics* **2007**, *26*, 1024–1030. [CrossRef]
16. Evans, K.J.; Campbell, C.L.; Haddow, M.F.; Luz, C.; Morton, P.A.; Mansell, S.M. Lithium Complexes with Bridging and Terminal NHC Ligands: The Decisive Influence of an Anionic Tether. *Eur. J. Inorg. Chem.* **2019**, *2019*, 4894–4901. [CrossRef]
17. Simler, T.; Karmazin, L.; Bailly, C.; Braunstein, P.; Danopoulos, A.A. Potassium and Lithium Complexes with Monodeprotonated, Dearomatized PNP and PNC NHC Pincer-Type Ligands. *Organometallics* **2016**, *35*, 903–912. [CrossRef]
18. Nesterov, V.; Reiter, D.; Bag, P.; Frisch, P.; Holzner, R.; Porzelt, A.; Inoue, S. NHCs in Main Group Chemistry. *Chem. Rev.* **2018**, *118*, 9678–9842. [CrossRef]
19. Tapu, D.; Dixon, D.A.; Roe, C. 13C NMR spectroscopy of "Arduengo-type" carbenes and their derivatives. *Chem. Rev.* **2009**, *109*, 3385–3407. [CrossRef] [PubMed]
20. Arduengo, A.J., III; Gamper, S.F.; Tamm, M.; Calabrese, J.C.; Davidson, F.; Craig, H.A. A Bis(carbene)-Proton Complex: Structure of a C-H-C Hydrogen Bond. *J. Am. Chem. Soc.* **1995**, *117*, 572–573. [CrossRef]
21. Herrmann, W.A.; Runte, O.; Artus, G. Synthesis and structure of an ionic beryllium-"carbene" complex. *J. Organomet. Chem.* **1995**, *501*, C1–C4. [CrossRef]
22. Simler, T.; Danopoulos, A.A.; Braunstein, P. N-Heterocyclic carbene-phosphino-picolines as precursors of anionic 'pincer' ligands with dearomatised pyridine backbones; transmetallation from potassium to chromium. *Chem. Commun.* **2015**, *51*, 10699–10702. [CrossRef] [PubMed]
23. Seyboldt, A.; Wucher, B.; Hohnstein, S.; Eichele, K.; Rominger, F.; Törnroos, K.W.; Kunz, D. Evidence for the Formation of Anionic Zerovalent Group 10 Complexes as Highly Reactive Intermediates. *Organometallics* **2015**, *34*, 2717–2725. [CrossRef]
24. Jürgens, E.; Kunz, D. A Rigid CNC Pincer Ligand Acting as a Tripodal Cp Analogue. *Eur. J. Inorg. Chem.* **2017**, *2017*, 233–236. [CrossRef]
25. Brookhart, M.; Green, M.L.H.; Parkin, G. Agostic interactions in transition metal compounds. *Proc. Natl. Acad. Sci. USA* **2007**, *104*, 6908–6914. [CrossRef] [PubMed]
26. Taniguchi, W.; Ito, J.; Yamashita, M. CNC-pincer iron complexes containing a bis(N-heterocyclic carbene)Amido ligand: Synthesis and application to catalytic hydrogenation of alkenes. *J. Organomet. Chem.* **2020**, *923*, 121436. [CrossRef]
27. Gusev, D.G.; Lough, A.J. Double C−H Activation on Osmium and Ruthenium Centers: Carbene vs Olefin Products. *Organometallics* **2002**, *21*, 2601–2603. [CrossRef]
28. Chatt, J.; Watson, H.R. 491. Complexes of zerovalent transition metals with the ditertiary phosphine, $Me_2P \cdot CH_2 \cdot CH_2 \cdot PMe_2$. *J. Chem. Soc.* **1962**, 2545–2549. [CrossRef]
29. Chatt, J.; Davidson, J.M. 154. The tautomerism of arene and ditertiary phosphine complexes of ruthenium(0), and the preparation of new types of hydrido-complexes of ruthenium(II). *J. Chem. Soc.* **1965**, 843–855. [CrossRef]
30. Kakiuchi, F.; Murai, S. Catalytic C-H/Olefin Coupling. *Acc. Chem. Res.* **2002**, *35*, 826–834. [CrossRef]
31. Arockiam, P.B.; Bruneau, C.; Dixneuf, P.H. Ruthenium(II)-catalyzed C-H bond activation and functionalization. *Chem. Rev.* **2012**, *112*, 5879–5918. [CrossRef] [PubMed]
32. Ackermann, L. Carboxylate-assisted transition-metal-catalyzed C-H bond functionalizations: Mechanism and scope. *Chem. Rev.* **2011**, *111*, 1315–1345. [CrossRef] [PubMed]
33. Crabtree, R.H. Organometallic alkane CH activation. *J. Organomet. Chem.* **2004**, *689*, 4083–4091. [CrossRef]
34. Zhou, X.; Malakar, S.; Zhou, T.; Murugesan, S.; Huang, C.; Emge, T.J.; Krogh-Jespersen, K.; Goldman, A.S. Catalytic Alkane Transfer Dehydrogenation by PSP-Pincer-Ligated Ruthenium. Deactivation of an Extremely Reactive Fragment by Formation of Allyl Hydride Complexes. *ACS Catal.* **2019**, *9*, 4072–4083. [CrossRef]
35. Gruver, B.C.; Adams, J.J.; Warner, S.J.; Arulsamy, N; Roddick, D.M. Acceptor Pincer Chemistry of Ruthenium: Catalytic Alkane Dehydrogenation by $(^{CF3}PCP)Ru(cod)(H)$. *Organometallics* **2011**, *30*, 5133–5140. [CrossRef]
36. Zhang, Y.; Yao, W.; Fang, H.; Hu, A.; Huang, Z. Catalytic alkane dehydrogenations. *Sci. Bull.* **2015**, *60*, 1316–1331. [CrossRef]
37. Chatt, J.; Hart, F.A.; Watson, H.R. 490. Complex compounds of ditertiary phosphines and arsines with nickel(0) and palladium(0). *J. Chem. Soc.* **1962**, 2537–2545. [CrossRef]
38. Al-Salem, N.A.; Empsall, H.D.; Markham, R.; Shaw, B.L.; Weeks, B. Formation of large chelate rings and cyclometallated products from diphosphines of type $Bu^t_2P(CH_2)_n PBu^t_2$ (n = 5–8) and $Ph_2P(CH_2)_5PPh_2$ with palladium and platinum chlorides: Factors affecting the stability and conformation of large chelate rings. *J. Chem. Soc. Dalton Trans.* **1979**, 1972–1982. [CrossRef]
39. Rousseaux, S.; Gorelsky, S.I.; Chung, B.K.W.; Fagnou, K. Investigation of the mechanism of C(sp3)-H bond cleavage in Pd(0)-catalyzed intramolecular alkane arylation adjacent to amides and sulfonamides. *J. Am. Chem. Soc.* **2010**, *132*, 10692–10705. [CrossRef] [PubMed]

40. Gottlieb, H.E.; Kotlyar, V.; Nudelman, A. NMR Chemical Shifts of Common Laboratory Solvents as Trace Impurities. *J. Org. Chem.* **1997**, *62*, 7512–7515. [CrossRef] [PubMed]
41. Fulmer, G.R.; Miller, A.J.M.; Sherden, N.H.; Gottlieb, H.E.; Nudelman, A.; Stoltz, B.M.; Bercaw, J.E.; Goldberg, K.I. NMR Chemical Shifts of Trace Impurities: Common Laboratory Solvents, Organics, and Gases in Deuterated Solvents Relevant to the Organometallic Chemist. *Organometallics* **2010**, *29*, 2176–2179. [CrossRef]
42. Hübschle, C.B.; Sheldrick, G.M.; Dittrich, B. ShelXle: A Qt graphical user interface for SHELXL. *J. Appl. Crystallogr.* **2011**, *44*, 1281–1284. [CrossRef]
43. Sheldrick, G.M. Recent developments in SHELX. *Acta Crystallogr. A Found. Crystallogr.* **2013**, *69*, s74. [CrossRef]
44. Sheldrick, G.M. Crystal structure refinement with SHELXL. *Acta Crystallogr. C Struct. Chem.* **2015**, *71*, 3–8. [CrossRef]
45. Spek, A.L. Platon Squeeze: A tool for the calculation of the disordered solvent contribution to the calculated structure factors. *Acta Crystallogr. Sect. C Cryst. Struct. Commun.* **2015**, *71*, 9–18. [CrossRef]
46. Becke, A.D. Density-functional exchange-energy approximation with correct asymptotic behavior. *Phys. Rev. A Gen. Phys.* **1988**, *38*, 3098–3100. [CrossRef] [PubMed]
47. Perdew, J.P. Density-functional approximation for the correlation energy of the inhomogeneous electron gas. *Phys. Rev. B Condens. Matter* **1986**, *33*, 8822–8824. [CrossRef]
48. Schäfer, A.; Horn, H.; Ahlrichs, R. Fully optimized contracted Gaussian basis sets for atoms Li to Kr. *J. Chem. Phys.* **1992**, *97*, 2571–2577. [CrossRef]
49. Schäfer, A.; Huber, C.; Ahlrichs, R. Fully optimized contracted Gaussian basis sets of triple zeta valence quality for atoms Li to Kr. *J. Chem. Phys.* **1994**, *100*, 5829–5835. [CrossRef]
50. Weigend, F.; Ahlrichs, R. Balanced basis sets of split valence, triple zeta valence and quadruple zeta valence quality for H to Rn: Design and assessment of accuracy. *Phys. Chem. Chem. Phys.* **2005**, *7*, 3297–3305. [CrossRef]
51. Weigend, F. Accurate Coulomb-fitting basis sets for H to Rn. *Phys. Chem. Chem. Phys.* **2006**, *8*, 1057–1065. [CrossRef]
52. Steffen, C.; Thomas, K.; Huniar, U.; Hellweg, A.; Rubner, O.; Schroer, A. TmoleX—A graphical user interface for TURBOMOLE. *J. Comput. Chem.* **2010**, *31*, 2967–2970. [CrossRef]
53. University of Karlsruhe and Forschungszentrum Karlsruhe GmbH. TURBOMOLE. 2011. Available online: https://www.turbomole.org/ (accessed on 21 January 2021).
54. Treutler, O.; Ahlrichs, R. Efficient molecular numerical integration schemes. *J. Chem. Phys.* **1995**, *102*, 346–354. [CrossRef]
55. von Arnim, M.; Ahlrichs, R. Performance of parallel TURBOMOLE for density functional calculations. *J. Comput. Chem.* **1998**, *19*, 1746–1757. [CrossRef]
56. van Wüllen, C. Shared-memory parallelization of the TURBOMOLE programs AOFORCE, ESCF, and EGRAD: How to quickly parallelize legacy code. *J. Comput. Chem.* **2011**, *32*, 1195–1201. [CrossRef] [PubMed]
57. Deglmann, P.; Furche, F.; Ahlrichs, R. An efficient implementation of second analytical derivatives for density functional methods. *Chem. Phys. Lett.* **2002**, *362*, 511–518. [CrossRef]
58. Deglmann, P.; Furche, F. Efficient characterization of stationary points on potential energy surfaces. *J. Chem. Phys.* **2002**, *117*, 9535–9538. [CrossRef]
59. Ahlrichs, R.; Bär, M.; Häser, M.; Horn, H.; Kölmel, C. Electronic structure calculations on workstation computers: The program system turbomole. *Chem. Phys. Lett.* **1989**, *162*, 165–169. [CrossRef]
60. Armbruster, M.K.; Weigend, F.; van Wüllen, C.; Klopper, W. Self-consistent treatment of spin-orbit interactions with efficient Hartree-Fock and density functional methods. *Phys. Chem. Chem. Phys.* **2008**, *10*, 1748–1756. [CrossRef] [PubMed]
61. Peng, D.; Middendorf, N.; Weigend, F.; Reiher, M. An efficient implementation of two-component relativistic exact-decoupling methods for large molecules. *J. Chem. Phys.* **2013**, *138*, 184105. [CrossRef]
62. Eichkorn, K.; Treutler, O.; Öhm, H.; Häser, M.; Ahlrichs, R. Auxiliary basis sets to approximate Coulomb potentials. *Chem. Phys. Lett.* **1995**, *240*, 283–290. [CrossRef]
63. Eichkorn, K.; Treutler, O.; Öhm, H.; Häser, M.; Ahlrichs, R. Auxiliary basis sets to approximate Coulomb potentials (Chem. Phys. Letters 240 (1995) 283–290). *Chem. Phys. Lett.* **1995**, *242*, 652–660. [CrossRef]
64. Deglmann, P.; May, K.; Furche, F.; Ahlrichs, R. Nuclear second analytical derivative calculations using auxiliary basis set expansions. *Chem. Phys. Lett.* **2004**, *384*, 103–107. [CrossRef]
65. Weigend, F. A fully direct RI-HF algorithm: Implementation, optimised auxiliary basis sets, demonstration of accuracy and efficiency. *Phys. Chem. Chem. Phys.* **2002**, *4*, 4285–4291. [CrossRef]
66. Sierka, M.; Hogekamp, A.; Ahlrichs, R. Fast evaluation of the Coulomb potential for electron densities using multipole accelerated resolution of identity approximation. *J. Chem. Phys.* **2003**, *118*, 9136–9148. [CrossRef]
67. Eichkorn, K.; Weigend, F.; Treutler, O.; Ahlrichs, R. Auxiliary basis sets for main row atoms and transition metals and their use to approximate Coulomb potentials. *Theor. Chem. Acc. Theory Comput. Modeling (Theor. Chim. Acta)* **1997**, *97*, 119–124. [CrossRef]
68. Grimme, S.; Antony, J.; Ehrlich, S.; Krieg, H. A consistent and accurate ab initio parametrization of density functional dispersion correction (DFT-D) for the 94 elements H-Pu. *J. Chem. Phys.* **2010**, *132*, 154104. [CrossRef]
69. Grimme, S.; Ehrlich, S.; Goerigk, L. Effect of the damping function in dispersion corrected density functional theory. *J. Comput. Chem.* **2011**, *32*, 1456–1465. [CrossRef] [PubMed]

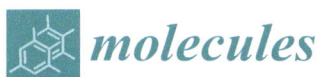

Article

Unsaturated and Benzannulated *N*-Heterocyclic Carbene Complexes of Titanium and Hafnium: Impact on Catalysts Structure and Performance in Copolymerization of Cyclohexene Oxide with CO_2

Lakshmi Suresh [1,†], Ralte Lalrempuia [1,2,†], Jonas B. Ekeli [1,†], Francis Gillis-D'Hamers [1,†], Karl W. Törnroos [1], Vidar R. Jensen [1,*] and Erwan Le Roux [1,*]

1 Department of Chemistry, University of Bergen, Allégaten 41, N-5007 Bergen, Norway; Lakshmi.Suresh@uib.no (L.S.); lalrempuia.ralte@dcu.ie (R.L.); Jonas.Ekeli@student.uib.no (J.B.E.); Francis.gillis567@gmail.com (F.G.-D.); Karl.Tornroos@uib.no (K.W.T.)
2 School of Chemical Sciences, Dublin City University, Dublin 9, Ireland
* Correspondence: Vidar.Jensen@kj.uib.no (V.R.J.); Erwan.LeRoux@uib.no (E.L.R.)
† These authors contributed equally to this work.

Academic Editor: Yves Canac
Received: 4 September 2020; Accepted: 21 September 2020; Published: 23 September 2020

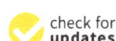

Abstract: Tridentate, bis-phenolate *N*-heterocyclic carbenes (NHCs) are among the ligands giving the most selective and active group 4-based catalysts for the copolymerization of cyclohexene oxide (CHO) with CO_2. In particular, ligands based on imidazolidin-2-ylidene (saturated NHC) moieties have given catalysts which exclusively form polycarbonate in moderate-to-high yields even under low CO_2 pressure and at low copolymerization temperatures. Here, to evaluate the influence of the NHC moiety on the molecular structure of the catalyst and its performance in copolymerization, we extend this chemistry by synthesizing and characterizing titanium complexes bearing tridentate bis-phenolate imidazol-2-ylidene (unsaturated NHC) and benzimidazol-2-ylidene (benzannulated NHC) ligands. The electronic properties of the ligands and the nature of their bonds to titanium are studied using density functional theory (DFT) and natural bond orbital (NBO) analysis. The metal–NHC bond distances and bond strengths are governed by ligand-to-metal σ- and π-donation, whereas back-donation directly from the metal to the NHC ligand seems to be less important. The NHC π-acceptor orbitals are still involved in bonding, as they interact with THF and isopropoxide oxygen lone-pair donor orbitals. The new complexes are, when combined with [PPN]Cl co-catalyst, selective in polycarbonate formation. The highest activity, albeit lower than that of the previously reported Ti catalysts based on saturated NHC, was obtained with the benzannulated NHC-Ti catalyst. Attempts to synthesize unsaturated and benzannulated NHC analogues based on Hf invariably led, as in earlier work with Zr, to a mixture of products that include zwitterionic and homoleptic complexes. However, the benzannulated NHC-Hf complexes were obtained as the major products, allowing for isolation. Although these complexes selectively form polycarbonate, their catalytic performance is inferior to that of analogues based on saturated NHC.

Keywords: *N*-heterocyclic carbene; titanium; hafnium; copolymerization of epoxide with CO_2; density functional theory; natural bond orbitals

---

1. Introduction

In the past few decades, *N*-heterocyclic carbenes (NHCs) have emerged as privileged ancillary ligands that, in particular, have been explored in combination with low-to-medium valent late-transition-metals due to their strong σ-donor capacity, structural diversity, and their successful use in organometallic catalysis [1–8]. In contrast, high-valent early-transition-metal NHC complexes have received much less attention [9–15], which to a large extent is due to their ease of dissociation from these metal centers [2,5,9,11,12,14]. However, their dissociation from oxophilic metals was partially prevented by designing multidentate anionic carbon, nitrogen, and oxygen-functionalized NHC ligands [5,13,15–17]. Anchoring such functionalized NHC ligands to oxophilic metals has proved to be a successful approach for developing catalysts, notably of group 4 metals, for the (oligo-)polymerization of olefins [18–29], hydroamination/cyclization of aminoalkenes [30–36], controlled ring-opening polymerization of rac-lactide [37–40], and more recently, for the copolymerization of epoxides with CO_2 [41–45].

Although most of the highly selective and active catalyst systems for the copolymerization of epoxides with CO_2 are based on divalent (Mg, Co, Zn) and trivalent (Cr, Co, Al) metals bearing ligands such as β-diketiminates, salens, porphyrins, and multidentate phenolate macrocycles [46–52], the group 4 metals have emerged as a new class of catalyst for this reaction, combining decent catalytic activity with high selectivity towards the formation of polycarbonates [41–45,53–66]. NHC-based catalysts of this kind have appeared to be particularly promising under relatively mild copolymerization conditions [41–45]. However, so far the tetravalent titanium, zirconium and hafnium complexes for the CO_2/cyclohexene oxide (CHO) copolymerization that have selectively given the desired poly(cyclohexene carbonate) (PCHC), without cyclohexene carbonate (CHC) or homopolymer of CHO (PCHO) as side products, have exclusively been based on tridentate bis-phenolate NHC-type ligands with saturated backbones (Scheme 1) [41–45]. Previous attempts to substitute the saturated-NHC backbone of zirconium catalysts by unsaturated- or benzannulated-NHC backbones in order to evaluate the effects on the copolymerization catalysis have irremediably led to a catalytically inactive isolable mixture of zwitterionic and heteroleptic zirconium compounds (Scheme 1) [44]. This suggests that strong σ-donation from the NHC ligand to the metal is vital for CO_2/CHO copolymerization.

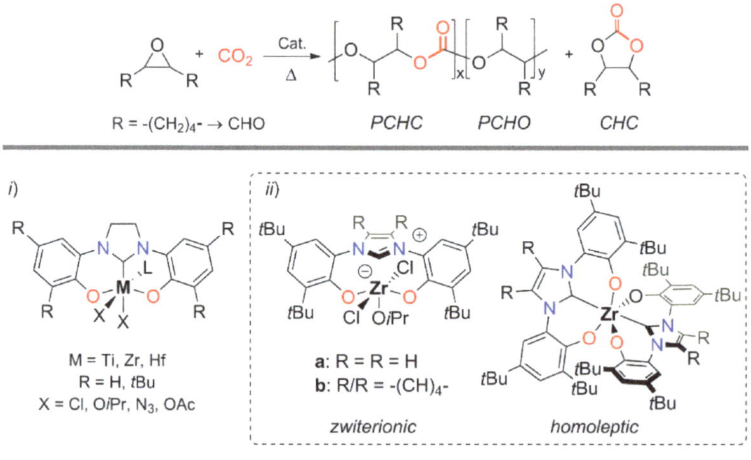

Scheme 1. Previously obtained complexes containing (*i*) saturated NHC with group 4, and (*ii*) unsaturated and benzannulated NHCs ligands (**a** and **b**, respectively) with zirconium.

We have continued our efforts to synthesize catalysts based on unsaturated NHC ligands, and present here, for the first time, bis-phenolate unsaturated- and benzannulated-NHC complexes of titanium and hafnium. The performance of these complexes in CO_2/CHO copolymerization is compared to those of saturated NHC ligands. Finally, with the help of density functional theory (DFT) and natural bond orbital (NBO) analysis, the structural and electronic property differences of these complexes are presented, and the potential impact of these differences on CO_2/CHO copolymerization is discussed.

2. Results and Discussion

2.1. Synthesis of Bis-Phenolate NHC Complexes of Titanium and Hafnium

The *N,N'*-di(2-hydroxy-3,5-di-*tert*-butylphenyl) imidazolium chloride (**a**) and *N,N'*-di(2-hydroxy-3,5-di-*tert*-butylphenyl) benzoimidazolium chloride (**b**) proligands were prepared according to previously reported procedures [26,67,68]. The alcohol elimination route involving the direct and slow addition of proligands **a** and **b** to a solution of Ti(O*i*Pr)$_4$ in THF at −30 °C was found to be the most appropriate protocol for the synthesis of both ([κ^3-O,C,O]-^{I}NHC)TiCl(O*i*Pr)(THF) **1a** and ([κ^3-O,C,O]-^{Bz}NHC)TiCl(O*i*Pr) **1b** complexes, respectively, in good yields and without the formation of side compounds, such as the homoleptic and zwitterionic complexes (Scheme 2). This protocol slightly diverges from the previously reported one in which *N,N'*-di(2-hydroxy-3,5-di-*tert*-butylphenyl) imidazolidinium chloride salt (**c**) was used as proligand and the addition was carried out at room temperature, leading quantitatively to ([κ^3-O,C,O]-^{Is}NHC)TiCl(O*i*Pr)(THF) **1c** [38].

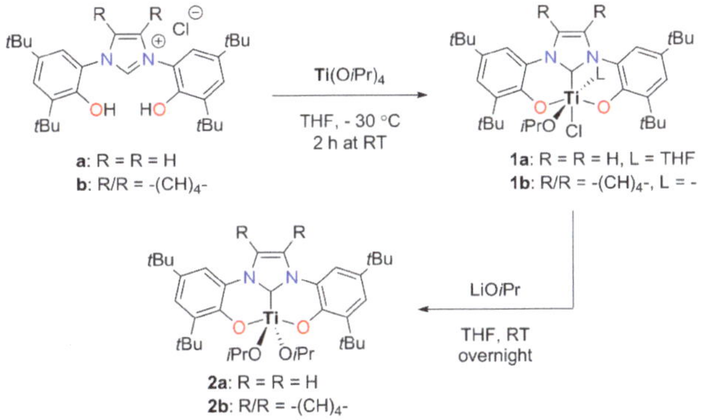

Scheme 2. Synthesis of NHC-Ti complexes **1a**, **1b**, **2a** and **2b**.

The ^{1}H and ^{13}C-NMR spectra show that the proligands are fully deprotonated with the concomitant disappearance of both OH and H$_{imidazolium}$ protons and all chemical resonances are shifted downfield in agreement with the bonding of bis-phenolate NHC ligands to the titanium metal center for both **1a** and **1b** compounds (Supplementary Figures S1–S4). The only immediately observed difference between these two compounds is that the THF molecule in complex **1b** is very labile and can easily be removed under prolonged vacuum. The ^{13}C-NMR spectra of both compounds **1a** and **1b** encompass typical imidazol-2-ylidene and benzimidazolin-2-ylidene NHC-C$_{carbene}$ resonances at δ 184.0 and 195.2 ppm (Supplementary Figures S2 and S4) [14,69], respectively, which are shifted upfield compared to that of the structurally analogous bis-phenolate saturated NHC complex of titanium ([κ^3-O,C,O]-^{Is}NHC)TiCl(O*i*Pr)(THF) **1c** (δ 198.6 ppm) [38].

As indicated above, the order of addition of the reagents is crucial here, contrasting the case of the Zr(O*i*Pr)$_4$(HO*i*Pr) precursor with either **a** or **b** proligands in which the homoleptic and zwitterionic compounds are observed independently of the addition order [44]. For instance, the addition of Ti(O*i*Pr)$_4$ to proligand **b** in THF at room temperature leads to a mixture of compounds containing at least complex **1b** (unambiguously deduced from by ^{1}H-NMR analysis, cf. Figure S5) along with the zwitterionic ([κ^2-O,O]-^{Bz}NHC-H)TiCl$_2$(O*i*Pr) **1b'** and homoleptic ([κ^3-O,C,O]-^{Bz}NHC)$_2$Ti **1b''** as minor products (9% and 5%, respectively). Consistent with the observations made earlier for the ^{Bz}NHC-Zr analogue [44], formation of zwitterionic **1b'** was further confirmed by single-crystal X-ray diffraction (SCXRD) analysis of a crystal sampled from the reaction mixture in toluene at −30 °C (Supplementary Figure S6 and Table S1).

Similarly, the molecular structures of **1a** and the THF-adduct of **1b** (**1b-THF**) were both confirmed by SCXRD analysis (Figure 1a,b). Selected bond lengths, angles and torsion angles are shown in Table 1. Further crystallographic information and data for **1a** and **1b-THF** are given in Table S2.

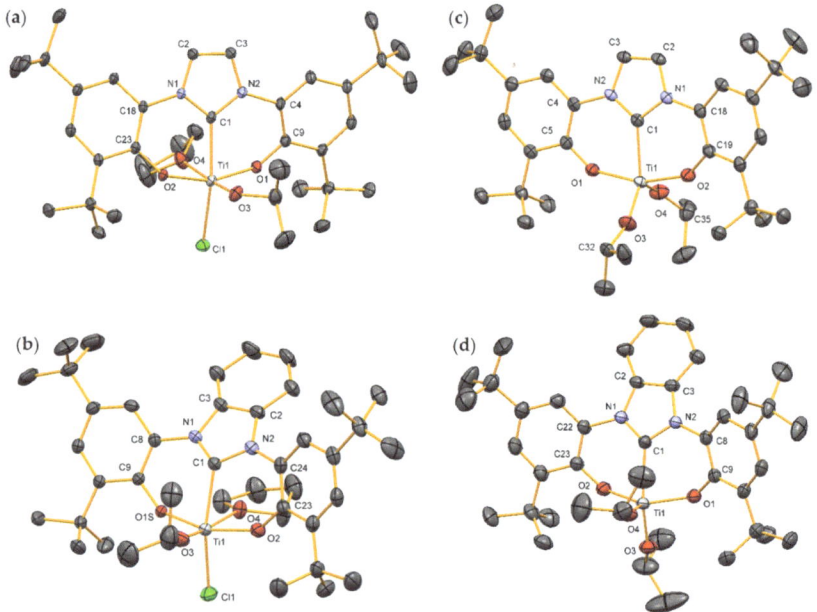

Figure 1. Molecular structures of (**a**) **1a**, (**b**) **1b-THF** (isomer A), (**c**) **2a** and (**d**) **2b**. Hydrogen atoms and solvent molecules are omitted for clarity. Anisotropic displacement parameters (ADP's) are given at the 50% pobability level.

Table 1. Interatomic distances, angles, and torsion angles from SCXRD data and from DFT-optimized geometries.

	(^{I}NHC)TiCl(OiPr)(THF) (**1a**)	(^{Bz}NHC)TiCl(OiPr)(THF) (**1b-THF**) ^{a}	(^{Is}NHC)TiCl(OiPr)(THF) (**1c**) ^{b}
	Bond Length (Å)^c		
Ti-C$_{carbene}$	2.1310(13)/2.144	2.221(2)/2.214	2.166(3)/2.180
Ti-Cl	2.3739(4)/2.337	2.3459(8)/2.325	2.383(1)/2.336
Ti-OiPr	1.7671(11)/1.785	1.758(2)/1.789	1.779(2)/1.774
Ti-THF	2.2573(11)/2.318	2.2865(2)/2.347	2.272(2)/2.351
	Angle (°)^c		
∠O$_{Ar}$-Ti-O$_{Ar}$	159.14(4)/157.93	159.18(8)/158.70	159.19(9)/158.23
∠Ti-O-C$_{iPr}$	139.95(9)/143.18	160.5(3)/140.92	154.7(3)/160.48
∠N-C$_{carbene}$-N	105.22(11)/105.40	106.0(2)/106.20	108.8(2)/108.91
	Torsion Angle (°)^c		
∠O$_{Ar}$-C$_{Ar}$-N-C$_{carbene}$	5.86/8.02	27.04/22.78	3.35/4.61
∠O$_{Ar}$-C$_{Ar}$-N-C$_{carbene}$	6.89/9.71	−25.40/−25.67	3.51/5.54

^{a} Selected bond distances (Å), angles, and torsion angles (°) for **1b-THF-isomer A** and for **1b-THF-isomer B**: Ti-C$_{carbene}$ = 2.212(2), Ti-Cl = 2.3422(8), Ti-OiPr = 1.7685(18), Ti-THF = 2.2867(19),: ∠O$_{Ar}$-Ti-O$_{Ar}$ = 155.38(8), ∠Ti-O-C$_{iPr}$ = 165.57(19), ∠N-C$_{carbene}$-N = 106.5(2), ∠O$_{Ar}$-C$_{Ar}$-N-C$_{carbene}$ = 24.50, ∠O$_{Ar}$-C$_{Ar}$-N-C$_{carbene}$ = −26.06. ^{b} Ref. [38]. ^{c} SCXRD structure/DFT-optimized structure.

Both **1a** and **1b-THF** show a slightly distorted octahedral geometry around the Ti(IV) center as a result of the *mer*-coordination of the tridentate NHC ligand, with ∠O$_{Ar}$-Ti-O$_{Ar}$ bite angles of 159.14(4)° and 159.18(8)°, respectively. This ligand coordination is similar to that observed earlier for other bis-phenolate NHC-Ti complexes [20,29,38,40,42,70].

The principal structural features of both **1a** and **1b-THF** include (i) a *mer*-NHC chelate deviating from planarity, with torsion angles ∠O$_{Ar}$-C$_{Ar}$-N-C$_{carbene}$ of 5.86/6.89° and 27.04/−25.40°, respectively, (ii) *trans*-dispositioning of the carbene moiety and the Cl atom, and (iii) *trans*-dispositioning of the O*i*Pr and the THF ligand. Compared to the corresponding titanium complex bearing a saturated NHC, ([κ^3-O,C,O]-^{Is}NHC)TiCl(O*i*Pr)(THF) **1c**, the torsion angles ∠O$_{Ar}$-C$_{Ar}$-N-C$_{carbene}$ are similar for **1a** but far more distorted from planarity for **1b-THF** (Table 1) [38]. The Ti–C$_{carbene}$ bond length (2.221(2) Å) in complex **1b-THF** is longer than that of 1c (2.166(3) Å), reflected in a shorter Ti-Cl bond distance (2.3459(8) Å) *trans* to the NHC. This is consistent with a weaker *trans* influence from the presumably less electron-donating benzimidazolin-2-ylidene moiety [2,71–73]. Less electron donation from the latter ligand and its deviation from planarity might help explain the relatively short Ti-O*i*Pr bond and the tendency toward *sp*^{2} hybridization, suggested by the relatively wide ∠Ti-O-C$_{iPr}$ angle (160.5(3)°, 165.57(19)° for isomer B), for this oxygen atom. The more *sp*^{2}-like hybridization may bring about increased π-donation from the O*i*Pr moiety and thus explain the apparent greater *trans* influence and the more weakly bound THF molecule in **1b-THF** (Ti-THF$_{avg}$ ≈ 2.28 Å) and **1c** than in **1a** (Table 1).

The latter complex has the shortest Ti-C$_{carbene}$ bond distance (2.1310(13) Å) of all reported NHC-Ti complexes of functionalized NHC ligands (Ti-C$_{carbene}$ = 2.14–2.33 Å) [12,14,29]. As expected, the short Ti–C$_{carbene}$ bond is, due to *trans* influence, reflected in a Ti–Cl$_{trans}$ bond that is longer than in **1b-THF** and only slightly shorter than in **1c**. Whereas ligands based on the imidazolidin-2-ylidene moiety are often reported to be more electron donating than those of the imidazol-2-ylidene moiety [2,71–73], the short Ti-C$_{carbene}$ bond distance of **1a** seems to suggest otherwise. The components of the Ti-C$_{carbene}$ bonds of the three ligands have thus been studied and compared using DFT and NBO analysis (vide infra). Furthermore, the relatively sharp ∠Ti-O-C$_{iPr}$ angle (139.95(5)°) of **1a** seems to suggest more *sp*^{3}-like hybridization and less π-donation of the O*i*Pr ligand. The sharp ∠Ti-O-C$_{iPr}$ angle appears not to be caused by steric repulsion between the imidazol-2-ylidene and O*i*Pr moieties, since the NHC in **1a** is only slightly less planar than that in **1c**. Thus, the presumed weaker π-donation from O*i*Pr in **1a** is consistent with the short Ti-THF bond (2.2573(11) Å) which, in turn, is consistent with the *trans* influence of O*i*Pr being weaker in **1a** than in **1b-THF** and **1c**.

To further investigate the structural differences of the complexes and their relation to the electronic properties of the NHC ligands, we studied the ligands and the complexes using DFT and NBO analyses. First, the DFT calculations predict the experimentally obtained bond distances accurately, to within 0.01–0.02 Å (Table 1). More importantly, the trend in calculated Ti-C$_{carbene}$ bond distances between the complexes faithfully reproduces that obtained in X-ray crystallographic analysis. The large variation in Ti-C$_{carbene}$ bond distances (up to 9 pm when comparing the X-ray structures) are thus not the result of crystal-packing effects but must instead originate from the carbenes themselves. The experimentally and computationally obtained Ti-C$_{carbene}$ distances thus suggest that the strength of the interaction between the metal and the carbene diminishes in the order **a** > **c** > **b** for the three NHC ligands (Table 1). Valence and torsional angles are also well reproduced, except for the ∠Ti-O-C$_{iPr}$ angle. However, this angle varies by more than 20° between the three complexes, presumably reflecting a very shallow bending potential.

Regarding the Ti–ligand bond energies and interactions, the bond "snapping" energies (Table 2), i.e., the bond energies calculated by dissociating the tridentate ligands heterolytically to frozen-geometry [TiCl(O*i*Pr)(THF)]$^{2+}$ fragments **M1a–c** and dianionic NHC ligands **Ma–c** (Supplementary Scheme S1), are consistent with the trend in Ti-C$_{carbene}$ bond distances. Orbital interactions between these pairs of fragments might thus reveal the origin of the trends in both Ti-C$_{carbene}$ bond distances and bond energies. The calculated ligand-to-metal net electron donations (Table 2) are essentially identical for the three complexes, showing that further resolution is necessary for uncovering the factors determining the differences in bond distances and energies.

To uncover these factors, we performed NBO [74] analyses of the individual fragments **M1a–c** and **Ma–c** as well as of the metal-ligand orbital interactions in the three complexes. The most important fragment and complex orbitals obtained in these analyses are shown in Figures 2 and 3.

Table 2. NHC binding energies, natural charges, and net electron donation to Ti.

Complex	Ti-NHC Snapping Energy [a] (kcal mol^{-1})	NHC Fragment Charge [b] (e^{-})	NHC→Ti Net Donation [c] (№ of e^{-})
1a	597.3	−0.76	0.57
1b-THF	587.3	−0.78	0.58
1c	592.7	−0.76	0.58

[a] The Ti-NHC bond energies, or bond snapping energies, were calculated from the DFT total energies (i.e., not the free energies; see Table S2) by dissociating the tridentate ligands heterolytically to frozen-geometry fragments **M1a–c** and **Ma–c**. [b] The NHC fragment charge is the sum of all the natural atomic charges of the tridentate NHC ligand. [c] The NHC→Ti net donation is estimated as the number of electrons needed to reach neutrality for a NHC fragment in which the atomic charges of the two oxygen atoms have been subtracted (Table S3).

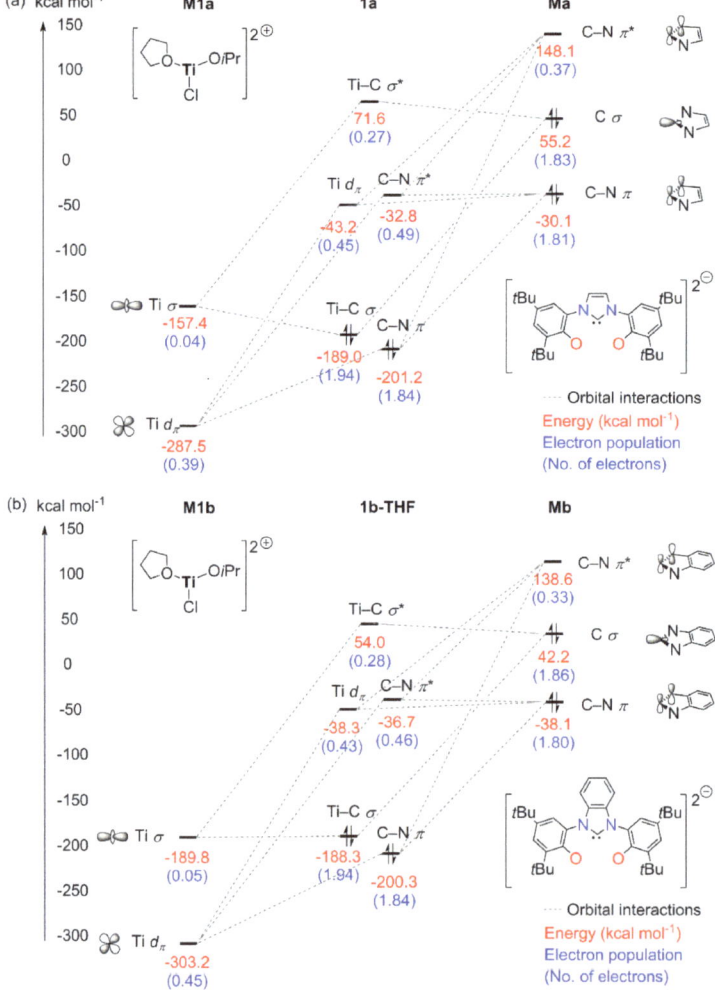

Figure 2. (a) Natural orbitals calculated for the **M1a** and **Ma** fragments and the **1a** complex. (b) Natural orbitals calculated for the **M1b** and **Mb** fragments and the **1b-THF** complex. The interactions between fragment orbitals leading to hybrid, bonding, or antibonding orbitals of the complexes are indicated by dashed lines.

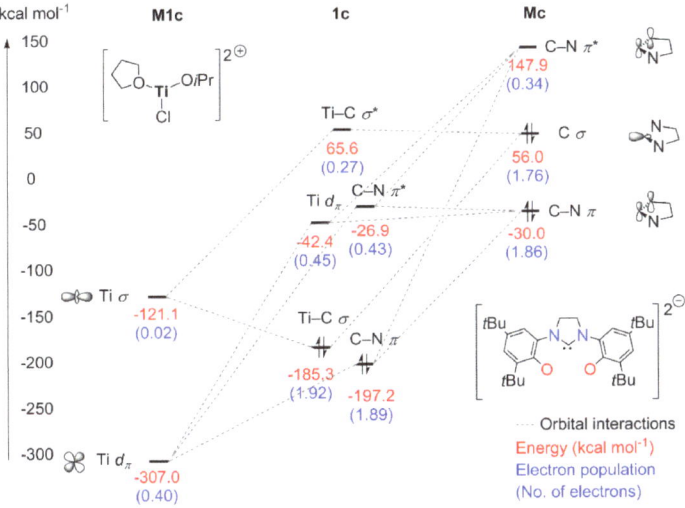

Figure 3. Natural orbitals calculated for the **M1c** and **Mc** fragments and the **1c** complex. The interactions between fragment orbitals leading to hybrid, bonding, or antibonding orbitals of the complex are indicated by dashed lines.

Insight is offered, for example, by the calculated energies of the C σ orbitals of the three OH-containing free-carbene ligands **Ma–cH$_2$** (Table 3 and Supplementary Scheme S1), which suggest that the σ-donating capacity should be greatest for **c**, followed by **a** and **b**. Whereas this ranking is consistent with the relative Ti-C$_{carbene}$ bond distances of **1a** and **1b-THF**, additional factors must explain why this distance is shorter in **1a** than in **1c**. An explanation might be offered by the interaction between the π-orbital of the ligand (C-N π) and a metal d-orbital of the same symmetry (Ti d_π).

Table 3. Absolute energies and electron populations of ligand natural orbitals important for the Ti-NHC interaction.

Orbital [a]			MaH$_2$ [b]	MbH$_2$	McH$_2$
C σ		Population (№ of electrons)	1.71	1.74	1.69
		Energy (kcal mol^{-1})	−136.2	−142.0	−133.3
C-N π		Population (№ of electrons)	1.85	1.86	1.90
		Energy (kcal mol^{-1})	−200.4	−200.3	−198.3
C-N π*		Population (№ of electrons)	0.49	0.45	0.42
		Energy (kcal mol^{-1})	−37.4	−37.4	−33.9

[a] The backbone of the NHC shown in the orbital figures is unsaturated for **MaH$_2$**, benzannulated for **MbH$_2$** and saturated for **McH$_2$**, see Scheme S1. [b] **MaH$_2$**, **MbH$_2$** and **McH$_2$** are the neutral, model, OH-containing free-carbene ligands of the complexes **1a**, **1b-THF** and **1c**.

The calculated second-order perturbative estimate of the donor-acceptor interaction between these two orbitals is largest for **1a**, followed by **1c**, and **1b-THF** (Table 4 and Supplementary Table S4), consistent with the trend in bond distances and bond energies. In other words, π-donation from the ligand to the metal is suggested to be stronger for **a** and to modify the trend offered by the ligand σ-donating capacity suggested by the C σ energies in Table 3. The importance of ligand-to-metal π-donation has already been noted for NHC complexes of early transition metals [75–79].

Table 4. Second-order perturbative estimates of donor-acceptor interactions in the NBO basis of **1a**, **1b-THF** and **1c**.

Complex	Donor Orbital [a]	Acceptor Orbital	E2 (kcal mol^{-1})
	C-N π	Ti d_π	2.95
1a	O$_{iPr}$ LP	C-N π*	1.01
	O$_{THF}$ LP	C-N π*	1.26
	C-N π	Ti d_π	2.44
1b-THF	O$_{iPr}$ LP	C-N π*	0.30
	O$_{THF}$ LP	C-N π*	3.28
	C-N π	Ti d_π	2.75
1c	C-N π	C-N π*	0.83
	O$_{iPr}$ LP	C-N π*	0.39
	O$_{THF}$ LP	C-N π*	1.42

[a] LP refers to lone pair.

Whereas the above-described donation from largely filled ligand π-orbitals to largely empty d_π-orbitals of the metal is estimated to contribute significantly to the Ti-NHC bonding, the low occupations of metal *d*-orbitals of early transition-metal complexes (see, e.g., Figures 2 and 3) suggest that π-back donation from titanium to the NHC is much less important for the present complexes than for complexes of mid-to-late transition metals [71,75]. The metal *d*-orbitals are considered to be "lone vacant" orbitals in the NBO analysis (Figures 2 and 3), and direct back-donation from the metal to the C-N π* orbitals does not appear in the analysis and is likely to be small.

In contrast, the C-N π* orbitals are reported to sometimes accept electrons from lone pairs of anionic ligands of early transition metals [76–79]. Weak contributions of this kind, between isopropoxide oxygen lone pairs and the C-N π* orbitals, are seen also in the present three complexes (Table 4). In addition, the second-order perturbation analysis also identifies analogous interactions between the THF oxygen lone pairs and C-N π*. The strongest of these interactions is in **1b-THF**, where it is likely to be one of the driving forces behind the tilting of the NHC ligand toward the THF.

In conclusion, the calculations show that the strength of the interactions between the metal and the NHC follows the trend portrayed by the calculated and experimental Ti-NHC bond distances (**a** > **c** > **b**). Although the ligand-to-metal σ-donation is predicted to be stronger for ligand **c** (followed by **a**, and **b**), the π-donation from **a** is stronger and contributes to giving the overall trend in metal-ligand interaction strength and bond distances. Whereas back-donation from the metal to the NHC seems to be unimportant, weak donor-acceptor interactions from THF and OiPr lone pairs to the C-N π* orbitals contribute and are probably involved in the tilting of the NHC seen in **1b-THF**.

Due to their potential application in polymerization of CHO with CO_2 [29,41–43], the bis-isopropoxide ^{I}NHC- and ^{Bz}NHC-titanium complexes **2a** and **2b** were also synthesized and were found to be readily accessible, in quantitative yields (Scheme 2), via salt metathesis of LiOiPr with complex **1a** and **1b**, respectively, similarly to the saturated NHC-titanium analogue [38].

The NMR spectra of **2a** and **2b** contain resonances typical of five-coordinate ([κ^3-O,C,O]-NHC)TiX$_2$ complexes including a doublet resonance originating from the Me groups of the two OiPr moieties (Supplementary Figures S7–S10), which are consistent with C_{2v}-symmetric structures in solution for both complexes [38,42,43]. The corresponding ^{13}C NMR spectra confirm the chelation of the NHC ligand to Ti center with typical chemical resonances at δ 183.7 and 198.1 ppm

(Supplementary Figures S8 and S10) [14,69], respectively, shifted upfield compared to the saturated ([κ^3-O,C,O]-^{Is}NHC)Ti(OiPr)$_2$ complex **2c** [38]. Furthermore, the complete molecular structures of **2a** and **2b** were confirmed by SCXRD analysis, showing that these complexes are five-coordinate and adopt a distorted square-pyramidal geometry according to the Addison and Reedijk geometric parameter (τ_5 = 0.49 for **2a** and 0.27 for **2b**), with one of the OiPr moieties in apical position (Figure 1; see Supplementary Table S6 for crystallographic data) [80]. Both geometries differ from that of saturated ([κ^3-O,C,O]-^{Is}NHC)Ti(OiPr)$_2$ complex **2c** in which the five-coordinate Ti metal center adopt a trigonal-bipyramidal geometry (τ_5 = 0.51) [38]. The overall structural data for **2a** and **2b** resemble those previously observed for **1a** and **1b-THF**, with the following main particularities: (i) an even more pronounced deviation from planarity for the *mer*-NHC chelate, with torsion angles ∠O$_{Ar}$-C$_{Ar}$-N-C$_{carbene}$ of −12.88/19.19° for **2a** and −28.95/30.36° for **2b**, (ii) a shorter Ti–C$_{carbene}$ bond length for **2a** compared to **2b** and to the saturated ([κ^3-O,C,O]-^{Is}NHC)Ti(OiPr)$_2$ complex, and (iii) ∠Ti-O-C$_{iPr}$ angles approaching linearity (162.7(3) for **2a** and 158.0(3)° for **2b**) for the OiPr co-ligand, indicating enhanced π-donation from this ligand for **2a** compared to **2b** and to the saturated-NHC analogue **2c** (Supplementary Table S6) [38]. The sharper ∠O$_{Ar}$-Ti-O$_{Ar}$ angle (138.19(8)°) observed for **2b** compared to **1b-THF** is most likely a result of steric interactions between the *t*Bu and OiPr moieties (Supplementary Table S6).

Aiming to further explore NHC-hafnium compounds as precursors for the copolymerization of epoxide with CO_2, attempts to synthesize ([κ^3-O,C,O]-^{I}NHC)HfCl(OiPr)(THF) **3a** complex via addition of proligand **a** to Hf(OiPr)$_4$(HOiPr) under the same reaction conditions as for titanium, invariably gave a mixture of unidentifiable compounds. Only when the addition of **a** to Hf(OiPr)$_4$(HOiPr) was performed overnight at room temperature and extended reaction time did the ^{1}H NMR spectrum of the reaction mixture showed three distinct sets of signals attributable to three different compounds (in ratio ≈ 2:1:0.8), which unfortunately could not be further separated or isolated. The most intense signal set was tentatively attributed to ([κ^3-O,C,O]-^{I}NHC)HfCl(OiPr)(THF) **3a**, and the two others to the zwitterionic ([κ^2-O,O]-^{Bz}NHCH)HfCl$_2$(OiPr) **3b'** and the homoleptic ([κ^3-O,C,O]-^{I}NHC)$_2$Hf **3a"** (Scheme 3).

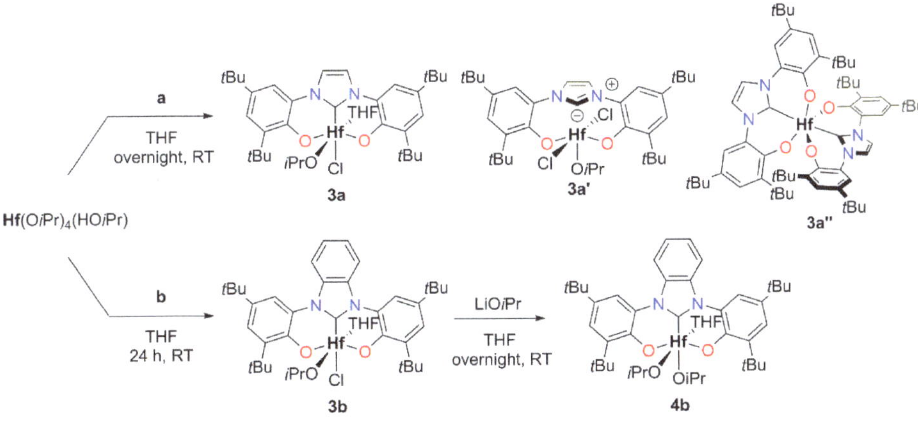

Scheme 3. Preparation of NHC-Hf complexes **3a**, **3a'**, **3a"**, **3b** and **4b**.

Similarly, addition of proligand **b** to Hf(OiPr)$_4$(HOiPr) under identical conditions led to a mixture of compounds, among which ([κ^3-O,C,O]-^{Bz}NHC)Hf(OiPr)(THF) **3b** is identified to be the major product according to ^{1}H NMR (estimated yield 86%, Supplementary Figure S11) and ^{13}C-NMR spectra (with a typical Hf-C$_{carbene}$ at δ 201.8 ppm) [14,69]. The minor side-products presumably are the zwitterionic **3b'** and the homoleptic **3b"** (Scheme 3). As previously observed for the reactivity of proligands **a** and **b** with the Zr-alkoxide precursor, the formation of the homoleptic complex cannot be completely avoided, most likely due to the reaction of a second proligand with the large metal ions such as Hf^{4+}. In contrast, the smaller Ti^{4+} leads to release of HCl, which, in turn, cleaves off the M-C$_{carbene}$ bond in the ([κ^3-O,C,O]-NHC)MCl(OiPr)(THF) complex and thus to the formation zwitterionic species [44]. Even if **3b** could not be further purified, the molecular structure was established by the recovery of single crystals of **3b** suitable for SCXRD analysis from a solution of unpurified **3b** in pentane at −30 °C (Figure 4). A crystallographic summary for **3b** is included with the selected bond lengths, angles, and torsion angles in the electronic supplementary information (Tables S5 and S7). As expected, complex **3b** exhibits structural features closely related to those of **1b-THF**. Similar observations can be made when **3b** is structurally compared to its saturated analogue ([κ^3-O,C,O]-^{Is}NHC)HfCl(OiPr)(THF) **3c** than between NHC-Ti complexes of **1b-THF** and **1c** [45]. The only exception is the angle ∠Hf-O-C$_{iPr}$, which is sharper in the case of **3b** than in **3c** (162.4(3)° vs. 171.1(3)°), indicating slightly diminished π-donation from the OiPr moiety.

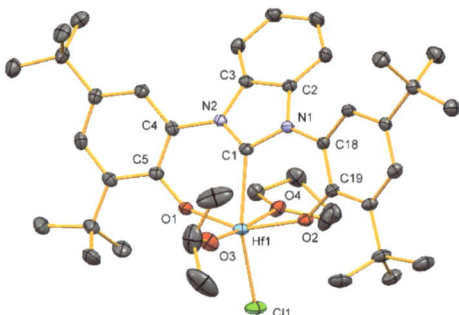

Figure 4. Molecular structure of **3b**. Hydrogen atoms and pentane solvent molecule are omitted for clarity. ADP's are given at the 50% probability level.

As previously reported for the bis-isopropoxide ^{Bz}NHC-titanium complex **2b**, the Hf analogue **4b** was also synthesized via salt metathesis from the reaction of LiOiPr with complex **3b** (Scheme 3). Although many attempts to isolate the **4b** in its pure form were unsuccessful, the NMR data unambiguously allowed identification of **4b** as the major product (Supplementary Figure S12).

2.2. Copolymerization of CHO with CO$_2$

The copolymerization of CHO and CO$_2$ was investigated by using unsaturated and benzannulated NHC-titanium and hafnium complexes in combination with 1 equiv. of bis(triphenylphosphine)iminium chloride ([PPN]Cl) as ionic co-catalyst in neat CHO (CHO:M = 1250:1) under mild conditions (P_{CO2} = 2 bar, at 65 °C) for 24 h (Table 5).

The results were compared with the benchmark saturated-NHC complexes ([κ^3-O,C,O]-^{Is}NHC)TiCl(OiPr)(THF) **1c** and ([κ^3-O,C,O]-^{Is}NHC)HfCl(OiPr)(THF) **3c** (Table 5) [41–43,45]. As for the benchmark binary catalyst systems, all NHC-Ti and NHC-Hf catalysts gave completely alternating PCHC selectively (99% in carbonate linkage) without concomitant formation of CHC or PCHO. Another characteristic feature of the new catalysts was that they all produced PCHCs of molecular weights below 4.5 kg mol^{-1}, with bimodal distributions and relatively narrow polydispersities (Đ < 1.6), indicating a controlled polymerization (entries 1–5 and 7–8, Table 5). A noticeable trend among the NHC-Ti catalysts is that the unsaturated NHC-Ti **1–2a**/[PPN]Cl systems are less active and productive than the benzannulated NHC-Ti **1–2b**/[PPN]Cl systems (entries 1–3 and 5, Table 5). To allow for a direct comparison with the benchmark saturated NHC-Ti **1c** catalyst, the reaction time was shortened to 5 h for avoiding recurrent mass transfer issues about half conversion in neat CHO [41]. It was found that saturated catalyst system **5**/[PPN]Cl is twice as active as the benzannulated NHC-Ti **1b**/[PPN]Cl system (entries 4 and 6, TOFs 62 h^{-1} vs. 116 h^{-1}, respectively). Even more pronounced differences in activity were observed when comparing the benzannulated NHC-Hf **3b** and **4b**/[PPN]Cl and the saturated NHC-Hf **3c** (entries 7–9; TOFs 6–7 h^{-1} vs. 116 h^{-1}).

Table 5. Copolymerization of CHO-CO$_2$ catalyzed by titanium and hafnium NHC complexes.

Entry	Precursor [a,b]	Yield (%) [c]	Productivity (g$_{PCHC}$ mol$_M^{-1}$ h^{-1})	TOF (h^{-1}) [d]	M_n (kg mol^{-1}) [e]	Đ [e]
1	1a	37	2745	22	1.8	1.59
2	2a	26	1940	15	- [g]	- [g]
3	1b	49	3618	28	4.5	1.43
4	1b [f]	19	6709	62	1.2	1.54
5	2b	48	3557	24	4.0	1.44
6	1c [f]	52	18,572	116	5.9	1.41
7	3b	10	770	6	- [g]	- [g]
8	4b	12	897	7	- [g]	- [g]
9	3c [f]	49	17,426	116	9.0	1.18

[a] Catalyst preformation: addition of 1 equiv. of [PPN]Cl to the precursor in CH$_2$Cl$_2$ at 30 °C for 15 min and dried 30 min under vacuum. [b] Copolymerization conditions: 0.08 mol%$_M$, 10 mmol of CHO, P_{CO_2} = 2 bar at 65 °C for 24 h. [c] Determined by gravimetry. [d] Turnover frequency. [e] Determined by GPC-SEC in THF at 30 °C against polystyrene standards. [f] 5 h. [g] Not determined. Note: For all runs, the carbonate linkages are ≥99% and the selectivity in PCHC are >99% without by-products and determined by ^{1}H-NMR spectroscopy in CDCl$_3$.

The trend in catalytic activity (**1c** > **1b-THF** > **1a**) might originate from the inherent stability of the complexes and might also, at least in part, originate from the lability of the THF molecule and the ease with which this ligand is displaced to form the putative anionic six-coordinate intermediate upon activation with [PPN]Cl, as previously shown with the anionic catalysts [([κ^3-O,C,O]-^{Is}NHC)HfCl$_3$]$^-$ [45] and [([κ^4-N,O,O,O]-ATP)TiCl(OiPr)]$^-$ (ATP = amino-tris(phenolate)) [62]. The more active catalysts **1c** and **1b-THF** have, according to SCXRD and DFT, longer Ti-THF bonds than **1a**, which indicate a weakly bonded THF ligand and a higher rate of formation of the active species and/or, by analogy to other catalytic systems [46–50,52,81], a faster dissociation of the growing polymer chains during the copolymerization. The length of the Ti-THF bond, in turn, does not correlate in a straightforward fashion with the net electron donation from the NHC moiety to the metal center (which are very similar; see Table 2) or with the length or strength of the Ti-NHC bond. The latter bond appears to influence the lability of the THF ligand more indirectly, via the Ti-OiPr bond *trans* to the THF. For example, the long Ti-C$_{carbene}$ bond in **1b-THF** results in a short Ti-OiPr bond and, due to *trans* influence, a long and presumably weak Ti-THF bond.

3. Materials and Methods

3.1. Experimental Details

All operations were performed with rigorous exclusion of moisture and air, using standard Schlenk-line system and glovebox techniques under argon atmosphere (MB Braun MB200B-G, <1 ppm O$_2$ and <1 ppm H$_2$O). Hexane, toluene, THF and dichloromethane were purified, by using Grubbs columns (MBraun solvent purification system). Pentane, C$_6$D$_6$, CDCl$_3$, and CHO were degassed and dried overnight over sodium or CaH$_2$, back transferred and then employing the freeze-pump-thaw procedure. All chemicals were obtained from Sigma-Aldrich/Merck and used as received. Proligands **a**, **b**, and **c** [26,67,68,82,83], compounds ([κ^3-O,C,O]-^{Is}NHC)TiCl(OiPr)(THF) **1c** [38] and ([κ^3-O,C,O]-^{Is}NHC)HfCl(OiPr)(THF) **3c** [25,45] were prepared according to the literature procedures. [PPN]Cl was recrystallized prior to use [84]. Carbon dioxide purity grade (99.999%) was purified through copper oxide on alumina and molecular sieves (3 Å).

The NMR spectra (Bruker, Billerica, MA, USA) of air and moisture sensitive compounds were recorded by using J. Young valve NMR tubes at 25 °C on a Bruker-BIOSPIN-AV500 ultrashield 500 plus

(5 mm BBO with z-gradient BTO, ^{1}H: 500.13 MHz; ^{13}C: 125.75 MHz), and a Bruker Ascend AV850 III HD (5 mm triple resonance CryoProbe, ^{1}H: 850.13 MHz; ^{13}C: 213.77 MHz). ^{1}H and ^{13}C shifts are referenced to internal solvent resonances and reported in parts per million relative to TMS. DRIFT spectra (Thermo Nicolet, Madison, WI, USA) were recorded by using a Nicolet protégé 460 ESP FTIR spectrometer and a DRIFT cell (KBr window) under argon atmosphere. The spectra were averaged over 64 scans; the resolution was ± 4 cm^{-1}. Elemental analysis of C, H and N elements was performed on an Elementar Vario EL III. GPC-SEC (Viscotek-Malvern, Worcestershire, UK) was measured, to determine M_n and M_w of the PCHC polymers obtained from the catalytic testing, from Viscotek. Narrow polystyrene PS-99K (M_w = 99.284 kg mol^{-1}, M_n = 97.381 kg mol^{-1} and IV = 0.477 dL g^{-1}) and all calibration standards were obtained from Malvern PolyCAL. Approx. 30 mg of each polymer, obtained from the catalytic testing, were dissolved in exactly 10 mL THF (containing 250 ppm BHT inhibitor). The sample solutions (≈ 3.0 mg mL^{-1} in THF) were filtered through syringe filter Whatmann (0.45 μm pore size) prior to injection. Chromatographic separation was performed at a column temperature of 30 °C with a flow rate of 1 mL min^{-1}. SEC was performed with a pump supplied by Viscotek (GPCmax), employing two ViscoGel columns. Signals were detected by means of a triple detection array (TDA 302) and calibrated against polystyrene standards (Đ < 1.2, from 0.12–940 kg mol^{-1}).

3.2. Synthesis of ([κ^3-O,C,O]-^{I}NHC)TiCl(OiPr)(THF) 1a

In a glovebox, to a stirred solution of Ti(OiPr)$_4$ (28 mg, 0.098 mmol) in 7 mL THF precooled at −30 °C was added dropwise a solution of one equiv. of **a** (50 mg, 0.098 mmol) in THF (12 mL) at −30 °C. The colorless mixture immediately turned yellow-orange upon addition of Ti(OiPr)$_4$ and was stirred 2 h at room temperature, then dried under vacuum. The yellow solid was washed with small fraction of hexane (3 × 2 mL) and all volatiles were removed under vacuum affording yellow powder **1a**. Yield = 86%. Yellow crystals of **1a** suitable for SCXRD analysis (Bruker-AXS, Madison, WI, USA) could be obtained from THF: hexane (1:3) at −30 °C after one week. Anal. Calcd for C$_{38}$H$_{57}$N$_2$O$_4$Ti: C, 66.22; H, 8.34; N, 4.06%. Found: C, 65.69; H, 7.82; N, 4.01%. Despite several attempts, no better elemental analysis data could be obtained. ^{1}H NMR (500.13 MHz, C$_6$D$_6$, 25 °C): δ, 7.60 (d, J = 2.2 Hz, 2H, Ar-H), 7.17 (d, J = 2.2 Hz, 2H, Ar-H), 6.99 (s, 2H, NCH), 4.76 (sept, J = 6.1 Hz, 1H, O-CH(CH$_3$)$_2$), 3.58 (m, 4H, THF), 1.93 (s, 18H, tBu), 1.41 (m, 4H, THF), 1.35 (s, 18H, tBu), 0.94 (d, J = 6.1 Hz, 6H, O-CH(CH$_3$)$_2$) ppm. ^{13}C{^{1}H} NMR (125.77 MHz, C$_6$D$_6$, 25 °C): δ, 184.0 (NCN), 151.8 (C$_q$, Ar), 141.5 (C$_q$, Ar), 139.9 (C$_q$, Ar), 127.1 (C$_q$, Ar), 122.7 (CH-Ar), 116.2 (NCH), 112.3 (CH-Ar), 84.0 (O-CH(CH$_3$)$_2$), 67.9 (THF), 36.3 (C$_q$, tBu), 34.7 (C$_q$, tBu), 31.8 (CH, tBu), 30.4 (CH, tBu), 26.0 (O-CH(CH$_3$)$_2$), 25.8 (THF) ppm. DRIFT (KBr, ν/cm^{-1}, [4000–400]): 2958vs, 2930s, 2906s, 2867m, 1477s, 1447s, 1390vw, 1361w, 1322s, 1270m, 1253w, 1115s, 1105m, 1009m, 923vw, 861s, 844w, 773w, 764vw, 571m, 454w.

3.3. Synthesis of ([κ^3-O,C,O]-^{Bz}NHC)TiCl(OiPr) 1b

In a glovebox, to a stirred solution of Ti(OiPr)$_4$ (50.5 mg, 0.178 mmol) in 5 mL THF precooled at −30 °C was added dropwise a solution of one equiv. of **b** (100 mg) in THF (12 mL) at −30 °C. The colorless mixture immediately turned yellow upon addition of Ti(OiPr)$_4$ and was stirred 2 h at room temperature, then dried under vacuum. The yellow solid was washed with small fraction of hexane (3 × 2 mL) and all volatiles were removed under vacuum affording yellow powder **1b**. Yield = 84%. Yellow crystals of THF adduct of **1b** (**1b-THF**) suitable for SCXRD analysis could be obtained from a mixture of THF:pentane (1:3) at −30 °C after 2 days. Anal. Calcd for C$_{42}$H$_{59}$ClN$_2$O$_4$Ti: C, 68.24; H, 8.04; N, 3.79%. Found: 68.36; H, 8.08; N, 4.15%. ^{1}H NMR (500.13 MHz, C$_6$D$_6$, 25 °C): δ, 7.90 (m, 2H, Ar$_{bz}$-H), 7.73 (d, J = 2.3 Hz, 2H, Ar-H), 7.62 (d, J = 2.3 Hz, 2H, Ar-H), 7.00 (m, 2H, Ar$_{bz}$-H), 4.35 (sept, J = 6.2 Hz, 1H, O-CH(CH$_3$)$_2$), 1.93 (s, 18H, tBu), 1.33 (s, 18H, tBu), 0.80 (d, J = 6.2 Hz, 6H, O-CH(CH$_3$)$_2$) ppm. ^{13}C{^{1}H} NMR (125.77 MHz, C$_6$D$_6$, 25 °C): δ, 195.2 (NCN), 152.9 (C$_q$, Ar), 141.3 (C$_q$, Ar), 139.6 (C$_q$, Ar), 133.3 (C$_q$, Ar), 126.2 (C$_q$, Ar), 125.3 (CH-Ar), 122.9 (CH-Ar), 116.2 (CH-Ar), 114.5 (CH-Ar), 86.4 (O-CH(CH$_3$)$_2$), 36.3 (C$_q$, tBu), 34.7 (C$_q$, tBu), 31.7 (CH$_3$, tBu), 30.3 (CH$_3$, tBu), 25.6 (O-CH(CH$_3$)$_2$) ppm. DRIFT (KBr, ν/cm^{-1}, [4000–400]): 2960vs, 2928s, 2869m, 1552m, 1483s, 1469m,

1441s, 1380m, 1364m, 1309m, 1291m, 1269m, 1256 m, 1202vw, 1119s, 1019m, 918w, 857s, 803vw, 752m, 701w, 637w, 576m, 495w, 418w.

3.4. Synthesis of [κ^3-O,C,O]-(^{I}NHC)Ti(OiPr)$_2$ 2a

To a solution of **1a** (26 mg, 0.037 mmol) in 5 mL THF precooled at −30 °C was added dropwise 1.1 equiv. of LiOiPr (2.7 mg, 0.041 mmol) dissolved in 3 mL THF. The solution was stirred at room temperature overnight, then dried under vacuum and extracted with hexane. The bright yellow solution mixture was centrifuged, filtered, and then dried under vacuum affording a pale-yellow powder **2a**. Yield = 78%. Orange crystal of **2a** suitable for SCXRD analysis could be obtained from hexane at −30 °C after 2 days. Anal. Calcd for $C_{37}H_{56}N_2O_4Ti$: C, 69.36; H, 8.81; N, 4.37%. Found: C, 68.97; H, 8.54; N, 4.00%. ^{1}H NMR (500.13 MHz, C_6D_6, 25 °C): δ, 7.61 (br d, J = 2.3 Hz, 2H, ArH), 7.18 (br d, J = 2.3 Hz, overlapping with benzene signal, ArH), 7.01 (s, overlapping with spinning side band, NCH), 5.07 (sept, J = 6.0 Hz, 2H, O-CH(CH$_3$)$_2$), 1.92 (s, 18H, tBu), 1.39 (s, 18H, tBu), 1.31 (d, J = 6.0 Hz, 12H, O-CH(CH_3)$_2$) ppm. ^{13}C{^{1}H} NMR (213.77 MHz, C_6D_6, 25 °C): δ, 183.6 (NCN), 152.7 (C_q, Ar), 141.5 (C_q, Ar), 139.4 (C_q, Ar), 127.2 (C_q, Ar), 122.3 (CH-Ar), 116.3 (NCH), 112.9 (CH-Ar), 77.9 (O-CH(CH$_3$)$_2$), 36.3 (C_q, tBu), 34.6 (C_q, tBu), 31.9 (CH$_3$, tBu), 30.5 (CH$_3$, tBu), 26.9 (O-CH(CH$_3$)$_2$) ppm. DRIFT (KBr, ν/cm^{-1}, [4000–400]): 2957vs, 2918s, 2900s, 2861m, 1480vs, 1450s, 1391vw, 1361w, 1321s, 1272m, 1254w, 1197w, 1125m, 1007m, 922vw, 850m, 799vw, 771w, 722w, 662vw, 558w, 454w.

3.5. Synthesis of ([κ^3-O,C,O]-^{Bz}NHC)Ti(OiPr)$_2$ 2b

To a solution of **1b** (80 mg, 0.108 mmol) in 5 mL THF precooled at −30 °C was added dropwise 1.2 equiv. of LiOiPr (8.3 mg, 0.126 mmol) dissolved in 3 mL THF. The yellow solution was stirred at room for 2 h, then dried under vacuum and extracted with hexane. The pale orange solution mixture was centrifuged, filtered, and then dried under vacuum affording a pale-yellow powder **2b**. Yellow crystals of **2b** suitable for SCXRD analysis could be obtained from hexane at −30 °C after 2 days. Yield = 94%. Anal. Calcd for $C_{41}H_{58}N_2O_4Ti·1/2THF$: C, 70.19; H, 8.63; N, 3.81%. Found: C, 69.64; H, 8.63; N, 3.79%. ^{1}H NMR (500.13 MHz, C_6D_6, 25 °C): δ, 7.87 (m, 2H, Ar$_{bz}$-H), 7.75 (d, J = 2.3 Hz, 2H, Ar-H), 7.64 (d, J = 2.3 Hz, 2H, Ar-H), 6.96 (m, 2H, Ar$_{bz}$-H), 4.94 (sept, J = 6.1 Hz, 1H, O-CH(CH$_3$)$_2$), 1.92 (s, 18H, tBu), 1.37 (s, 18H, tBu), 1.27 (d, J = 6.1 Hz, 6H, O-CH(CH_3)$_2$) ppm. ^{13}C{^{1}H} NMR (125.77 MHz, C_6D_6, 25 °C): δ, 198.1 (NCN), 153.7 (C_q, Ar), 139.5 (C_q, Ar), 139.0 (C_q, Ar), 133.6 (C_q, Ar), 126.9 (C_q, Ar), 124.5 (CH-Ar), 122.3 (CH-Ar), 116.8 (CH-Ar), 114.2 (CH-Ar), 78.9 (O-CH(CH$_3$)$_2$), 36.3 (C_q, tBu), 34.6 (C_q, tBu), 31.9 (CH, tBu), 30.4 (CH, tBu), 26.5 (O-CH(CH$_3$)$_2$) ppm. DRIFT (KBr, ν/cm^{-1}, [4000–400]): 2960vs, 2928s, 2865m, 1566m, 1485s, 1465m, 1431s, 1370m, 1362m, 1309m, 1325w, 1289m, 1269m, 1256m, 1236w, 1226w, 1198vw, 1163m, 1123s, 1013s, 922vw, 878w, 853s, 797vw, 766w, 752m, 695w, 641w, 616w, 592w, 560m, 485w.

3.6. Synthesis of ([κ^3-O,C,O]-^{Bz}NHC)HfCl(OiPr)(THF) 3b

In a glovebox, Hf(OiPr)$_4$(HOiPr) (76.4 mg, 0.160 mmol) in 7 mL THF was added dropwise over one hour to ligand **b** (80 mg, 0.142 mmol) dissolved in 20 mL THF at room temperature. The solution immediately turned pale yellow and then completely colorless after stirring for 24 h. The reaction mixture was dried under vacuum and extracted with hexane. The colorless solution mixture was centrifuged, filtered, washed with pentane, and then dried under vacuum affording a yellow-white powder corresponding to compound **3b** along with side products. Yield ≈ 86% (based on ^{1}H NMR data). Colorless crystals of **3b** suitable for SCXRD analysis could be obtained from pentane at −30 °C after 3 days. This compound could never be isolated in pure form even after repeated washings with hydrocarbon solvents. Major compound **3b**: ^{1}H NMR (500.13 MHz, C_6D_6, 25 °C): δ, 8.01 (m, 2H, Ar$_{bz}$-H), 7.72 (d, J = 2.4 Hz, 2H, Ar-H), 7.68 (d, J = 2.4 Hz, 2H, Ar-H), 7.01 (m, 2H, Ar$_{bz}$-H), 4.56 (sept, J = 6.1 Hz, 1H, O-CH(CH$_3$)$_2$), 3.47 (m, 4H, THF), 1.89 (s, 18H, tBu), 1.36 (s, 18H, tBu), 1.10 (d, J = 6.1 Hz, 6H, O-CH(CH_3)$_2$), 0.67 (br s, 4H, THF) ppm. ^{13}C{^{1}H} NMR (213.77 MHz, C_6D_6, 25 °C): δ, 201.8 (NCN), 152.2 (C_q, Ar), 141.1 (C_q, Ar), 139.3 (C_q, Ar), 134.2 (C_q, Ar), 126.9 (C_q, Ar), 124.7 (CH-Ar), 123.2 (CH-Ar), 117.9

(CH-Ar), 114.0 (CH-Ar), 73.7 (THF), 70.7 (O-CH(CH$_3$)$_2$), 36.2 (C$_q$, tBu), 34.6 (C$_q$, tBu), 31.8 (CH$_3$, tBu), 30.4 (CH$_3$, tBu), 27.0 (O-CH(CH$_3$)$_2$), 25.0 (THF) ppm.

3.7. Synthesis of ([κ^3-O,C,O]-^{Bz}NHC)Hf(OiPr)$_2$(THF) 4b

In a glovebox, to a solution of **3b** (37.2 mg, 0.043 mmol) in 10 mL THF was added dropwise 1.1 equiv. LiOiPr (3.1 mg, 0.047 mmol) dissolved in 5 mL THF. The solution immediately turned yellow and then completely colorless after stirring at room temperature for 24 h. The reaction mixture was dried under vacuum and extracted with hexane. The colorless solution mixture was centrifuged, filtered, washed with pentane, and then dried under vacuum affording a white powder corresponding to compound **4b** as major compound in quantitative yield along with minor unidentified side compounds. This compound could never be isolated in pure form even after repeated washings with hydrocarbon solvents. Major compound **4b**: ^{1}H-NMR (500.13 MHz, C$_6$D$_6$, 25 °C): δ, 7.98 (m, 2H, Ar$_{bz}$-H), 7.72 (d, J = 2.7 Hz, 2H, Ar-H), 7.68 (d, J = 2.7 Hz, 2H, Ar-H), 7.01 (m, 2H, Ar$_{bz}$-H), 4.63 (br m, 2H, O-CH(CH$_3$)$_2$), 3.42 (br m, 4H, THF), 1.90 (s, 18H, tBu), 1.37 (s, 18H, tBu), 1.31 (6H, O-CH(CH_3)$_2$), 1.07 (br m, 4H, THF) ppm. ^{13}C{^{1}H} NMR (213.77 MHz, C$_6$D$_6$, 25 °C): δ, 206.2 (NCN), 153.1 (C$_q$, Ar), 140.7 (C$_q$, Ar), 138.7 (C$_q$, Ar), 134.5 (C$_q$, Ar$_{bz}$), 127.1 (C$_q$, Ar), 124.2 (CH-Ar$_{bz}$), 122.7 (CH-Ar), 118.2 (CH-Ar), 113.8 (CH-Ar$_{bz}$), 71.5 (O-CH(CH$_3$)$_2$), 69.1 (THF), 36.3 (C$_q$, tBu), 34.5 (C$_q$, tBu), 31.9 (CH$_3$, tBu), 30.4 (CH$_3$, tBu), 28.0 (O-CH(CH$_3$)$_2$), 25.2 (THF) ppm.

3.8. Copolymerization of CHO and CO$_2$

A detailed copolymerization procedure is described as a typical example (Table 5, Entry 1). In a glovebox, an reaction tube for low-pressure reactions equipped with a magnetic stirring bar, a solution of the [PPN]Cl cocatalyst (8 µmol) in dichloromethane (ca. 1 mL) was added under vigorous stirring to a solution of complex **1a** (8 µmol) in dichloromethane (ca. 1 mL). The mixture was stirred at ambient temperature for 15 min and the solvent was removed under vacuum (30 min). The resulting solid was then dissolved in a precooled (−30 °C) solution of CHO (10 mmol). Then to the reaction tube was added 2 bar of CO$_2$ and the reaction mixture was heated to 65 °C. After 24 h, the reaction was cooled down and the pressure was released. An aliquot of the solution was taken for characterization of crude material by ^{1}H-NMR spectroscopy in CDCl$_3$. Then, the reaction mixture was quenched with 1 mL of acidic methanol, precipitated with methanol, and dried for several hours at 80 °C until constant weight. The yield was determined gravimetrically.

3.9. X-ray Crystallographic Details

Suitable crystals for diffraction experiments were selected in a glovebox and mounted in a minimum of Parabar 10,312 oil (Hampton Research) in a nylon loop and then mounted under a nitrogen cold stream from an Oxford Cryosystems 700 series open-flow cryostat. Data collection was done on a Bruker AXS TXS rotating anode system with an APEXII Pt^{135} CCD detector (Bruker-AXS, Madison, WI, USA) using graphite-monochromated Mo Kα radiation (λ = 0.710 73 Å). Data collection and data processing were done using APEX2 [85], SAINT [86], and SADABS [87] version 2012/1, whereas structure solution and final model refinement were done using SHELXS [88] version 2013/1 or SHELXT [89] version 2014/4 and SHELXL [90] version 2014/7. Details of the crystallographic analyses for **1a**, **2a**, **1b-THF**, **1b'**, **2b**, and **3b** are given in Supplementary Tables S1 and S5 and in CIF files (CCDC reference codes 2026401-2026406). These data can be obtained free of charge via www.ccdc.cam.ac.uk/data_request/cif, or by emailing data_request@ccdc.cam.ac.uk, or by contacting The Cambridge Crystallographic Data Centre, 12 Union Road, Cambridge CB2 1EZ, UK, fax: +44 223 336033.

3.10. Computational Methods

All density functional theory (DFT) calculations were performed with the Gaussian 16 suite of programs [91].

3.10.1. Geometry Optimization

Geometry optimization was performed using the Gaussian 16 implementation of the generalized-gradient approximation (GGA) functional of Perdew, Burke and Ernzerhof (PBE) [92] including Grimme's D3 empirical dispersion term [93] with revised Becke-Johnson damping parameters [94] (overall labelled PBE-D3M(BJ) for brevity). All atoms except titanium were described by Dunning's correlation-consistent valence triple-ζ plus polarization basis sets (termed cc-pVTZ) [95,96], as retrieved from the EMSL basis set exchange database [97,98]. Titanium was described by the Stuttgart 10-electron relativistic effective core potential (termed ECP10MDF) in conjunction with its accompanying primitive basis set (8s7p6d2f1g) contracted to [6s5p3d2f1g]. Both the effective core potential and the accompanying basis set were retrieved from the Stuttgart/Cologne group website [99]. Numerical integrations were performed using the Gaussian 16 (99,590) "ultrafine" grid (keyword int = ultrafine), a pruned grid consisting of 99 radial shells and 590 angular points per shell, except when solving the coupled-perturbed Hartree-Fock equations (part of the analytical second-derivatives calculations) for which the pruned (75,302 grid) "fine" grid was used (keyword CPHF=(Grid=Fine)). Geometries were optimized using tight convergence criteria (max. force 1.5×10^{-5} a.u., RMS force 1.0×10^{-5} a.u., max. force 6.0×10^{-5} a.u., RMS force 4.0×10^{-5} a.u.), without symmetry constraints, using convergence criteria for the self-consistent field (SCF) optimization procedure that were tightened tenfold compared to the default settings. The tightened criteria were RMS change in density matrix $< 1.0 \times 10^{-9}$ and max. change in density matrix $< 1.0 \times 10^{-7}$. All stationary points were characterized by the eigenvalues of the analytically calculated Hessian matrix and confirmed to be minima.

3.10.2. Single-Point Energy Calculations

All single-point energy calculations were performed with the same PBE-D3M(BJ) functional as described above for geometry optimization. For titanium, carbon, and hydrogen atoms, the basis sets were also the same as those used in the geometry optimizations. All other atoms (N, O and Cl) were described by correlation-consistent valence triple-ζ plus polarization basis sets augmented by diffuse functions (EMSL: aug-cc-pVTZ) [95,97,98,100]. Numerical integrations were performed with the "ultrafine" grid of Gaussian 16, and the SCF density-based convergence criterion was set to 10^{-5} (RMS change in density matrix $< 1.0 \times 10^{-5}$, max. change in density matrix $= 1.0 \times 10^{-3}$).

3.10.3. Natural Bond Orbital Calculations

All natural bond orbital calculations were performed with the NBO7 program [74], using the wavefunction produced by the Gaussian 16 single-point energy calculation as input. Keywords used in the NBO7 job include "bndidx", which requests the print-out of the NAO-Wiberg Bond Index array, "NBO" which requests the calculation and printing of NBO's, and "DMNAO" which requests the natural atomic orbital density matrix. To get a comparable set of orbitals among the complexes, the Lewis structures were explicitly restricted to those shown in Supplementary Scheme S2 via the $CHOOSE input section.

4. Conclusions

A series of titanium and hafnium complexes bearing unsaturated and benzannulated tridentate, bis-phenolate NHC ligands have been synthesized and characterized. The Ti-C$_{carbene}$ distances with which these ligands bind to the metal vary considerably (by 9 pm), and these differences manifest themselves, via *trans* influence and other "ripple effects", in significant variations also in the other metal-ligand bond distances. These structural differences and their relation to the metal-NHC bonds and the electronic properties of the ligands have been studied for titanium complexes **1a**, **1b-THF**, and **1c** using DFT and NBO analyses. The shorter Ti-C$_{carbene}$ distance in **1a** than in the other two complexes seems to originate from stronger ligand-to-metal π-donation, whereas the corresponding σ-donation is weaker than in **1c**. In contrast, back-donation directly from the metal to the NHC ligand seems to be unimportant in these d^0 complexes. Still, the C-N π* NHC orbitals are involved in bonding as they interact with THF and isopropoxide oxygen lone-pair donor orbitals, an interaction that appears to contribute to the tilting of the NHC ligand toward the THF in **1b-THF**.

The new complexes catalyze the copolymerization of CHO with CO_2 under mild reaction conditions (P_{CO2} = 2 bar and 65 °C) to exclusively give poly(cyclohexene carbonate) product, albeit with low-to-moderate yields. Among the new complexes, the benzannulated-NHC-coordinated titanium complex (**1b-THF**) gives the most active catalyst upon activation with [PPN]Cl. Including previously reported complexes, the order among the NHC ligands in terms of catalytic activity is as follows: imidazolidin-2-ylidene (saturated) > benzimidazolin-2-ylidene (benzannulated) > imidazolin-2-ylidene (unsaturated). Although further mechanistic studies are needed to uncover the factors governing this order, it might be influenced by the inherent stability of the complexes and possibly also the lability of the THF ligand, as suggested by the variation in Ti-THF distance among the complexes.

Supplementary Materials: The following are available online at, Figure S1: ^{1}H-NMR spectrum of complex **1a**; Figure S2: ^{13}C NMR spectrum of complex **1a**; Figure S3: ^{1}H NMR spectrum of complex **1b**; Figure S4: ^{13}C NMR spectrum of complex **1b**; Figure S5: ^{1}H NMR spectrum of **1b**, **1b′** and **1b″**; Figure S6: Molecular structure of zwitterionic compound **1b′**; Table S1: Crystal structure and refinement data for **1a**, **1b-THF** and **1b′**; Scheme S1: Complexes and ligands that have been subjected to DFT calculations; Table S2: DFT energies at the single-point level of theory; Table S3: Natural atomic charges of complexes **1a**, **1b-THF** and **1c**; Table S4: Second-order perturbative estimates of donor-acceptor interactions in the NBO basis of **1a**, **1b-THF** and **1c**; Figure S7: ^{1}H NMR spectrum of complex **2a**; Figure S8: ^{13}C NMR spectrum of complex **2a**; Figure S9: ^{1}H NMR spectrum of complex **2b**; Figure S10: ^{13}C NMR spectrum of complex **2b**; Table S5: Crystal structure and refinement data for **2a**, **2b** and **3b**; Figure S11: ^{1}H NMR spectrum of complex **3b**, **3b′** and **3b″**; Figure S12: ^{1}H NMR spectrum of complex **4b**; Table S6: Interatomic distances, angles and torsion angles for 5-coordinate complexes **2a**, **2b** and **2c**; Table S7: Interatomic distances, angles and torsion angles for 6-coordinate complexes **3b** and **3c**; Scheme S2: Lewis structures used in the NBO analyses; and list of Cartesian coordinates. The following are available online, Supporting Information (pdf) containing crystal data. CIF files containing crystal data for complexes **1a**, **2a**, **1b-THF**, **1b′**, **2b**, and **3b**.

Author Contributions: Synthesis of NHC ligands and complexes, R.L., L.S., F.G.-D., and E.L.R.; polymerization, L.S. and E.L.R.; inorganic characterization, L.R., L.S., F.G.-D., and E.L.R.; computational investigations, J.B.E. and V.R.J.; polymer characterization, L.S. and E.L.R.; crystallography, K.W.T.; writing—original draft preparation, R.L., L.S., J.B.E., F.G.-D., V.R.J., and E.L.R.; writing—review and editing, L.S., R.L., J.B.E., K.W.T., V.R.J., and E.L.R.; resources/funding acquisition, V.R.J. and E.L.R.; supervision of all contributions, V.R.J. and E.L.R. All authors have read and agreed to the published version of the manuscript.

Funding: This research was funded by Research Council of Norway (FRINATEK program: grant no. 240333 and NNP program: grant no. 226244) and University of Bergen. The Article Processing Charge was funded by the University of Bergen.

Acknowledgments: L.S. and J.B.E. acknowledge the University of Bergen for their respective doctoral fellowships.

Conflicts of Interest: The authors declare no conflict of interest. The funders had no role in the design of the study; in the collection, analyses, or interpretation of data; in the writing of the manuscript, or in the decision to publish the results.

References

1. Herrmann, W.A. N-Heterocyclic Carbenes: A New Concept in Organometallic Catalysis. *Angew. Chem. Int. Ed.* **2002**, *41*, 1290–1309. [CrossRef]
2. Díez-González, S.; Nolan, S.P. Stereoelectronic Parameters Associated with N-heterocyclic Carbene (NHC) Ligands: A Quest for Understanding. *Coord. Chem. Rev.* **2007**, *251*, 874–883. [CrossRef]
3. Díez-González, S.; Marion, N.; Nolan, S.P. N-Heterocyclic Carbenes in Late Transition Metal Catalysis. *Chem. Rev.* **2009**, *109*, 3612–3676. [CrossRef]
4. Lin, J.C.Y.; Huang, R.T.W.; Lee, C.S.; Bhattacharyya, A.; Hwang, W.S.; Lin, I.J.B. Coinage Metal–N-heterocyclic Carbene Complexes. *Chem. Rev.* **2009**, *109*, 3561–3598. [CrossRef]
5. Poyatos, M.; Mata, J.A.; Peris, E. Complexes with Poly(N-heterocyclic carbene) Ligands: Structural Features and Catalytic Applications. *Chem. Rev.* **2009**, *109*, 3677–3707. [CrossRef]

6. Hopkinson, M.N.; Richter, C.; Schedler, M.; Glorius, F. An Overview of *N*-heterocyclic Carbenes. *Nature* **2014**, *510*, 485–496. [CrossRef]
7. Riener, K.; Haslinger, S.; Raba, A.; Högerl, M.P.; Cokoja, M.; Herrmann, W.A.; Kühn, F.E. Chemistry of Iron *N*-Heterocyclic Carbene Complexes: Syntheses, Structures, Reactivities, and Catalytic Applications. *Chem. Rev.* **2014**, *114*, 5215–5272. [CrossRef]
8. Nasr, A.; Winkler, A.; Tamm, M. Anionic *N*-Heterocyclic Carbenes: Synthesis, Coordination Chemistry and Applications in Homogeneous Catalysis. *Coord. Chem. Rev.* **2016**, *316*, 68–124. [CrossRef]
9. Liddle, S.T.; Edworthy, I.S.; Arnold, P.L. Anionic Tethered *N*-heterocyclic Carbene Chemistry. *Chem. Soc. Rev.* **2007**, *36*, 1732–1744. [CrossRef]
10. Pugh, D.; Danopoulos, A.A. Metal Complexes with 'Pincer'-type Ligands Incorporating *N*-Heterocyclic Carbene Functionalities. *Coord. Chem. Rev.* **2007**, *251*, 610–641. [CrossRef]
11. McGuinness, D. Alkene Oligomerisation and Polymerisation with Metal-NHC Based Catalysts. *Dalton Trans.* **2009**, *2009*, 6915–6923. [CrossRef] [PubMed]
12. Bellemin-Laponnaz, S.; Dagorne, S. Group 1 and 2 and Early Transition Metal Complexes Bearing *N*-Heterocyclic Carbene Ligands: Coordination Chemistry, Reactivity, and Applications. *Chem. Rev.* **2014**, *114*, 8747–8774. [CrossRef]
13. Hameury, S.; de Fremont, P.; Braunstein, P. Metal Complexes with Oxygen-functionalized NHC Ligands: Synthesis and Applications. *Chem. Soc. Rev.* **2017**, *46*, 632–733. [CrossRef]
14. Zhang, D.; Zi, G. *N*-Heterocyclic Carbene (NHC) Complexes of Group 4 Transition Metals. *Chem. Soc. Rev.* **2015**, *44*, 1898–1921.
15. Romain, C.; Bellemin-Laponnaz, S.; Dagorne, S. Recent Progress on NHC-stabilized Early Transition Metal (group 3–7) Complexes: Synthesis and Applications. *Coord. Chem. Rev.* **2020**, *422*, 213411.
16. Kuhl, O. The Chemistry of Functionalised *N*-Heterocyclic Carbenes. *Chem. Soc. Rev.* **2007**, *36*, 592–607. [CrossRef]
17. Charra, V.; de Frémont, P.; Braunstein, P. Multidentate *N*-Heterocyclic Carbene Complexes of the 3d Metals: Synthesis, Structure, Reactivity and Catalysis. *Coord. Chem. Rev.* **2017**, *341*, 53–176.
18. Aihara, H.; Matsuo, T.; Kawaguchi, H. Titanium *N*-Heterocyclic Carbene Complexes Incorporating an Imidazolium-linked Bis(phenol). *Chem. Commun.* **2003**, 2204–2205. [CrossRef]
19. McGuinness, D.S.; Gibson, V.C.; Steed, J.W. Bis(carbene)pyridine Complexes of the Early to Middle Transition Metals: Survey of Ethylene Oligomerization and Polymerization Capability. *Organometallics* **2004**, *23*, 6288–6292. [CrossRef]
20. Zhang, D.; Liu, N. Titanium Complexes Bearing Bisaryloxy-*N*-heterocyclic Carbenes: Synthesis, Reactivity, and Ethylene Polymerization Study. *Organometallics* **2009**, *28*, 499–505. [CrossRef]
21. Bocchino, C.; Napoli, M.; Costabile, C.; Longo, P. Synthesis of Octahedral Zirconium Complex Bearing [NHC-O] Ligands, and its Behavior as Catalyst in the Polymerization of Olefins. *J. Polym. Sci. Part A Polym. Chem.* **2011**, *49*, 862–870. [CrossRef]
22. El-Batta, A.; Waltman, A.W.; Grubbs, R.H. Bis-ligated Ti and Zr Complexes of Chelating *N*-Heterocyclic Carbenes. *J. Organomet. Chem.* **2011**, *696*, 2477–2481. [CrossRef]
23. Larocque, T.G.; Badaj, A.C.; Dastgir, S.; Lavoie, G.G. New Stable Aryl-substituted Acyclic Imino-*N*-heterocyclic Carbene: Synthesis, Characterisation and Coordination to Early Transition Metals. *Dalton Trans.* **2011**, *40*, 12705–12712. [CrossRef]
24. Larocque, T.G.; Lavoie, G.G. Coordination and Reactivity Study of Titanium Phenoxo Complexes Containing a Bulky Bidentate Imino-*N*-heterocyclic Carbene Ligand. *J. Organomet. Chem.* **2012**, *715*, 26–32. [CrossRef]
25. Dagorne, S.; Bellemin-Laponnaz, S.; Romain, C. Neutral and Cationic *N*-Heterocyclic Carbene Zirconium and Hafnium Benzyl Complexes: Highly Regioselective Oligomerization of 1-Hexene with a Preference for Trimer Formation. *Organometallics* **2013**, *32*, 2736–2743. [CrossRef]
26. Despagnet-Ayoub, E.; Henling, L.M.; Labinger, J.A.; Bercaw, J.E. Addition of a Phosphine Ligand Switches an *N*-Heterocyclic Carbene-zirconium Catalyst from Oligomerization to Polymerization of 1-Hexene. *Dalton Trans.* **2013**, *42*, 15544–15547. [CrossRef]
27. Despagnet-Ayoub, E.; Takase, M.K.; Henling, L.M.; Labinger, J.A.; Bercaw, J.E. Mechanistic Insights on the Controlled Switch from Oligomerization to Polymerization of 1-Hexene Catalyzed by an NHC-Zirconium Complex. *Organometallics* **2015**, *34*, 4707–4716. [CrossRef]

28. Wan, L.; Zhang, D. Brønsted Base-Induced Rearrangement and Nucleophilic Addition of O/N-Functionalized NHCs and Relative Group 4 Metal Complexes for Ethylene Polymerization Catalysis. *Organometallics* **2016**, *35*, 138–150. [CrossRef]
29. Quadri, C.C.; Lalrempuia, R.; Frøystein, N.Å.; Törnroos, K.W.; Le Roux, E. Steric Factors on Unsymmetrical *O*-Hydroxyaryl *N*-Heterocyclic Carbene Ligands Prevailing the Stabilization of Single Stereoisomer of bis-Ligated Titanium Complexes. *J. Organomet. Chem.* **2018**, *860*, 106–116. [CrossRef]
30. Cho, J.; Hollis, T.K.; Helgert, T.R.; Valente, E.J. An Improved Method for the Synthesis of Zirconium (CCC-*N*-Heterocyclic Carbene) Pincer Complexes and Applications in Hydroamination. *Chem. Commun.* **2008**, 5001–5003. [CrossRef]
31. Cho, J.; Hollis, T.K.; Valente, E.J.; Trate, J.M. CCC–*N*-Heterocyclic Carbene Pincer Complexes: Synthesis, Characterization and Hydroamination Activity of a Hafnium Complex. *J. Organomet. Chem.* **2011**, *696*, 373–377. [CrossRef]
32. Helgert, T.R.; Hollis, T.K.; Valente, E.J. Synthesis of Titanium CCC-NHC Pincer Complexes and Catalytic Hydroamination of Unactivated Alkenes. *Organometallics* **2012**, *31*, 3002–3009. [CrossRef]
33. Barroso, S.; de Aguiar, S.R.M.M.; Munha, R.F.; Martins, A.M. New Zirconium Complexes Supported by *N*-Heterocyclic Carbene (NHC) Ligands: Synthesis and Assessment of Hydroamination Catalytic Properties. *J. Organomet. Chem.* **2014**, *760*, 60–66. [CrossRef]
34. Clark, W.D.; Cho, J.; Valle, H.U.; Hollis, T.K.; Valente, E.J. Metal and Halogen Dependence of the Rate Effect in Hydroamination/Cyclization of Unactivated Aminoalkenes: Synthesis, Characterization, and Catalytic Rates of CCC-NHC Hafnium and Zirconium Pincer Complexes. *J. Organomet. Chem.* **2014**, *751*, 534–540. [CrossRef]
35. Clark, W.D.; Leigh, K.N.; Webster, C.E.; Hollis, T.K. Experimental and Computational Studies of the Mechanisms of Hydroamination/Cyclisation of Unactivated α,ω-Amino-alkenes with CCC-NHC Pincer Zr Complexes*. *Aust. J. Chem.* **2016**, *69*, 573–582. [CrossRef]
36. Valle, H.U.; Akurathi, G.; Cho, J.; Clark, W.D.; Chakraborty, A.; Hollis, T.K. CCC-NHC Pincer Zr Diamido Complexes: Synthesis, Characterisation, and Catalytic Activity in Hydroamination/Cyclisation of Unactivated Amino-Alkenes, -Alkynes, and Allenes. *Aust. J. Chem.* **2016**, *69*, 565–572. [CrossRef]
37. Patel, D.; Liddle, S.T.; Mungur, S.A.; Rodden, M.; Blake, A.J.; Arnold, P.L. Bifunctional Yttrium(III) and Titanium(IV) NHC Catalysts for Lactide Polymerisation. *Chem. Commun.* **2006**, 1124–1126. [CrossRef]
38. Romain, C.; Brelot, L.; Bellemin-Laponnaz, S.; Dagorne, S. Synthesis and Structural Characterization of a Novel Family of Titanium Complexes Bearing a Tridentate Bis-phenolate-*N*-Heterocyclic Carbene Dianionic Ligand and Their Use in the Controlled ROP of *rac*-Lactide. *Organometallics* **2010**, *29*, 1191–1198. [CrossRef]
39. Romain, C.; Heinrich, B.; Laponnaz, S.B.; Dagorne, S. A Robust Zirconium *N*-Heterocyclic Carbene Complex for the Living and Highly Stereoselective Ring-opening Polymerization of *rac*-Lactide. *Chem. Commun.* **2012**, *48*, 2213–2215. [CrossRef]
40. Zhao, N.; Hou, G.; Deng, X.; Zi, G.; Walter, M.D. Group 4 Metal Complexes with New Chiral Pincer NHC-ligands: Synthesis, Structure and Catalytic Activity. *Dalton Trans.* **2014**, *43*, 8261–8272. [CrossRef]
41. Quadri, C.C.; Le Roux, E. Copolymerization of Cyclohexene Oxide with CO_2 Catalyzed by Tridentate *N*-Heterocyclic Carbene Titanium(IV) Complexes. *Dalton Trans.* **2014**, *43*, 4242–4246. [PubMed]
42. Hessevik, J.; Lalrempuia, R.; Nsiri, H.; Tornroos, K.W.; Jensen, V.R.; Le Roux, E. Sterically (un)Encumbered *mer*-Tridentate *N*-heterocyclic Carbene Complexes of Titanium(IV) for the Copolymerization of Cyclohexene Oxide with CO_2. *Dalton Trans.* **2016**, *45*, 14734–14744. [PubMed]
43. Quadri, C.C.; Lalrempuia, R.; Hessevik, J.; Törnroos, K.W.; Le Roux, E. Structural Characterization of Tridentate N-Heterocyclic Carbene Titanium(IV) Benzyloxide, Silyloxide, Acetate, and Azide Complexes and Assessment of Their Efficacies for Catalyzing the Copolymerization of Cyclohexene Oxide with CO_2. *Organometallics* **2017**, *36*, 4477–4489.
44. Lalrempuia, R.; Breivik, F.; Törnroos, K.W.; Le Roux, E. Coordination Behavior of Bis-phenolate Saturated and Unsaturated *N*-Heterocyclic Carbene Ligands to Zirconium: Reactivity and Activity in the Copolymerization of Cyclohexene Oxide with CO_2. *Dalton Trans.* **2017**, *46*, 8065–8076.
45. Lalrempuia, R.; Underhaug, J.; Törnroos, K.W.; Le Roux, E. Anionic Hafnium Species: An Active Catalytic Intermediate for the Coupling of Epoxides with CO_2? *Chem. Commun.* **2019**, *55*, 7227–7230.
46. Coates, G.W.; Moore, D.R. Discrete Metal-Based Catalysts for the Copolymerization of CO_2 and Epoxides: Discovery, Reactivity, Optimization, and Mechanism. *Angew. Chem. Int. Ed.* **2004**, *43*, 6618–6639.

47. Darensbourg, D.J.; Mackiewicz, R.M.; Phelps, A.L.; Billodeaux, D.R. Copolymerization of CO_2 and Epoxides Catalyzed by Metal Salen Complexes. *Acc. Chem. Res.* **2004**, *37*, 836–844.
48. Darensbourg, D.J. Making Plastics from Carbon Dioxide: Salen Metal Complexes as Catalysts for the Production of Polycarbonates from Epoxides and CO_2. *Chem. Rev.* **2007**, *107*, 2388–2410.
49. Kember, M.R.; Buchard, A.; Williams, C.K. Catalysts for CO_2/Epoxide Copolymerisation. *Chem. Commun.* **2011**, *47*, 141–163.
50. Klaus, S.; Lehenmeier, M.W.; Anderson, C.E.; Rieger, B. Recent Advances in CO_2/Epoxide Copolymerization—New Strategies and Cooperative Mechanisms. *Coord. Chem. Rev.* **2011**, *255*, 1460–1479.
51. Paul, S.; Zhu, Y.; Romain, C.; Brooks, R.; Saini, P.K.; Williams, C.K. Ring-opening Copolymerization (ROCOP): Synthesis and Properties of Polyesters and Polycarbonates. *Chem. Commun.* **2015**, *51*, 6459–6479.
52. Kozak, C.M.; Ambrose, K.; Anderson, T.S. Copolymerization of Carbon Dioxide and Epoxides by Metal Coordination Complexes. *Coord. Chem. Rev.* **2018**, *376*, 565–587.
53. Le Roux, E. Chapter 6 Titanium-based Catalysts for Polymer Synthesis. In *Sustainable Catalysis: With Non-endangered Metals, Part 1*; The Royal Society of Chemistry: Cambridge, UK, 2015; pp. 116–139.
54. Le Roux, E. Recent Advances on Tailor-made Titanium Catalysts for Biopolymer Synthesis. *Coord. Chem. Rev.* **2016**, *306*, 65–85.
55. Mandal, M. Group 4 Complexes as Catalysts for the Transformation of CO_2 into Polycarbonates and Cyclic Carbonates. *J. Organomet. Chem.* **2020**, *907*, 121067.
56. Nakano, K.; Kobayashi, K.; Nozaki, K. Tetravalent Metal Complexes as a New Family of Catalysts for Copolymerization of Epoxides with Carbon Dioxide. *J. Am. Chem. Soc.* **2011**, *133*, 10720–10723.
57. Wang, Y.; Qin, Y.; Wang, X.; Wang, F. Coupling Reaction Between CO_2 and Cyclohexene Oxide: Selective Control from Cyclic Carbonate to Polycarbonate by Ligand Design of Salen/Salalen Titanium Complexes. *Catal. Sci. Technol.* **2014**, *4*, 3964–3972.
58. Wang, Y.; Qin, Y.; Wang, X.; Wang, F. Trivalent Titanium Salen Complex: Thermally Robust and Highly Active Catalyst for Copolymerization of CO_2 and Cyclohexene Oxide. *ACS Catal.* **2015**, *5*, 393–396.
59. Mandal, M.; Chakraborty, D. Group 4 Complexes Bearing Bis(salphen) Ligands: Synthesis, Characterization, and Polymerization Studies. *J. Polym. Sci. Part A Polym. Chem.* **2016**, *54*, 809–824.
60. Mandal, M.; Monkowius, U.; Chakraborty, D. Synthesis and Structural Characterization of Titanium and Zirconium Complexes Containing Half-salen Ligands as Catalysts for Polymerization Reactions. *New J. Chem.* **2016**, *40*, 9824–9839.
61. Garden, J.A.; White, A.J.P.; Williams, C.K. Heterodinuclear Titanium/Zinc Catalysis: Synthesis, Characterization and Activity for CO_2/Epoxide Copolymerization and Cyclic Ester Polymerization. *Dalton Trans.* **2017**, *46*, 2532–2541.
62. Raman, S.K.; Deacy, A.C.; Pena Carrodeguas, L.; Reis, N.V.; Kerr, R.W.F.; Phanopoulos, A.; Morton, S.; Davidson, M.G.; Williams, C.K. Ti(IV)–tris(phenolate) Catalyst Systems for the Ring-opening Copolymerization of Cyclohexene Oxide and Carbon Dioxide. *Organometallics* **2020**, *39*, 1619–1627. [CrossRef] [PubMed]
63. Su, C.K.; Chuang, H.J.; Li, C.Y.; Yu, C.Y.; Ko, B.T.; Chen, J.D.; Chen, M.J. Oxo-Bridged Bimetallic Group 4 Complexes Bearing Amine-bis(benzotriazole phenolate) Derivatives as Bifunctional Catalysts for Ring-opening Polymerization of Lactide and Copolymerization of Carbon Dioxide with Cyclohexene Oxide. *Organometallics* **2014**, *33*, 7091–7100. [CrossRef]
64. Chuang, H.J.; Ko, B.T. Facilely Synthesized Benzotriazole Phenolate Zirconium Complexes as Versatile Catalysts for Copolymerization of Carbon Dioxide with Cyclohexene Oxide and Lactide Polymerization. *Dalton Trans.* **2015**, *44*, 598–607. [CrossRef] [PubMed]
65. Mandal, M.; Chakraborty, D.; Ramkumar, V. Zr(IV) Complexes Containing Salan-type Ligands: Synthesis, Structural Characterization and Role as Catalysts Towards the Polymerization of ε-Caprolactone, *rac*-Lactide, Ethylene, Homopolymerization and Copolymerization of Epoxides with CO_2. *RSC Adv.* **2015**, *5*, 28536–28553. [CrossRef]
66. Mandal, M.; Ramkumar, V.; Chakraborty, D. Salen Complexes of Zirconium and Hafnium: Synthesis, Structural Characterization and Polymerization Studies. *Polym. Chem.* **2019**, *10*, 3444–3460. [CrossRef]
67. Borré, E.; Dahm, G.; Aliprandi, A.; Mauro, M.; Dagorne, S.; Bellemin-Laponnaz, S. Tridentate Complexes of Group 10 Bearing Bis-aryloxide N-Heterocyclic Carbene Ligands: Synthesis, Structural, Spectroscopic, and Computational Characterization. *Organometallics* **2014**, *33*, 4374–4384. [CrossRef]

68. Harris, C.F.; Bayless, M.B.; van Leest, N.P.; Bruch, Q.J.; Livesay, B.N.; Bacsa, J.; Hardcastle, K.I.; Shores, M.P.; de Bruin, B.; Soper, J.D. Redox-Active Bis(phenolate) N-Heterocyclic Carbene [OCO] Pincer Ligands Support Cobalt Electron Transfer Series Spanning Four Oxidation States. *Inorg. Chem.* **2017**, *56*, 12421–12435. [CrossRef]
69. Tapu, D.; Dixon, D.A.; Roe, C. ^{13}C NMR Spectroscopy of "Arduengo-type" Carbenes and Their Derivatives. *Chem. Rev.* **2009**, *109*, 3385–3407. [CrossRef]
70. Zhang, D. Dinuclear Titanium(IV) Complexes Bearing Phenoxide-Tethered N-Heterocyclic Carbene Ligands with cisoid Conformation through Control of Hydrolysis. *Eur. J. Inorg. Chem.* **2007**, *2007*, 4839–4845.
71. Occhipinti, G.; Bjørsvik, H.R.; Jensen, V.R. Quantitative Structure–Activity Relationships of Ruthenium Catalysts for Olefin Metathesis. *J. Am. Chem. Soc.* **2006**, *128*, 6952–6964. [CrossRef]
72. Nelson, D.J.; Nolan, S.P. Quantifying and Understanding the Electronic Properties of N-Heterocyclic Carbenes. *Chem. Soc. Rev.* **2013**, *42*, 6723–6753. [CrossRef] [PubMed]
73. Huynh, H.V. Electronic Properties of N-Heterocyclic Carbenes and Their Experimental Determination. *Chem. Rev.* **2018**, *118*, 9457–9492. [CrossRef]
74. Glendening, E.D.; Badenhoop, K.; Reed, A.E.; Carpenter, J.E.; Bohmann, J.A.; Morales, C.M.; Karafiloglou, P.; Landis, C.R.; Weinhold, F. *NBO 7.0*; Theoretical Chemistry Institute, University of Wisconsin: Madison, WI, USA, 2018.
75. Jacobsen, H.; Correa, A.; Poater, A.; Costabile, C.; Cavallo, L. Understanding the M(NHC) (NHC = N-heterocyclic carbene) Bond. *Coord. Chem. Rev.* **2009**, *253*, 687–703. [CrossRef]
76. Shukla, P.; Johnson, J.A.; Vidovic, D.; Cowley, A.H.; Abernethy, C.D. Amine Elimination Synthesis of a Titanium(IV) N-heterocyclic Carbene Complex with Short Intramolecular Cl···C$_{carbene}$ contacts. *Chem. Commun.* **2004**, 360–361. [CrossRef]
77. Jacobsen, H.; Correa, A.; Costabile, C.; Cavallo, L. π-Acidity and π-Basicity of N-Heterocyclic Carbene Ligands. A Computational Assessment. *J. Organomet. Chem.* **2006**, *691*, 4350–4358. [CrossRef]
78. Tonner, R.; Heydenrych, G.; Frenking, G. Bonding Analysis of N-Heterocyclic Carbene Tautomers and Phosphine Ligands in Transition-Metal Complexes: A Theoretical Study. *Chem. Asian J.* **2007**, *2*, 1555–1567. [CrossRef]
79. Horrer, G.; Krahfuß, M.J.; Lubitz, K.; Krummenacher, I.; Braunschweig, H.; Radius, U. N-Heterocyclic Carbene and Cyclic (Alkyl)(amino)carbene Complexes of Titanium(IV) and Titanium(III). *Eur. J. Inorg. Chem.* **2020**, *2020*, 281–291. [CrossRef]
80. Addison, A.W.; Rao, T.N.; Reedijk, J.; van Rijn, J.; Verschoor, G.C. Synthesis, Structure, and Spectroscopic Properties of Copper(II) Compounds Containing Nitrogen-sulphur Donor Ligands; the Crystal and Molecular Structure of Aqua[1,7-bis(N-methylbenzimidazol-2′-yl)-2,6-dithiaheptane]copper(II) Perchlorate. *J. Chem. Soc. Dalton Trans.* **1984**, 1349–1356. [CrossRef]
81. Darensbourg, D.J. Chemistry of Carbon Dioxide Relevant to Its Utilization: A Personal Perspective. *Inorg. Chem.* **2010**, *49*, 10765–10780. [CrossRef]
82. Bellemin-Laponnaz, S.; Welter, R.; Brelot, L.; Dagorne, S. Synthesis and Structure of V(V) and Mn(III) NHC Complexes Supported by a Tridentate Bis-aryloxide-N-heterocyclic Carbene Ligand. *J. Organomet. Chem.* **2009**, *694*, 604–606. [CrossRef]
83. Romain, C.; Specklin, D.; Miqueu, K.; Sotiropoulos, J.M.; Fliedel, C.; Bellemin-Laponnaz, S.; Dagorne, S. Unusual Benzyl Migration Reactivity in NHC-Bearing Group 4 Metal Chelates: Synthesis, Characterization, and Mechanistic Investigations. *Organometallics* **2015**, *34*, 4854–4863. [CrossRef]
84. Martinsen, A.; Songstad, J. Preparation and Properties of Some Bis(triphenylphosphine)-iminium Salts, [[Ph$_3$P)$_2$N]X. *Acta Chem. Scand.* **1977**, *31*, 645–650. [CrossRef]
85. *APEX2. Version 2014.11-0*; Bruker-AXS, Inc.: Madison, WI, USA, 2014.
86. *SAINT. Version 7.68A*; Bruker-AXS, Inc.: Madison, WI, USA, 2010.
87. Krause, L.; Herbst-Irmer, R.; Sheldrick, G.M.; Stalke, D. Comparison of Silver and Molybdenum Microfocus X-ray Sources for Single-crystal Structure Determination. *J. Appl. Crystallogr.* **2015**, *48*, 3–10. [CrossRef] [PubMed]
88. Sheldrick, G.M. *XS. Version 2013/1*; Georg-August-Universität Göttingen: Göttingen, Germany, 2013.
89. Sheldrick, G.M. SHELXT—Integrated Space-group and Crystal-structure Determination. *Acta Crystallogr. Sect. A Found. Adv.* **2015**, *71*, 3–8. [CrossRef]
90. Sheldrick, G.M. Crystal Structure Refinement with SHELXL. *Acta Crystallogr. Sect. C Cryst. Struct. Chem.* **2015**, *71*, 3–8. [CrossRef]

91. Frisch, M.J.; Trucks, G.W.; Schlegel, H.B.; Scuseria, G.E.; Robb, M.A.; Cheeseman, J.R.; Scalmani, G.; Barone, V.; Petersson, G.A.; Nakatsuji, H.; et al. *Gaussian 16, Revision C.01*; Gaussian, Inc.: Wallingford, CT, USA, 2016.
92. Perdew, J.P.; Burke, K.; Ernzerhof, M. Generalized Gradient Approximation Made Simple. *Phys. Rev. Lett.* **1996**, *77*, 3865–3868, Erratum in **1977**, *78*, 1396. [CrossRef]
93. Grimme, S.; Ehrlich, S.; Goerigk, L. Effect of the Damping Function in Dispersion Corrected Density Functional Theory. *J. Comput. Chem.* **2011**, *32*, 1456–1465. [CrossRef]
94. Smith, D.G.A.; Burns, L.A.; Patkowski, K.; Sherrill, C.D. Revised Damping Parameters for the D3 Dispersion Correction to Density Functional Theory. *J. Phys. Chem. Lett.* **2016**, *7*, 2197–2203. [CrossRef]
95. Dunning, T.H. Gaussian Basis Sets for Use in Correlated Molecular Calculations. I. The Atoms Boron through Neon and Hydrogen. *J. Chem. Phys.* **1989**, *90*, 1007–1023. [CrossRef]
96. Woon, D.E.; Dunning, T.H. Gaussian Basis Sets for Use in Correlated Molecular Calculations. III. The Atoms Aluminum through Argon. *J. Chem. Phys.* **1993**, *98*, 1358–1371. [CrossRef]
97. Feller, D. The Role of Databases in Support of Computational Chemistry Calculations. *J. Comput. Chem.* **1996**, *17*, 1571–1586. [CrossRef]
98. Schuchardt, K.L.; Didier, B.T.; Elsethagen, T.; Sun, L.; Gurumoorthi, V.; Chase, J.; Li, J.; Windus, T.L. Basis Set Exchange: A Community Database for Computational Sciences. *J. Chem. Inf. Model.* **2007**, *47*, 1045–1052. [CrossRef] [PubMed]
99. Peterson, K.A.; Figgen, D.; Dolg, M.; Stoll, H. Energy-consistent Relativistic Pseudopotentials and Correlation Consistent Basis Sets for the 4d Elements Y–Pd. *J. Chem. Phys.* **2007**, *126*, 124101. [CrossRef]
100. Kendall, R.A.; Dunning, T.H.; Harrison, R.J. Electron Affinities of the First-row Atoms Revisited. Systematic Basis Sets and Wave Functions. *J. Chem. Phys.* **1992**, *96*, 6796–6806. [CrossRef]

Sample Availability: Not available.

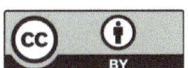

© 2020 by the authors. Licensee MDPI, Basel, Switzerland. This article is an open access article distributed under the terms and conditions of the Creative Commons Attribution (CC BY) license (http://creativecommons.org/licenses/by/4.0/).

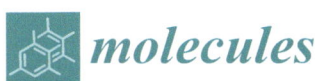 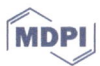

Article

Mercury(II) Complexes of Anionic *N*-Heterocyclic Carbene Ligands: Steric Effects of the Backbone Substituent

Chandrakanta Dash *,†, Animesh Das ‡ and H. V. Rasika Dias *

Department of Chemistry and Biochemistry, The University of Texas at Arlington, Arlington, TX 76019, USA; adas@iitg.ac.in
* Correspondence: ckdash@curaj.ac.in (C.D.); dias@uta.edu (H.V.R.D.)
† Current address: Department of Chemistry, School of Chemical Sciences and Pharmacy, Central University of Rajasthan, Bandar Sindri, Ajmer-305817, Rajasthan, India.
‡ Current address: Department of Chemistry, Indian Institute of Technology Guwahati, Guwahati-781039, Assam, India.

Academic Editor: Yves Canac
Received: 27 July 2020; Accepted: 13 August 2020; Published: 16 August 2020

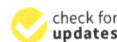

Abstract: Mercury(II) complexes (Me-maloNHC$_{Dipp}$)HgCl (**1b**), (*t*-Bu-maloNHC$_{Dipp}$)HgCl (**2b**) and (*t*-Bu-maloNHC$_{Dipp}$)HgMe (**2c**) supported by anionic *N*-heterocyclic carbenes have been obtained in good yields from the reaction of the potassium salt of *N*-heterocyclic carbene ligand precursors and mercury(II) salts, HgCl$_2$ and MeHgI. These molecules have been characterized by ^{1}H-NMR, ^{13}C-NMR and IR spectroscopy and elemental analysis. X-ray crystal structures of **1b** and **2b** are also presented. Interestingly, complex **1b** is polymeric {(Me-maloNHC$_{Dipp}$)HgCl}$_n$ in the solid state, as a result of inter-molecular Hg-O contacts, and features rare three coordinate mercury sites with a T-shaped arrangement, whereas the (*t*-Bu-maloNHC$_{Dipp}$)HgCl (**2b**) is monomeric and has a linear, two-coordinate mercury center. The formation of T-shaped structure and the aggregation of complex **1b** is attributable to the reduced steric demand of the *N*-heterocyclic carbene ligand backbone substituent.

Keywords: ligands; *N*-heterocyclic carbene; mercury(II) complex; X-ray; T-shaped

---

1. Introduction

During the past three decades, considerable attention has been given to the chemistry of metal complexes of *N*-heterocyclic carbenes [1–9]. *N*-heterocyclic carbenes are versatile ligands with extensive applications in coordination chemistry and catalysis, as well as in bioinorganic chemistry [10–17]. Though traditional *N*-heterocyclic carbenes (NHCs) are neutral "L" type ligands, NHCs bearing tethered anionic donor sites (e.g., alkoxide, aryloxide, amido etc.) have also been reported, along with their metal complexes [18–27]. In contrast, *N*-heterocyclic carbene ligands with remote anionic functional groups/moieties within the heterocyclic ligand backbone have been less widely investigated [12,28,29]. Reactions of these anionic NHCs with transition metals afford corresponding zwitterionic complexes. Anionic, six-membered ring NHCs based on a malonate unit (maloNHC), introduced by Cesar, Lavigne and co-workers [30], are particularly interesting as they are attractive ligands to stabilize late transition metal ion complexes such as those involving Ag^I, Au^I, Rh^I, Cu^I [30–35], as well as Fe^{II} [36].

The first known metal-NHC complex was a mercury(II) compound reported by Wanzlick and Schonherr in 1968 [37]. The mercury(II)-NHC complexes have played an important role in the development of *N*-heterocyclic carbene chemistry, but are still less explored compared to other metals of the d-block [38–48]. Furthermore, to our knowledge, mercury(II) complexes of anionic *N*-herterocyclic carbene ligands, such as maloNHC, have not been investigated. As a continuation of our interest in the NHCs and their metal chemistry [49–60], we have set out to probe the use of anionic N-heterocyclic carbene ligands in mercury chemistry. In particular, we describe the synthesis and spectroscopic data of three new mercury(II) complexes (Figure 1), (Me-maloNHC$_{Dipp}$)HgCl (**1b**), (*t*-Bu-maloNHC$_{Dipp}$)HgCl (**2b**) and (*t*-Bu-maloNHC$_{Dipp}$)HgMe (**2c**), involving a bulkier maloNHC. We have also studied the effects of backbone substituent in heterocyclic ring (malonate unit), on the structure of the mercury complexes **1b** and **2b**.

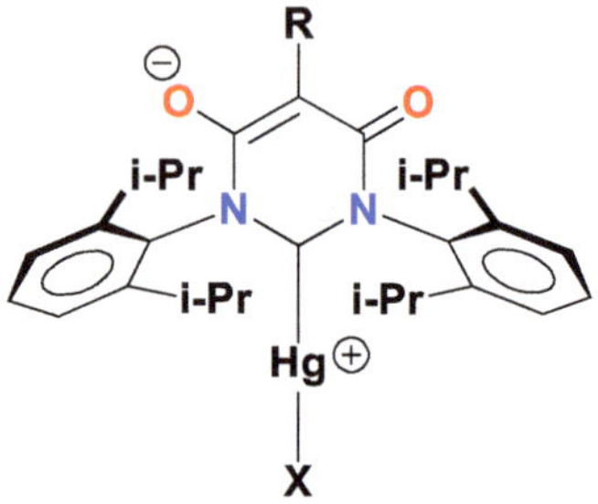

R = Me, X = Cl (**1b**)
R = *t*-Bu, X = Cl (**2b**)
R = *t*-Bu, X = Me (**2c**)

Figure 1. Mercury(II) complexes supported by anionic N-heterocyclic carbenes [Me-maloNHC$_{Dipp}$]$^-$ and [*t*-Bu-maloNHC$_{Dipp}$]$^-$.

2. Results and Discussion

Synthesis and Characterization

The anionic, six-membered N-heterocyclic carbene ligand precursor **1a** has been reported earlier [32]. The anionic-NHC ligand precursors **1a** and **2a** were synthesized using the strategy reported by César et al. (from the condensation of N,N'-bis(2,6-diisopropylphenyl)formamidine and monosubstituted malonic acid) [30]. Moreover, ^{1}H NMR spectrum of **2a** in CDCl$_3$ at room temperature exhibits a signal corresponding to the NCHN proton at the δ 8.07 ppm (compare for **1a**: δ 8.06 ppm [32]). The mercury(II) complexes, (Me-maloNHC$_{Dipp}$)HgCl (**1b**) and (*t*-Bu-maloNHC$_{Dipp}$)HgCl (**2b**), were prepared from in situ generated anionic N-heterocyclic carbene ligand, by using KHMDS as the base and HgCl$_2$ as the mercury source (Scheme 1). The complexes **1b** and **2b** are yellow crystalline solids, which were characterized by NMR, IR spectroscopy, elemental analysis and X-ray crystallography. They are air and light stable solids, and soluble in dichloromethane, THF and chloroform. The ^{1}H NMR spectra of **1b** and **2b** in CDCl$_3$ at room temperature showed the absence of NCHN resonance of the starting precursors (**1a** or **2a**). The ^{13}C{^{1}H} NMR spectrum showed the appearance of a highly downfield shifted mercury bound carbene carbon resonance at δ 180.9 and 179.9 ppm, for **1b** and **2b**, respectively. We did not observe Hg-C$_{carbene}$ coupling in the ^{13}C NMR spectrum, although large C$_{carbene}$-Hg coupling in the range 2700–3300 Hz has been reported in the literature [61,62]. Yellow crystals of these molecules could be obtained from dichloromethane solution layering with hexane at −10 °C.

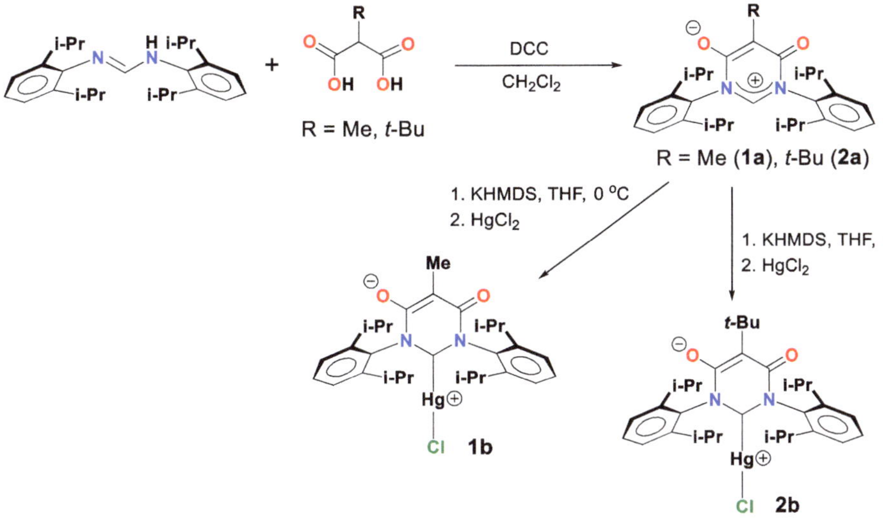

Scheme 1. Synthesis of mercury(II) complexes **1b** and **2b** supported by anionic NHC.

The molecular structures of the complexes **1b** and **2b** are illustrated in Figures 2 and 3. The complex **1b** crystallizes in P-1 space group with two chemically similar molecules of **1b** in the asymmetric unit. X-ray structure of **1b** shows the presence of three coordinated mercury atoms (and zig-zag polymeric chains resulting from bridging Hg-O contacts involving neighboring molecules) having a distorted T-shaped geometry with bond angles of 86.68(7)°, 157.34(12)°, 115.97(13)° at Hg1 and 86.52(7)°, 156.92(12)°, 116.55(13)° at Hg2. The inter-molecular Hg-O bond distances of 2.537(3) and 2.529(3) Å are shorter than the sum of van der Waals radii of the respective elements, which is 3.07 Å for an Hg···O interaction. For comparison, interactions of similar magnitude have been observed in the complex $C_6F_5HgCl·DMSO$ [Hg-O = 2.542(2) Å], reported by the Gabbai group [63]. The average Hg-$C_{carbene}$ bond distance in **1b** is 2.091(4) Å, which is in good agreement with the five membered imidazole based mercury carbene complexes, i.e., [(IDipp)HgCl$_2$] [2.090(4) Å], [(IMes)HgCl$_2$] [2.084(6) Å] [64]. The average Hg-Cl bond distance in **1b** (2.3154(11) Å) is comparable to the other three coordinated, T-shaped mercury complexes, namely, [2-(Me$_2$NCH$_2$)C$_6$H$_4$]HgCl [2.319(2) Å], $C_6F_5HgCl·DMSO$ [2.322(2) Å] [63,65].

The complex (*t*-Bu-maloNHC$_{Dipp}$)HgCl (**2b**) crystallizes in P-1 space group with two independent molecules of (*t*-Bu-maloNHC$_{Dipp}$)HgCl in the asymmetric unit. In contrast to the complex **1b**, the mercury complex **2b** has a two-coordinate linear mercury center with $C_{carbene}$-Hg-Cl bond angles of 177.50(15)° and 177.74(15)° for the two molecules. This is likely a result of having a bulky *t*-Bu moiety in the six-membered ring at the remote, apical carbon, in addition to the bulky N-aryl group, which inhibit the interaction of mercury atom with oxygen atom in an adjacent molecule. We should note here that electronic donor properties at the carbene center have been modulated by using electrophiles to interact with oxygen atoms of remote malonate group of Me-maloNHC$_{Mes}$ and *t*-Bu-maloNHC$_{Mes}$ in rhodium complexes [35]. The linear geometry at mercury of (*t*-Bu-maloNHC$_{Dipp}$)HgCl is commonly found in Hg-NHC complexes involving five membered neutral NHCs. The average $C_{carbene}$-Hg bond distance in **2b** (2.059(5) Å) is similar to those observed in the other mercury complexes reported in the literature. The Hg-Cl distances in **2b** 2.2558(15) and 2.235(2) Å are shorter than in those found in complex **1b** [2.3158(10) Å]. This is not surprising, as complex **1b** has three coordinate mercury sites, whereas they are two-coordinate in **2b**.

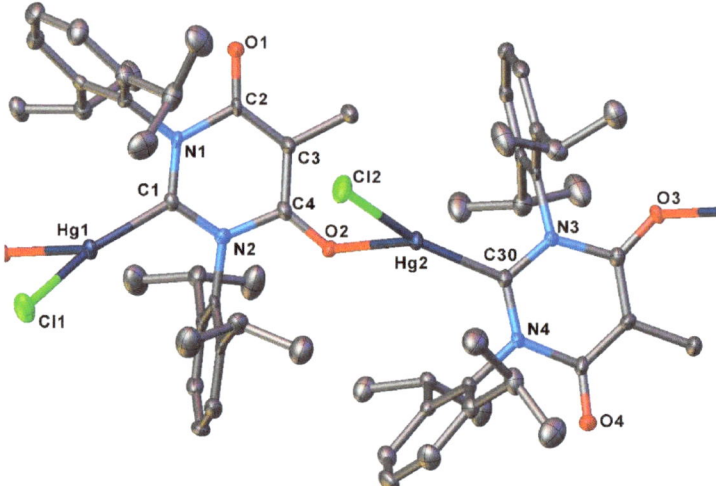

Figure 2. Molecular structure of (Me-maloNHC$_{Dipp}$)HgCl (**1b**). Hydrogen atoms have been omitted for clarity. Selected bond distances (Å) and angles (°): Hg1-Cl1 2.3157(11), Hg1-O3 2.537(3), Hg1-C1 2.090(4), Hg2-Cl2 2.3152(11), Hg2-O2 2.529(3), Hg2-C30 2.092(4), O1-C2 1.228(5), O2-C4 1.262(5), O3-C31 1.256(5), O4-C33 1.227(5); Cl1-Hg1-O3[1] 86.68(7); C1-Hg1-Cl1 157.34(12), C1-Hg1-O3 [1] 115.97(13), Cl2-Hg2-O2 86.52(7), C30-Hg2-Cl2 156.92(12), C30-Hg2-O2 116.55(13), C4-O2-Hg2 116.7(3), C31-O3-Hg1 [2] 117.3(3), where [1] +X, 1 + Y,+Z; [2] +X, −1 + Y, +Z.

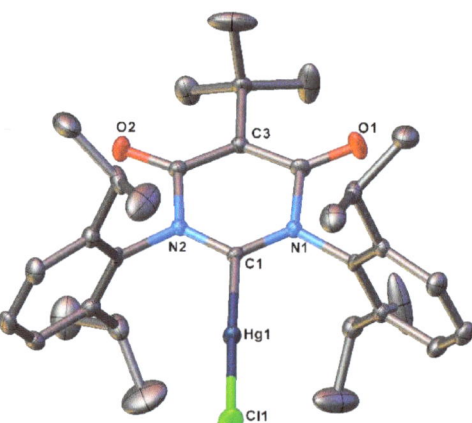

Figure 3. Molecular structure of (*t*-Bu-maloNHC$_{Dipp}$)HgCl (**2b**). The second molecule in the asymmetric unit and hydrogen atoms have been omitted for clarity. Selected bond distances (Å) and angles (°): Molecule 1, Hg1-Cl1 2.2558(15), Hg1-C1 2.056(5), O1-C4 1.221(7), O2-C2 1.232(7); C1-Hg1-Cl1 177.50(15); Molecule 2 (not shown), Hg2-Cl2 2.235(2), Hg2-C33 2.062(5), O3-C34 1.229(7), O4-C36 1.220(7), C33-Hg2-Cl2 177.74(15).

The mercury(II) complex, (*t*-Bu-maloNHC$_{Dipp}$)HgMe (**2c**) was synthesized from a reaction between in situ generated anionic *N*-heterocyclic carbene ligand and MeHgI as the metal precursor (Scheme 2) in THF. It was isolated as a yellow colored solid in 70% yield. The ^{13}C resonance of the mercury(II)-bound carbene carbon (NCN) of (*t*-Bu-maloNHC$_{Dipp}$)HgMe (**2c**) in CDCl$_3$ was observed as a singlet at δ 205.8 ppm. We have not attempted to obtain crystalline materials of **2c** for an X-ray crystallographic study.

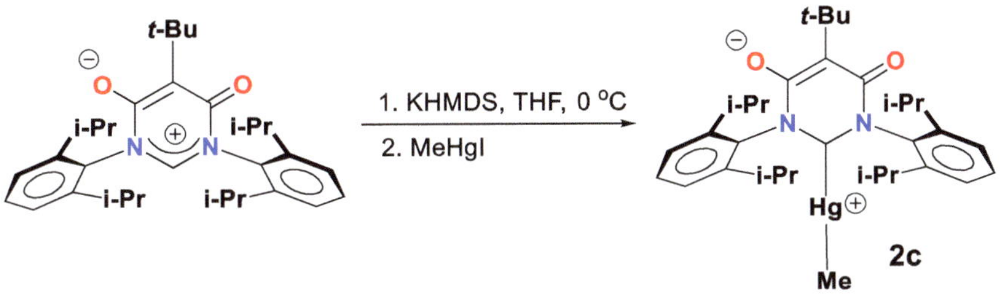

Scheme 2. Synthesis of mercury(II) complex (*t*-Bu-maloNHC$_{Dipp}$)HgMe (**2c**).

3. Experimental Sections

3.1. Materials and General Methods

All manipulations were carried out under an atmosphere of dry nitrogen, using standard Schlenk techniques, or in a glove box. Solvents were purchased from commercial sources, purified using an Innovative Technology SPS-400 PureSolv solvent drying system (Innovative Technology, Inc., Galway, Ireland), degassed by the freeze-pump-thaw method twice prior to use. Glassware was oven-dried at 150 °C overnight. NMR spectra were recorded at 298 K on JEOL Eclipse 500 and 300 spectrometers (Jeol Ltd., Tokyo, Japan). NMR annotations used: br. = broad, d = doublet, m = multiplet, s = singlet, t = triplet, sept = septet. Infrared spectra were recorded on a JASCO FT-IR 410 spectrometer (Jasco, Tokyo, Japan) operating at 2 cm^{-1} spectral resolution. IR spectroscopic data were collected using KBr pellets. Herein, we use abbreviations based on IUPAC guidelines, that is, ν for frequency and $\bar{\nu}$ for wavenumber. Elemental analyses were performed using a Perkin Elmer Series II CHNS/O analyzer. Methylmalonic acid, DCC were purchased from Sigma-Aldrich and used without further purification. *N,N'*-bis(2,6-diisopropylphenyl)formamidine [66] and *tert*-butylmalonic acid [67] were synthesized as reported, and anionic-NHC ligand precursor (**1a**) [32] was obtained via a modified literature procedure (noted below). The data of NMR spectrum can be found in the Supplementary Materials.

3.1.1. Synthesis of 1,3-Bis(2,6-diisopropylphenyl)-5-methyl-6-oxo-6H-pyrimidinium-4-olate (**1a**)

A mixture of *N,N'*-bis(2,6-diisopropylphenyl)formamidine (1.81 g, 4.96 mmol) and *N,N'*-dicyclohexylcarbodiimide (DCC) (2.04 g, 9.92 mmol) in dichloromethane (ca. 35 mL) was placed in a 50 mL Schlenk flask. To this mixture, methylmalonic acid (0.586 g, 4.96 mmol) was added as a solid at room temperature. The reaction mixture was stirred for 5 h. The solution was filtered and the solvents were evaporated. The residue was purified by flash chromatography (SiO$_2$, 30% EtOAc in hexane), to obtain a yellow crystalline solid (1.62 g, 73% yield). The analytical data agree with the reported values [32].

3.1.2. Synthesis of 1,3-Bis(2,6-diisopropylphenyl)-5-tert-butyl-6-oxo-6H-pyrimidinium-4-olate (**2a**)

A mixture of *N,N'*-bis(2,6-diisopropylphenyl)formamidine (5.18 g, 14.2 mmol) and *N,N'*-dicyclohexylcarbodiimide (DCC) (5.86 g, 28.4 mmol) in dichloromethane (ca. 50 mL) was taken in a 100 mL Schlenk flask. To this mixture, *tert*-butylmalonic acid (2.27 g, 14.2 mmol) was then added as a solid at room temperature. The reaction mixture was stirred for 6 h. The solution was filtered and the solvents were evaporated. The residue was purified by chromatography (SiO$_2$, 10% EtOAc in hexane) to give a yellow crystalline solid (4.71 g, 68% yield). Mp: 255–260 °C. ^{1}H NMR (CDCl$_3$, 500.16 MHz, 298 K): δ 8.07 (s, 1H, NCHN), 7.42 (t, 2H, $^3J_{HH}$ = 8.0 Hz, C$_6$H$_3$), 7.25 (d, 4H, $^3J_{HH}$ = 8.0 Hz, C$_6$H$_3$), 2.80 (sept, 4H, $^3J_{HH}$ = 6.9 Hz, CH(CH$_3$)$_2$), 1.46 (s, 9H, C(CH$_3$)$_3$), 1.30 (d, 12H, $^3J_{HH}$ = 6.9 Hz, CH(CH$_3$)$_2$), 1.20 (d, 12H, $^3J_{HH}$ = 6.9 Hz, CH(CH$_3$)$_2$). ^{13}C{^{1}H} NMR (CDCl$_3$, 125.77 MHz, 298 K): δ 158.3 (C-O), 146.9, 145.7, 132.5, 130.6, 124.2, 104.2, 34.5, 30.0, 29.2, 24.1, 23.9. IR (KBr) cm^{-1}: 3068, 2991, 2856, 1926, 1778, 1760, 1687, 1598, 1581, 1462, 1425, 1387, 1364, 1351, 1327, 1304, 1282, 1258,

1218, 1183, 1149, 1107, 1059, 1018, 981, 937, 875, 803, 761, 741. Anal. Calcd. for $C_{32}H_{44}N_2O_2$: C, 78.65; H, 9.07; N, 5.73. Found: C, 79.01; H, 9.03; N, 6.04%.

3.1.3. Synthesis of (Me-maloNHC$_{Dipp}$)HgCl (1b)

To a solution of **1a** (0.491 g, 1.10 mmol) in THF (30 mL), KHMDS (0.5 M in toluene, 2.2 mL, 1.10 mmol, 1.0 equiv.) was added dropwise at 0 °C (ice bath). After 30 min at 0 °C, HgCl$_2$ (0.299 g, 1.10 mmol) was added as a solid. The reaction mixture was stirred at room temperature for 6 h. The solvent was removed under vacuum, and the crude residue was dissolved in dichloromethane (30 mL). The mixture was filtered through a pad of Celite, and the filtrate was evaporated under vacuum to obtain a yellow solid. The compound was further washed with hexane and vacuum dried (0.405 g, 54% yield). Mp: 287 °C. ^{1}H NMR (CDCl$_3$, 500.16 MHz, 298 K): δ 7.53 (t, 2H, $^3J_{HH}$ = 8.0 Hz, C$_6$H$_3$), 7.33 (d, 4H, $^3J_{HH}$ = 8.0 Hz, C$_6$H$_3$), 2.80 (sept, 4H, $^3J_{HH}$ = 6.9 Hz, CH(CH$_3$)$_2$), 2.02 (s, 3H, CH$_3$), 1.27 (d, 12H, $^3J_{HH}$ = 6.9 Hz, CH(CH$_3$)$_2$), 1.22 (d, 12H, $^3J_{HH}$ = 6.9 Hz, CH(CH$_3$)$_2$). ^{13}C{^{1}H} NMR (CDCl$_3$, 125.77 MHz, 298 K): δ 180.9 (Hg-NCN), 160.1 (C-O), 146.2, 136.7, 131.8, 125.4, 94.4, 29.1, 24.6, 24.4, 10.1. IR (KBr) cm^{-1}: 2963, 2928, 2871, 1727, 1678, 1645, 1610, 1546, 1466, 1447, 1386, 1365, 1345, 1322, 1259, 1222, 1181, 1147, 1107, 1062, 1039, 934, 795, 755. Anal. Calcd. for $C_{29}H_{37}N_2O_2HgCl$•THF: C, 52.58; H, 6.02; N, 3.72. Found: C, 52.63; H, 5.81; N, 4.13%.

3.1.4. (t-Bu-maloNHC$_{Dipp}$)HgCl (2b)

To a solution of **2a** (0.752 g, 1.54 mmol) in THF (30 mL), KHMDS (0.5 M in toluene, 3.4 mL, 1.70 mmol, 1.1 equiv.) was added dropwise at 0 °C (ice bath). After 30 min at 0 °C, HgCl$_2$ (0.418 g, 1.54 mmol) was added as a solid. The reaction mixture was stirred at room temperature for 6 h. The solvent was removed under vacuum, and the crude residue was dissolved in dichloromethane (40 mL). The mixture was filtered through a pad of Celite, and the filtrate was evaporated under vacuum to obtain a yellow solid. The compound was further washed with hexane and vacuum dried (0.657 g, 59% yield). Mp: 250 °C. ^{1}H NMR (CDCl$_3$, 500.16 MHz, 298 K): δ 7.51 (t, 2H, $^3J_{HH}$ = 8 Hz, C$_6$H$_3$), 7.33 (d, 4H, $^3J_{HH}$ = 8 Hz, C$_6$H$_3$), 2.85 (sept, 4H, $^3J_{HH}$ = 6.9 Hz, CH(CH$_3$)$_2$), 1.45 (s, 9H, C(CH$_3$)$_3$), 1.31 (d, 12H, $^3J_{HH}$ = 6.9 Hz, CH(CH$_3$)$_2$), 1.26 (d, 12H, $^3J_{HH}$ = 6.9 Hz, CH(CH$_3$)$_2$). ^{13}C{^{1}H} NMR (CDCl$_3$, 125.77 MHz, 298 K): δ 179.9 (Hg-NCN), 159.1 (C-O), 146.1, 136.9, 131.6, 125.3, 104.1, 34.5, 30.0, 29.2, 24.4, 24.3. IR (KBr) cm^{-1}: 3069, 2990, 2863, 1644, 1465, 1410, 1387, 1365, 1345, 1325, 1301, 1257, 1215, 1181, 1148, 1111, 1056, 1014, 979, 936, 879, 797, 759, 749. Anal. Calcd. for $C_{32}H_{43}N_2O_2HgCl$: C, 53.11; H, 5.99; N, 3.87. Found: C, 53.41; H, 6.52; N, 3.87%.

3.1.5. Synthesis of (t-Bu-maloNHC$_{Dipp}$)HgMe (2c)

To a solution of 1,3-diisopropyl-5-*tert*-butyl-6-oxo-6H-pyrimidinium-4-olate (0.376 g, 0.77 mmol) in THF (20 mL), KHMDS (0.5 M in toluene, 1.92 mL, 0.96 mmol, 1.25 equiv.) was added dropwise at 0 °C (ice bath). After 30 min at 0 °C, MeHgI (0.264 g, 0.77 mmol) was added as a solid. The reaction mixture was stirred at room temperature for 12 h. The solvent was removed under vacuum, and the crude residue was dissolved in dichloromethane (20 mL). The mixture was filtered through a pad of Celite, and the filtrate was evaporated under vacuum to obtain a yellow solid. The compound was washed with hexane and vacuum dried (0.380 g, 70% yield). ^{1}H NMR (CDCl$_3$, 500.16 MHz, 298 K): δ 7.43 (t, 2H, $^3J_{HH}$ = 8 Hz, C$_6$H$_3$), 7.27 (d, 4H, $^3J_{HH}$ = 7.5 Hz, C$_6$H$_3$), 2.88 (sept, 4H, $^3J_{HH}$ = 6.9 Hz, CH(CH$_3$)$_2$), 1.45 (s, 9H, C(CH$_3$)$_3$), 1.29 (d, 12H, $^3J_{HH}$ = 6.9 Hz, CH(CH$_3$)$_2$), 1.21 (d, 12H, $^3J_{HH}$ = 6.9 Hz, CH(CH$_3$)$_2$), 0.21 (s, 3H, CH$_3$). ^{13}C{^{1}H} NMR (CDCl$_3$, 125.77 MHz, 298 K): δ 205.8 (HgNCN), 160.3 (C-O), 146.3, 136.2, 130.5, 124.6, 104.0, 34.5, 30.2, 29.0, 24.3, 24.2, 4.9 (HgCH$_3$). Anal. Calcd. for $C_{33}H_{46}N_2O_2$IHg: C, 56.35; H, 6.59; N, 3.98. Found: C, 55.98; H, 6.37; N, 4.11%.

3.2. Crystallographic Data Collection and Refinement

A suitable crystal covered with a layer of hydrocarbon/Paratone-N oil was selected and mounted with in a Cryo-loop, and immediately placed in the low-temperature nitrogen stream. Diffraction data were collected at T = 100(2) K. The data sets were collected on a Bruker SMART APEX II CCD detector diffractometer with graphite monochromated Mo Kα radiation (λ = 0.71073 Å). The cell parameters were obtained from a least-squares refinement of the spots (from 60 collected frames), using the SMART program. Intensity data were processed using the Bruker ApexII program suite. Absorption corrections were applied by using SADABS. Initial atomic positions were located by direct methods using XS, and the structures of the compounds were refined by the least-squares method using SHELXL [68]. All the hydrogen atoms were refined anisotropically. Hydrogen positions were input and refined in a riding manner, along with the attached carbons. X-ray structural figures were generated using Olex2 [69]. The CCDC 2019022–2019023 contains the supplementary crystallographic data. These data can be obtained free of charge via http://www.ccdc.cam.ac.uk/conts/retrieving.html or from the Cambridge Crystallographic Data Centre (CCDC) (12 Union Road, Cambridge, CB2 1EZ, UK).

Crystal data for (Me-maloNHC$_{Dipp}$)HgCl (**1b**): $C_{58}H_{74}Cl_2Hg_2N_4O_4$ (M = 1363.29 g/mol): triclinic, space group $P\bar{1}$ (no. 2), a = 10.7845(8) Å, b = 13.9152(11) Å, c = 19.1697(15) Å, α = 106.9910(10)°, β = 91.2040(10)°, γ = 90.0910(10)°, V = 2750.5(4) Å^3, Z = 2, T = 100.15 K, μ(MoKα) = 5.721 mm^{-1}, D_{calc} = 1.646 g/cm^3, 22,195 reflections measured (3.06° ≤ 2Θ ≤ 50.996°), 10,213 unique (R_{int} = 0.0257, R_{sigma} = 0.0369), which were used in all calculations. The final R_1 was 0.0313 (I > 2σ(I)) and wR_2 was 0.0797 (all data).

Crystal data for (*t*-Bu-maloNHC$_{Dipp}$)HgCl (**2b**): $C_{32}H_{43}ClHgN_2O_2$ (M = 723.72 g/mol): triclinic, space group $P\bar{1}$ (no. 2), a = 10.9912(9) Å, b = 14.9118(13) Å, c = 19.9787(17) Å, α = 99.9700(10)°, β = 98.6110(10)°, γ = 90.2430(10)°, V = 3187.1(5) Å^3, Z = 4, T = 100.15 K, μ(MoKα) = 4.942 mm^{-1}, D_{calc} = 1.508 g/cm^3, 27,908 reflections measured (2.774° ≤ 2Θ ≤ 53.464°), 13,462 unique (R_{int} = 0.0260, R_{sigma} = 0.0407), which were used in all calculations. The final R_1 was 0.0405 (I > 2σ(I)) and wR_2 was 0.1067 (all data).

4. Conclusions

In summary, we report the isolation of three new mercury(II) complexes supported by anionic maloNHC ligands. Solid state structures of **1b** and **2b** illustrate the effects of backbone substituent in maloNHC, supplemented by the N-aryl substituent steric demands have on the aggregation of these mercury complexes. The (Me-maloNHC$_{Dipp}$)HgCl (**1b**) bearing methyl substituent in the malonate unit forms a polymeric mercury(II) complex, with a rare, distorted T-shaped structure, whereas (*t*-Bu-maloNHC$_{Dipp}$)HgCl (**2b**) having a *t*-butyl substituent on the ligand backbone, remains monomeric. The [*t*-Bu-maloNHC$_{Dipp}$]$^-$ is a sterically demanding and useful supporting ligand to stabilize low-coordinate metal complexes.

Supplementary Materials: The following are available online. Crystal data, structure refinement, bond distances and angles for (Me-maloNHCDipp)HgCl (**1b**) and (*t*-Bu-maloNHCDipp)HgCl (**2b**), additional figures, and NMR spectra of new molecules.

Author Contributions: Conceptualization, H.V.R.D.; funding acquisition, H.V.R.D.; Data curation, C.D., A.D.; Methodology, C.D. and A.D.; writing and editing, C.D. and H.V.R.D.; All authors have read and agreed to the published version of the manuscript.

Funding: This research was supported by the Robert A. Welch Foundation (Grant Y-1289).

Acknowledgments: We thank Muhammed Yousufuddin for collecting the X-ray data.

Conflicts of Interest: The authors declare no conflict of interest.

References

1. Hopkinson, M.N.; Richter, C.; Schedler, M.; Glorius, F. An overview of N-heterocyclic carbenes. *Nature* **2014**, *510*, 485–496. [CrossRef] [PubMed]
2. Díez-González, S.; Marion, N.; Nolan, S.P. N-Heterocyclic carbenes in late transition metal catalysis. *Chem. Rev.* **2009**, *109*, 3612–3676. [CrossRef] [PubMed]

3. Doddi, A.; Peters, M.; Tamm, M. N-Heterocyclic carbene adducts of main group elements and their use as ligands in transition metal chemistry. *Chem. Rev.* **2019**, *119*, 6994–7112. [CrossRef] [PubMed]
4. Zhao, Q.; Meng, G.; Nolan, S.P.; Szostak, M. N-Heterocyclic carbene complexes in C–H activation reactions. *Chem. Rev.* **2020**, *120*, 1981–2048. [CrossRef] [PubMed]
5. Peris, E. Smart N-heterocyclic carbene ligands in catalysis. *Chem. Rev.* **2017**, *118*, 9988–10031. [CrossRef]
6. Wang, W.; Cui, L.; Sun, P.; Shi, L.; Yue, C.; Li, F. Reusable N-heterocyclic carbene complex catalysts and beyond: A perspective on recycling strategies. *Chem. Rev.* **2018**, *118*, 9843–9929. [CrossRef]
7. Cheng, J.; Wang, L.; Wang, P.; Deng, L. High-Oxidation-State 3d metal (Ti–Cu) complexes with N-heterocyclic carbene ligation. *Chem. Rev.* **2018**, *118*, 9930–9987. [CrossRef]
8. Weskamp, T.; Böhm, V.P.; Herrmann, W.A. N-Heterocyclic carbenes: State of the art in transition-metal-complex synthesis. *J. Organomet. Chem.* **2000**, *600*, 12–22. [CrossRef]
9. Herrmann, W.A.; Elison, M.; Fischer, J.; Köcher, C.; Artus, G.R.J. Metal complexes of N-heterocyclic carbenes—A new structural principle for catalysts in homogeneous catalysis. *Angew. Chem. Int. Ed.* **1995**, *34*, 2371–2374. [CrossRef]
10. Hahn, F.E.; Jahnke, M.C. Heterocyclic carbenes: Synthesis and coordination chemistry. *Angew. Chem. Int. Ed.* **2008**, *47*, 3122–3172. [CrossRef]
11. Herrmann, W.A. N-Heterocyclic carbenes: A new concept in organometallic catalysis. *Angew. Chem. Int. Ed.* **2002**, *41*, 1290–1309. [CrossRef]
12. Nasr, A.; Winkler, A.; Tamm, M. Anionic N-heterocyclic carbenes: Synthesis, coordination chemistry and applications in homogeneous catalysis. *Coord. Chem. Rev.* **2016**, *316*, 68–124. [CrossRef]
13. Peris, E.; Crabtree, R.H. Recent homogeneous catalytic applications of chelate and pincer N-heterocyclic carbenes. *Coord. Chem. Rev.* **2004**, *248*, 2239–2246. [CrossRef]
14. Mercs, L.; Albrecht, M. Beyond catalysis: N-heterocyclic carbene complexes as components for medicinal, luminescent, and functional materials applications. *Chem. Soc. Rev.* **2010**, *39*, 1903–1912. [CrossRef]
15. Zou, T.; Lok, C.-N.; Wan, P.-K.; Zhang, Z.-F.; Fung, S.-K.; Che, C.-M. Anticancer metal- N-heterocyclic carbene complexes of gold, platinum and palladium. *Curr. Opin. Chem. Biol.* **2018**, *43*, 30–36. [CrossRef]
16. Ibáñez, S.; Poyatos, M.; Peris, E. N-heterocyclic carbenes: A door open to supramolecular organometallic chemistry. *Acc. Chem. Res.* **2020**, *53*, 1401–1413. [CrossRef]
17. Santini, C.; Pellei, M.; Gandin, V.; Porchia, M.; Tisato, F.; Marzano, C. Advances in copper complexes as anticancer agents. *Chem. Rev.* **2013**, *114*, 815–862. [CrossRef]
18. Aihara, H.; Matsuo, T.; Kawaguchi, H. Titanium N-heterocyclic carbene complexes incorporating an imidazolium-linked bis(phenol). *Chem. Commun.* **2003**, *17*, 2204–2205. [CrossRef]
19. Arduengo, A.J., III; Dolphin, J.S.; Gurău, G.; Marshall, W.J.; Nelson, J.C.; Petrov, V.A.; Runyon, J.W. Synthesis and complexes of fluoroalkoxy carbenes. *Angew. Chem. Int. Ed.* **2013**, *52*, 5110–5114. [CrossRef]
20. Arnold, P.L.; Mungur, S.A.; Blake, A.J.; Wilson, C. Anionic amido N-heterocyclic carbenes: Synthesis of covalently tethered lanthanide–carbene complexes. *Angew. Chem. Int. Ed.* **2003**, *42*, 5981–5984. [CrossRef]
21. Arnold, P.L.; Rodden, M.; Wilson, C. Thermally stable potassium N-heterocyclic carbene complexes with alkoxide ligands, and a polymeric crystal structure with distorted, bridging carbenes. *Chem. Commun.* **2005**, *13*, 1743–1745. [CrossRef] [PubMed]
22. Arnold, P.L.; Scarisbrick, A.C. Di- and trivalent Ruthenium complexes of chelating, anionic N-heterocyclic carbenes. *Organometallics* **2004**, *23*, 2519–2521. [CrossRef]
23. Asay, M.; Donnadieu, B.; Baceiredo, A.; Soleilhavoup, M.; Bertrand, G. Cyclic (amino)[bis(ylide)]carbene as an anionic bidentate ligand for transition-metal complexes. *Inorg. Chem.* **2008**, *47*, 3949–3951. [CrossRef] [PubMed]
24. Hameury, S.; de Frémont, P.; Breuil, P.-A.R.; Olivier-Bourbigou, H.; Braunstein, P. Synthesis and characterization of palladium(II) and nickel(II) alcoholate-functionalized NHC complexes and of mixed nickel(II)–lithium(I) complexes. *Inorg. Chem.* **2014**, *53*, 5189–5200. [CrossRef] [PubMed]
25. Ketz, B.E.; Cole, A.P.; Waymouth, R.M. Structure and reactivity of an allylpalladium N-heterocyclic carbene enolate complex. *Organometallics* **2004**, *23*, 2835–2837. [CrossRef]
26. Legault, C.Y.; Kendall, C.; Charette, A.B. Structure and reactivity of a new anionic N-heterocyclic carbene silver(i) complex. *Chem. Commun.* **2005**, *30*, 3826–3828. [CrossRef]

27. Spencer, L.P.; Beddie, C.; Hall, M.B.; Fryzuk, M.D. Synthesis, reactivity, and DFT studies of tantalum complexes incorporating diamido-*N*-heterocyclic carbene ligands. facile endocyclic C−H bond activation. *J. Am. Chem. Soc.* **2006**, *128*, 12531–12543. [CrossRef]
28. Forster, T.D.; Krahulic, K.E.; Tuononen, H.M.; McDonald, R.; Parvez, M.; Roesler, R. A σ-donor with a planar six-π-electron B2N2C2 framework: Anionic *N*-heterocyclic carbene or heterocyclic terphenyl anion? *Angew. Chem. Int. Ed.* **2006**, *45*, 6356–6359. [CrossRef]
29. Vujkovic, N.; César, V.; Lugan, N.; Lavigne, G. An ambidentate janus-type ligand system based on fused carbene and imidato functionalities. *Chem. Eur. J.* **2011**, *17*, 13151–13155. [CrossRef]
30. César, V.; Lugan, N.; Lavigne, G. A Stable Anionic *N*-heterocyclic carbene and its zwitterionic complexes. *J. Am. Chem. Soc.* **2008**, *130*, 11286–11287. [CrossRef]
31. Bastin, S.; Barthes, C.; Lugan, N.; Lavigne, G.; César, V. Anionic *N*-heterocyclic carbene complexes of gold(I) as precatalysts for silver-free cycloisomerization of enynes. *Eur. J. Inorg. Chem.* **2015**, *13*, 2216–2221. [CrossRef]
32. César, V.; Barthes, C.; Farré, Y.C.; Cuisiat, S.V.; Vacher, B.Y.; Brousses, R.; Lugan, N.; Lavigne, G. Anionic and zwitterionic copper(I) complexes incorporating an anionic *N*-heterocyclic carbene decorated with a malonate backbone: Synthesis, structure and catalytic applications. *Dalton Trans.* **2013**, *42*, 7373–7385. [CrossRef] [PubMed]
33. Hobbs, M.G.; Knapp, C.J.; Welsh, P.T.; Borau-Garcia, J.; Ziegler, T.; Roesler, R. Anionic *N*-heterocyclic carbenes with N,N′-bis(fluoroaryl) and N,N′-bis(perfluoroaryl) substituents. *Chem. Eur. J.* **2010**, *16*, 14520–14533. [CrossRef] [PubMed]
34. Chotard, F.; Romanov, A.S.; Hughes, D.L.; Linnolahti, M.; Bochmann, M. Zwitterionic mixed-carbene coinage metal complexes: Synthesis, structures, and photophysical studies. *Eur. J. Inorg. Chem.* **2019**, *2019*, 4234–4240. [CrossRef]
35. César, V.; Lugan, N.; Lavigne, G. Electronic Tuning of a carbene center via remote chemical induction, and relevant effects in catalysis. *Chem. Eur. J.* **2010**, *16*, 11432–11442. [CrossRef] [PubMed]
36. César, V.; Misal Castro, L.C.; Dombray, T.; Sortais, J.-B.; Darcel, C.; Labat, S.; Miqueu, K.; Sotiropoulos, J.-M.; Brousses, R.; Lugan, N.; et al. (Cyclopentadienyl)iron(II) complexes of *N*-heterocyclic carbenes Bearing a malonate or imidate backbone: Synthesis, structure, and catalytic potential in hydrosilylation. *Organometallics* **2013**, *32*, 4643–4655. [CrossRef]
37. Wanzlick, H.-W.; Schönherr, H.-J. Direct synthesis of a mercury salt-carbene complex. *Angew. Chem. Int. Ed.* **1968**, *7*, 141–142. [CrossRef]
38. Yu, M.-H.; Yang, H.-H.; Gu, Y.-C.; Wang, B.-H.; Liu, F.-C.; Lin, I.J.; Lee, G.-H. Formation of anionic NHC complexes through the reaction of benzimidazoles with mercury chloride. Subsequent protonation and transmetallation reactions. *J. Organomet. Chem.* **2019**, *887*, 12–17. [CrossRef]
39. Baker, M.V.; Brown, D.H.; Haque, R.A.; Simpson, P.V.; Skelton, B.W.; White, A.H.; Williams, C.C. Mercury complexes of *N*-heterocyclic carbenes derived from imidazolium-linked cyclophanes: Synthesis, structure, and reactivity. *Organometallics* **2009**, *28*, 3793–3803. [CrossRef]
40. Haque, R.A.; Budagumpi, S.; Choo, S.Y.; Choong, M.K.; Lokesh, B.E.; Sudesh, K. Nitrile-functionalized Hg(II)- and Ag(I)- *N*-heterocyclic carbene complexes: Synthesis, crystal structures, nuclease and DNA binding activities. *Appl. Organomet. Chem.* **2012**, *26*, 689–700. [CrossRef]
41. Budagumpi, S.; Haque, R.A.; Salman, A.W.; Ghdhayeb, M.Z. Mercury(II)- and silver(I)-*N*-heterocyclic carbene complexes of CNC pincer-type ligands: Synthesis, crystal structures and Hofmann-type elimination studies. *Inorg. Chim. Acta* **2012**, *392*, 61–72. [CrossRef]
42. Budagumpi, S.; Endud, S. Group XII metal–*N*-heterocyclic carbene complexes: Synthesis, structural diversity, intramolecular interactions, and applications. *Organometallics* **2013**, *32*, 1537–1562. [CrossRef]
43. Scheele, U.J.; Dechert, S.; Meyer, F. Bridged dinucleating *N*-heterocyclic carbene ligands and their double helical mercury(II) complexes. *Inorg. Chim. Acta* **2006**, *359*, 4891–4900. [CrossRef]
44. Lee, K.-M.; Chen, J.C.; Lin, I.J. Helical mono and dinuclear mercury(II) *N*-heterocyclic carbene complexes. *J. Organomet. Chem.* **2001**, *617*, 364–375. [CrossRef]
45. Liu, Q.-X.; Yin, L.-N.; Feng, J.-C. New *N*-heterocyclic carbene silver(I) and mercury(II) 2-D supramolecular layers by the π–π stacking interactions. *J. Organomet. Chem.* **2007**, *692*, 3655–3663. [CrossRef]
46. Haque, R.A.; Salman, A.W.; Guan, T.S.; Abdallah, H.H. New *N*-heterocyclic carbene mercury(II) complexes: Close mercury–arene interaction. *J. Organomet. Chem.* **2011**, *696*, 3507–3512. [CrossRef]
47. Liu, Y.; Wan, X.; Xu, F. An arene−mercury(II) *N*-heterocyclic carbene complex. *Organometallics* **2009**, *28*, 5590–5592. [CrossRef]

48. Liu, Q.-X.; Yin, L.-N.; Wu, X.-M.; Feng, J.-C.; Guo, J.; Song, H.-B. New *N*-heterocyclic carbene mercury(II) and silver(I) complexes. *Polyhedron* **2008**, *27*, 87–94. [CrossRef]
49. Adiraju, V.A.K.; Jin, W.; Yousufuddin, M.; Dias, H.V. Copper(I) complexes of anionic tridentate CNC pincer ligands. *Z. Anorg. Allg. Chem.* **2020**, *646*, 215–219. [CrossRef]
50. Dash, C.; Wang, G.; Muñoz-Castro, A.; Ponduru, T.T.; Zacharias, A.O.; Yousufuddin, M.; Dias, H.V.R. Organic azide and auxiliary-ligand-free complexes of coinage metals supported by *N*-heterocyclic carbenes. *Inorg. Chem.* **2019**, *59*, 2188–2199. [CrossRef]
51. Wang, G.; Pecher, L.; Frenking, G.; Dias, H.V. Vinyltrifluoroborate complexes of silver supported by *N*-heterocyclic carbenes. *Eur. J. Inorg. Chem.* **2018**, *2018*, 4142–4152. [CrossRef]
52. Adiraju, V.A.K.; Yousufuddin, M.; Dias, H.V. Copper(I), silver(I) and gold(I) complexes of *N*-heterocyclic carbene-phosphinidene. *Dalton Trans.* **2015**, *44*, 4449–4454. [CrossRef]
53. Dash, C.; Yousufuddin, M.; Cundari, T.R.; Dias, H.V.R. Gold-mediated Expulsion of dinitrogen from organic azides. *J. Am. Chem. Soc.* **2013**, *135*, 15479–15488. [CrossRef] [PubMed]
54. Dash, C.; Das, A.; Yousufuddin, M.; Dias, H.V.R. Isolable, copper(I) dicarbonyl complexes supported by *N*-heterocyclic carbenes. *Inorg. Chem.* **2013**, *52*, 1584–1590. [CrossRef] [PubMed]
55. Dash, C.; Kroll, P.; Yousufuddin, M.; Dias, H.V.R. Isolable, gold carbonyl complexes supported by *N*-heterocyclic carbenes. *Chem. Commun.* **2011**, *47*, 4478–4480. [CrossRef] [PubMed]
56. Arduengo, A.J.; Dias, H.V.R.; Harlow, R.L.; Kline, M. Electronic stabilization of nucleophilic carbenes. *J. Am. Chem. Soc.* **1992**, *114*, 5530–5534. [CrossRef]
57. Arduengo, A.J.; Davidson, F.; Dias, H.V.R.; Goerlich, J.R.; Khasnis, D.; Marshall, W.J.; Prakasha, T.K. An Air stable carbene and mixed carbene "dimers". *J. Am. Chem. Soc.* **1997**, *119*, 12742–12749. [CrossRef]
58. Arduengo, A.J.; Dias, H.V.R.; Dixon, D.A.; Harlow, R.L.; Klooster, W.T.; Koetzle, T.F. Electron distribution in a stable carbene. *J. Am. Chem. Soc.* **1994**, *116*, 6812–6822. [CrossRef]
59. Dias, H.V.R.; Jin, W. A stable tridentate carbene ligand. *Tetrahedron Lett.* **1994**, *35*, 1365–1366. [CrossRef]
60. Arduengo, A.J.; Dias, H.V.R.; Calabrese, J.C.; Davidson, F. Homoleptic carbene-silver(I) and carbene-copper(I) complexes. *Organometallics* **1993**, *12*, 3405–3409. [CrossRef]
61. Buron, C.; Stelzig, L.; Guerret, O.; Gornitzka, H.; Romanenko, V.; Bertrand, G. Synthesis and structure of 1,2,4-triazol-2-ium-5-ylidene complexes of Hg(II), Pd(II), Ni(II), Ni(0), Rh(I) and Ir(I). *J. Organomet. Chem.* **2002**, *664*, 70–76. [CrossRef]
62. Arduengo, A.J., III; Harlow, R.L.; Marshall, W.J.; Prakasha, T.K. Investigation of a mercury(II) carbene complex: Bis(1,3-dimethylimidazol-2-ylidene) mercury chloride. *Heteroat. Chem.* **1996**, *7*, 421–426. [CrossRef]
63. Tschinkl, M.; Schier, A.; Riede, J.; Gabbaï, F.P. Complexation of DMF and DMSO by a monodentate organomercurial lewis acid. *Organometallics* **1999**, *18*, 2040–2042. [CrossRef]
64. Pelz, S.; Mohr, F. "Oxide route" for the preparation of mercury(II) *N*-heterocyclic carbene complexes. *Organometallics* **2011**, *30*, 383–385. [CrossRef]
65. Bumbu, O.; Silvestru, C.; Gimeno, M.C.; Laguna, A. New organomercury(II) compounds containing intramolecular N→Hg interactions: Crystal and molecular structure of [2-(Me$_2$NCH$_2$)C$_6$H$_4$]HgCl and [2-(Me$_2$NCH$_2$)C$_6$H$_4$]Hg[S(S)PPh$_2$]. *J. Organomet. Chem.* **2004**, *689*, 1172–1179. [CrossRef]
66. Kolychev, E.L.; Portnyagin, I.A.; Shuntikov, V.V.; Khrustalev, V.N.; Nechaev, M.S. Six- and seven-membered ring carbenes: Rational synthesis of amidinium salts, generation of carbenes, synthesis of Ag(I) and Cu(I) complexes. *J. Organomet. Chem.* **2009**, *694*, 2454–2462. [CrossRef]
67. Leung-Toung, R.; Wentrup, C. Flash vacuum pyrolysis of tert-butyl β-ketoesters: Sterically protected α-oxoketenes. *Tetrahedron* **1992**, *48*, 7641–7654. [CrossRef]
68. Sheldrick, G.M. A short history of SHELX. *Acta Crystallogr. Sect. A Found. Crystallogr.* **2007**, *64*, 112–122. [CrossRef]
69. Dolomanov, O.V.; Bourhis, L.J.; Gildea, R.J.; Howard, J.A.K.; Puschmann, H. OLEX2: A complete structure solution, refinement and analysis program. *J. Appl. Crystallogr.* **2009**, *42*, 339–341. [CrossRef]

Sample Availability: Samples of the compounds are not available from the authors.

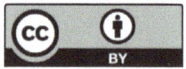

© 2020 by the authors. Licensee MDPI, Basel, Switzerland. This article is an open access article distributed under the terms and conditions of the Creative Commons Attribution (CC BY) license (http://creativecommons.org/licenses/by/4.0/).

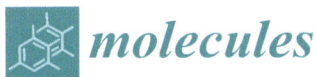

Article

Syntheses and Reactivity of New Zwitterionic Imidazolium Trihydridoborate and Triphenylborate Species

Maura Pellei [1], Riccardo Vallesi [1], Luca Bagnarelli [1], H. V. Rasika Dias [2,*] and Carlo Santini [1,*]

[1] School of Science and Technology, Chemistry Division, University of Camerino, via S. Agostino 1, 62032 Camerino, Macerata, Italy; maura.pellei@unicam.it (M.P.); riccardo.vallesi@unicam.it (R.V.); luca.bagnarelli@unicam.it (L.B.)
[2] Department of Chemistry and Biochemistry, The University of Texas at Arlington, Arlington, TX 76019-0065, USA
* Correspondence: dias@uta.edu (H.V.R.D.); carlo.santini@unicam.it (C.S.); Tel.: +390737402213 (C.S.); Fax: +390737637345 (C.S.)

Academic Editor: Yves Canac
Received: 18 June 2020; Accepted: 10 July 2020; Published: 13 July 2020

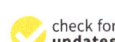

Abstract: In this study, four new N-(alkyl/aryl)imidazolium-borates were prepared, and their deprotonation reactions were investigated. Addition of $BH_3 \bullet THF$ to N-benzylimidazoles and N-mesitylimidazoles leads to imidazolium-trihydridoborate adducts. Ammonium tetraphenylborate reacts with benzyl- or mesityl-imidazoles with the loss of one of the phenyl groups yielding the corresponding imidazolium-triphenylborates. Their authenticity was confirmed by CHN analysis, ^{1}H-NMR, ^{13}C-NMR, ^{11}B-NMR, FT-IR spectroscopy, and electrospray ionization mass spectrometry (ESI-MS). 3-Benzyl-imidazolium-1-yl)trihydridoborate, $(HIm^{Bn})BH_3$, and (3-mesityl-imidazolium-1-yl)trihydridoborate, $(HIm^{Mes})BH_3$, were also characterized by X-ray crystallography. The reactivity of these new compounds as carbene precursors in an effort to obtain borate-NHC complexes was investigated and a new carbene-borate adduct (which dimerizes) was obtained via a microwave-assisted procedure.

Keywords: N-heterocyclic carbenes; imidazole; spectroscopy; X-ray

1. Introduction

N-heterocyclic carbenes (NHCs) [1–3] are an extremely useful and versatile class of ligands [4–10] with donor properties similar to phosphanes [11–14]. By tuning the steric and electronic properties around the carbene center, several carbenes featuring various σ-donating and π-accepting properties have been developed to date [15–17]. Their chemical versatility not only implies a wide variety of structural diversity and coordination modes, but also a capability to form stable complexes with a large number of transition metals with different oxidation states [6,7,18–20] and labile ligands [21–26]. Metal-NHCs complexes gained considerable interest in recent years because of their application in material chemistry [27], in catalysis [19,28–37], in carbene transfer reactions [38,39], and in medicinal inorganic chemistry [40–49].

In the last thirty years, several carbenes based on the imidazol-2-ylidene (Scheme 1a) as well as the imidazolin-2-ylidene [50] and the chain-like carbene compound have been reported [51]. Such NHCs compounds have in common the presence of only organic substituents attached to the nitrogen atoms, whereas carbenes with other main-group elements as substituents (Scheme 1b) are scarce [52–56]. Substitution of one of the groups attached to nitrogen by a borane would result in the generation of carbene-borate anions NHC-BR$_3^-$ (Scheme 1c), as anionic analogs of the neutral imidazol-2-ylidenes.

To the best of our knowledge, only few examples of monoanionic carbenes such as the on in Scheme 1c have been published as yet [53,57–63].

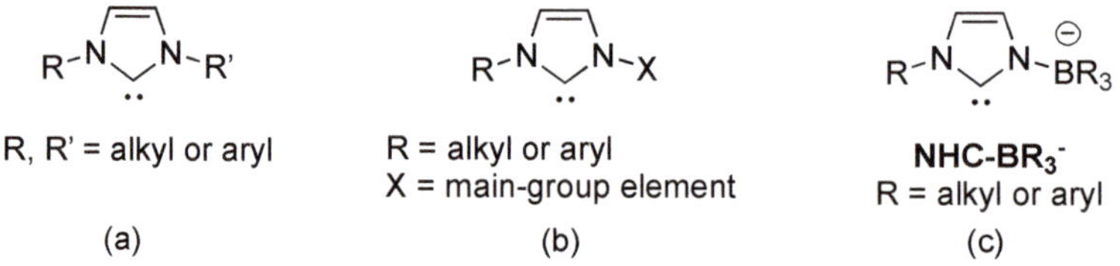

R−N⌒N−R' R,R' = alkyl or aryl (a)

R−N⌒N−X R = alkyl or aryl X = main-group element (b)

R−N⌒N−BR$_3$ ⊖ NHC-BR$_3^-$ R = alkyl or aryl (c)

Scheme 1. Structure of carbenes based on the imidazol-2-ylidene moieties: (**a**) with alkyl and aryl substituents; (**b**) with a main-group element substituent; (**c**) with a borate moiety substituent.

In 1998 and 2002, Siebert and co-workers reported that deprotonation of imidazole-borane complexes or imidazolium-borate species (Scheme 2a) with BuLi leads to the formation of the carbene-borate anions NHC-BH$_3^-$ [59,64]. These kinds of nucleophilic carbenes allowed the formation of neutral manganese complexes and anionic iron compounds by reactions with BrMn(CO)$_5$ and Fe(CO)$_5$, respectively [59]. The analogous reaction with [(C$_7$H$_{11}$)Fe(CO)$_2$Br], Cp$_2$TiCl, VCl$_3$, and ScCl$_3$ yielded the corresponding metal complexes [64]. Bis(imidazolyl) compounds with BH$_3$ or BEt$_3$ (Scheme 2b) and their behavior towards treatment with butyllithium to give dianionic chelating dicarbene-diborate ligands have also been reported [53]. Among them, the dianionic bis(imidazol-2-ylidene) species obtained from b2 (Scheme 2) reacted with Cp$_2$TiCl$_2$ and Cp$_2$ZrCl$_2$ allowing the formation of the corresponding carbene-borate complexes [53]. Isomerization to the 2-borate imidazole forms by 1,2-BR$_3$ migration [65], intramolecular addition/elimination or dimerization reactions may or may not occur on deprotonation [57–61,66]. For example, deprotonation of the triethylborane adduct (Scheme 2c) produced the isomerized N-heterocyclic carbene-borate species (Scheme 2d) [59]. Attempts to synthesize the carbene-borate anions by deprotonation of the parent imidazole (Scheme 2(e1,e2)) and benzimidazole (Scheme 2(e3)) adducts, have invariably resulted in the formation of isomers (Scheme 2f) [57,67] by ring-closure due to a rapid intramolecular nucleophilic aromatic substitution. On the other hand, Contreras et al. [60,66] reported the imidazaboles (Scheme 2(g1,g2)), by elimination of H$_2$ from the (N-alkylimidazolium)borate species with iodine at 270 °C. Okada et al. [61] reported the synthesis of analogous imidazaboles (Scheme 2(g3,g4)), from reaction of the parent (N-alkylimidazolium)borates with organolithium reagents. Recently, Chiu and coworkers [65] reported that dimerization of 2-borylimidazoles through B−N coordination yielded the head-to-tail dimers g5 and g6 (Scheme 2). Compound g7 is the only isolable product of the reaction of [Ph$_2$B(Im^{t}Bu)$_2$Br] and [Ca{N(SiMe$_3$)$_2$}$_2$(THF)$_2$] [68].

Functionalized imidazole-based NHCs have attracted special interest because they can be utilized to tune the environment and properties at the coordinated metal [4,69]. Whereas there are many studies describing the coordination of chelate and pincer N-heterocyclic carbene ligands, the use of anionic NHC-borates is still scarce [52,63]. Recently, significant research efforts have been devoted to the development of ionic liquids based on (N-alkylimidazolium)borate as new potential hypergolic fuels owing to their excellent physiochemical properties including and unique hypergolic reactivity [70]. The first chelating tricarbene ligand with the topology of Trofimenko's tris(pyrazolyl)borates [71,72], tris(3-methylimidazolin-2-ylidene-1-yl)borate, in which the carbene units are connected via a BH group, was introduced in 1995 by Fehlhammer and co-workers [54] together with its hexacarbene iron(III) and cobalt(III) complexes [73,74]. The synthesis of monoanionic chelating dicarbene bis(imidazol-2-ylidene-1-yl)borates and their use as ligands in various homoleptic and heteroleptic metal complexes has been described [75,76] and recently reviewed [15,52].

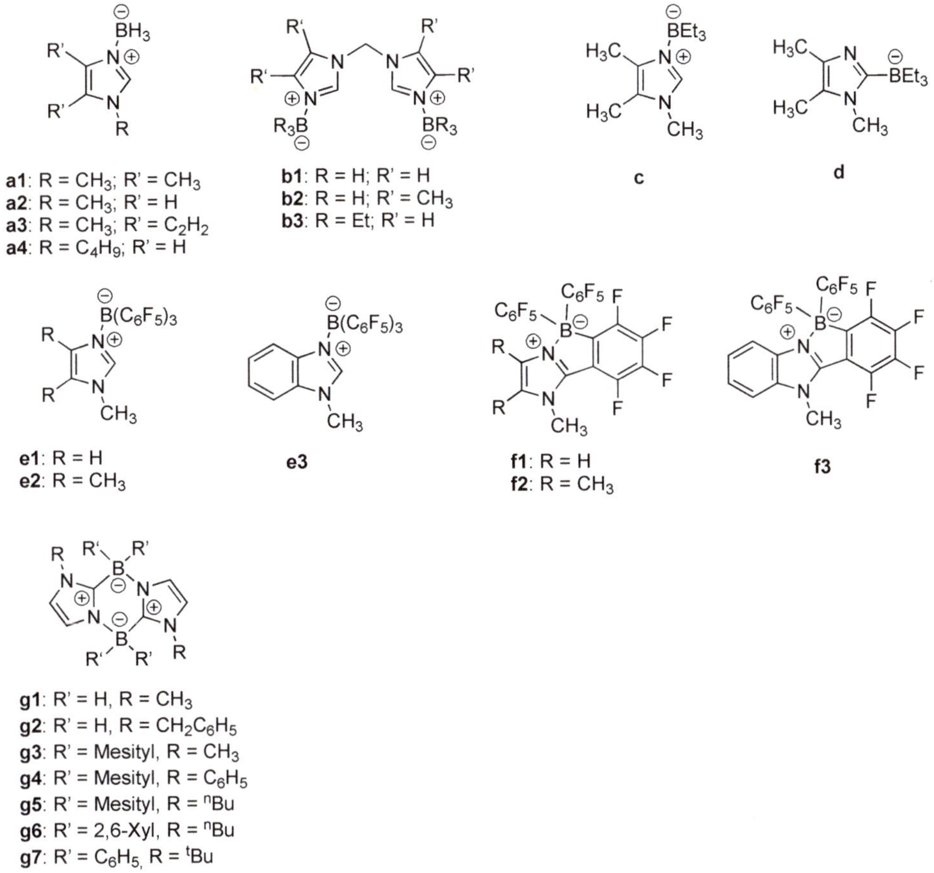

a1: R = CH₃; R' = CH₃
a2: R = CH₃; R' = H
a3: R = CH₃; R' = C₂H₂
a4: R = C₄H₉; R' = H

b1: R = H; R' = H
b2: R = H; R' = CH₃
b3: R = Et; R' = H

c

d

e1: R = H
e2: R = CH₃

e3

f1: R = H
f2: R = CH₃

f3

g1: R' = H, R = CH₃
g2: R' = H, R = CH₂C₆H₅
g3: R' = Mesityl, R = CH₃
g4: R' = Mesityl, R = C₆H₅
g5: R' = Mesityl, R = ⁿBu
g6: R' = 2,6-Xyl, R = ⁿBu
g7: R' = C₆H₅, R = ᵗBu

Scheme 2. Structure of: (**a**) imidazolium trihydridoborate species; (**b**) bis(imidazolium)borate species; (**c**) imidazolium triethylborate species; (**d**) 2-substituted imidazolylborate species; (**e**) imidazolium and benzimidazolium triarylborate species; (**f**) ring-closed imidazolium and benzimidazolium triarylborate species; (**g**) imidazaboles.

In the last years, we developed several classes of coinage metal NHCs complexes obtained from the chelating precursors [HB(RImH)₃]Br₂ (R = Benzyl, Mesityl and t-Butyl) [77], [H₂B(HTz^{Bn})₂]Br [78], H₂C(HTz^R)₂, and H₂C(HIm^R)₂ (HTz = 1,2,4-triazole; HIm = imidazole; R = (CH₂)₃SO₃⁻ or (CH₂)₂COO⁻) [79]. Recently, we have focused the research work on the development of new group 11 metal-NHCs complexes obtained from the water-soluble precursors HIm^{1R,3R}Cl (R = COOCH₃, COOCH₂CH₃, or CON(CH₂CH₃)₂) [80,81] or the zwitterionic water-soluble precursor NaHIm^{1R,3R} (R = (CH₂)₃SO₃⁻) [82].

Despite the impressive chemistry based on parent poly(azolyl)borate, the analogous mono(azolyl)borate have received very little attention in recent years [83,84]. Recently, we prepared trihydro(pyrazolyl)borates such as Na[H₃B(5-(CF₃)pz)] and Na[H₃B(3-(NO₂)pz)] and related copper(I) and silver(I) phosphane complexes [85,86].

Here, we present the synthesis of (N-(alkyl/aryl)imidazolium)borate-based systems (Scheme 3) and their reactivity as carbene precursors in the effort to obtain borate-NHCs silver(I) complexes.

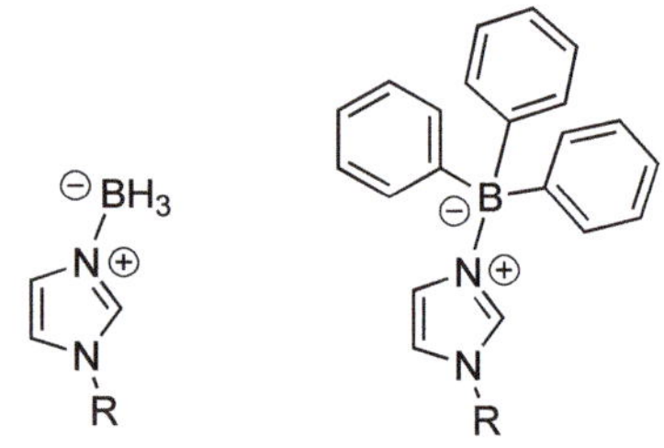

1: R = benzyl
2: R = mesityl

3: R = CH_3
4: R = benzyl

Scheme 3. Chemical structures of (*N*-(alkyl/aryl)imidazolium)borates **1–4**.

2. Result and Discussion

Synthesis and Characterization

The *N*-(alkyl/aril)imidazolium-borate adducts **1–4** were synthesized in one step by two different routes (Scheme 4).

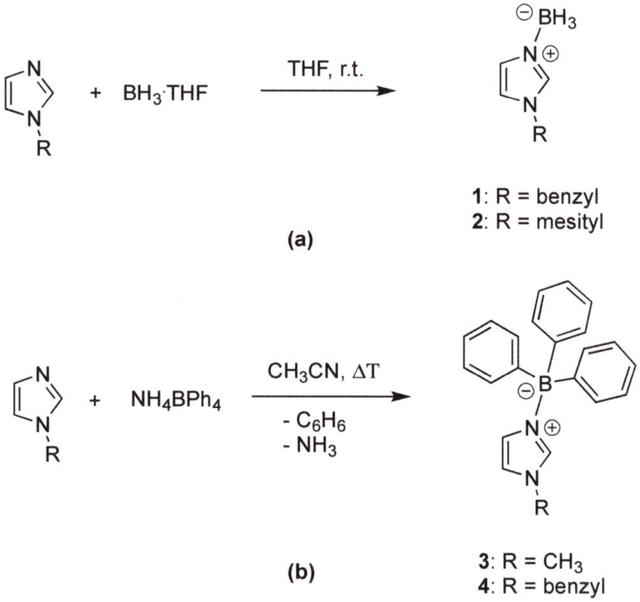

Scheme 4. Synthesis of: (**a**) imidazolium trihydridoborates **1** and **2**; (**b**) imidazolium triphenyborates **3** and **4**.

The addition of one equivalent of BH_3•THF to a solution of *N*-benzylimidazole or *N*-mesitylimidazole at room temperature yields the colorless imidazolium-borate adducts **1** or **2**, respectively, in nearly quantitative yields (Scheme 4a). By dissolving the crude ligands **1** and **2** in $CHCl_3$ and $CHCl_3$/THF solution, respectively, single crystals suitable for X-ray diffraction analysis were obtained.

Compounds **3** and **4** were prepared by addition of NH_4BPh_4 to an acetonitrile solution of methylimidazole or benzylimidazole under reflux conditions. It is known that under acidic conditions the tetraphenylborate anion has limited stability producing triphenylboranes [87], and when heated with alkylammonium salts can lose a phenyl ring to form a B–N bond with the ammonium compound [88]. This kind of displacement was observed in our studies: the loss of a phenyl ring and the formation of imidazolium-triphenylborate species occurred in good yields, volatile benzene and ammonia being also produced. Compound **3** was previously obtained as a crystalline byproduct of the reaction mixture of [ReO$_2$(1-MeIm)$_4$]$^+$ complex and NaBPh$_4$ in acidic conditions [89].

Derivatives **1** and **2** are white and brownish solids, respectively, both soluble in CH$_3$OH, CHCl$_3$, CH$_2$Cl$_2$, THF, DMSO, and acetone. Derivatives **3** and **4** are white solids, both soluble in THF, CH$_2$Cl$_2$, CHCl$_3$, CH$_3$CN, DMSO, and acetone.

The authenticity of compounds **1–4** was confirmed by CHN analysis, ^{1}H-NMR, ^{13}C-NMR, ^{11}B-NMR, FT-IR spectroscopy, and electrospray ionization mass spectrometry (ESI-MS). Compounds **1** and **2** were also characterized by X-ray crystallography.

The (HIm^{Bn})BH$_3$ (**1**) crystallizes in the Orthorhombic P2$_1$2$_1$2$_1$ space group. The molecular structure is illustrated in Figure 1. It is monomeric in the solid state and C1-N1 distance is slightly longer than the C1-N2 distance.

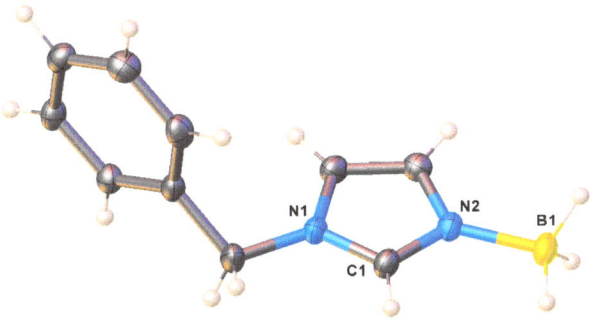

Figure 1. Molecular structure of (HIm^{Bn})BH$_3$ (**1**). Selected bond distances (Å) and angles (°): N1-C1 1.343(2), N2-C1 1.323(2), N2-B1 1.587(2), N1-C4 1.474(2), N1-C1-N2 110.29(14), C1-N2-B1 126.58(14).

The molecular structure of (HIm^{Mes})BH$_3$ (**2**) is shown in Figure 2. It crystallizes in the Monoclinic P2$_1$/n space group with two chemically similar but crystallographically different molecules in the asymmetric unit. Structural features of **2** are similar to those observed for **1**.

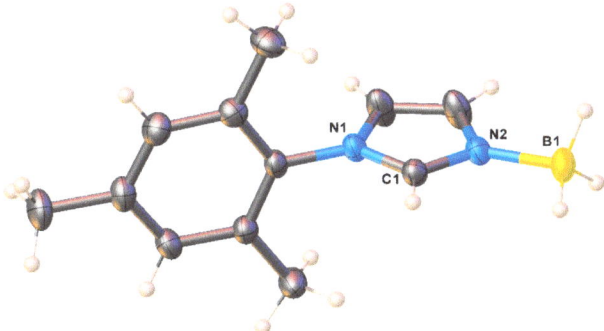

Figure 2. Molecular structure of (HIm^{Mes})BH$_3$ (**2**). There are two chemical similar but crystallographically different molecules of (HIm^{Mes})BH$_3$ in the asymmetric unit but only one is shown here. Selected bond distances (Å) and angles (°): N1-C1 1.3442(14), N2-C1 1.3207(14), N2-B1 1.5836(16), N1-C4 1.4465(14), N1-C1-N2 110.36(10), C1-N2-B1 127.91(10).

The FT-IR spectra of Compounds **1–4** showed weak absorptions in the range 3010–3177 cm^{-1}, due to the azolyl ring C-H stretching and the presence of the BH$_3$ moiety in Compounds **1** and **2** was detected by intense absorptions at 2255–2374 cm^{-1}.

The ^{1}H- and ^{13}C-NMR spectra of **1** and **2** were recorded in CDCl$_3$ and CD$_3$OD, while the spectra of **3** and **4** were recorded in DMSO solution. Compounds **1–4** showed a single set of resonances for the imidazolium rings. The ^{1}H NMR spectra of Compounds **1** and **2** at the 2-CH position does not show any reduced intensity after two days in CD$_3$OD solution at room temperature, suggesting the absence of fast H-D exchange and therefore lack of deuteration at this position.

The ^{11}B-NMR spectra showed a quartet at δ −19.38 and −19.21 ppm for Compounds **1** and **2**, respectively, in CDCl$_3$ solution, indicating a coordination of the imidazole rings at the BH$_3$ group [62,90]. The single broad ^{11}B resonances observed at δ −6.52 ppm for Compound **3** and at δ −6.37 ppm for Compound **4**, in (CD$_3$)$_2$CO and CDCl$_3$ solutions, respectively, are indicative of a four-coordinate boron center; they are in the range observed for analogously triphenylborate species [91], being considerably shifted in comparison with the triphenylborane one, which is observed at δ −60.2 ppm [92].

In the ESI(+)-MS spectra of **1** and **2** we observed peaks at m/z 195 and 223, due to the molecular specie [(HIm^{Bn})BH$_3$ + Na]$^+$ and [(HIm^{Mes})BH$_3$ + Na]$^+$, respectively. In addition the ESI(+)MS spectra displayed peaks due to the fragmentation species [HIm^R + H]$^+$ and to the aggregates [(HIm^R)$_2$BH$_2$]$^+$ (R = Bn or Mes). Analogously, the ESI(+)-MS spectra of Compounds **3** and **4** were dominated by the peaks at m/z 83 and 159 due to the [HIm^{CH3} + H]$^+$ and [HIm^{Bn} + H]$^+$, respectively, along with a fragment at m/z 247 ([(HIm^{CH3})BPh$_2$]$^+$, 25%) and an aggregate at 481 ([(Im^{Bn})$_2$BPh$_2$]$^+$, 45%), in **3** and **4** respectively.

Our aim was to synthesize new N-(alkyl/aryl)imidazolium-borates and study their reactivity and investigate their reactivity as carbene precursors in an effort to obtain borate-NHCs silver(I) complexes. However, treatment of Compounds **1–4** with ^{n}BuLi to yield the imidazol-2-ylidenes always led to decomposition species. Further direct reactions of **1–4** with Ag$_2$O, in different reaction conditions (r.t. or reflux; reaction times = 5, 24, 48, and 120 h; solvent = THF, CH$_2$Cl$_2$, CH$_3$OH, and CH$_3$CN), or with silver acetate (in CH$_3$OH or CH$_3$CN) to give silver carbene complexes were unsuccessful: only mixtures of unreacted or decomposition products were detected. The only partially isolable product of the reaction of **4** and Ag$_2$O in CH$_3$CN was the imidazabole species **5**. After these efforts, we found that the direct synthesis of imidazaboles [60,61,66] could be achieved by using microwave-assisted procedure [93], following a pre-set heating ramp of 1 h up to 80 °C, in technical-grade CH$_3$CN and in the presence of Ag$_2$O (Scheme 5). Unfortunately, this methodology was only successful for Compound **5**, and mixtures of products were obtained by using microwave-assisted procedure employing Compounds **1–3** as starting materials.

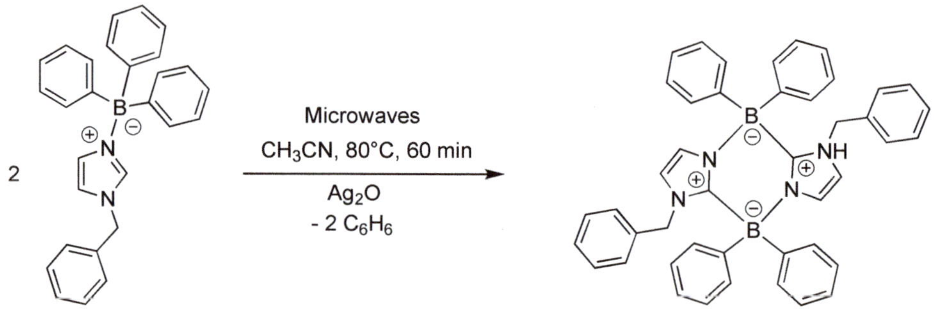

Scheme 5. Microwave-assisted synthesis of Compound **5**.

Compound **5** is an oil soluble in CH$_3$OH, CH$_3$CN and DMSO. Its formation can be explained by the abstraction of proton at 2-position of the imidazolium-triphenylborate and the successive bimolecular condensation of the produced anions with elimination of two benzene molecules (Scheme 5) [65].

Compound **5** has a framework of 1,4-diazonia-2,5-diboratacyclohexa-3,6-diene, which can also be regarded as an intramolecular carbene-borate adduct [59,60].

NMR spectra showed significant changes going from Compound **4** to the corresponding imidazabole species **5**. In particular, the ^{1}H-NMR spectrum of **5** recorded in deuterated DMSO showed the disappearance of the diagnostic 2-C*H* imidazolium signal of **4** at 8.37 ppm upon cyclization. Analogously, in the ^{13}C-NMR spectrum, the 2-CH imidazolium signal of **4** at 136.33 ppm was no longer observed in the spectrum of **5** that instead showed a new, albeit poorly intense, 2-C signal at 159.18 ppm indicative of the carbene-borate formation [94]. The remaining ^{13}C-NMR data are very similar to those of **4**. The ^{11}B-NMR spectrum contains a singlet at δ 1.43. The decreased ^{11}B-NMR nuclear shielding in **5** as compared to **4** (δ^{11}B −6.37) points towards lower delocalization of the positive charge in the imidazabole system [95].

Isomerization to the 2-borate imidazole forms by 1,2-BR$_3$ migration [65], intramolecular addition/elimination or dimerization reactions may occur on deprotonation [57–61,66], presumably involving intermediates such as in Scheme 6A,B.

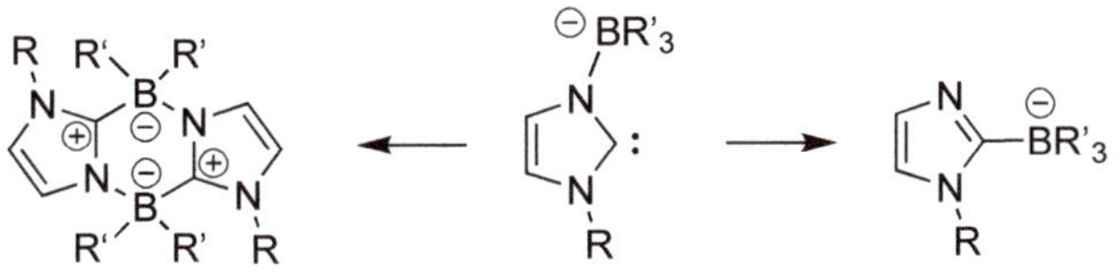

Scheme 6. Rearrangement species (**B**,**C**) by isomerization or dimerization of the NHC-borate form (**A**).

DFT studies by Vagedes et al. [57] suggested that direct interconversion of such anions by 1,2-migration is very unlikely. The borate substituent thermodynamically prefers to be bound to C-2 of the anionic heterocyclic moiety. Presumably, the Lewis acidic borane compensates the negative charge much more efficiently when bound to the carbon atom than when bound to the nitrogen atom, but their interconversion was precluded by a very high barrier of the respective 1,2-BR$_3$ shift [57]. In particular, for Compound **5**, the probably initially generated "anionic Arduengo carbene" product **A** is proved unstable under the reaction conditions and it must be assumed that the rearrangement, experimentally observed to yield species C, is likely to have proceeded intermolecularly by two successive nucleophilic substitutions or by radical pathway as recently proposed by Chiu et al. [65].

As demonstrated in the BR$_3$-functionalized NHC, the incorporation of anionic borate functionality enhances the donating ability of NHC [96,97]. However, we must conclude that the *N*-borato carbene anion A could exhibit its characteristic NHC chemistry when prepared or generated under conditions precluding intermolecular rearrangement pathways to their thermodynamically favored C(2)-borated imidazole isomers or head-to-tail imidazabole dimers.

3. Experimental Section

3.1. Materials and General Methods

All syntheses and handling were carried out under an atmosphere of dry oxygen-free dinitrogen, using standard Schlenk techniques or a glove box. Glassware was dried with a heat-gun under high vacuum. Solvents were purchased from commercial sources and purified by conventional methods prior to use. Elemental analyses (C, H, N, and S) were performed with a Fisons Instruments EA-1108 CHNS-O Elemental Analyzer (Thermo Fisher Scientific Inc., Waltham, MA, USA). Melting points were taken on an SMP3 Stuart Scientific Instrument (Bibby Sterilin Ltd., London, UK). IR spectra were recorded from 4000 to 400 cm^{-1} on a PerkinElmer Frontier FT-IR instrument (Perkin Elmer Inc., Waltham, MA, USA), equipped with single reflection universal diamond ATR top-plate. IR annotations used were as follows: br = broad, m = medium, mbr = medium broad, s = strong, sbr = strong broad, sh = shoulder, vs = very strong, w = weak, wbr = weak broad. ^{1}H-, ^{13}C-, and ^{11}B-NMR spectra were recorded with an Oxford AS400 Varian spectrometer (400.4 MHz for ^{1}H, 100.1 MHz for ^{13}C, and 128.4 MHz for ^{11}B) (Oxford Instruments, MA, USA) or with a 500 Bruker Ascend (500.1 MHz for ^{1}H, 125 MHz for ^{13}C, and 160.5 MHz for ^{11}B) (Bruker BioSpin Corporation, 15 Fortune Drive, Billerica, MA, USA). Referencing was relative to tetramethylsilane (TMS) (^{1}H and ^{13}C) and BF$_3$.Et$_2$O (^{11}B). NMR annotations used were as follows: br = broad; d = doublet, m = multiplet, s = singlet. Syntheses under microwave irradiation were performed by means of a Flexible Microwave Platform FlexSynth Milestone apparatus (Milestone Srl, Via Fatebenefratelli, Sorisole (BG), Italy). The reactions were performed in a 100-mL PTFE vessel, sealed using a Teflon crimp top. Electrospray mass spectra (ESI-MS) were obtained in positive—(ESI(+)MS) or negative-ion (ESI(−)MS) mode on an Agilent Technologies Series 1100 LC/MSD Mass Spectrometer (Agilent Technologies Inc, Santa Clara, CA, USA), using a methanol or acetonitrile mobile phase. The compounds were added to reagent grade methanol to give approximately 0.1 mM solutions, injected (1 µL) into the spectrometer via a Hewlett Packard 1090 Series II UV-Visible HPLC system (Agilent Technologies Inc, Santa Clara, CA, USA) fitted with an autosampler. The pump delivered the solutions to the mass spectrometer source at a flow rate of 300 mL min^{-1}, and nitrogen was employed both as a drying and nebulizing gas. Capillary voltages were typically 4000 and 3500 V for the ESI(+)MS and ESI(−)MS modes, respectively. Confirmation of all major species in this ESI-MS study was supported by comparison of the observed and predicted isotope distribution patterns, the latter calculated using the IsoPro 3.1 computer program (T-Tech Inc., Norcross, GA, USA). 1-Benzylimidazole, 1-methylimidazole, BH$_3$•THF complex, ammonium tetraphenylborate, and silver oxide were purchased from Sigma-Aldrich (Merck Life Science S.r.l., Via Monte Rosa, Milano, Italy). The 1-mesitylimidazole was synthesized in accordance with the literature method [98].

Caution! The materials used and synthesized in this study are energetic. They should be handled in quantities not exceeding the millimolar scale. Manipulations should be carried out behind blast shields and with adequate personal safety gear.

3.1.1. Synthesis of (HIm^{Bn})BH$_3$ (**1**)

1-Benzylimidazole (1.840 g, 11.631 mmol) was dissolved in dry THF (50 mL) under N$_2$ atmosphere and BH$_3$•THF complex (12.0 mL, 1M) was added drop by drop. The reaction mixture was stirred at room temperature for 24 h. Then, the volatiles were removed under reduced pressure to give a colorless oil. It was re-crystallized by CHCl$_3$/diethyl ether/n-hexane (1/3/3) solution to obtain a white precipitate; it was filtered, washed with diethyl ether, and dried under reduced pressure to give **1** in 80% yield (1.601 g). Single crystals of **1** suitable for X-ray analysis were obtained by slow evaporation of a CHCl$_3$ solution of **1**. Melting point: 92–94 °C. IR (cm^{-1}): 3159w, 3135m, 3061w, 3038w (C-H); 2352m, 2297m, 2255m (B-H); 1540m, 1533m (C=C/C=N). ^{1}H-NMR (CDCl$_3$, 293 K): δ 2.2 (br, 3H, BH$_3$), 5.13 (s, 2H, CH$_2$Ph), 6.91 (s, 1H, 4-CH or 5-CH), 7.14 (s, 1H, 4-CH or 5-CH), 7.23–7.44 (m, 5H, C$_6$H$_5$), 7.79 (s, 1H, 2-CH). ^{1}H-NMR (CD$_3$OD, 293 K): δ 2.2 (qbr, 3H, BH$_3$), 5.24 (s, 2H, CH$_2$Ph), 7,03 (s, 1H, 4-CH or 5-CH), 7.19 (s, 1H, 4-CH or 5-CH), 7.26–7.43 (m, 5H, C$_6$H$_5$), 8.13 (s, 1H, 2-CH). ^{13}C{^{1}H}-NMR (CDCl$_3$, 293 K): δ 52.35 (CH$_2$Ph), 119.94, 127.98, 128.21, 129.33, 129.47, 133.46 (CH), 136.33 (2-CH). ^{11}B{^{1}H}-NMR (CDCl$_3$, 293 K): δ −19.38 (s, BH$_3$). ^{11}B-NMR (CDCl$_3$, 293 K): δ −19.38 (q, BH$_3$, J$_{B-H}$ = 96 Hz). ESI-MS (major positive-ions, CH$_3$OH), m/z (%): 159 (40) [HIm^{Bn} + H]$^+$, 181 (40) [HIm^{Bn} + Na]$^+$, 195 (90) [(HIm^{Bn})BH$_3$ + Na]$^+$, 329 (100) [(HIm^{Bn})$_2$BH$_2$]$^+$. Anal. Calcd. for C$_{10}$H$_{13}$BN$_2$: C 69.82, H 7.62, N 16.28%. Found: C 69.52, H 7.30, N 15.91%.

3.1.2. Synthesis of (HIm^{Mes})BH$_3$ (**2**)

1-mesityl-imidazole (0.930 g, 5.000 mmol) was dissolved in dry THF (30 mL) under N$_2$ atmosphere and BH$_3$•THF complex (5.2 mL, 1M) was added drop by drop. The reaction mixture was stirred at room temperature for 24 h. Then, the volatiles were removed under reduced pressure to give a brown oil. It was re-crystallized by CHCl$_3$/diethyl ether/n-hexane (1/3/3) solution to obtain a brown precipitate; it was filtered, washed with diethyl ether, and dried under reduced pressure to give **1** in

68% yield (0.680 g). Single crystals of **2** suitable for X-ray analysis were obtained by slow evaporation of a CHCl$_3$/THF solution of **2**. Melting point: 109–111 °C. IR (cm^{-1}): 3177w, 3155w, 3132w, 3061w, 3028w (C-H); 2374m, 2338m, 2323m, 2300m, 2259m (B-H); 1526s (C=C/C=N). ^{1}H-NMR (CDCl$_3$, 293 K): δ 2.03 (s, 6H, CH$_3{}^{Mes}$), 2.3 (br, 3H, BH$_3$), 2.37 (s, 3H, CH$_3{}^{Mes}$), 6.90 (s, 1H, 4-CH or 5-CH), 7.02 (s, 2H, CH^{Mes}), 7.31 (s, 1H, 4-CH or 5-CH), 7.75 (s, 1H, 2-CH). ^{1}H-NMR (CD$_3$OD, 293 K): δ 2.04 (s, 6H, CH$_3{}^{Mes}$), 2.1 (br, 3H, BH$_3$), 2.35 (s, 3H, CH$_3{}^{Mes}$), 7.08 (s, 2H, CH^{Mes}), 7.23 (s, 1H, 4-CH or 5-CH), 7.25 (s, 1H, 4-CH or 5-CH), 8.14 (s, 1H, 2-CH). ^{13}C{^{1}H}-NMR (CDCl$_3$, 293 K): δ 17.33, 21.06 (CH$_3{}^{Mes}$), 121.25, 128.12, 129.49, 131.71, 134.86, 136.85 (CH), 140.34 (2-CH). ^{11}B-NMR (CDCl$_3$, 293 K): δ −19.21 (dbr, BH$_3$). ESI-MS (major positive-ions, CH$_3$OH), *m/z* (%): 187 (15) [HIm^{Mes} + H]$^+$, 223 (55) [(HIm^{Mes})BH$_3$ + Na]$^+$, 385 (100) [(HIm^{Mes})$_2$BH$_2$]$^+$. Anal. Calcd. for C$_{12}$H$_{17}$BN$_2$: C 72.03, H 8.56, N 14.00%. Found: C 71.81, H 8.25, N 13.60%.

3.1.3. Synthesis of (HIm^{CH3})BPh$_3$ (**3**)

A large excess of 1-methylimidazole (0.603 g, 7.344 mmol) was dissolved in acetonitrile (CH$_3$CN, 60 mL). Then, ammonium tetraphenylborate (NH$_4$BPh$_4$, 1.770 g, 5.248 mmol) was added to the solution. A white precipitate was formed, but the solution became limpid after 1 h. The reaction proceeded for 70 h at reflux under magnetic stirring. At the end, the solution was dried at reduced pressure, obtaining a white solid. Et$_2$O was added to the round-bottom flask to purify the residue from the starting materials that did not react. The resulting suspension was filtered, dried under reduced pressure, and furthe purified with CHCl$_3$ to precipitate the excess of NH$_4$BPh$_4$. The mixture was filtered and the mother liquors were dried at reduced pressure to give the white ligand (HIm^{CH3})BPh$_3$ (**3**) in 76% yield (1.293 g). Melting point: 209–212 °C. IR (cm^{-1}): 3158m, 3133m, 3085w, 3064m, 3054mbr, 3010mbr (C-H); 1546m, 1531m, 1483mbr (C=C/C=N). ^{1}H-NMR (DMSO-d_6, 293 K): δ 3.79 (s, 3H, NCH$_3$), 6.90 (d, 1H, 4-CH or 5-CH), 7.03–7.15 (m, 15H, CH), 7.44 (d, 1H, 4-CH or 5-CH), 8.09 (s, 1H, 2-CH). ^{13}C{^{1}H}-NMR (DMSO-d_6, 293 K): δ 35.13 (NCH$_3$), 122.34, 124.85, 126.42, 127.02, 134.49, 138.58 (CH). ^{11}B-NMR (Acetone-d_6, 293 K): δ −6.52 (s, BPh$_3$). ESI-MS (major positive ions, CH$_3$CN), *m/z* (%): 83 (100) [HIm^{CH3} + H]$^+$, 247 (25) [(HIm^{CH3})BPh$_2$]$^+$. Anal. Calcd. for C$_{22}$H$_{21}$BN$_2$: C 81.50, H 6.53, N 8.64. Found: C 81.14, H 6.56, N 8.38.

3.1.4. Synthesis of (HIm^{Bn})BPh$_3$ (**4**)

A large excess of 1-benzylimidazole (0.633 g, 4.000 mmol) was dissolved in CH$_3$CN (60 mL). Then, NH$_4$BPh$_4$ (0.961 g, 2.850 mmol) was added to the solution. A white precipitate was formed, but the solution became limpid after 1 h. The reaction proceeded for 70 h at reflux under magnetic stirring. At the end, the solution was dried at reduced pressure, obtaining a white solid. EtOH was added to the round-bottom flask to purify the residue from the starting materials that did not react. The resulting suspension was filtered and dried at reduced pressure to give the white ligand (HIm^{Bn})BPh$_3$ (**4**) in 50% yield (0.570 g). Melting point: 175–178 °C. IR (cm^{-1}): 3163m, 3140m, 3125m, 3064mbr, 3023m (C-H); 1531mbr, 1506m, 1489mbr (C=C/C=N). ^{1}H-NMR (DMSO-d_6, 293 K): δ 5.39 (s, 2H, CH$_2$Ph), 6.91 (s, 1H, 4-CH or 5-CH), 7.04–7.43 (m, 20H, C$_6$H$_5$), 7.49 (s, 1H, 4-CH or 5-CH), 8.37 (s, 1H, 2-CH). ^{13}C{^{1}H}-NMR (DMSO-d_6, 293 K): δ 51.24 (CH$_2$Ph), 121.25, 124.90, 127.23, 128.21, 129.33, 129.47, 133.46 (CH), 136.33 (2-CH). ^{11}B-NMR (CDCl$_3$, 293 K): δ −6.37 (s, BPh$_3$). ESI-MS (major positive ions, CH$_3$CN), *m/z* (%): 91 (80) [C$_7$H$_7$]$^+$, 159 (100) [HIm^{Bn} + H]$^+$, 242 (50) [BPh$_3$ + H]$^+$, 481 (45) [(Im^{Bn})$_2$BPh$_2$]$^+$. Anal. Calcd. for C$_{28}$H$_{25}$BN$_2$: C 84.01, H 6.29, N 7.00. Found: C 83.72, H 6.03, N 7.06.

3.1.5. Synthesis of (Im^{Bn}BPh$_2$)$_2$ (**5**)

In a 100-mL PTFE vessel equipped with a magnetic stir bar, Compound **4** (0.360 g, 0.900 mmol), silver oxide (Ag$_2$O, 0.104 g, 0.450 mmol), and CH$_3$CN (25 mL) were added. The reaction mixture was heated in the microwave reactor following a pre-set heating ramp, up to 80 °C. Once the temperature was reached, the reaction proceeded for 1 h and then it was cooled following a pre-set cooling ramp, to room temperature. All the steps were performed always under magnetic stirring. At the end, the mixture was filtered and the obtained mother liquors were dried at reduced pressure to give the oily brownish residue (Im^{Bn}BPh$_2$)$_2$ (**5**) in 54% yield (0.157 g). IR (cm^{-1}): 3161m, 3143m, 3113sh, 3087m, 3064m, 3038m, 3024m, 3010m, 2999m, 2972m, 2938wbr (C-H); 1600m, 1587m, 1571m, 1534s, 1509s, 1496sbr (C=C/C=N). ^{1}H-NMR (DMSO-d_6, 293 K): δ 5.18 (s, 2H, CH$_2$), 6.91 (s, 1H, 4-CH or 5-CH), 7.18–7.36 (m, 15H, ArH), 7.77 (s, 1H, 4-CH or 5-CH). ^{1}H-NMR (CDCl$_3$, 293 K): δ 5.13 (s, 2H, CH$_2$), 6.92 (s, 1H, 4-CH or 5-CH), 7.11–7.44 (m, 15H, ArH), 7.67 (s, 1H, 4-CH or 5-CH). ^{13}C{^{1}H}-NMR (DMSO-d_6, 293 K): δ 50.04 (CH$_2$Ph), 120.14, 127.98, 128.28, 128.79, 128.94, 129.17, 130.56, 134.47 (CH), 159.18 (2-C). ^{11}B-NMR (DMSO-d_6, 293 K): δ 1.43 (s). ESI-MS (major positive ions, CH$_3$CN), m/z (%): 91 (95) [C$_7$H$_7$]$^+$, 159 (100) [HIm^{Bn} + H]$^+$. Elemental analysis for C$_{29}$H$_{27}$AgBN$_2$ (%): calculated: H 5.94, C 82.01, N 8.69; found: H 6.04, C 81.27, N 8.89.

3.2. Crystallographic Data Collection and Refinement

A suitable crystal covered with a layer of hydrocarbon/Paratone-*N* oil was selected and mounted on a Cryo-loop and immediately placed in the low temperature nitrogen stream. X-ray intensity data were measured at 100(2) K on a Bruker SMART APEX II CCD area detector system equipped with an Oxford Cryosystems 700 series cooler, a graphite monochromator, and a Mo Kα fine-focus sealed tube (λ = 0.71073 Å). Intensity data were processed using the Bruker ApexII program suite. Absorption corrections were applied by using SADABS. Initial atomic positions were located by direct methods using XS, and the structures of the compounds were refined by the least-squares method using SHELXL [99]. All the non-hydrogen atoms were refined anisotropically. The hydrogen atoms attached to boron (B-H) were located in difference Fourier maps, included and refined freely with isotropic displacement parameters. All the other hydrogen atoms were placed at calculated positions and refined using a riding model. X-ray structural figures were generated using Olex2 [100]. The CCDC 2010217–2010218 contain the supplementary crystallographic data. These data can be obtained free of charge via http://www.ccdc.cam.ac.uk/conts/retrieving.html or from the Cambridge Crystallographic Data Centre (CCDC), 12 Union Road, Cambridge, CB2 1EZ, UK).

4. Conclusions

Two imidazolium-trihydridoborate adducts were obtained by addition of BH$_3$•THF to *N*-benzyl- and *N*-mesitylimidazoles. In addition, two imidazolium-triphenylborates were obtained by displacement of one phenyl group of ammonium tetraphenylborate reacting with methyl- or benzyl-imidazoles. 3-Benzyl-imidazolium-1-yl)trihydridoborate and (3-mesityl-imidazolium-1-yl)trihydridoborate were also characterized by X-ray crystallography. The reactivity of these new compounds as carbene precursors was investigated and a new dimeric carbene-borate adduct was obtained via a microwave-assisted procedure. The intermolecular rearrangement pathway to the head-to-tail imidazabole dimer prevented the isolation of this type of compounds and the development of their characteristic NHC chemistry.

Author Contributions: Conceptualization, C.S.; Data curation, R.V. and H.V.R.D.; Formal analysis, L.B. and H.V.R.D.; Investigation, M.P.; Methodology, M.P.; Supervision, M.P. and C.S.; Writing – original draft, M.P., H.V.R.D. and C.S. All authors have read and agreed to the published version of the manuscript.

Funding: This research was supported by the University of Camerino (FAR 2019). H.V.R.D. is thankful for the financial support by the Robert A. Welch Foundation (Grant Y-1289).

Acknowledgments: We are grateful to CIRCMSB (Consorzio Interuniversitario di Ricerca in Chimica dei Metalli nei Sistemi Biologici).

Conflicts of Interest: The authors declare no conflict of interest.

References

1. Arduengo, A.J.; Dias, H.V.R.; Harlow, R.L.; Kline, M. Electronic stabilization of nucleophilic carbenes. *J. Am. Chem. Soc.* **1992**, *114*, 5530–5534. [CrossRef]
2. Igau, A.; Grutzmacher, H.; Baceiredo, A.; Bertrand, G. Analogous.alpha.,.alpha.'-bis-carbenoid, triply bonded species: Synthesis of a stable.lambda.3-phosphino carbene-.lambda.5-phosphaacetylene. *J. Am. Chem. Soc.* **1988**, *110*, 6463–6466. [CrossRef]
3. Arduengo, A.J.; Harlow, R.L.; Kline, M. A stable crystalline carbene. *J. Am. Chem. Soc.* **1991**, *113*, 361–363. [CrossRef]
4. Hopkinson, M.N.; Richter, C.; Schedler, M.; Glorius, F. An overview of N-heterocyclic carbenes. *Nature* **2014**, *510*, 485–496. [CrossRef]
5. Martin, C.D.; Soleilhavoup, M.; Bertrand, G. Carbene-Stabilized Main Group Radicals and Radical Ions. *Chem. Sci.* **2013**, *4*, 3020–3030. [CrossRef] [PubMed]
6. Hahn, F.E.; Jahnke, M.C. Heterocyclic Carbenes: Synthesis and Coordination Chemistry. *Angew. Chem. Int. Ed.* **2008**, *47*, 3122–3172. [CrossRef] [PubMed]
7. Nolan, S.P. *N-Heterocyclic Carbenes in Synthesis*; Wiley-VCH Verlag GmbH & Co. KGaA: Weinheim, Germany, 2006.
8. Dröge, T.; Glorius, F. The Measure of All Rings-N-Heterocyclic Carbenes. *Angew. Chem. Int. Ed.* **2010**, *49*, 6940–6952. [CrossRef]
9. Hahn, F.E. Heterocyclic Carbenes. *Angew. Chem. Int. Ed.* **2006**, *45*, 1348–1352. [CrossRef]
10. Díez-González, S. *N-Heterocyclic Carbenes: From Laboratory Curiosities to Efficient Synthetic Tools: Edition 2*; Royal Society of Chemistry: Cambridge, UK, 2017.
11. Öfele, K.; Herrmann, W.A.; Mihalios, D.; Elison, M.; Herdtweck, E.; Scherer, W.; Mink, J. Multiple bonds between Main-Group elements and transition metals. CXXVI. Heterocyclene-carbenes as phosphine-analog ligands in metal complexes. *J. Organomet. Chem.* **1993**, *459*, 177–184. [CrossRef]
12. Kühl, O. *Functionalised N-Heterocyclic Carbene Complexes*; John Wiley & Sons Ltd.: Chichester, UK, 2010.
13. Zeng, X.; Soleilhavoup, M.; Bertrand, G. Gold-Catalyzed Intermolecular Markovnikov Hydroamination of Allenes with Secondary Amines. *Org. Lett.* **2009**, *11*, 3166–3169. [CrossRef]
14. Crabtree, R.H. NHC ligands versus cyclopentadienyls and phosphines as spectator ligands in organometallic catalysis. *J. Organomet. Chem.* **2005**, *690*, 5451–5457. [CrossRef]
15. Nesterov, V.; Reiter, D.; Bag, P.; Frisch, P.; Holzner, R.; Porzelt, A.; Inoue, S. NHCs in Main Group Chemistry. *Chem. Rev.* **2018**, *118*, 9678–9842. [CrossRef] [PubMed]
16. Arduengo, A.J.; Bertrand, G. Carbenes Introduction. *Chem. Rev.* **2009**, *109*, 3209–3210. [CrossRef] [PubMed]
17. Doddi, A.; Peters, M.; Tamm, M. N-Heterocyclic Carbene Adducts of Main Group Elements and Their Use as Ligands in Transition Metal Chemistry. *Chem. Rev.* **2019**, *119*, 6994–7112. [CrossRef]
18. Arnold, P.L.; Casely, I.J. F-Block N-Heterocyclic Carbene Complexes. *Chem. Rev.* **2009**, *109*, 3599–3611. [CrossRef]
19. Cazin, C.S.J. *N-Heterocyclic Carbenes in Transition Metal Catalysis and Organocatalysis*; Springer Science & Business Media: Dordrecht, The Netherlands, 2011; Volume 32.
20. Lin, J.C.Y.; Huang, R.T.W.; Lee, C.S.; Bhattacharyya, A.; Hwang, W.S.; Lin, I.J.B. Coinage Metal–N-Heterocyclic Carbene Complexes. *Chem. Rev.* **2009**, *109*, 3561–3598. [CrossRef]
21. Dash, C.; Kroll, P.; Yousufuddin, M.; Dias, H.V.R. Isolable, gold carbonyl complexes supported by N-heterocyclic carbenes. *Chem. Commun.* **2011**, *47*, 4478. [CrossRef]
22. Celik, M.A.; Dash, C.; Adiraju, V.A.; Das, A.; Yousufuddin, M.; Frenking, G.; Dias, H.V.R. End-On and Side-On π-Acid Ligand Adducts of Gold(I): Carbonyl, Cyanide, Isocyanide, and Cyclooctyne Gold(I) Complexes Supported by N-Heterocyclic Carbenes and Phosphines. *Inorg. Chem.* **2012**, *52*, 729–742. [CrossRef]
23. Dash, C.; Das, A.; Yousufuddin, M.; Dias, H.V.R. Isolable, Copper(I) Dicarbonyl Complexes Supported by N-Heterocyclic Carbenes. *Inorg. Chem.* **2013**, *52*, 1584–1590. [CrossRef]
24. Dash, C.; Yousufuddin, M.; Cundari, T.R.; Dias, H.V.R.; Dias, H.V.R. Gold-Mediated Expulsion of Dinitrogen from Organic Azides. *J. Am. Chem. Soc.* **2013**, *135*, 15479–15488. [CrossRef]
25. Wang, G.; Ponduru, T.T.; Wang, Q.; Zhao, L.; Frenking, G.; Dias, H.V.R. Heterobimetallic Complexes Featuring Fe(CO)5 as a Ligand on Gold. *Chem. - A Eur. J.* **2017**, *23*, 17222–17226. [CrossRef] [PubMed]

26. Dash, C.; Wang, G.; Muñoz-Castro, A.R.; Ponduru, T.T.; Zacharias, A.O.; Yousufuddin, M.; Dias, H.V.R. Organic Azide and Auxiliary-Ligand-Free Complexes of Coinage Metals Supported by N-Heterocyclic Carbenes. *Inorg. Chem.* **2019**, *59*, 2188–2199. [CrossRef] [PubMed]
27. Smith, C.A.; Narouz, M.R.; Lummis, P.A.; Singh, I.; Nazemi, A.; Li, C.H.; Crudden, C.M. N-Heterocyclic Carbenes in Materials Chemistry. *Chem. Rev.* **2019**, *119*, 4986–5056. [CrossRef] [PubMed]
28. Rovis, T.; Nolan, S.P. Stable Carbenes: From 'Laboratory Curiosities' to Catalysis Mainstays. *Synlett* **2013**, *24*, 1188–1189. [CrossRef]
29. Schaper, L.-A.; Hock, S.J.; Herrmann, W.A.; Kuehn, F.E. Synthesis and Application of Water-Soluble NHC Transition-Metal Complexes. *Angew. Chem. int. Ed.* **2013**, *44*, 270–289. [CrossRef]
30. He, Y.; Lv, M.-F.; Cai, C. A simple procedure for polymer-supported N-heterocyclic carbene silver complex via click chemistry: An efficient and recyclable catalyst for the one-pot synthesis of propargylamines. *Dalton Trans.* **2012**, *41*, 12428–12433. [CrossRef]
31. Li, Y.; Chen, X.; Song, Y.; Fang, L.; Zou, G. Well-defined N-heterocyclic carbene silver halides of 1-cyclohexyl-3-arylmethylimidazolylidenes: Synthesis, structure and catalysis in A3-reaction of aldehydes, amines and alkynes. *Dalton Trans.* **2011**, *40*, 2046. [CrossRef]
32. Herrmann, W.A. N-heterocyclic carbenes: A new concept in organometallic catalysis. *Angew. Chem. Int. Ed.* **2002**, *41*, 1290–1309. [CrossRef]
33. Glorius, F.; Glorius, F. *N-Heterocyclic Carbenes in Transition Metal Catalysis*; Springer-Verlag Berlin Heidelberg: Heidelberg, Germany, 2007.
34. Marion, N.; Nolan, S.P.; Díez-González, S. N-Heterocyclic Carbenes as Organocatalysts. *Angew. Chem. Int. Ed.* **2007**, *46*, 2988–3000. [CrossRef]
35. Izquierdo, J.; Hutson, G.E.; Cohen, D.T.; Scheidt, K.A. A continuum of progress: Applications of N-heterocyclic carbene catalysis in total synthesis. *Angew. Chem. Int. Ed.* **2012**, *51*, 11686–11698. [CrossRef]
36. Bugaut, X.; Glorius, F. Organocatalytic umpolung: N-heterocyclic carbenes and beyond. *Chem. Soc. Rev.* **2012**, *41*, 3511. [CrossRef] [PubMed]
37. Díez-González, S.; Marion, N.; Nolan, S.P. N-Heterocyclic Carbenes in Late Transition Metal Catalysis. *Chem. Rev.* **2009**, *109*, 3612–3676. [CrossRef] [PubMed]
38. Kantchev, E.A.B.; O'Brien, C.J.; Organ, M.G. Palladium Complexes of N-Heterocyclic Carbenes as Catalysts for Cross-Coupling Reactions — A Synthetic Chemist's Perspective. *Angew. Chem. Int. Ed.* **2007**, *38*, 2768–2813. [CrossRef] [PubMed]
39. Wang, H.M.J.; Lin, I.J.B. Facile Synthesis of Silver(I)–Carbene Complexes. Useful Carbene Transfer Agents. *Organometallics* **1998**, *17*, 972–975. [CrossRef]
40. Mjos, K.D.; Orvig, C. Metallodrugs in Medicinal Inorganic Chemistry. *Chem. Rev.* **2014**, *114*, 4540–4563. [CrossRef] [PubMed]
41. Aher, S.B.; Muskawar, P.N.; Thenmozhi, K.; Bhagat, P.R. Recent developments of metal N-heterocyclic carbenes as anticancer agents. *Eur. J. Med. Chem.* **2014**, *81*, 408–419. [CrossRef] [PubMed]
42. Ceresa, C.; Bravin, A.; Cavaletti, G.; Pellei, M.; Santini, C. The combined therapeutical effect of metal-based drugs and radiation therapy: The present status of research. *Curr. Med. Chem.* **2014**, *21*, 2237–2265. [CrossRef]
43. Budagumpi, S.; Haque, R.A.; Endud, S.; Rehman, G.U.; Salman, A.W. Biologically Relevant Silver(I)-N-Heterocyclic Carbene Complexes: Synthesis, Structure, Intramolecular Interactions, and Applications. *Eur. J. Inorg. Chem.* **2013**, *2013*, 4367–4388. [CrossRef]
44. Liu, W.; Gust, R. Metal N-heterocyclic carbene complexes as potential antitumor metallodrugs. *Chem. Soc. Rev.* **2013**, *42*, 755–773. [CrossRef]
45. Monteiro, D.C.F.; Phillips, R.M.; Crossley, B.D.; Fielden, J.; Willans, C.E. Enhanced cytotoxicity of silver complexes bearing bidentate N-heterocyclic carbeneligands. *Dalton Trans.* **2012**, *41*, 3720. [CrossRef]
46. Hindi, K.M.; Panzner, M.J.; Tessier, C.A.; Cannon, C.L.; Youngs, W.J. The Medicinal Applications of Imidazolium Carbene–Metal Complexes. *Chem. Rev.* **2009**, *109*, 3859–3884. [CrossRef] [PubMed]
47. Teyssot, M.-L.; Jarrousse, A.-S.; Manin, M.; Chevry, A.; Roche, S.; Norre, F.; Beaudoin, C.; Morel, L.; Boyer, D.; Mahiou, R.; et al. Metal-NHC complexes: A survey of anti-cancer properties. *Dalton Trans.* **2009**, *35*, 6894. [CrossRef] [PubMed]
48. Hartinger, C.G.; Dyson, P.J. Bioorganometallic chemistry—from teaching paradigms to medicinal applications. *Chem. Soc. Rev.* **2009**, *38*, 391–401. [CrossRef] [PubMed]

49. Porchia, M.; Pellei, M.; Marinelli, M.; Tisato, F.; Del Bello, F.; Santini, C. New insights in Au-NHCs complexes as anticancer agents. *Eur. J. Med. Chem.* **2018**, *146*, 709–746. [CrossRef] [PubMed]
50. Arduengo, A.J.; Goerlich, J.R.; Marshall, W.J. A stable diaminocarbene. *J. Am. Chem. Soc.* **1995**, *117*, 11027–11028. [CrossRef]
51. Alder, R.W.; Allen, P.R.; Murray, M.; Orpen, A.G. Bis(diisopropylamino)carbene. *Angew. Chem. Int. Ed.* **1996**, *35*, 1121–1123. [CrossRef]
52. Santini, C.; Marinelli, M.; Pellei, M. Boron-Centered Scorpionate-Type NHC-Based Ligands and Their Metal Complexes. *Eur. J. Inorg. Chem.* **2016**, *2016*, 2312–2331. [CrossRef]
53. Weiss, A.; Pritzkow, H.; Siebert, W. Synthesis, Structures and Reactivity ofN-Borane-Protected 1,1′-Bisimidazoles with Different Bridging Functions. *Eur. J. Inorg. Chem.* **2002**, *2002*, 1607–1614. [CrossRef]
54. Kernbach, U.; Ramm, M.; Luger, P.; Fehlhammer, W.P. A Chelating Triscarbene Ligand and Its Hexacarbene Iron Complex. *Angew. Chem. Int. Ed.* **1996**, *35*, 310–312. [CrossRef]
55. Lapointe, R.E.; Roof, G.R.; Abboud, K.A.; Klosin, J. New Family of Weakly Coordinating Anions. *J. Am. Chem. Soc.* **2000**, *122*, 9560–9561. [CrossRef]
56. Asada, T.; Hoshimoto, Y.; Ogoshi, S. Rotation-Triggered Transmetalation on a Heterobimetallic Cu/Al N-Phosphine-Oxide-Substituted Imidazolylidene Complex. *J. Am. Chem. Soc.* **2020**, *142*, 9772–9784. [CrossRef]
57. Vagedes, D.; Kehr, G.; König, D.; Wedeking, K.; Fröhlich, R.; Erker, G.; Mück-Lichtenfeld, C.; Grimme, S. Formation of Isomeric BAr3 Adducts of 2-Lithio-N-methylimidazole. *Eur. J. Inorg. Chem.* **2002**, *2002*, 2015–2021. [CrossRef]
58. Wacker, A.; Pritzkow, H.; Siebert, W. Nucleophilic Substitution Reactions with the 3-Borane-1,4,5-trimethylimidazol-2-ylidene Anion. – Unexpected Formation of an Imidazabole Isomer. *Eur. J. Inorg. Chem.* **1999**, *5*, 789–793. [CrossRef]
59. Wacker, A.; Pritzkow, H.; Siebert, W. Borane-substituted imidazol-2-ylidenes. Syntheses, structures, and reactivity. *Eur. J. Inorg. Chem.* **1998**, *6*, 843–849. [CrossRef]
60. Padilla-Martínez, I.I.; Martínez-Martínez, F.J.; López-Sandoval, A.; Girón-Castillo, K.I.; Brito, M.A.; Contreras, R. New imidazabole derivatives: Dimers of carbene-borane adducts. *Eur. J. Inorg. Chem.* **1998**, *10*, 1547–1553.
61. Okada, K.; Suzuki, R.; Oda, M. Novel boron–nitrogen containing compounds from the reaction of organolithiums with complexes between dimesitylfluoroborane and six- or five-membered aza aromatic compounds. *J. Chem. Soc., Chem. Commun.* **1995**, *20*, 2069–2070. [CrossRef]
62. Padilla-Martínez, I.I.; Ariza-Castolo, A.; Contreras, R. NMR Study of isolobal N-CH3+, N-BH3 and N-BF3 imidazole derivatives. *Magn. Reson. Chem.* **1993**, *31*, 189–193. [CrossRef]
63. Nasr, A.; Winkler, A.; Tamm, M. Anionic N-heterocyclic carbenes: Synthesis, coordination chemistry and applications in homogeneous catalysis. *Coord. Chem. Rev.* **2016**, *316*, 68–124. [CrossRef]
64. Wacker, A.; Yan, C.G.; Kaltenpoth, G.; Ginsberg, A.; Arif, A.M.; Ernst, R.; Pritzkow, H.; Siebert, W. Metal complexes of anionic 3-borane-1-alkylimidazol-2-ylidene derivatives. *J. Organomet. Chem.* **2002**, *641*, 195–202. [CrossRef]
65. Liu, W.-C.; Liu, Y.-H.; Lin, T.-S.; Peng, S.-M.; Chiu, C.-W. 1,2-Migration of N-Diarylboryl Imidazol-2-ylidene through Intermolecular Radical Process. *Inorg. Chem.* **2017**, *56*, 10543–10548. [CrossRef]
66. Padilla-Martínez, I.I.; Rosalez-Hoz, M.D.J.; Contreras, R.; Kerschl, S.; Wrackmeyer, B. From Azole—Borane Adducts to Azaboles—Molecular Structure of an Imidazabole. *Eur. J. Inorg. Chem.* **1994**, *127*, 343–346. [CrossRef]
67. Vagedes, D.; Erker, G.; Kehr, G.; Bergander, K.; Kataeva, O.; Fröhlich, R.; Grimme, S.; Mück-Lichtenfeld, C. Tris(pentafluorophenyl)borane adducts of substituted imidazoles: Conformational features and chemical behavior upon deprotonation. *Dalton Trans.* **2003**, *7*, 1337–1344. [CrossRef]
68. Arrowsmith, M.; Heath, A.; Hill, M.S.; Hitchcock, P.B.; Kociok-Köhn, G. Tris(imidazolin-2-ylidene-1-yl)borate Complexes of the Heavier Alkaline Earths: Synthesis and Structural Studies. *Organometallics* **2009**, *28*, 4550–4559. [CrossRef]
69. Crudden, C.M.; Allen, D.P. Stability and reactivity of N-heterocyclic carbene complexes. *Co-ord. Chem. Rev.* **2004**, *248*, 2247–2273. [CrossRef]

70. Huang, S.; Zhang, W.; Liu, T.; Wang, K.; Qi, X.; Zhang, J.; Zhang, Q. TowardsN-Alkylimidazole Borane-based Hypergolic Fuels. *Chem. – Asian J.* **2016**, *11*, 3528–3533. [CrossRef]
71. Santini, C.; Pellei, M.; Gioia Lobbia, G.; Papini, G. Synthesis and properties of poly(pyrazolyl)borate and related boron-centered scorpionate ligands. Part A: Pyrazole-based systems. *Mini-Rev. Org. Chem.* **2010**, *7*, 84–124. [CrossRef]
72. Pellei, M.; Lobbia, G.G.; Papini, G.; Santini, C. Synthesis and Properties of Poly(pyrazolyl)borate and Related Boron-Centered Scorpionate Ligands. Part B: Imidazole-, Triazole- and Other Heterocycle-Based Systems. *Mini-Reviews Org. Chem.* **2010**, *7*, 173–203. [CrossRef]
73. Fränkel, R.; Birg, C.; Kernbach, U.; Habereder, T.; Noth, H.; Fehlhammer, W.P. A Homoleptic Carbene–Lithium Complex. *Angew. Chem., Int. Ed.* **2001**, *40*, 1907–1910. [CrossRef]
74. Frankel, R.; Kernbach, U.; Bakola-Christianopoulou, M.; Plaia, U.; Suter, M.; Ponikwar, W.; Noth, H.; Moinet, C.; Fehlhammer, W.P. Homoleptic carbene complexes. Part VIII. Hexacarbene complexes. *J. Organomet. Chem.* **2001**, 530–545. [CrossRef]
75. Fränkel, R.; Kniczek, J.; Ponikwar, W.; Noth, H.; Polborn, K.; Fehlhammer, W.P. Homoleptic carbene complexes: Part IX. Bis(imidazolin-2-ylidene-1-yl)borate complexes of palladium(II), platinum(II) and gold(I). *Inorg. Chim. Acta* **2001**, *312*, 23–39.
76. Nieto, I.; Bontchev, R.P.; Smith, J.M. Synthesis of a Bulky Bis(carbene)borate Ligand – Contrasting Structures of Homoleptic Nickel(II) Bis(pyrazolyl)borate and Bis(carbene)borate Complexes. *Eur. J. Inorg. Chem.* **2008**, *2008*, 2476–2480. [CrossRef]
77. Biffis, A.; Lobbia, G.G.; Papini, G.; Pellei, M.; Santini, C.; Scattolin, E.; Tubaro, C. Novel scorpionate-type triscarbene ligands and their silver and gold complexes. *J. Organomet. Chem.* **2008**, *693*, 3760–3766. [CrossRef]
78. Papini, G.; Bandoli, G.; Dolmella, A.; Lobbia, G.G.; Pellei, M.; Santini, C. New homoleptic carbene transfer ligands and related coinage metal complexes. *Inorg. Chem. Commun.* **2008**, *11*, 1103–1106. [CrossRef]
79. Papini, G.; Pellei, M.; Lobbia, G.G.; Burini, A.; Santini, C. Sulfonate- or carboxylate-functionalized N-heterocyclic bis-carbene ligands and related water soluble silver complexes. *Dalton Trans.* **2009**, 6985. [CrossRef]
80. Giorgetti, M.; Aquilanti, G.; Pellei, M.; Gandin, V. The coordination core of Ag(i) N-heterocyclic carbene (NHC) complexes with anticancer properties as revealed by synchrotron radiation X-ray absorption spectroscopy. *J. Anal. At. Spectrom.* **2014**, *29*, 491–497. [CrossRef]
81. Pellei, M.; Gandin, V.; Marinelli, M.; Marzano, C.; Yousufuddin, M.; Dias, H.V.R.; Santini, C. Synthesis and Biological Activity of Ester- and Amide-Functionalized Imidazolium Salts and Related Water-Soluble Coinage Metal N-Heterocyclic Carbene Complexes. *Inorg. Chem.* **2012**, *51*, 9873–9882. [CrossRef]
82. Gandin, V.; Pellei, M.; Marinelli, M.; Marzano, C.; Dolmella, A.; Giorgetti, M.; Santini, C. Synthesis and in vitro antitumor activity of water soluble sulfonate- and ester-functionalized silver(I) N-heterocyclic carbene complexes. *J. Inorg. Biochem.* **2013**, *129*, 135–144. [CrossRef]
83. Maria, L.; Paulo, A.; Santos, I.C.; Santos, I.; Kurz, P.; Spingler, B.; Alberto, R. Very Small and Soft Scorpionates: Water Stable Technetium Tricarbonyl Complexes Combining a Bis-agostic (k3-H, H, S) Binding Motif with Pendant and Integrated Bioactive Molecules. *J. Am. Chem. Soc.* **2006**, *128*, 14590–14598. [CrossRef]
84. Lu, D.; Tang, H. Theoretical survey of the ligand tunability of poly(azolyl)borates. *Phys. Chem. Chem. Phys.* **2015**, *17*, 17027–17033. [CrossRef]
85. Pellei, M.; Papini, G.; Lobbia, G.G.; Ricci, S.; Yousufuddin, M.; Dias, H.V.R.; Santini, C.; Dias, H.V.R. Scorpionates bearing nitro substituents: Mono-, bis- and tris-(3-nitro-pyrazol-1-yl)borate ligands and their copper(i) complexes. *Dalton Trans.* **2010**, *39*, 8937. [CrossRef]
86. Dias, H.V.R.; Alidori, S.; Lobbia, G.G.; Papini, G.; Pellei, M.; Santini, C.; Dias, H.V.R. Small Scorpionate Ligands: Silver(I)-Organophosphane Complexes of 5-CF3-Substituted Scorpionate Ligand Combining a B–H··Ag Coordination Motif. *Inorg. Chem.* **2007**, *46*, 9708–9714. [CrossRef] [PubMed]
87. Meisters, M.; VandeBerg, J.T.; Cassaretto, F.P.; Posvic, H.; Moore, C.E. Studies in the tetraarylborates: Part V. The influence of substituents on the stability of tetraarylborates. *Anal. Chim. Acta* **1970**, *49*, 481–485. [CrossRef]
88. Bakshi, P.K.; Linden, A.; Vincent, B.R.; Roe, S.P.; Adhikesavalu, D.; Cameron, T.S.; Knop, O. Crystal chemistry of tetraradial species. Part 4. Hydrogen bonding to aromatic π systems: Crystal structures of fifteen tetraphenylborates with organic ammonium cations. *Can. J. Chem.* **1994**, *72*, 1273–1293. [CrossRef]

89. Belanger, S.; Beauchamp, A.L. (1-Methylimidazole- N 3)triphenylboron. *Acta Crystallogr. Sect. C Cryst. Struct. Commun.* **1998**, *54*, IUC9800057. [CrossRef]
90. Bélanger-Chabot, G.; Kaplan, S.M.; Deokar, P.; Szimhardt, N.; Haiges, R.; Christe, K.O. Synthesis and Characterization of Nitro-, Trinitromethyl-, and Fluorodinitromethyl-Substituted Triazolyl- and Tetrazolyl-trihydridoborate Anions. *Chem. - A Eur. J.* **2017**, *23*, 13087–13099. [CrossRef]
91. Ridlen, S.G.; Kulkarni, N.; Dias, H.V.R. Monoanionic, Bis(pyrazolyl)methylborate [(Ph3B)CH(3,5-(CH3)2Pz)2)]−as a Supporting Ligand for Copper(I)-ethylene, cis-2-Butene, and Carbonyl Complexes. *Inorg. Chem.* **2017**, *56*, 7237–7246. [CrossRef] [PubMed]
92. Good, C.D.; Ritter, D.M. Alkenylboranes. II. Improved Preparative Methods and New Observations on Methylvinylboranes. *J. Am. Chem. Soc.* **1962**, *84*, 1162–1166. [CrossRef]
93. Winkelmann, O.H.; Navarro, O. Microwave-Assisted Synthesis of N-Heterocyclic Carbene- Palladium(II) Complexes. *Adv. Synth. Catal.* **2010**, *352*, 212–214. [CrossRef]
94. Curran, D.P.; Solovyev, A.; Brahmi, M.M.; Fensterbank, L.; Malacria, M.; Lacôte, E. Synthesis and Reactions of N-Heterocyclic Carbene Boranes. *Angew. Chem. Int. Ed.* **2011**, *50*, 10294–10317. [CrossRef]
95. Wrackmeyer, B. Nuclear Magnetic Resonance Spectroscopy of Boron Compounds Containing Two-, Three- and Four-Coordinate Boron. *Annual Reports on NMR Spectroscopy* **1988**, *20*, 61–203. [CrossRef]
96. Kronig, S.; Theuergarten, E.; Daniliuc, C.; Jones, P.G.; Tamm, M. Anionic N-Heterocyclic Carbenes That Contain a Weakly Coordinating Borate Moiety. *Angew. Chem. Int. Ed.* **2012**, *51*, 3240–3244. [CrossRef] [PubMed]
97. Kolychev, E.L.; Kronig, S.; Brandhorst, K.; Freytag, M.; Jones, P.G.; Tamm, M. Iridium(I) Complexes with Anionic N-Heterocyclic Carbene Ligands as Catalysts for the Hydrogenation of Alkenes in Nonpolar Media. *J. Am. Chem. Soc.* **2013**, *135*, 12448–12459. [CrossRef]
98. Liu, J.; Chen, J.; Zhao, J.; Zhao, Y.; Li, L.; Zhang, H. A Modified Procedure for the Synthesis of 1-Arylimidazoles. *Synthesis* **2003**, *17*, 2661–2666. [CrossRef]
99. Sheldrick, G.M. A short history of SHELX. *Acta Crystallogr. Sect. A Found. Crystallogr.* **2007**, *64*, 112–122. [CrossRef]
100. Dolomanov, O.; Bourhis, L.J.; Gildea, R.; Howard, J.A.; Puschmann, H. OLEX2: A complete structure solution, refinement and analysis program. *J. Appl. Crystallogr.* **2009**, *42*, 339–341. [CrossRef]

Sample Availability: Samples of the compounds are available from the authors.

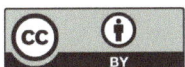

© 2020 by the authors. Licensee MDPI, Basel, Switzerland. This article is an open access article distributed under the terms and conditions of the Creative Commons Attribution (CC BY) license (http://creativecommons.org/licenses/by/4.0/).

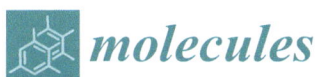

Article

N-Heterocyclic Carbene Platinum(IV) as Metallodrug Candidates: Synthesis and ^{195}Pt NMR Chemical Shift Trend

Mathilde Bouché [1], Bruno Vincent [2], Thierry Achard [1] and Stéphane Bellemin-Laponnaz [1,*]

[1] Institut de Physique et Chimie des Matériaux de Strasbourg, Université de Strasbourg-CNRS UMR7504, 23 rue du Loess, BP 43 CEDEX 2, 67034 Strasbourg, France; mathilde.bouche9@gmail.com (M.B.); thierry.achard@ipcms.unistra.fr (T.A.)

[2] Service de RMN, Fédération de Chimie Le Bel, Université de Strasbourg, CNRS FR2010, 1 rue Blaise Pascal, BP 296R8, CEDEX, 67008 Strasbourg, France; bvincent@unistra.fr

* Correspondence: bellemin@unistra.fr; Tel.: +33-388107166

Academic Editor: Yves Canac
Received: 19 June 2020; Accepted: 8 July 2020; Published: 9 July 2020

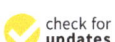

Abstract: A series of octahedral platinum(IV) complexes functionalized with both N-heterocyclic carbene (NHC) ligands were synthesized according to a straightforward procedure and characterized. The coordination sphere around the metal was varied, investigating the influence of the substituted NHC and the amine ligand in trans position to the NHC. The influence of those structural variations on the chemical shift of the platinum center were evaluated by ^{195}Pt NMR. This spectroscopy provided more insights on the impact of the structural changes on the electronic density at the platinum center. Investigation of the in vitro cytotoxicities of representative complexes were carried on three cancer cell lines and showed IC$_{50}$ values down to the low micromolar range that compare favorably with the benchmark cisplatin or their platinum(II) counterparts bearing NHC ligands.

Keywords: N-heterocyclic carbene; platinum; metal complexes; ^{195}Pt NMR

1. Introduction

In the treatment of solid tumors, platinum-based chemotherapy remains a top-notch drug thanks to its high anticancer efficiency and high remission rates in selected cancers, up to 90% in patients suffering testicular cancer [1]. However, the severe systemic toxicity and poor selectivity for tumors, with only 1% of the injected dose of cisplatin actually reaching their target, stress the importance to explore new strategies to stabilize the platinum center and prevent off-target interactions [2]. Lot of efforts have focused on adjusting the coordination sphere of the platinum or oxidizing the well established Pt(II) center into redox-activable Pt(IV) pro-drugs [3–5]. In particular, platinum complexes functionalized with N-heterocyclic carbenes have appeared as promising alternatives to cisplatin, as possible chemotherapeutics targeting the mitochondria [6–9]. In addition to investigating the redox potential of Pt(IV) complexes, ^{195}Pt NMR is a valuable technique for the fast and standardized characterization of platinum complexes to complement routine characterization [10–15]. Moreover, investigating the chemical shift in ^{195}Pt NMR is a prerequisite to further enable mechanistic and pharmacokinetic investigations of the platinum complex and its metabolites using ^{195}Pt spectroscopy [16], as an alternative to LA-ICP-MS [17] or X-ray-based techniques [18–21]. Of note, Huynh et al. recently suggested the direct correlation of the platinum chemical shift in ^{195}Pt NMR to both the electronic density at the platinum center and the electronic donation of the coordination sphere, in particular in the case of N-heterocyclic carbene (NHC)-platinum complexes [22–24]. Moreover, a linear correlation of the ^{195}Pt NMR chemical shift with the in vitro anticancer activity (IC$_{50}$) has been noted in azido-Pt(IV) complexes [25]. The chemistry in the solution of cisplatin and its derivatives have been studied by ^{195}Pt NMR spectroscopy. In particular, they have been used to characterize related complexes with aqua, chloro, nitrato, sulfato, acetate, and phosphate ligands [26,27]. Therefore, we report herein a series of NHC-Pt(IV) complexes and a few examples of their Pt(II) metabolites possibly formed in vitro, that were synthesized and characterized using routine techniques. In vitro activities against three cancer cell lines of representative NHC-Pt(IV) complexes are also presented. Moreover, the shift in the platinum resonance signal in ^{195}Pt NMR is investigated and discussed as a function of tuning their oxidation degree and coordination sphere.

2. Results and Discussion

2.1. Synthesis of the Platinum(II) and Platinum(IV) Complexes

All NHC-Pt complexes were prepared using standard synthetic procedures as previously reported. The general scheme for the synthesis of the Pt(II) and Pt(VI) complexes is described in Scheme 1. First, platinum(II) NHC pyridine complexes were synthesized involving the in situ deprotonation of the imidazolium salt with K_2CO_3 and the coordination of the carbene to the $PtCl_2$ precursor in dry amine with excess NaI overnight ((1), first step, Scheme 1) [28]. Chemical variation was then possible by the ligand substitution of the pyridine with various nitrogen-based ligands as shown in (1), second step, Scheme 1. The obtained (NHC)PtI$_2$(pyridine) and (NHC)PtI$_2$(amine) complexes could further be oxidized according to a procedure previously reported by us [9]. The aforementioned Pt(II) complexes were reacted with a 10-fold excess of bromine at 0 °C to obtain the corresponding (NHC)PtBr$_4$(L) complexes ((2), Scheme 1). The reaction proceeded very quickly and cleanly to give the expected corresponding Pt(IV) species after only 5 min of reaction. The chlorinated complexes ((NHC)PtCl$_4$L) were obtained by direct oxidation using a 2-fold excess of freshly prepared hypervalent iodine reagent PhICl$_2$ ((3), Scheme 1). The reaction was complete after 1 h at 0 °C. All the platinum(IV) complexes were easily isolated by precipitation with pentane. They were usually obtained in high chemical yield and were stable under air in the solid state or in chlorinated solvents and showed increasing solubility in organic solvents in respect to the length of alkyl chains on the NHC or amine ligand.

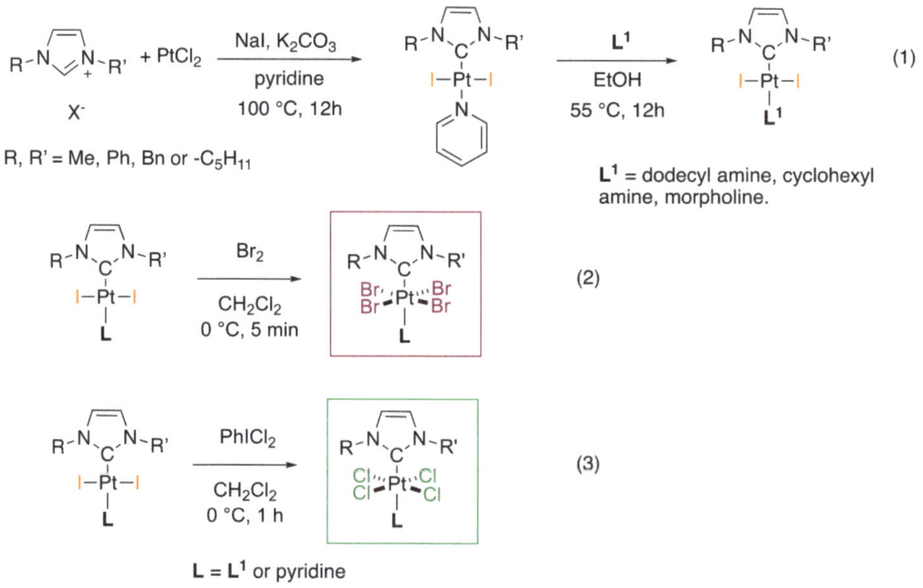

Scheme 1. General synthesis of the platinum (II) and platinum (IV) complexes.

Scheme 2 displays the molecular structures of the five platinum(II) NHC complexes used either as precursors for the Pt(IV) syntheses, or as a reference for the studies discussed here. The (NHC)Pt(II)(DMSO) complexes **3** and **4** were obtained by a transmetallation route from the bis(benzyl)imidazol-2-ylidene silver(I) bromide precursor reacted with platinum salt as previously published by us [7]. The NHC Pt(II) complexes **2** and **5** were obtained using the procedure described in (1), Scheme 1 using the corresponding salt NaBr or NaCl respectively.

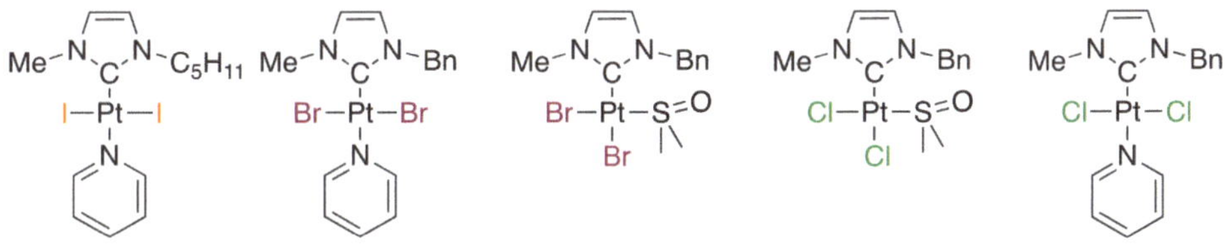

Scheme 2. Molecular structure of the *N*-heterocyclic carbene (NHC)-Pt(II) references.

Scheme 3 displays all the platinum(IV) that were synthesized and characterized. A series of (NHC)PtBr$_4$(amine) complexes bearing a (methyl-, benzyl-)NHC, were obtained in a 99% yield with various trans amine ligands, i.e., dodecylamine, cyclohexylamine, morpholine and pyridine, corresponding to complexes **6**, **8**, **12** and **18**, respectively. Identically, the (NHC)PtCl$_4$(amine) complexes with varying amine ligands were obtained in good yields, the corresponding amine ligand being a cyclohexylamine for **22**, a morpholine for **23** and a pyridine for **26**. The versatile synthesis tolerated the NHC structural variations among the (NHC)PtBr$_4$(amine) family, with *N*-substituents being a CH$_2$-*tert*-butylacetate for **14**, *p*-nitro-benzyl for **15**, *p*-benzaldehyde for **16**, a pentyl for **19**, a cyclopentyl for **20** and a phenyl for **21**, all obtained in 99% yield. The functionalization of the positions 4 and 5 of the NHC ligand did not hamper the oxidation reaction, and the (NHC)PtBr$_4$(amine) complexes **9**, **11**, **13** and **17** were isolated in high yield, corresponding respectively to a benzimidazole, 4-metyl- and 5-aldehyde, 4-methylester, and 4,5-dichloro-NHC. Similarly, the (NHC)PtCl$_4$(amine) complexes **24** bearing a 4,5-dichloro-NHC and **25** functionalized with a pentyl-*N*-substituted NHC were obtained also in a yield up to 99%. The characterization by the ^{1}H NMR showed that all the proton signals displayed a shift to a lower field compared to their imidazolium precursors which proved typical for such complexes. Overall, the NHC-Pt(IV) complexes showed a signal duplication typically observed for all the protons in up to the ^{5}J position to the platinum center, suggesting an enhanced coupling with the ^{195}Pt isotope compared to their NHC-Pt(II) precursors. Of note, the very low solubility of (NHC)PtBr$_4$(pyridine) complexes prevented the successful acquisition of the ^{13}C NMR of complexes **4**, **5**, **11**, **20** and **26**, or rendered the carbenic carbon signal not visible. However, in the case of more lipophilic complexes, coupling between the carbenic carbon and the platinum center was observed in ^{13}C NMR. Such a trend was found typical throughout all the NHC-Pt(IV) complexes, the carbenic carbon signal appearing as a singlet and doublet system, possibly due to the heavy atom effect of platinum [29]. Moreover, chemical shifts to a higher field of the carbenic carbon were also observed by ^{13}C NMR spectroscopy, ca. δ 109–120 ppm in the case of NHC-Pt(IV) complexes, while (NHC)PtI$_2$(amine) complexes previously reported by us [30,31] and others [32,33] typically show a signal shift at least 30 ppm greater.

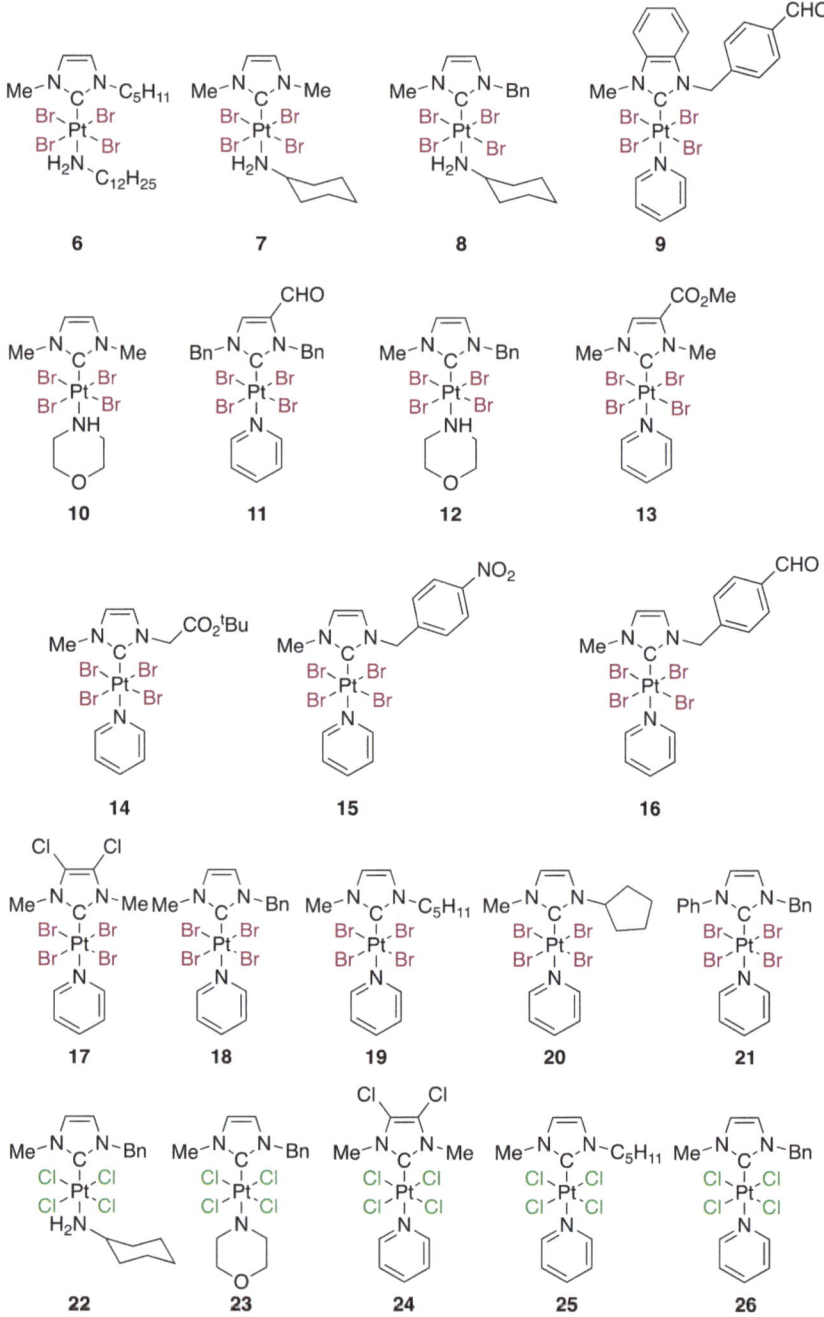

Scheme 3. Molecular structure of the NHC-Pt(IV) complexes.

Among these Pt(IV) complexes, the molecular structure of the (NHC)PtBr₄(amine) complex **15** was determined by X-ray diffraction and is presented in Figure 1. The platinum center shows an octahedral geometry with bromine ligands forming a distorted square planar shape in equatorial position, comparable to other (NHC)PtBr$_4$(amine) complexes previously reported by us [6,7]. The pyridine ligand is located in trans position to the NHC with a platinum-pyridine length of 2.128(6) Å while the NHC-platinum bond is found to be 2.057(8) Å. The molecular structure of the (NHC)PtCl$_4$(amine) complex **23** revealed a comparable geometry with overall shorter bonds between the platinum center and the ligands, reflective of the influence of the coordination sphere on platinum's electronic density, exemplified by the NHC-platinum length of 2.034(3) Å, and the chloride-platinum bonds in the range of 2.327(3)–2.336(3) Å [7].

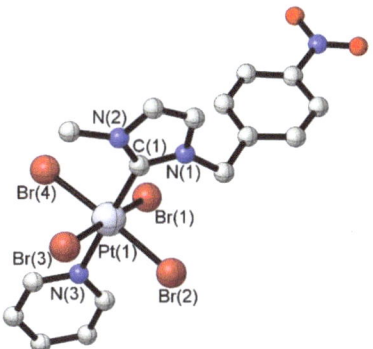

Figure 1. Molecular structure of complex **15**. Selected bond distances (Å) and angles (deg): C(1)-Pt(1), 2.057(8); Br(1)-Pt(1), 2.4882(8); Br(2)-Pt(1), 2.4657(8); Br(3)-Pt(1), 2.4615(8); Br(4)-Pt, 2.4839(8); N(3)-Pt(1), 2.128(6); C(1)-Pt(1)-N(3), 179.2(3); C(1)-Pt(1)-Br(3), 92.9(2); N(3)-Pt(1)-Br(3), 87.10(16); Br(2)-Pt(1)-Br(3), 86.10(3); Br(1)-Pt(1)-Br(4), 177.05(3).

2.2. In Vitro Activities against Cancer Cell Lines

Among the series of NHC-platinum complexes herein, a series of the most soluble complexes were selected for the evaluation of their in vitro anticancer activities. Overall, most NHC-Pt(IV) complexes were found to display comparable IC$_{50}$ values to cisplatin in the range of 0.5–23 µM. Contrastingly, the complex **16** showed disparate anticancer activities depending on the cancer cell line with the IC$_{50}$ values of 5.42 µM and 81.09 µM against the PC3 or HCT116 respectively (Table 1). Of note, the low solubility of this complex in aqueous media might explain the low IC$_{50}$ values observed in this study. The series of the (NHC)PtBr$_4$(amine) complexes **6**, **8**, **12** and **19** show potencies that compare favorably with the NHC-Pt(II) complexes which are expected to be the species released upon their redox activation. Such a result is in line with our previous findings suggesting their rapid reduction and release of the active species [6,7]. Remarkably, the (NHC)PtCl$_4$(amine) complexes **22** and **25** show the most promising in vitro potencies with IC$_{50}$ values in the low micromolar range against the three tested cancer cell lines.

Table 1. Half-inhibitory concentrations IC$_{50}$ (μM) of the selected complexes toward the HCT116, MCF7 and PC3 cancer cells.

Complex Number	Structure	IC$_{50}$ (μM) HCT116 [1]	IC$_{50}$ (μM) MCF7 [1]	IC$_{50}$ (μM) PC3 [1]
Cisplatin	(NH$_3$)$_2$PtCl$_2$	3.57 ± 0.1	4.15 ± 0.7	3.10 ± 0.2
2	(NHC)PtBr$_2$(pyr)	5.44 ± 1	7.73 ± 1	5.35 ± 1.6
3	(NHC)PtBr$_2$(DMSO)	>100	>100	>100
4	(NHC)PtCl$_2$(DMSO)	63 ± 5	80 ± 13	65 ± 6
5	(NHC)PtCl$_2$(pyr)	3.78 ± 0.1	3.48 ± 1	4.40 ± 0.9
6		7.5 ± 0.3	23 ± 5	10 ± 1
8		14 ± 2	5 ± 1	5 ± 1
12	(NHC)PtBr$_4$(amine)	11 ± 0.3	3 ± 0.7	2 ± 0.5
16		81.09 ± 2	17.22 ± 1.8	5.42 ± 0.5
19		5 ± 1	4 ± 0.2	5 ± 1
22		0.5 ± 0.03	0.5 ± 0.09	1 ± 0.1
25	(NHC)PtCl$_4$(amine)	1.48 ± 0.2	1.78 ± 0.6	1.31 ± 0.2

[1] HCT116, colon cancer cells; MCF7, breast carcinoma; PC3, prostate adenocarcinoma. (After 72 h of incubation; stock solutions in DMSO for all complexes; stock solution in H$_2$O for cisplatin).

2.3. ^{195}Pt NMR Spectroscopy

The NHC-platinum complexes were further characterized using a ^{1}H detection inverse NMR spectroscopy sequence which was preferred to direct the ^{195}Pt measurement in regard of shorter acquisition time and enhanced sensibility. This was supported by a test experiment using complex 8 as a reference, comparing spectra obtained in direct ^{195}Pt NMR or indirect HMQC ^{1}H-^{195}Pt NMR, and both showed a signal peak at δ_{Pt} = −2168 ppm irrespective of the sequence used. Table 2 displays the ^{195}Pt chemical shift NMR of all the complexes and carbenic carbon signal in the ^{13}C NMR, when observed. The most significant variation in the platinum chemical shift was found as a function of the oxidation state of the platinum center. All the (NHC)PtBr$_4$(amine) complexes 6–21 displayed a platinum chemical shift in the range of δ_{Pt} −1901 to −2196 ppm while the (NHC)PtCl$_4$(amine) complexes 22–26 were observed at δ_{Pt} −883 to −795 ppm and all other NHC-Pt(II) complexes 1–5 displayed a chemical shift below −3304 ppm.

Of note, the use of ^{1}H detection inverse spectroscopy proved of high interest for most complexes to observe the $^4J_{H-Pt}$ long-range couplings between the platinum center and C$_3$, C$_4$ protons on the NHC backbone as well as the protons on the N-substituents of the NHC. This strong chemical coupling suggests a high electronic delocalization from the platinum center to the substituents of the NHC ligand which yet does not seem to significantly affect the chemical shift in ^{195}Pt NMR. Thus, the series of NHC-Pt(IV) complexes 14–16, 19 and 20 show a platinum chemical shift decrease from δ_{Pt} = −2032 to −2070 ppm with the N-substituents following the trend Cy > C$_5$H$_{11}$ > Bn > CH$_2$CO$_2$^{t}Bu. Similarly, the functionalization of C$_3$ and C$_4$ positions on the NHC backbone of the NHC-Pt(IV) complexes is shown to have a negligible effect on the platinum shift with $\Delta\delta_{Pt}$ = 2 ppm between complexes 13 and 11. Moreover, a large platinum chemical shift variation $\Delta\delta_{Pt}$ = 64 ppm was observed between the imidazolin-2-ylidene ligand in 16 (δ_{Pt} −2063 ppm) and the benzimidazolin-2-ylidene ligand in 9 (δ_{Pt} −2127 ppm), which was found to correlate with the $\Delta\delta_C$ = 23.1 ppm of their carbenic carbon observed by ^{13}C NMR. Among the series of the NHC-Pt(IV) complexes, the variation of the trans amine ligand shows a trend in the platinum chemical shift that follows the amine's basicity from δ_{Pt} −2040 ppm for complex 18 to δ_{Pt} −2196 ppm for complex 6. Thus, the trend in the platinum chemical shift is found to be 18 > 12 > 8 > 6, corresponding to a trans ligand being pyridine > morpholine > cyclohexylamine > dodecylamine. Of note, the same trend is visible while comparing their carbenic carbon shift as complex 18 bearing a pyridine shows a δ_C of 109.3 ppm while its cyclohexylamine counterpart 8 shows a shift up to 115.2 ppm. Moreover, the (NHC)PtCl$_4$(amine) complexes follow the same trend with platinum chemical shifts being 26 > 23 > 22, corresponding to the trans amine ligand pyridine > morpholine > cyclohexylamine.

Table 2. Chemical shift evolution of the Pt signal as a function of the metal oxidation state, the coordination sphere of the metal and the NHC substituents (external reference for ^{195}Pt: H_2PtCl_6 in D_2O: δ_{Pt} = 0 ppm).

Complex	Ox. State	δ_{Pt} (ppm) ^{195}Pt NMR	δ_C (ppm) ^{13}C NMR
1	+II	−4313	125.1
2	+II	−3814	138.2
3	+II	−3356	154.7
4	+II	−3351	n.o. [1]
5	+II	−3304	n.o.
6	+IV	−2196	n.o.
7	+IV	−2168	113.4
8	+IV	−2168	115.2
9	+IV	−2167	133.9
10	+IV	−2083	124.6
11	+IV	−2081	n.o.
12	+IV	−2080	112.7
13	+IV	−2079	115.4
14	+IV	−2070	n.o.
15	+IV	−2067	n.o.
16	+IV	−2063	110.8
17	+IV	−2058	110.7
18	+IV	−2048	109.3
19	+IV	−2040	109.2
20	+IV	−2032	n.o.
21	+IV	−1901	n.o.
22	+IV	−883	n.o.
23	+IV	−853	n.o.
24	+IV	−825	112.9
25	+IV	−810	111.5
26	+IV	−795	n.o.

[1] n.o.: not observed.

3. Materials and Methods

All the manipulations of the air- and moisture-sensitive compounds were carried out using standard Schlenk techniques under an argon atmosphere and the solvents were purified and degassed following standard procedures. All the reagents were purchased from commercial chemical suppliers (Acros (Illkirch, France), Alfa Aesar (Lancashire, UK), and TCI Europe (Paris, France)) and used without further purification. ^{1}H and ^{13}C nuclear magnetic resonance (NMR) spectra were recorded on a Brucker AVANCE 300 or Bruker AVANCE 500 spectrometer (Bruker, Wissembourg, France) using the residual solvent peak as a reference ($CDCl_3$: δ_H = 7.26 ppm; δ_C = 77.16 ppm) at 295 K. The HMQC ^{1}H-^{195}Pt spectra were recorded on a Bruker AVANCE 600 spectrometer using the residual solvent peak as reference for the ^{1}H calibration and an external reference for the ^{195}Pt (H_2PtCl_6 in D_2O: δ_{Pt} = 0 ppm) at the Institut de Chimie NMR Facility of the University of Strasbourg. Positive mode electrospray ionization mass spectra (ESI-HRMS) analyses were carried out on microTOF, Bruker Daltonics (Bruker, Wissembourg, France).

All the syntheses and characterizations are available in the Supplementary Materials.

4. Conclusions

In the present work, a series of N-heterocyclic carbene-coordinated platinum(IV) complexes were synthesized in high yield according to a versatile procedure. All the complexes were found stable in the air and in chlorinated solvents for months. Some representative examples of these NHC-Pt(IV) complexes were selected for the in vitro evaluation of their cancer inhibitory properties and compared to their possible Pt(II) metabolites formed in the biological environment. Overall, the lipophilic (NHC)PtCl$_4$(amine) complex **22** was found to induce the greater in vitro potencies toward selected cancer cell lines with IC$_{50}$ values in the low micromolar range.

In the development of platinum-based metallodrugs, numerous parameters have to be considered in addition to the apparent electronic density at the platinum center that may be reflected by the ^{195}Pt NMR chemical shift, namely lipophilicity and pharmacological properties and so forth. Moreover, the balance between the stability of the platinum drugs in the blood stream and their ability to form metabolites and interact with DNA is difficult to anticipate by finetuning the coordination sphere of the platinum. However, the ^{195}Pt NMR has proved to be a helpful probe in investigating the biological activity of platinum-based drugs. For example, a recent study involving the monitoring of carboplatin after subcutaneous injection in rats was studied using ^{195}Pt NMR [34]. Thus, all the complexes presented here were characterized with standard techniques and the influence of structural variations, i.e., on one hand the coordination sphere and on the other hand the NHC ligand's functionalization, were correlated to their chemical shift in ^{195}Pt NMR. All the (NHC)PtBr$_4$(amine) complexes displayed platinum chemical shifts in the range of δ_{Pt} −1900 to −2200 ppm while the (NHC)PtCl$_4$(amine) complexes were observed at δ_{Pt} −900 to −800 ppm. All other NHC–Pt(II) complexes displayed a chemical shift below −3304 ppm. The ^{195}Pt NMR spectroscopy could then be used to monitor the kinetics and the mechanism of such platinum complexes with biological substances.

Supplementary Materials: The following are available online. ^{195}Pt NMR spectra and characterization for all compounds.

Author Contributions: S.B.-L. designed the research. M.B., T.A. and S.B.-L. conceived, designed and performed the chemical experiments. B.V. performed the NMR experiments. S.B.-L. and M.B. wrote the paper and T.A. and B.V. participated in manuscript writing. All authors have read and agreed to the published version of the manuscript.

Funding: This research was funded by the University of Strasbourg/CNRS-Program IDEX Interdisciplinaire. M.B. was granted by the French "Ministère de la Recherche".

Acknowledgments: The authors gratefully acknowledge the Ministère de l'Enseignement Supérieur et de la Recherche for Ph.D. grants to M.B. Biological evaluations of cell proliferation inhibition have been performed at the Ciblothèque Cellulaire ICSN (Gif sur Yvette, France). The authors also thank Michel Sigrist for technical assistance.

Conflicts of Interest: The authors declare no conflict of interest.

References

1. Gietema, J.A.; Meinardi, M.T.; Messerschmidt, J.; Gelevert, T.; Alt, F.; Uges, D.; Seijfer, D.T. Circulating plasma platinum more than 10 years after cisplatin treatment for testicular cancer. *Lancet* **2000**, *355*, 1075–1076. [CrossRef]
2. Cheff, D.M.; Hall, M.D. A Drug of Such Damned Nature. 1 Challenges and Opportunities in Translational Platinum Drug Research: Miniperspective. *J. Med. Chem.* **2017**, *60*, 4517–4532. [CrossRef] [PubMed]
3. Um, I.S.; Armstrong-Gordon, E.; Moussa, Y.E.; Gnjidic, D.; Wheate, N.J. Platinum drugs in the Australian cancer chemotherapy healthcare setting: Is it worthwhile for chemists to continue to develop platinums? *Inorg. Chim. Acta* **2019**, *492*, 177–181. [CrossRef]
4. Gibson, D. Multi-action Pt (IV) anticancer agents; do we understand how they work? *J. Inorg. Biochem.* **2019**, *191*, 77–84. [CrossRef]
5. Hall, M.D.; Hambley, T.W. Platinum (IV) antitumour compounds: Their bioinorganic chemistry. *Coord. Chem. Rev.* **2002**, *232*, 49–67. [CrossRef]
6. Bouché, M.; Bonnefont, A.; Achard, T.; Bellemin-Laponnaz, S. Exploring diversity in platinum (IV) N-heterocyclic carbene complexes: Synthesis, characterization, reactivity and biological evaluation. *Dalton Trans.* **2018**, *33*, 11491–11502. [CrossRef]
7. Bouché, M.; Dahm, G.; Wantz, M.; Fournel, S.; Achard, T.; Bellemin-Laponnaz, S. Platinum (IV) N-heterocyclic carbene complexes: Their synthesis, characterisation and cytotoxic activity. *Dalton Trans.* **2016**, *45*, 11362–11368. [CrossRef]

8. Chardon, E.; Dahm, G.; Guichard, G.; Bellemin-Laponnaz, S. Derivatization of preformed platinum N-heterocyclic carbene complexes with amino acid and peptide ligands and cytotoxic activities toward human cancer cells. *Organometallics* **2012**, *31*, 7618–7621. [CrossRef]
9. Bellemin-Laponnaz, S. N-Heterocyclic Carbene Platinum Complexes: A Big Step Forward for Effective Antitumor Compounds. *Eur. J. Inorg. Chem.* **2020**, *2020*, 10–20. [CrossRef]
10. Priqueler, J.R.L.; Butler, I.S.; Rochon, D.D. High selectivity of colorimetric detection of p-nitrophenol based on Ag nanoclusters. *Appl. Spectrosc. Rev.* **2006**, *41*, 185–226. [CrossRef]
11. Höfer, D.; Varbaniv, H.P.; Hejl, M.; Jakupec, M.A.; Roller, A.; Galanski, M.; Keppler, B.K. Impact of the equatorial coordination sphere on the rate of reduction, lipophilicity and cytotoxic activity of platinum (IV) complexes. *J. Inorg. Biochem.* **2017**, *174*, 119–129. [CrossRef] [PubMed]
12. Johnstone, T.C.; Suntharalingam, K.; Lippard, S.J. The next generation of platinum drugs: Targeted Pt (II) agents, nanoparticle delivery, and Pt (IV) prodrugs. *Chem. Rev.* **2016**, *116*, 3436–3486. [CrossRef] [PubMed]
13. Johnstone, T.C.; Alexander, S.M.; Wilson, J.J.; Lippard, S.J. Oxidative halogenation of cisplatin and carboplatin: Synthesis, spectroscopy, and crystal and molecular structures of Pt (IV) prodrugs. *Dalton Trans.* **2015**, *44*, 119–129. [CrossRef] [PubMed]
14. Bokach, N.A.; Kukushkin, V.Y.; Kuznetsov, M.L.; Garnovskii, D.A.; Natile, G.; Pombeiro, A.J.L. Direct addition of alcohols to organonitriles activated by ligation to a platinum (IV) center. *Inorg. Chem.* **2002**, *41*, 2041–2053. [CrossRef]
15. Still, B.M.; Anil Kumar, P.G.; Aldrich-Wright, J.R.; Price, W.S. 195Pt NMR—Theory and application. *Chem. Soc. Rev.* **2007**, *36*, 665–686. [CrossRef]
16. Hu, D.; Yang, C.; Lok, C.-N.; Xing, F.; Lee, P.-Y.; Fung, Y.M.E.; Jiang, H.; Che, C.-M. An Antitumor Bis (N-Heterocyclic Carbene) Platinum (II) Complex That Engages Asparagine Synthetase as an Anticancer Target. *Angew. Chem. Int. Ed.* **2019**, *58*, 10914–10918. [CrossRef]
17. Matczuk, M.; Ruzik, L.; Alekssanko, S.S.; Keppler, B.K.; Jarosz, M.; Timerbaev, A.R. Analytical methodology for studying cellular uptake, processing and localization of gold nanoparticles. *Anal. Chim. Acta* **2019**, *1052*, 1–9. [CrossRef]
18. Galvez, L.; Theiner, S.; Grabarics, M.; Kowol, C.R.; Keppler, B.K.; Hann, S.; Koellensperger, G. Critical assessment of different methods for quantitative measurement of metallodrug-protein associations. *Anal. Bioanal. Chem.* **2018**, *410*, 7211–7220. [CrossRef]
19. Ahmad, S. Kinetic aspects of platinum anticancer agents. *Polyhedron* **2017**, *138*, 109–124. [CrossRef]
20. Hall, M.D.; Daly, H.L.; Zhang, J.Z.; Zhang, M.; Alderden, R.A.; Pursche, D.; Foran, G.J.; Hambley, T.W. Quantitative measurement of the reduction of platinum (IV) complexes using X-ray absorption near-edge spectroscopy (XANES). *Metallomics* **2012**, *4*, 568–575. [CrossRef]
21. Czapla-Masztafiak, J.; Kubas, A.; Kayser, Y.; Fernandes, D.L.A.; Kwiatek, W.M.; Lipiec, E.; Deacon, G.B.; Al-Jorani, K.; Wood, B.R.; Szlachetko, J.; et al. Mechanism of hydrolysis of a platinum (IV) complex discovered by atomic telemetry. *J. Inorg. Biochem.* **2018**, *187*, 56–61. [CrossRef] [PubMed]
22. Huynh, H.V. *The Organometallic Chemistry of N-heterocyclic Carbenes*; John Wiley & Sons: Hoboken, NJ, USA, 2017.
23. Teng, Q.Q.; Huynh, H.V. A Unified Ligand Electronic Parameter Based on 13 C NMR Spectroscopy of N-heterocyclic Carbene Complexes. *Dalton Trans.* **2017**, *46*, 614–627. [CrossRef]
24. Teng, Q.Q.; Ng, P.S.; Leung, J.N.; Huynh, H.V. Donor strengths determination of pnictogen and chalcogen ligands by the Huynh electronic parameter and its correlation to sigma Hammett constants. *Chem. Eur. J.* **2019**, *25*, 13956–13963. [CrossRef]
25. Tsipis, A.C.; Karapetsas, I.N. Prediction of 195Pt NMR of photoactivable diazido- and azine-Pt(IV) anticancer agents by DFT computational protocols. *Magn. Reson. Chem.* **2017**, *55*, 145–153. [CrossRef]
26. Appleton, T.G.; Berry, R.D.; Davis, C.A.; Hall, J.R.; Kimlin, H.A. Reactions of platinum(II) aqua complexes. I: Multinuclear (195Pt, 15N, and 31P) NMR study of reactions between the cis-diamminediaquaplatinum(II) cation and the oxygen-donor ligands hydroxide, perchlorate, nitrate, sulfate, phosphate, and acetate. *Inorg. Chem.* **1984**, *23*, 3514–3531. [CrossRef]
27. Appleton, T.G.; Hall, J.R.; Ralph, S.F.; Thompson, C.S.M. Reactions of platinum(II) aqua complexes. 2. Platinum-195 NMR study of reactions between the tetraaquaplatinum(II) cation and chloride, hydroxide, perchlorate, nitrate, sulfate, phosphate, and acetate. *Inorg. Chem.* **1984**, *23*, 3521–3525. [CrossRef]
28. Benhamou, L.; Chardon, E.; Lavigne, G.; Bellemin-Laponnaz, S.; César, V. Synthetic routes to N-heterocyclic carbene precursors. *Chem. Rev.* **2009**, *111*, 2705–2733. [CrossRef] [PubMed]

29. Sutter, K.; Autschbach, J. Computational study and molecular orbital analysis of NMR shielding, spin–spin coupling, and electric field gradients of azido platinum complexes. *J. Am. Chem. Soc.* **2012**, *134*, 13374–13385. [CrossRef]
30. Dahm, D.; Bailly, C.; Karmazin, L.; Bellemin-Laponnaz, S. Synthesis, structural characterization and in vitro anti-cancer activity of functionalized N-heterocyclic carbene platinum and palladium complexes. *J. Organomet. Chem.* **2015**, *794*, 115–124. [CrossRef]
31. Chardon, E.; Puleo, G.-L.; Dahm, G.; Guichard, G.; Bellemin-Laponnaz, S. Direct functionalisation of group 10 N-heterocyclic carbene complexes for diversity enhancement. *Chem. Commun.* **2011**, *47*, 5864–5866. [CrossRef]
32. Chtchigrovsky, M.; Eloy, L.; Jullien, H.; Saker, L.; Ségal-Bendirdjian, E.; Poupon, J.; Bombard, S.; Cresteil, T.; Retailleau, P.; Marinetti, A. Antitumor trans-N-Heterocyclic Carbene–Amine–Pt(II) Complexes: Synthesis of Dinuclear Species and Exploratory Investigations of DNA Binding and Cytotoxicity Mechanisms. *J. Med. Chem.* **2013**, *56*, 2074–2086. [CrossRef] [PubMed]
33. Skander, M.; Retailleau, P.; Bourri, B.; Schio, L.; Mailliet, P.; Marinetti, A. N-heterocyclic carbene-amine Pt (II) complexes, a new chemical space for the development of platinum-based anticancer drugs. *J. Med. Chem.* **2010**, *53*, 2146–2154. [CrossRef] [PubMed]
34. Becker, M.; Port, R.E.; Zabel, H.-J.; Zeller, W.J.; Bachert, P. Monitoring Local Disposition Kinetics of Carboplatin in Vivo after Subcutaneous Injection in Rats by Means of ^{195}Pt NMR. *J. Magn. Reson.* **1998**, *133*, 115–122. [CrossRef] [PubMed]

Sample Availability: Not available.

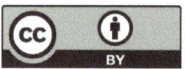

© 2020 by the authors. Licensee MDPI, Basel, Switzerland. This article is an open access article distributed under the terms and conditions of the Creative Commons Attribution (CC BY) license (http://creativecommons.org/licenses/by/4.0/).

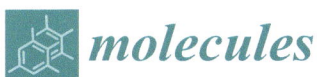

Article

Hybrid Gold(I) NHC-Artemether Complexes to Target Falciparum Malaria Parasites

Manel Ouji [1,2,†], **Guillaume Barnoin** [1,†], **Álvaro Fernández Álvarez** [1], **Jean-Michel Augereau** [1,2], **Catherine Hemmert** [1,*], **Françoise Benoit-Vical** [1,2,3,*] **and Heinz Gornitzka** [1,*]

1. CNRS, Laboratoire de Chimie de Coordination (LCC), Université de Toulouse, UPS, INPT, 205 route de Narbonne, BP 44099, F-31077 Toulouse CEDEX 4, France; manel.ouji@lcc-toulouse.fr (M.O.); guillaume.barnoin@gmail.com (G.B.); alvaritocanada@yahoo.es (Á.F.Á.); jean-michel.augereau@lcc-toulouse.fr (J.-M.A.)
2. Institut de Pharmacologie et de Biologie Structurale, IPBS, Université de Toulouse, CNRS, UPS, 31077 Toulouse, France
3. INSERM, Institut National de la Santé et de la Recherche Médicale, 31024 Toulouse, France
* Correspondence: catherine.hemmert@lcc-toulouse.fr (C.H.); francoise.benoit-vical@lcc-toulouse.fr (F.B.-V.); heinz.gornitzka@lcc-toulouse.fr (H.G.); Tel.: +33-561333187/+33-561553003 (C.H.); +33-561333161/+33-561553003 (H.G.)
† These authors contributed equally to this work.

Academic Editor: Yves Canac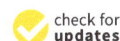
Received: 20 May 2020; Accepted: 17 June 2020; Published: 18 June 2020

Abstract: The emergence of *Plasmodium falciparum* parasites, responsible for malaria disease, resistant to antiplasmodial drugs including the artemisinins, represents a major threat to public health. Therefore, the development of new antimalarial drugs or combinations is urgently required. In this context, several hybrid molecules combining a dihydroartemisinin derivative and gold(I) N-heterocyclic carbene (NHC) complexes have been synthesized based on the different modes of action of the two compounds. The antiplasmodial activity of these molecules was assessed in vitro as well as their cytotoxicity against mammalian cells. All the hybrid molecules tested showed efficacy against *P. falciparum*, in a nanomolar range for the most active, associated with a low cytotoxicity. However, cross-resistance between artemisinin and these hybrid molecules was evidenced. These results underline a fear about the risk of cross-resistance between artemisinins and new antimalarial drugs based on an endoperoxide part. This study thus raises concerns about the use of such molecules in future therapeutic malaria policies.

Keywords: malaria; *Plasmodium falciparum*; gold; NHC-ligands; hybrid molecules; drug resistance

1. Introduction

Plasmodium falciparum, the protozoan parasite causing malaria, was responsible for 228 million cases with 405,000 deaths in 2018, mainly in Sub-Saharan Africa where about 90% of the deaths affect children under five [1]. The current malaria treatments recommended by the WHO are artemisinin-based combination therapies (ACTs) combining an artemisinin derivative with one or two other antimalarial drugs with the particularity of having different modes of action and different pharmacokinetic properties. The use of these drug combinations has contributed to a significant decrease in malaria mortality in all endemic regions these last 20 years. However, since 2008, resistance of *P. falciparum* to artemisinins and partner drugs has widely spread in South-East Asia, resulting in a loss of efficacy of many antimalarial drugs to treat patients [2–4]. This situation is a major threat to global public health [5] and imposes a need to accelerate the discovery of new compounds able to eliminate resistant parasites. Among the strategies followed to improve the efficacy of artemisinin both directly against the parasite or for pharmacokinetic and pharmacodynamic enhancements, the synthesis of artemisinin dimers is proposed [6–8]. One of the aims was to amplify oxidative stress through increased production of reactive oxygen species (ROS) to kill the parasites. However, although some of these compounds show antiplasmodial activities in the nanomolar range, they have not been evaluated in an artemisinin resistance framework needing particular assays. Indeed, because artemisinin resistance is based on a quiescence mechanism corresponding to a cell cycle arrest of a small number of parasites during artemisinins treatment and resumption of their growth when the drug is eliminated [9–11], specific compounds have to be designed. Artemisinin resistance is also associated with mutations in the propeller domain of the gene *pfk13* linked to a complex combination of different biochemical pathways [10,12,13]. It is to note that, at the quiescent state, the parasite's metabolism is greatly downregulated. However, apicoplast and mitochondrion seem still active in quiescent parasites [14]. Targeting these two organelles appears thus as a very promising avenue to kill quiescent artemisinin-resistant parasites. In this context, we have recently synthetized and evaluated hybrid gold(I) N-heterocyclic carbene (NHC) complexes based on triclosan targeting mitochondrion and apicoplast, respectively [12]. These novel hybrids showed a strong antiplasmodial activity, however a cross-resistance trend with artemisinins was noted [12]. Interestingly, we showed that there is no cross-resistance between a gold(I) complex and artemisinins [12]. This is in accordance with former studies showing that atovaquone, a mitochondrial electron transfer inhibitor, was efficient not only on proliferating parasites but also on artemisinin-pretreated and dormant parasites [15,16].

Here, we focused our investigations on the second organelle involved in the quiescence mechanism: the parasite mitochondrion. In addition to its role as an energy supplier, mitochondrion contains a wide variety of additional processes notably the two major antioxidant defence systems: thioredoxin (Trx) and glutathione systems, Trx being essential for the erythrocytic *P. falciparum* cycle [17].

Our chemical research is mainly focused on the design of bioactive gold(I) NHC complexes for parasitic diseases, *P. falciparum* [18–20] and *Leishmania infantum* [21,22], and anticancer applications [23–25]. Moreover, in the field of anticancer metal-based agents, the ubiquitous selenoenzyme thioredoxin reductase (TrxR), responsible for cell homeostasis regulation, is considered as one of the most relevant targets for gold(I) complexes and inhibition of TrxR could lead to apoptosis though a mitochondrial pathway [24–26]. Considering that artemisinins—and dihydroartemisinin, the active metabolite of all artemisinin derivatives—are active against all erythrocytic stages of *P. falciparum* and are still the best antiplasmodial drugs on the field, we designed hybrid complexes combining an ether derivative of dihydroartemisinin (called here DHA) with a gold(I) cation, covalently integrated in our NHC ligand systems. This approach aims to firstly eliminate most of the parasite stages thanks to the highly active DHA part, thereafter, the remaining resistant quiescent parasites will be treated by the gold(I) moiety. The goal of this work is to determine the activity of these hybrid molecules against *P. falciparum*, then to evaluate the efficacy of the most active hybrids in a context of artemisinin resistance.

2. Results and Discussion

2.1. Chemistry

The gold(I) complexes designed here are divided in three series depending on the length of the spacers between the carbene and the pharmacophore derivative. In order to fuse DHA and NHCs precursors we used aliphatic linkers containing 3 to 5 carbon atoms. The synthetic pathway involves three steps (Scheme 1). First, etherification of DHA with a bromoalcohol in the presence of boron trifluoride etherate catalyst [27,28] gave after purification the single β-isomers **DHA-C3** to **DHA-C5**. The next step was the quaternization of a substituted imidazole, either commercially available (Me, *i*Pr and Bn) or previously described in the literature (Mes, Quin) [22,29], to obtain the corresponding carbene precursors **Ln-R(1–13)** in yields ranging from 35 to 98%. They were classically characterized by ^{1}H- and ^{13}C-NMR spectroscopy, mass spectrometry and elemental analysis. The most notable features in the ^{1}H- and ^{13}C-NMR spectra of the imidazolium salts are the resonances for the imidazolium protons (H2) located between 10.07 and 12.15 ppm, the upfield value being attributed to the proligands containing a quinoline group and the corresponding imidazolium carbons (C2) in the range of 135.7–138.7 ppm. The formation of the target gold(I) complexes was achieved by direct metalation involving K$_2$CO$_3$ as base and **Au(SMe$_2$)Cl**, in a ratio 2:1 for the cationic **Aubis(n-R)** complexes **15–26** and in a ratio 1:1 for the neutral **Au(n-R)Cl** ones (**27** and **28**). Complexes **Aubis(L3-Me)** (**14**), was synthetized by the convenient transmetalation route involving the mild base Ag$_2$O, followed by an ion exchange with AgNO$_3$ and subsequent addition of **Au(SMe$_2$)Cl** [28]. The neutral complex **Au(3-Quin)Cl** (**29**) was obtained as a byproduct from the purification by column chromatography of **Aubis(3-Quin)** (**18**). The gold(I) complexes **15–26** were isolated after purification as white solids with yields of 31 to 92%. All compounds were characterized by ^{1}H- and ^{13}C-NMR spectroscopy, high-resolution mass spectrometry and elemental analysis. ^{13}C-NMR spectroscopy unequivocally evidences the formation of the cationic gold(I) complexes **Aubis(n-R)** (**15–26**) with resonance of the carbenic carbons located at 181.8-183.9 ppm. In the case of mono-NHC complexes **Au(n-R)Cl** (**27–29**), the most characteristic features in ^{13}C NMR spectra are the C2 peaks at 173.3, 174.5 and 173.7 ppm for **Au(3-iPr)Cl** (**27**), **Au(3-Bn)Cl** (**28**) and **Au(3-Quin)Cl** (**29**), respectively. The elemental analysis for the gold(I) complexes correspond to the general formula [AuL$_2$][Cl] (except for **Aubis(L3-Me)** (**14**) with nitrate anion) for the bis(NHC) complexes **Aubis(n-R)** (**15–26**) and AuLCl for the mono(NHC) complexes **Au(n-R)Cl** (**27–29**). The high resolution mass spectra (ESI$^+$) HRMS spectra of all gold(I) complexes exhibit the classical peak *m/z* for the cationic fragment [M–X$^-$]$^+$.

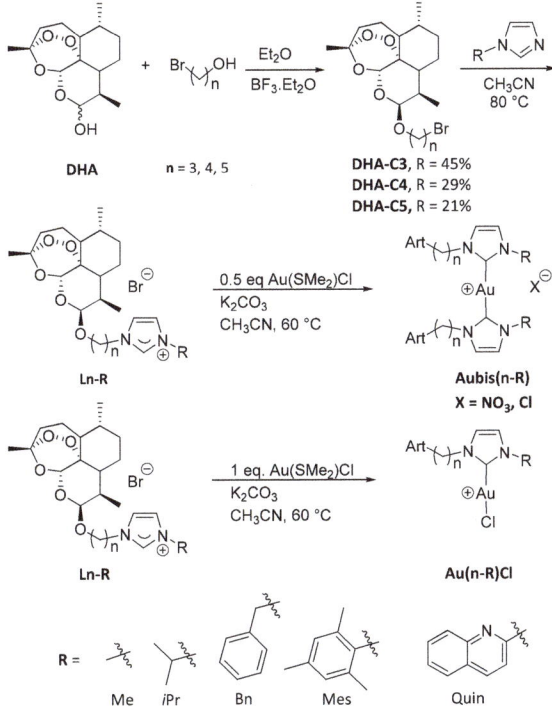

Scheme 1. *Cont.*

Entry	Proligand	n	R	Yield (%)	Entry	Complex	n	R	Yield (%)
1*	L3-Me	3	Me	65	14 *,§	Aubis(3-Me)	3	Me	84
2	L3-iPr	3	iPr	47	15	Aubis(3-iPr)	3	iPr	83
3	L3-Bn	3	Bn	87	16	Aubis(3-Bn)	3	Bn	65
4	L3-Mes	3	Mes	76	17	Aubis(3-Mes)	3	Mes	52
5	L3-Quin	3	Quin	84	18	Aubis(3-Quin)	3	Quin	86
6*	L4-Me	4	Me	98	19*	Aubis(4-Me)	4	Me	80
7	L4-Bn	4	Bn	73	20	Aubis(4-Bn)	4	Bn	92
8	L4-Mes	4	Mes	62	21	Aubis(4-Mes)	4	Mes	89
9	L4-Quin	4	Quin	58	22	Aubis(4-Quin)	4	Quin	92
10*	L5-Me	5	Me	35	23*	Aubis(5-Me)	5	Me	32
11	L5-Bn	5	Bn	52	24	Aubis(5-Bn)	5	Bn	45
12	L5-Mes	5	Mes	60	25	Aubis(5-Mes)	5	Mes	74
13	L5-Quin	5	Quin	66	26	Aubis(5-Quin)	5	Quin	47
					27	Au(3-iPr)Cl	3	Me	42
					28	Au(3-Bn)Cl	3	Bn	81
					29	Au(3-Quin)Cl	3	Quin	-

Scheme 1. Synthesis of proligands **Ln-R** (**1–13**) and gold(I) complexes **Aubis(n-R)** and **Au(n-R)Cl** complexes (**14–29**).

2.2. Antiplasmodial Activity and Selectivity

The proligands (**Ln-R**) and the complexes (**Aubis(n-R)** and **Au(n-R)Cl**) as well as reference molecules, artemisinin, artemether, auranofin and the proligand precursor **DHA-C3**, were screened in vitro against the *P. falciparum* strain F32-Tanzania and the cytotoxicity on Vero cells was evaluated to determine the selectivity of the most active compounds (Table 1). Globally, the results are extremely interesting, with IC_{50} values against *Plasmodium* ranging from 9 to 935 nM for the proligands and the gold(I) complexes. The DHA-ether derivative used for the synthesis of the proligands containing a C3 lateral chain, **DHA-C3**, has an IC_{50} value of 8.5 nM comparable to that of the antimalarial reference drug artemether (IC_{50} = 6.1 nM). Surprisingly, for the imidazolium salts obtained by addition of a substituted imidazole moiety to **DHAC3-C5** precursors, a significant loss of the antimalarial activity was observed (IC_{50} = 98–935 nM, entries 5–9, 18-21 and 26–29). In contrast, the presence of the gold(I) cation in the corresponding complexes greatly improved the antiplasmodial efficacy (IC_{50} = 9–104 nM, entries 10–17, 22–25 and 30–33) compared to the corresponding proligands. The antiplasmodial activity was notable, with IC_{50} values below 100 nM for two proligands in the C5 series (**L5-Bn** (**11**) and **L5-Mes** (**12**) and for the majority of the cationic and neutral gold(I) complexes. By comparison, auranofin, a gold-based reference molecule used for the treatment of rheumatoid arthritis, was not active against *P. falciparum* parasites with a higher IC_{50} value of 1.5 µM.

Moreover, ten complexes are highly efficient, with IC_{50} values lower than 50 nM, including nine cationic gold(I) bis(NHC) complexes and one neutral NHC-Art complex, namely **Au(3-iPr)Cl** (**27**). Among them, five complexes, namely **Aubis(3-iPr)** (**15**), **Aubis(3-Bn)** (**16**), **Aubis(3-Quin)** (**18**), **Aubis(4-Me)** (**19**) and **Aubis(5-Me)** (**23**) have an antiplasmodial activity comparable (an IC_{50} between 9 and 23 nM) to the reference antimalarial drugs artemisinin (IC_{50} = 18 nM) and artemether (IC_{50} = 6.1 nM). Regarding structure activity relationship, the potency of the complexes containing methyl (**14**, **19** and **23**) or benzyl (**16**, **20** and **24**) groups on the NHCs increased with the length of the spacer whereas, no correlation was highlighted for the mesityl and the quinoline series (**17**, **21**, **25**, and **18**, **22**, **26**, respectively). Surprisingly while artemether and **DHA-C3** had the same antiplasmodial activity, the selectivity indexes (SI) were largely higher for artemether (SI = 35,000) than for **DHA-C3** (SI = 294) demonstrating that the C3 moiety seems less selective. The selectivity indexes for the tested proligands and gold(I) complexes were between 8 and 255, the best value being obtained for the proligand **L5-Mes** (**12**, IC_{50} = 98 nM). Interestingly, regardless of the number of carbons in the spacer, hybrid molecules with aliphatic R groups (Me, iPr) have the best selectivities with SI values of 143 and 178 for **Aubis(3-Me)** (**14**) and **Au(3-iPr)Cl** (**27**), respectively, 62 for **Aubis(4-Me)** (**19**) and 111 for **Aubis(5-Me)** (**23**), in comparison with aromatic groups.

Table 1. Antimalarial and cytotoxic activities of proligands and gold(I) complexes.

Entry	Compounds		Antiplasmodial Activity on P. falciparum IC$_{50}$ ± SEM (nM)	Cytotoxicity on Vero Cells IC$_{50}$ ± SEM (nM)	Selectivity Index Vero Cells/P. falciparum
1	Auranofin		$1.5 \times 10^3 \pm 0.1 \times 10^3$	130×10^3	7 000
2	Artemisinin		18 ± 2	$214 \times 10^3 \pm 29 \cdot 10^3$	35 000
3	Artemether		6.1 ± 1	-	-
4	DHA-C3		8.5 ± 3	$2.5 \times 10^3 \pm 0.1 \times 10^3$	294
5	L3-Me	1	935 ± 117	-	-
6	L3-iPr	2	335 ± 28	-	-
7	L3-Bn	3	351 ± 56	-	-
8	L3-Mes	4	655 ± 53	-	-
9	L3-Quin	5	330 ± 69	-	-
10	Aubis(3-Me)	14	35 ± 8	$5 \times 10^3 \pm 1.5 \times 10^3$	143
11	Aubis(3-iPr)	15	13 ± 5	$0.7 \times 10^3 \pm 0.2 \times 10^3$	54
12	Au(3-iPr)Cl	27	45 ± 8	$8 \times 10^3 \pm 10^3$	178
13	Aubis(3-Bn)	16	22 ± 3	$0.3 \times 10^3 \pm 0.005 \times 10^3$	14
14	Au(3-Bn)Cl	28	104 ± 24	$8 \times 10^3 \pm 2.3 \times 10^3$	77
15	Aubis(3-Mes)	17	61 ± 37	$0.5 \times 10^3 \pm 0.1 \times 10^3$	8
16	Aubis(3-Quin)	18	23 ± 8	$1.2 \times 10^3 \pm 0.5 \times 10^3$	52
17	Au(3-Quin)Cl	29	90 ± 9	-	-
18	L4-Me	6	840 ± 64	-	-
19	L4-Bn	7	326 ± 44	-	-
20	L4-Mes	8	219 ± 18	-	-
21	L4-Quin	9	330 ± 37	-	-
22	Aubis(4-Me)	19	13 ± 3	$0.8 \times 10^3 \pm 0.2 \times 10^3$	62
23	Aubis(4-Bn)	20	40 ± 21	$0.7 \times 10^3 \pm 0.2 \times 10^3$	18
24	Aubis(4-Mes)	21	38 ± 3	$0.7 \times 10^3 \pm 0.1 \times 10^3$	18
25	Aubis(4-Quin)	22	83 ± 31	-	-
26	L5-Me	10	172 ± 22	-	-
27	L5-Bn	11	98 ± 26	$10^3 \pm 0.1 \times 10^3$	10
28	L5-Mes	12	98 ± 24	$25 \times 10^3 \pm 10 \times 10^3$	255
29	L5-Quin	13	226 ± 29	-	-
30	Aubis(5-Me)	23	9 ± 0.9	$10^3 \pm 0.5 \times 10^3$	111
31	Aubis(5-Bn)	24	72 ± 14	$0.6 \times 10^3 \pm 0.1 \times 10^3$	8
32	Aubis(5-Mes)	25	100 ± 12	-	-
33	Aubis(5-Quin)	26	38 ± 9	$2 \times 10^3 \pm 0.7 \times 10^3$	53

Values of the 50% inhibitory concentration (IC$_{50}$) against Plasmodium falciparum were obtained using both SYBR Green and radioactivity assays. Cytotoxic activities of the compounds were determined against the Vero cell line. The antiplasmodial control drugs, artemether and artemisinin were routinely tested.

2.3. In Vitro Cross-Resistance between Hybrid Molecules and Artemisinin

Three hybrid molecules with the best selectivity indexes in each series, i.e., **Aubis(3-Me) (14)**, **Aubis(4-Me) (19)** and **Aubis(5-Me) (23)**, were evaluated in vitro for their efficacy in a context of resistance to artemisinins. For that, the comparison of the recovery capacity between the strain F32-ART, artemisinin-resistant, and its twin artemisinin-sensitive F32-TEM was evaluated after 48 h-treatment with the molecule to be tested via the recrudescence assay [9,15]. When ring-stage resistant parasites are exposed to artemisinin, most of them die, but a small sub-set of parasites is able to escape the treatment by a cell cycle arrest, called quiescence mechanism. This phenomenon is characterized by a halt of DNA synthesis, which explains the very low IC_{50} values obtained with all artemisinins even for the artemisinin-resistant strain F32-ART [9,15,30]. Therefore, the standard in vitro chemosensitivity assay, based on the measurement of DNA levels to estimate the inhibition of the parasite proliferation, is irrelevant to study the resistance to artemisinins and evaluate possible cross-resistances.

The validation of the test was here done thanks to the results obtained after 18 μM artemisinin treatment and demonstrating that F32-ART is able to recrudesce faster than F32-TEM with a difference to reach the initial parasitemia between the two strains of 9.7 days (Table 2). For the three hybrid molecules tested, namely **Aubis(3-Me) (14)**, **Aubis(4-Me) (19)** and **Aubis(5-Me) (23)**, Table 2 showed a difference of recrudescence between F32-ART and F32-TEM. Whatever the hybrid tested, the differences of recrudescence between both strains rise at the higher doses confirming that increase the doses of the molecules to be tested allows a better discrimination of the recrudescence capacity between the artemisinin-resistant and the -sensitive strains [9]. According to the obtained results, a cross-resistance between artemisinin and the hybrid molecules **Aubis(3-Me) (14)**, **Aubis(4-Me) (19)** and **Aubis(5-Me) (23)** was noted. This cross-resistance could be explained by the DHA part of the hybrid, responsible for the quiescence entrance of the parasites and the lack of activity of the NHC part at the mitochondrial level due to limited access or pharmacodynamic properties. These data are in accordance with previously obtained results which highlighted the risks of parasites cross-resistance between artemisinins and endoperoxide-based compounds [31,32].

Table 2. Recrudescence capacity of *Plasmodium falciparum* F32-ART and F32-TEM strains after 48h-drug exposure.

Complexes	Doses	Number of Experiments	Median (range) Recrudescence Days		Mean ± SEM Difference of Recrudescence Days between F32-TEM and F32-ART
			F32-ART	F32-TEM	
Artemisinin	18 μM	6	9.5 (6–17)	18.5 (17–>30)	9.7 ± 0.3
Aubis(4-Me) (14)	100 nM	1	5	6	1
	500 nM	2	12.5 (11–14)	>30	>17.5 ± 1.5
	1 μM	1	16	30	14
Aubis(5-Me) (19)	100 nM	1	6	15	9
	500 nM	2	9.5 (8–11)	>25.5 (21–>30)	>16
	1 μM	1	9	30	21
Aubis(3-Me) (23)	200 nM	3	7 (7–13)	14 (11–16)	4.6 ± 1.2
	500 nM	1	8	24	16

Synchronized ring-stage parasites have undergone 48 h of drug treatment. After that, cultures were washed and parasitemia was monitored during 30 days or until reaching the initial parasitemia, defined as the recrudescence day. If no parasites were observed at the end of the experiment, the culture was classified as showing no recrudescence, and the recrudescence day was noted as >30.

3. Materials and Methods

3.1. Chemistry

3.1.1. General Information

All complexation reactions were performed under an inert atmosphere of dry nitrogen by using standard vacuum line and Schlenk tube techniques. Reactions involving silver compounds were performed with the exclusion of light. CH_3CN was dried over

CaH$_2$ and subsequently distilled. 10β-(20-Bromopropoxy)dihydroartemisinin (**DHA-C3**) [27], 10β-(21-bromobutoxy) dihydroartemisinin (**DHA-C4**), 10β-(22-bromopentoxy)dihydroartemisinin (**DHA-C5**), 3′-methyl-1′-[10β-(20-propoxy)-dihydroartemisinin]1H-imidazol-3-ium bromide (**L3-Me** (1)), 3′-methyl-1′-[10β-(21-butoxy)-dihydroartemisinin]1H-imidazol-3-ium bromide (**L4-Me** (2)), 3′-methyl-1′-[10β-(22-pentoxy)-dihydroartemisinin]1H-imidazol-3-ium bromide (**L5-Me** (3)), complexes **Aubis(3-Me)** (14), **Aubis(4-Me)** (19), **Aubis(5-Me)** (23) [28], 1-mesitylimidazole [29] and 2-(2H-imidazol-1-yl)quinoline [22] were synthetized according to the referenced literature procedures. All other reagents were used as received from commercial suppliers. ^{1}H- (300, 400 or 500 MHz) and ^{13}C-NMR spectra (75, 101 or 126 MHz) were recorded at 298 K on AV300, AV400 or Avance 500 spectrometers (Bruker, Billerica, MA) in CDCl$_3$ as solvent. All chemical shifts for ^{1}H and ^{13}C are relative to TMS using ^{1}H (residual) or ^{13}C chemical shifts of the solvent as a secondary standard. High Resolution Mass Spectrometry (HRMS) analysis were performed with a Xévo G2 QTOF spectrometer (Waters Corporation, Milford, MA) using electrospray ionization (ESI) by the "Service de Spectrométrie de Masse de Chimie UPS-CNRS (University of Toulouse, France)". Elemental analyses were carried out by the "Service de Microanalyse du Laboratoire de Chimie de Coordination (Toulouse, France)".

3.1.2. Synthesis of proligands (**Ln-R**) and gold(I) complexes **Aubis(n-R)** and **Au(n-R)Cl**

3′-Isopropyl-1′-[10β-(20-propoxy)dihydroartemisinin]1H-imidazol-3-ium bromide (**L3-iPr**, (1)). To a stirred solution of **DHA-C3** (164 mg, 0.4 mmol) in CH$_3$CN (10 mL), 1-isopropylimidazole (61.7 mg, 0.4 mmol) was added and the reaction mixture was stirred 1 day at 70 °C. Then, the solvent was evaporated under reduced pressure and the viscous residue was washed with diethylether to afford a yellow powder (97 mg, 47% yield). Anal. Calcd. for C$_{24}$H$_{39}$BrN$_2$O$_5$: C, 55.92; H, 7.63; N, 5.43. Found C, 55.85; H, 7.64; N, 5.89. ^{1}H-NMR (300 MHz, CDCl$_3$): δ 10.67 (s, 1H, H$_2$), 7.48 (d, J = 1.8 Hz, 1H, H$_4$), 7.40 (d, J = 1.8 Hz, 1H, H$_5$), 5.38 (s, 1H, H$_{Art}$), 4.93 (h, J = 6.6, 5.6 Hz, 1H, H$_{iPr}$), 4.78 (d, J = 3.2 Hz, 1H, H$_{Art}$), 4.52–4.46 (m, 2H, H$_{CH2}$), 3.92–3.84 (m, 1H, H$_{CH2}$), 3.54–3.46 (m, 1H, H$_{CH2}$), 2.71–2.57 (m, 1H, H$_{Art}$), 2.40–2.22 (m, 3H, H$_{Art}$, H$_{CH2}$), 2.07–1.97 (s, 2H, H$_{Art}$), 1.96–1.84 (m, 1H, H$_{Art}$), 1.81–1.69 (m, 2H, H$_{Art}$), 1.65 (s, 3H, H$_{iPr}$), 1.63 (s, 3H, H$_{iPr}$), 1.54–1.45 (m, 2H, H$_{Art}$), 1.41 (s, 3H, H$_{Art}$), 1.38–1.32 (m, 1H, H$_{Art}$), 1.29–1.20 (m, 1H, H$_{Art}$), 0.96 (d, J = 6.1 Hz, 3H, H$_{Art}$), 0.95–0.86 (m, 1H, H$_{Art}$), 0.92 (d, J = 7.4 Hz, 3H, H$_{Art}$). ^{13}C NMR (101 MHz, CDCl$_3$): δ 136.5 (1C, C$_2$), 122.3 (1C, C$_4$), 119.9 (1C, C$_5$), 104.2 (1C, C$_{Art}$), 102.2 (1C, C$_{Art}$), 88.0 (1C, C$_{Art}$), 80.9 (1C, C$_{Art}$), 64.7 (1C, C$_{CH2}$), 53.5 (1C, C$_{iPr}$), 52.4 (1C, C$_{Art}$), 47.4 (1C, C$_{CH2}$), 44.2 (1C, C$_{Art}$), 37.5 (1C, C$_{Art}$), 36.3 (1C, C$_{Art}$), 34.5 (1C, C$_{Art}$), 30.8 (1C, C$_{CH2}$), 30.7 (1C, C$_{Art}$), 26.1 (1C, C$_{Art}$), 24.6 (1C, C$_{Art}$), 24.6 (1C, C$_{Art}$), 23.2 (2C, C$_{iPr}$), 20.3 (1C, C$_{Art}$), 13.2 (1C, C$_{Art}$). HRMS (ESI$^+$): calcd. for C$_{24}$H$_{39}$N$_2$O$_5$ m/z = 435.2859, found 435.2856.

3′-Benzyl-1′-[10β-(20-propoxy)dihydroartemisinin]1H-imidazol-3-ium bromide (**L3-Bn**, (2)). To a stirred solution of **DHA-C3** (275 mg, 0.68 mmol) in CH$_3$CN (4 mL) heated at 70 °C, 1-benzylimidazole (107 mg, 0.68 mmol) was added and the reaction mixture was stirred 3 days. Then, the solvent was removed under reduced pressure and the crude product was dissolved in CH$_2$Cl$_2$ and precipitated with Et$_2$O. This treatment was repeated three times to afford a sticky white solid (286 mg, 87% yield). Anal. Calcd. for C$_{28}$H$_{39}$BrN$_2$O$_5$: C, 59.68; H, 6.98; N, 4.97. Found C, 59.57; H, 6.95; N, 4.90. ^{1}H-NMR (400 MHz, CDCl$_3$): δ 10.71 (s, 1H, H$_2$), 7.52 (m, 1H, H$_{Bn}$), 7.51 (d, J = 1.8 Hz, 1H, H$_4$), 7.40 (d, J = 1.8 Hz, 1H, H$_5$), 7.39 (m, 2H, H$_{Bn}$), 7.34 (d, J = 1.6 Hz, 2H, H$_{Bn}$), 5.64 (s, 2H, H$_{Bn}$), 5.37 (s, 1H, H$_{Art}$), 4.76 (d, J = 3.6 Hz, 1H, H$_{Art}$), 4.40-4.44 (m, 2H, H$_{CH2}$), 3.90–3.85 (m, 1H, H$_{CH2}$), 3.51–3.44 (m, 1H, H$_{CH2}$), 2.62–2.66 (m, 1H, H$_{Art}$), 2.40–2.32 (m, 1H, H$_{Art}$), 2.29–2.23 (m, 2H, H$_{CH2}$), 2.05 (m, 1H, H$_{Art}$), 2.01 (m, 1H, H$_{Art}$),1.92–1.86 (m, 1H, H$_{Art}$), 1.78–1.74 (m, 1H, H$_{Art}$), 1.69–1.63 (m, 2H, H$_{Art}$), 1.50–1.43 (m, 2H, H$_{Art}$), 1.41 (s, 3H, H$_{Art}$), 1.33–1.37 (m, 1H, H$_{Art}$), 1.28–1.24 (m, 1H, H$_{Art}$), 0.96 (d, J = 6.3 Hz, 3H, H$_{Art}$), 0.92 (m, 1H, H$_{Art}$), 0.89 (d, J = 7.4 Hz, 3H, H$_{Art}$). ^{13}C NMR (101 MHz, CDCl$_3$): δ 137.7 (1C, C$_2$), 132.7 (1C, C$_{Bn}$), 129.7 (2C, C$_{Bn}$), 129.5 (1C, C$_{Bn}$), 129.1 (2C, C$_{Bn}$), 122.1 (1C, C$_4$), 121.5 (1C, C$_5$), 104.3 (1C, C$_{Art}$), 102.3 (1C, C$_{Art}$), 88.0 (1C, C$_{Art}$), 80.9 (1C, C$_{Art}$), 64.6 (1C, C$_{CH2}$), 53.6 (1C, C$_{Bn}$), 52.4 (1C, C$_{Art}$), 47.6 (1C, C$_{CH2}$), 44.2 (1C, C$_{Art}$), 37.5 (1C, C$_{Art}$), 36.3 (1C, C$_{Art}$), 34.4 (1C, C$_{Art}$), 30.8 (1C, C$_{CH2}$), 30.5 (1C, C$_{Art}$), 26.1 (1C, C$_{Art}$),

24.7 (1C, C_{Art}), 24.6 (1C, C_{Art}), 20.3 (1C, C_{Art}), 13.1 (1C, C_{Art}). HRMS (ESI$^+$): calcd. for $C_{28}H_{39}N_2O_5$ m/z = 483.2855, found 483.2859.

3'-Mesityl-1'-[10β-(20-propoxy)dihydroartemisinin]1H-imidazol-3-ium bromide (**L3-Mes**, (**3**)). To a stirred solution of **DHA-C3** (251 mg, 0.62 mmol) in CH$_3$CN (4 mL) heated at 70 °C, 1-mesitylimidazole (115 mg, 0.62 mmol) was added and the reaction mixture was stirred for 3 days. The solvent was removed under reduced pressure and the crude product was dissolved in CH$_2$Cl$_2$ and precipitated with Et$_2$O. This treatment was repeated three times to afford a white solid (238 mg, 76% yield). Anal. Calcd. for $C_{30}H_{43}BrN_2O_5$: C, 60.91; H, 7.33; N, 4.74. Found C, 60.93; H, 7.27; N, 4.65. ^{1}H-NMR (300 MHz, CDCl$_3$): δ 10.49 (s, 1H, H$_2$), 7.76 (t, J = 1.8 Hz, 1H, H$_4$), 7.17 (t, J = 1.8 Hz, 1H, H$_4$), 7.03 (m, 2H, H$_{Mes}$), 5.45 (s, 1H, H$_{Art}$), 4.92 (m, 1H, H$_{Art}$), 4.87–4.76 (m, 2H, H$_{CH2}$), 3.90–3.83 (m, 1H, H$_{CH2}$), 3.65–3.54 (m, 1H, H$_{CH2}$), 2.71–2.66 (m, 1H, H$_{Art}$), 2.36 (s, 3H, H$_{Mes}$), 2.44–2.33 (m, 3H, H$_{Art}$), 2.11 (s, 6H, H$_{Mes}$), 2.06–2.00 (m, 1H, H$_{Art}$), 1.95–1.84 (m, 1H, H$_{Art}$), 1.83–1.78 (m, 1H, H$_{Art}$), 1.77–1.67 (m, 2H, H$_{Art}$), 1.65 (s, 1H, H$_{Art}$), 1.54–1.48 (m, 2H, H$_{Art}$), 1.45–1.36 (m, 1H, H$_{Art}$), 1.37 (s, 3H, H$_{Art}$), 1.32–1.26 (m, 1H, H$_{Art}$), 0.98 (d, J = 6.2 Hz, 3H, H$_{Art}$), 0.94 (m, 1H, H$_{Art}$), 0.93 (d, J = 7.4 Hz, 3H, H$_{Art}$). ^{13}C NMR (101 MHz, CDCl$_3$): δ 141.2 (1C, C_{Mes}), 137.7 (1C, C_2), 134.2 (2C, C_{Mes}), 130.7 (1C, C_{Mes}), 129.8 (2C, C_{Mes}), 123.6 (1C, C_4), 123.6 (1C, C_5), 104.2 (1C, C_{Art}), 102.2 (1C, C_{Art}), 87.9 (1C, C_{Art}), 81.0 (1C, C_{Art}), 64.7 (1C, C_{CH2}), 52.4 (1C, C_{Art}), 47.6 (1C, C_{CH2}), 44.2 (1C, C_{Art}), 37.4 (1C, C_{Art}), 36.3 (1C, C_{Art}), 36.1 (1C, C_{Art}), 34.4 (1C, C_{CH2}), 30.9 (1C, C_{Art}), 30.1 (1C, C_{Art}), 25.9 (1C, C_{Art}), 24.6 (1C, C_{Art}), 24.5 (1C, C_{Art}), 21.1 (1C, C_{Mes}), 20.3 (1C, C_{Art}), 17.6 (1C, C_{Mes}), 13.2 (1C, C_{Art}). HRMS (ESI$^+$): calcd. for $C_{30}H_{43}N_2O_5$ m/z = 511.3174, found 511.3172.

3'-Quinolin-2-yl-1'-[10β-(20-propoxy)dihydroartemisinin]1H-imidazol-3-ium bromide (**L3-Quin**, (**4**)). To a stirred solution of **DHA-C3** (292 mg, 0.72 mmol) in CH$_3$CN (3 mL) heated at 70)° C, 1-(quinolin-2-yl)-imidazole (140 mg, 0.72 mmol) was added and the reaction mixture was stirred for 3 days. Then, the solvent was removed under reduced pressure and the crude product was dissolved in CH$_2$Cl$_2$ and precipitated with Et$_2$O. This treatment was repeated three times to afford a yellow solid (315 mg, 84 % yield). Anal. Calcd. for $C_{30}H_{38}BrN_3O_5$: C, 60.00; H, 6.38; N, 7.00. Found C, 60.15; H, 6.42; N, 6.95. ^{1}H-NMR (400 MHz, CDCl$_3$): δ 12.15 (s, 1H, H$_2$), 8.71 (m, 1H, H$_{Quin}$), 8.56–8.53 (m, 2H, H$_4$, H$_{Quin}$), 8.06 (d, J = 8.5 Hz, 1H, H$_{Quin}$), 7.96 (d, J = 7.8 Hz, 1H, H$_{Quin}$), 7.84 (m, 1H, H$_{Quin}$), 7.68 (m, 1H, H$_{Quin}$), 7.54 (t, J = 1.7 Hz, 1H, H$_5$), 5.43 (s, 1H, H$_{Art}$), 4.83 (d, J = 3.6 Hz, 1H, H$_{Art}$), 4.75 (m, 2H, H$_{CH2}$), 4.78–4.70 (m, 2H, H$_{CH2}$), 4.02–3.96 (m, 1H, H$_{CH2}$), 3.65–3.60 (m, 1H, H$_{CH2}$), 2.68 (m, 1H, H$_{Art}$), 2.47–2.41 (m, 2H, H$_{CH2}$), 2.39–2.35 (m, 1H, H$_{Art}$), 2.08–2.02 (m, 1H, H$_{Art}$), 1.94–1.84 (m, 1H, H$_{Art}$), 1.82–1.77 (m, 1H, H$_{Art}$), 1.72–1.65 (m, 2H, H$_{Art}$), 1.56–1.45 (m, 2H, H$_{Art}$), 1.44 (s, 3H, H$_{Art}$), 1.40–1.34 (m, 1H, H$_{Art}$), 1.30–1.23 (m, 1H, H$_{Art}$), 0.97 (d, J = 6.4 Hz, 3H, H$_{Art}$), 0.95 (d, J = 7.4 Hz, 3H, H$_{Art}$), 0.91–0.85 (m, 1H, H$_{Art}$). ^{13}C NMR (101 MHz, CDCl$_3$): δ 146.1 (1C, C_{Quin}), 144.5 (1C, C_{Quin}), 141.7 (1C, C_{Quin}), 137.0 (1C, C_2), 131.5 (1C, C_{Quin}), 128.8 (1C, C_{Quin}), 128.3 (1C, C_{Quin}), 128.2 (2C, C_{Quin}), 122.4 (1C, C_4), 118.7 (1C, C_5), 112.7 (1C, C_{Quin}), 104.3 (1C, C_{Art}), 102.3 (1C, C_{Art}), 88.0 (1C, C_{Art}), 80.9 (1C, C_{Art}), 64.8 (1C, C_{CH2}), 52.4 (1C, C_{Art}), 49.2 (1C, C_{CH2}), 44.2 (1C, C_{Art}), 37.5 (1C, C_{Art}), 36.3 (1C, C_{Art}), 34.5 (1C, C_{Art}), 30.8 (1C, C_{CH2}), 30.8 (1C, C_{CH2}), 26.1 (1C, C_{Art}), 24.6 (1C, C_{Art}), 24.6 (1C, C_{Art}), 20.3 (1C, C_{Art}), 13.2 (1C, C_{Art}). HRMS (ESI$^+$): calcd. for $C_{30}H_{38}N_3O_5$ m/z = 520.2798, found 520.2811.

Complex **Aubis(3-iPr)** (**15**). Under a nitrogen atmosphere and protection of the light, **L3-iPr** (102 mg, 0.2 mmol) and Ag$_2$O (26 mg, 0.11 mmol) was dissolved in CH$_3$CN (3 mL) and stirred overnight at rt. Then, AgNO$_3$ (19 mg, 0.11 mmol) was added to the mixture followed 2 h later by addition of **Au(SMe$_2$)Cl** (32 mg, 0.11 mmol). After stirring 1 h at rt, the solution was filtered through a pad of celite and the solvent removed under reduced pressure to afford a white solid after centrifugation (95 mg, 83% yield). Anal. Calcd. For $C_{48}H_{76}AuClN_4O_{10}$: C, 52.34; H, 6.95; N, 5.09. Found C, 52.28; H, 6.85; N, 5.02. ^{1}H-NMR (400 MHz, CDCl$_3$): δ 7.31 (d, J = 1.9 Hz, 1H, H$_4$), 7.30 (s, 1H, H$_5$), 5.39 (s, 1H, H$_{Art}$), 4.95 (h, J = 6.9 Hz, 1H, H$_{iPr}$), 4.80 (d, J = 3.6 Hz, 1H, H$_{Art}$), 4.42–4.31 (m, 2H, H$_{CH2}$), 3.95–3.89 (m, 1H, H$_{CH2}$), 3.49–3.43 (m, 1H, H$_{CH2}$), 2.68–2.64 (m, 1H, H$_{Art}$), 2.39 (td, J = 14.0, 3.9 Hz, 1H, H$_{Art}$), 2.31–2.18 (m, 2H, H$_{CH2}$), 2.08–2.03 (m, 1H, H$_{Art}$), 1.94–1.89 (m, 1H, H$_{Art}$), 1.78–1.65 (m, 3H, H$_{Art}$), 1.62 (s, 3H, H$_{iPr}$), 1.60 (s, 3H, H$_{iPr}$), 1.52–1.47 (m, 2H, H$_{Art}$), 1.44 (s, 3H, H$_{Art}$), 1.36–1.25 (m, 2H, H$_{Art}$), 0.98

(d, J = 6.1 Hz, 3H, H$_{Art}$), 0.97–0.88 (m, 1H, H$_{Art}$), 0.93 (d, J = 7.3 Hz, 3H, Art). ^{13}C NMR (101 MHz, CDCl$_3$): δ 182.1 (1C, C$_2$), 122.3 (1C, C$_4$), 118.3 (1C, C$_5$), 104.2 (1C, C$_{Art}$), 102.0 (1C, C$_{Art}$), 88.0 (1C, C$_{Art}$), 80.9 (1C, C$_{Art}$), 64.8 (1C, C$_{CH2}$), 53.8 (1C, C$_{iPr}$), 52.4 (1C, C$_{Art}$), 48.9 (1C, C$_{CH2}$), 44.2 (1C, C$_{Art}$), 37.5 (1C, C$_{Art}$), 36.4 (1C, C$_{Art}$), 34.5 (1C, C$_{Art}$), 31.7 (1C, C$_{CH2}$), 30.8 (1C, C$_{Art}$), 26.1 (1C, C$_{Art}$), 24.7 (1C, C$_{Art}$), 24.6 (1C, C$_{Art}$), 23.8 (1C, C$_{iPr}$), 23.8 (1C, C$_{iPr}$), 20.3 (1C, C$_{Art}$), 13.2 (1C, C$_{Art}$). HRMS (ESI$^+$): calcd. for C$_{48}$H$_{76}$AuClN$_4$O$_{10}$ m/z = 1065.5227, found 1065.5220.

Complex **Aubis(3-Bn)** (**16**). Under a nitrogen atmosphere, K$_2$CO$_3$ (26 mg, 0.19 mmol) was added to **L3-Bn** (108 mg, 0.19 mmol) in dry CH$_3$CN (4 mL) and heated at 60 °C under stirring. Then, **Au(SMe$_2$)Cl** (28 mg, 0.096 mmol) was added and the mixture was stirred for 10 h. After cooling to room temperature, the solution was filtered through a pad of celite and the solvent removed under reduced pressure. The complex was purified by flash chromatography on silica with CH$_2$Cl$_2$-MeOH as eluent (100/0 to 100/10) to give a white solid (75 mg, 65 % yield). Anal. Calcd. for C$_{56}$H$_{76}$AuClN$_4$O$_{10}$: C, 56.16; H, 6.40; N, 4.48. Found C, 56.28; H, 6.55; N, 4.42. ^{1}H-NMR (500 MHz, CDCl$_3$): δ 7.34 (d, J = 1.9 Hz, 1H, H$_4$), 7.30 (m, 2H, H$_{Bn}$), 7.29 (m, 1H, H$_{Bn}$), 7.24 (m, 2H, H$_{Bn}$), 7.23 (d, J = 1.9 Hz, 1H, H$_5$), 5.39 (s, 2H, H$_{Bn}$), 4.74 (d, J = 3.5 Hz, 1H, H$_{Art}$), 4.28–4.24 (m, 2H, H$_{CH2}$), 3.87–3.81 (m, 1H, H$_{CH2}$), 3.41–3.36 (m, 1H, H$_{CH2}$), 2.64–2.60 (m, 1H, H$_{Art}$), 2.41–2.33 (m, 1H, H$_{Art}$), 2.11 (m, 2H, H$_{CH2}$), 2.07–2.01 (m, 1H, H$_{Art}$), 1.91–1.85 (m, 2H, H$_{Art}$), 1.74–1.69 (m, 2H, H$_{Art}$), 1.63–1.57 (m, 1H, H$_{Art}$), 1.41–1.46 (m, 2H, H$_{Art}$), 1.41 (s, 3H, H$_{Art}$), 1.33–1.26 (m, 2H, H$_{Art}$), 0.94 (d, J = 6.1 Hz, 3H, H$_{Art}$), 0.92 (m, 1H, H$_{Art}$), 0.87 (d, J = 7.3 Hz, 3H, H$_{Art}$). ^{13}C NMR (126 MHz, CDCl$_3$): δ 183.5 (1C, C$_2$), 135.7 (1C, C$_{Bn}$), 129.1 (2C, C$_{Bn}$), 128.6 (1C, C$_{Bn}$), 127.6 (2C, C$_{Bn}$), 122.5 (1C, C$_4$), 122.2 (1C, C$_5$), 104.2 (1C, C$_{Art}$), 102.0 (1C, C$_{Art}$), 87.9 (1C, C$_{Art}$), 80.9 (1C, C$_{Art}$), 64.7 (1C, C$_{CH2}$), 54.8 (1C, C$_{Bn}$), 52.5 (1C, C$_{Art}$), 48.6 (1C, C$_{CH2}$), 44.2 (1C, C$_{Art}$), 37.6 (1C, C$_{Art}$), 36.4 (1C, C$_{Art}$), 34.5 (1C, C$_{Art}$), 31.6 (1C, C$_{CH2}$), 30.7 (1C, C$_{Art}$), 26.2 (1C, C$_{Art}$), 24.7 (1C, C$_{Art}$), 24.5 (1C, C$_{Art}$), 20.3 (1C, C$_{Art}$), 13.1 (1C, C$_{Art}$). HRMS (ESI$^+$): calcd. for C$_{56}$H$_{76}$AuN$_4$O$_{10}$ m/z = 1161.5227, found 1161.5247.

Complex **Aubis(3-Mes)** (**17**). Under a nitrogen atmosphere, K$_2$CO$_3$ (24 mg, 0.17 mmol) was added to **L3-Mes** (104 mg, 0.17 mmol) in dry CH$_3$CN (4 mL). The mixture was then heated at 60 °C. After, **Au(SMe$_2$)Cl** (26 mg, 0.087 mmol) was added and the mixture was stirred for 10 h. After cooling to room temperature, the solution was filtered through a pad of celite and the solvent removed under reduced pressure. The complex was purified by flash chromatography on silica with CH$_2$Cl$_2$-MeOH as eluent (100/0 to 100/10) to give a yellow solid (58 mg, 52% yield). Anal. Calcd. for C$_{60}$H$_{84}$AuClN$_4$O$_{10}$: C, 57.48; H, 6.75; N, 4.47. Found C, 57.42; H, 6.68; N, 4.35. ^{1}H-NMR (500 MHz, CDCl$_3$): δ 7.59 (d, J = 1.9 Hz, 1H, H$_4$), 6.96 (m, 3H, H$_5$, H$_{Mes}$), 5.37 (s, 1H, H$_{Art}$), 4.73 (d, J = 3.5 Hz, 1H, H$_{1Art}$), 4.13 (m, 2H, H$_{CH2}$), 3.72 (m, 1H, H$_{CH2}$), 3.22 (m, 1H, H$_{CH2}$), 2.65 (m, 1H, H$_{Art}$), 2.37 (s, 3H, H$_{Mes}$), 2.41–2.33 (m, 1H, H$_{Art}$), 2.09–1.98 (m, 2H, H$_{CH2}$), 1.90 (m, 1H, H$_{Art}$), 1.85 (s, 3H, H$_{Mes}$), 1.83 (m, 3H, H$_{Mes}$), 1.83–1.65 (m, 4H, H$_{Art}$), 1.51–1.45 (m, 2H, H$_{Art}$), 1.43 (m, 1H, H$_{Art}$), 1.36–1.32 (m, 1H, H$_{Art}$), 1.29–1.25 (s, 1H, H$_{Art}$), 0.98 (d, J = 6.3 Hz, 3H, H$_{Art}$), 0.96–0.88 (m, 1H, H$_{Art}$), 0.94 (d, J = 7.2 Hz, 3H, H$_{Art}$). ^{13}C NMR (126 MHz, CDCl$_3$): δ 183.8 (1C, C$_2$), 139.6 (1C, C$_{Mes}$), 134.8 (2C, C$_{Mes}$), 134.7 (1C, C$_{Mes}$), 129.2 (2C, C$_{Mes}$), 123.0 (1C, C$_5$), 122.7 (1C, C$_4$), 104.1 (1C, C$_{Art}$), 102.0 (1C, C$_{Art}$), 87.9 (1C, C$_{Art}$), 81.0 (1C, C$_{Art}$), 64.8 (1C, C$_{CH2}$), 52.5 (1C, C$_{Art}$), 48.3 (1C, C$_{CH2}$), 44.2 (1C, C$_{Art}$), 37.7 (1C, C$_{Art}$), 36.4 (1C, C$_{Art}$), 34.6 (1C, C$_{Art}$), 31.6 (C$_{CH2}$), 30.9 (1C, C$_{Art}$), 26.1 (1C, C$_{Art}$), 24.7 (1C, C$_{Art}$), 24.6 (1C, C$_{Art}$), 21.2 (2C, C$_{Mes}$), 20.3 (1C, C$_{Art}$), 17.6 (1C, C$_{Mes}$), 13.3 (1C, C$_{Art}$). HRMS (ESI$^+$): calcd. for C$_{60}$H$_{74}$AuN$_6$O$_{10}$ m/z = 1235.5157, found 1235.5132.

Complex **Aubis(3-Quin)** (**18**). Under a nitrogen atmosphere, K$_2$CO$_3$ (24 mg, 0.17 mmol) was added to **L3-Quin** (100 mg, 0.17 mmol) in dry CH$_3$CN (4 mL). The stirred mixture was then heated at 60 °C. Then, **Au(SMe$_2$)Cl** (25 mg, 0.085 mmol) was added and the mixture was stirred for 10 h. After cooling to room temperature, the solution was filtered through a pad of celite and the solvent removed under reduced pressure to give a white solid (93 mg, 86% yield). Anal. Calcd. For C$_{60}$H$_{74}$AuClN$_6$O$_{10}$: C, 56.67; H, 5.87; N, 6.61. Found C, 56.62; H, 5.85; N, 6.54. ^{1}H-NMR (500 MHz, CDCl$_3$): δ 8.30 (d, J = 8.6 Hz, 1H, H$_{Quin}$), 8.13 (d, J = 8.7 Hz, 1H, H$_{Quin}$), 8.09 (d, J = 1.6 Hz, 1H, H$_4$), 7.80 (d, J = 8.4 Hz, 1H, H$_{Quin}$), 7.73 (d, J = 8.2 Hz, 1H, H$_{Quin}$), 7.62 (m, 1H, H$_{Quin}$), 7.51 (d, J = 2.0 Hz, 1H, H$_5$), 7.47 (m, 1H,

H$_{Quin}$), 5.34 (s, 1H, H$_{Art}$), 4.71 (d, *J* = 3.5 Hz, 1H, H$_{Art}$), 4.53–4.44 (m, 2H, H$_{CH2}$), 3.87–3.82 (m, 1H, H$_{CH2}$), 3.43–3.38 (m, 1H, H$_{Art}$), 2.61–2.56 (m, 1H, H$_{Art}$), 2.33 (td, *J* = 14.0, 4.0 Hz, 1H, H$_{Art}$), 2.26–2.18 (m, 2H, H$_{CH2}$), 2.02–1.97 (m, 1H, H$_{Art}$), 1.86–1.81 (m, 1H, H$_{Art}$), 1.67–1.62 (m, 2H, H$_{Art}$), 1.54–1.50 (m, 1H, H$_{Art}$), 1.46–1.35 (m, 2H, H$_{Art}$), 1.39 (m, 3H, H$_{Art}$), 1.30-1.16 (m, 2H, H$_{Art}$), 0.88 (d, *J* = 6.2 Hz, 3H, H$_{Art}$), 0.86–080 (m, 1H, H$_{Art}$), 0.83 (d, *J* = 7.2 Hz, 3H, H$_{Art}$). ^{13}C NMR (126 MHz, CDCl$_3$): δ 181.8 (1C, C$_2$), 148.9 (1C, C$_{Quin}$), 146.3 (1C, C$_{Quin}$), 139.9 (1C, C$_{Quin}$), 131.0 (1C, C$_{Quin}$), 128.4 (1C, C$_{Quin}$), 127.9 (1C, C$_{Quin}$), 127.6 (1C, C$_{Quin}$), 127.5 (1C, C$_{Quin}$), 122.9 (1C, C$_4$), 121.6 (1C, C$_5$), 115.7 (1C, C$_{Quin}$), 104.2 (1C, C$_{Art}$), 102.0 (1C, C$_{Art}$), 87.9 (1C, C$_{Art}$), 80.9 (1C, C$_{Art}$), 64.8 (1C, C$_{CH2}$), 52.4 (C1, C$_{Art}$), 49.8 (1C, C$_{CH2}$), 44.2 (1C, C$_{Art}$), 37.6 (1C, C$_{Art}$), 36.3 (1C, C$_{Art}$), 34.5 (1C, C$_{Art}$), 31.5 (1C, C$_{CH2}$), 30.7 (1C, C$_{Art}$), 26.1 (1C, C$_{Art}$), 24.6 (1C, C$_{Art}$), 24.5 (1C, C$_{Art}$), 20.3 (1C, C$_{Art}$), 13.1 (1C, C$_{Art}$). HRMS (ESI$^+$): calcd. for C$_{60}$H$_{74}$AuN$_6$O$_{10}$ *m/z* = 1235.5157, found 1235.5132.

Complex **Au(3-*i*Pr)Cl (27)**. Under a nitrogen atmosphere and protection of the light, **L3-*i*Pr** (21 mg, 0.04 mmol), K$_2$CO$_3$ (6 mg, 0.04 mmol) and **Au(SMe$_2$)Cl** (12 mg, 0.04 mmol) were dissolved in CH$_3$CN (3 mL) and stirred for 6 h at 60 °C. The solution was filtered through a syringe filter (0.2 µm) and the solvent removed under reduced pressure to afford a white powder (9.8 mg, 42% yield). Anal. Calcd. for C$_{24}$H$_{38}$AuClN$_2$O$_5$: C, 43.22; H, 5.74; N, 4.20. Found C, 43.32; H, 5.72; N, 4.15. ^{1}H-NMR (400 MHz, CDCl$_3$): δ 7.01 (d, *J* = 2.0 Hz, 1H, H$_4$), 6.97 (d, *J* = 1.9 Hz, 1H, H$_5$), 5.41 (s, 1H, H$_{Art}$), 5.10 (hept, *J* = 7.0 Hz, 1H, H$_{iPr}$), 4.81 (d, *J* = 3.4 Hz, 1H, H$_{Art}$), 4.26 (td, *J* = 7.1, 4.8 Hz, 2H, H$_{CH2}$), 3.95–3.86 (m, 1H, H$_{CH2}$), 3.48–3.40 (m, 1H, H$_{CH2}$), 2.73–2.63 (m, 1H, H$_{Art}$), 2.45–2.33 (m, 1H, H$_{Art}$), 2.23–2.13 (m, 2H, H$_{CH2}$), 2.06 (ddd, *J* = 14.0, 4.6, 2.9 Hz, 1H, H$_{Art}$), 1.95–1.83 (m, 2H, H$_{Art}$), 1.78–1.70 (m, 2H, H$_{Art}$), 1.60–1.52 (s, 2H, H$_{Art}$), 1.50 (s, 3H, H$_{iPr}$), 1.48 (s, 3H, H$_{iPr}$), 1.45 (s, 3H, H$_{iPr}$), 1.41–1.36 (m, 1H, H$_{Art}$), 1.30–1.24 (m, 1H, H$_{Art}$), 0.99 (d, *J* = 5.5 Hz, 3H, H$_{Art}$), 0.98 (d, *J* = 5.5 Hz, 3H, H$_{Art}$), 0.96–0.86 (m, 1H, H$_{Art}$). ^{13}C NMR (101 MHz, CDCl$_3$): δ 173.3 (1C, C$_2$), 120.9 (1C, C$_4$), 116.4 (1C, C$_5$), 104.2 (1C, C$_{Art}$), 102.2 (1C, C$_{Art}$), 88.0 (1C, C$_{Art}$), 81.0 (1C, C$_{Art}$), 64.8 (1C, C$_{CH2}$), 53.6 (1C, C$_{iPr}$), 52.5 (1C, C$_{Art}$), 48.7 (1C, C$_{CH2}$), 44.3 (1C, C$_{Art}$), 37.5 (1C, C$_{Art}$), 36.4 (1C, C$_{Art}$), 34.5 (1C, C$_{Art}$), 31.3 (1C, C$_{CH2}$), 30.9 (1C, C$_{Art}$), 29.7 (1C, C$_{Art}$), 26.2 (1C, C$_{Art}$), 24.7 (2C, C$_{Art}$), 23.4 (2C, C$_{iPr}$), 20.3 (1C, C$_{Art}$), 13.3 (1C, C$_{Art}$). HRMS (ESI$^+$): calcd. for C$_{24}$H$_{38}$AuN$_2$O$_5$ *m/z* = 631.2449, found 631.2446.

Complex **Au(3-Bn)Cl (28)**. Under a nitrogen atmosphere, K$_2$CO$_3$ (20 mg, 0.15 mmol) was added to **L3-Bn** (85 mg, 0.15 mmol) in dry CH$_3$CN (7 mL). The mixture was then heated at 60 °C. After, **Au(SMe$_2$)Cl** (44 mg, 0.15 mmol) was added and the mixture was stirred for 10 h. After cooling to room temperature, the solution was filtered through a pad of celite and the solvent was removed under reduced pressure to give a white solid (87 mg, 81% yield). Anal. Calcd. for C$_{28}$H$_{38}$AuClN$_2$O$_5$: C, 47.03; H, 5.36; N, 3.92. Found C, 47.12; H, 5.29; N, 3.91. ^{1}H-NMR (400 MHz, CDCl$_3$): δ 7.31–7.40 (m, 5H, H$_{Bn}$), 6.97 (d, *J* = 2.0 Hz, 1H, H$_4$), 6.89 (d, *J* = 1.9 Hz, 1H, H$_5$), 5.38 (s, 2H, H$_{Bn}$), 5.40 (s, 1H, H$_{Art}$), 4.79 (d, *J* = 3.5 Hz, 1H, H$_{Art}$), 4.31–4.24 (m, 2H, H$_{CH2}$), 3.92–3.87 (m, 1H, H$_{CH2}$), 3.46–4.40 (m, 1H, H$_{CH2}$), 2.68–2.63 (m, 1H, H$_{Art}$), 2.41–2.32 (ddd, *J* = 14.5, 13.4, 3.9 Hz, 1H, H$_{Art}$), 2.24–2.21 (m, 2H, H$_{CH2}$), 2.04 (ddd, *J* = 14.6, 4.8, 2.9 Hz, 1H, H$_{Art}$), 1.93–1.68 (m, 4H, H$_{Art}$), 1.55–1.44 (m, 2H, H$_{Art}$), 1.43 (s, 3H, H$_{Art}$), 1.39–1.33 (m, 1H, H$_{Art}$), 1.29–1.22 (m, 1H, H$_{Art}$), 0.97 (d, *J* = 6.1 Hz, 3H, H$_{Art}$), 0.95 (d, *J* = 7.3 Hz, 3H, H$_{Art}$), 0.94–0.88 (m, 1H, H$_{Art}$). ^{13}C NMR (101 MHz, CDCl$_3$): δ 174.5 (1C, C$_2$), 134.9 (1C, C$_{Bn}$), 129.1 (2C, C$_{Bn}$), 128.8 (2C, C$_{Bn}$), 128.1 (2C, C$_{Bn}$), 121.2 (1C, C$_4$), 120.2 (1C, C$_5$), 104.2 (1C, C$_{Art}$), 102.2 (1C, C$_{Art}$), 88.0 (1C, C$_{Art}$), 81.0 (1C, C$_{Art}$), 64.7 (1C, C$_{CH2}$), 55.2 (1C, C$_{Bn}$), 52.5 (1C, C$_{Art}$), 48.7 (1C, C$_{CH2}$), 44.3 (1C, C$_{Art}$), 37.5 (1C, C$_{Art}$), 36.4 (1C, C$_{Art}$), 34.5 (1C, C$_{Art}$), 31.2 (1C, C$_{CH2}$), 30.9 (1C, C$_{Art}$), 26.2 (1C, C$_{1Art}$), 24.7 (2C, C$_{Art}$), 20.3 (1C, C$_{Art}$), 13.3 (C$_{Art}$). HRMS (ESI$^+$): calcd. for C$_{28}$H$_{38}$AuN$_2$O$_5$ *m/z* = 679.2452, found 679.2446.

Complex **Au(3-Quin)Cl (29)** was obtained as a byproduct from the purification by column chromatography of **Aubis(3-Quin)** (8 mg). Anal. Calcd. For C$_{30}$H$_{37}$AuClN$_3$O$_5$: C, 47.91; H, 4.96; N, 5.59. Found C, 47.85; H, 5.08; N, 5.49. ^{1}H-NMR (400 MHz, CDCl$_3$): δ 8.78 (d, *J* = 8.7 Hz, 1H, H$_{Quin}$), 8.41 (d, *J* = 8.6 Hz, 1H, H$_{Quin}$), 8.07 (d, *J* = 8.2 Hz, 1H, H$_{Quin}$), 8.04 (d, *J* = 2.0 Hz, 1H, H$_4$), 7.93 (dd, *J* = 8.2, 1.4 Hz, 1H, H$_{Quin}$), 7.81 (ddd, *J* = 8.5, 6.9, 1.5 Hz, 1H, H$_{Quin}$), 7.64 (ddd, *J* = 8.1, 6.9, 1.2

Hz, 1H, H$_{Quin}$), 7.20 (d, J = 2.1 Hz, 1H, H$_5$), 5.44 (s, 1H, H$_{Art}$), 4.84 (d, J = 3.6 Hz, 1H, H$_{Art}$), 4.48–4.44 (m, 2H, H$_{CH2}$), 4.01–3.96 (m, 1H, H$_{CH2}$), 3.56–3.50 (m, 1H, H$_{CH2}$), 2.69 (m, 1H, H$_{Art}$), 2.44–2.36 (m, 1H, H$_{Art}$), 2.31–2.27 (m, 2H, H$_{CH2}$), 2.09–2.03 (m, 1H, H$_{Art}$), 1.93–1.85 (m, 2H, H$_{Art}$), 1.79–1.71 (m, 2H, H$_{Art}$), 1.55–1.45 (m, 2H, H$_{Art}$), 1.46 (s, 3H, H$_{Art}$), 1.41–1.26 (m, 2H, H$_{Art}$), 0.99 (d, J = 6.3 Hz, 3H, H$_{Art}$), 0.97 (d, J = 6.3 Hz, 3H, H$_{Art}$), 0.94–0.90 (m, 1H, H$_{Art}$). ^{13}C NMR (101 MHz, CDCl$_3$): δ 173.7 (1C, C$_2$), 149.1 (1C, C$_{Quin}$), 146.5 (1C, C$_{Quin}$), 139.6 (1C, C$_{Quin}$), 130.9 (1C, C$_{Quin}$), 128.9 (1C, C$_{Quin}$), 127.9 (1C, C$_{Quin}$), 127.9 (1C, C$_{Quin}$), 127.5 (1C, C$_{Quin}$), 121.2 (1C, C$_5$), 120.6 (1C, C$_4$), 115.4 (C$_{Quin}$), 104.2 (1C, C$_{Art}$), 102.2 (1C, C$_{Art}$), 88.0 (1C, C$_{Art}$), 81.0 (1C, C$_{Art}$), 64.8 (1C, C$_{CH2}$), 52.5 (1C, C$_{Art}$), 49.7 (1C, C$_{CH2}$), 44.3 (1C, C$_{Art}$), 37.5 (1C, C$_{Art}$), 36.4 (1C, C$_{Art}$), 34.5 (1C, C$_{Art}$), 31.3 (1C, C$_{CH2}$), 30.9 (1C, C$_{Art}$), 26.2 (1C, C$_{Art}$), 24.7 (2C, C$_{Art}$), 20.3 (1C, C$_{Art}$), 13.3 (1C, C$_{Art}$). HRMS (ESI$^+$): calcd. for C$_{30}$H$_{37}$AuN$_3$O$_5$ m/z = 716.2399, found 716.2418.

3'-Benzyl-1'-[10β-(21-butoxy)dihydroartemisinin]1H-imidazol-3-ium bromide (**L4-Bn** (**7**)). To a stirred solution of **DHA-C4** (109 mg, 0.26 mmol) in CH$_3$CN (4 mL) heated at 70 °C, 1-benzylimidazole (41 mg, 0.26 mmol) was added and the reaction mixture was stirred 3 days. Then, the solvent was removed under reduced pressure and the crude product was dissolved in CH$_2$Cl$_2$ and precipitated with Et$_2$O. This treatment was repeated three times to afford a white solid (109 mg, 73% yield). Anal. Calcd. for C$_{29}$H$_{41}$BrN$_2$O$_5$: C, 60.31; H, 7.16; N, 4.85. Found C, 60.26; H, 7.07; N, 4.79. ^{1}H-NMR (300 MHz, CDCl$_3$): δ 11.19 (sl, 1H, H$_2$), 7.50–7.43 (m, 5H, H$_{Bn}$), 7.23–7.02 (m, 1H, H$_4$, H$_5$), 5.62 (s, 2H, H$_{Bn}$), 5.38 (s, 1H, H$_{Art}$), 5.17 (s, 2H, H$_{CH2}$), 4.78 (d, J = 3.5 Hz, 1H, H$_{Art}$), 4.52–4.41 (m, 4H, H$_{CH2}$), 3.81 (t, J = 5.6 Hz, 1H, H$_{CH2}$), 3.50 (d, J = 10.0 Hz, 2H, H$_{CH2}$), 2.65 (s, 1H, H$_{Art}$), 2.21–2.09 (m, 1H, H$_{Art}$), 2.09–2.00 (m, 2H, H$_{Art}$), 1.66–1.64 (m, 6H, H$_{Art}$), 1.45 (s, 2H, H$_{Art}$), 1.35 (sl, 1H, H$_{Art}$), 1.25 (t, J = 7.0 Hz, 1H, H$_{Art}$), 0.98 (d, J = 6.1 Hz, 3H, H$_{Art}$), 0.96–0.94 (m, 1H, H$_{Art}$), 0.91 (d, J = 7.4 Hz, 3H, H$_{Art}$). ^{13}C NMR (101 MHz, CDCl$_3$): δ 137.3 (1C, C$_2$), 129.7 (2C, C$_{Bn}$), 129.1 (2C, C$_{Bn}$), 128.6 (1C, C$_{Bn}$), 122.1 (1C, C$_4$), 121.4 (1C, C$_5$), 120.6 (1C, C$_{Bn}$), 102.1 (1C, C$_{Art}$), 94.0 (1C, C$_{Art}$), 87.9 (1C, C$_{Art}$), 61.1 (1C, C$_{Art}$), 56.5 (1C, C$_{CH2}$), 53.6 (1C, C$_{Bn}$), 51.7 (1C, C$_{Art}$), 50.0 (1C, C$_{Art}$), 45.3 (1C, C$_{Art}$), 41.2 (1C, C$_{Art}$), 40.3 (1C, C$_{Art}$), 34.5 (1C, C$_{Art}$), 30.3 (1C, C$_{Art}$), 30.0 (1C, C$_{CH2}$), 29.5 (1C, C$_{CH2}$), 28.3 (1C, C$_{Art}$), 27.5 (1C, C$_{Art}$), 20.5 (1C, C$_{CH2}$), 20.0 (1C, C$_{Art}$), 11.1 (1C, C$_{Art}$). HRMS (ESI$^+$): calcd. for C$_{29}$H$_{41}$N$_2$O$_5$ m/z = 497.3010, found 497.3007.

3'-Mesityl-1'-[10β-(21-butoxy)dihydroartemisinin]1H-imidazol-3-ium bromide (**L4-Mes** (**8**)). To a stirred solution of **DHA-C4** (189 mg, 0.45 mmol) in CH$_3$CN (4 mL) heated at 70 °C, 1-mesitylimidazole (142 mg, 0.76 mmol) was added and the reaction mixture was stirred for 3 days. The solvent was removed under reduced pressure and the crude product was dissolved in CH$_2$Cl$_2$ and precipitated with Et$_2$O. This treatment was repeated three times to afford a white solid (168 mg, 62% yield). Anal. Calcd. for C$_{31}$H$_{45}$BrN$_2$O$_5$: C, 61.48; H, 7.49; N, 4.63. Found C, 62.21; H, 7.66; N, 4.36. ^{1}H-NMR (300 MHz, CDCl$_3$): δ 10.55 (t, J = 1.4 Hz, 1H, H$_2$), 7.68 (t, J = 1.9 Hz, 1H, H$_4$), 7.15 (t, J = 1.9 Hz, 1H, H$_5$), 7.03 (s, 2H, H$_{Mes}$), 5.42 (s, 1H, H$_{Art}$), 5.02 (s, 1H, H$_{Art}$), 4.86 (d, J = 3.3 Hz, 2H, H$_{CH2}$), 3.94 (dt, J = 9.7, 6.2 Hz, 1H, H$_{CH2}$), 3.63 (dt, J = 9.7, 6.2 Hz, 1H, H$_{CH2}$), 2.37 (s, 3H, H$_{Mes}$), 2.36–2.24 (m, 1H, H$_{Art}$), 2.19 (s, 1H, H$_{Art}$), 2.11 (s, 6H, H$_{Mes}$), 2.10–2.01 (m, 1H, H$_{Art}$), 1.95–1.87 (m, 1H, H$_{CH2}$), 1.80–1.75 (m, 2H, H$_{CH2}$), 1.72–1.66 (m, 2H, H$_{Art}$), 1.64–1.60 (m, 3H, H$_{Art}$), 1.57–1.52 (m, 1H, H$_{CH2}$), 1.50–1.43 (m, 1H, H$_{Art}$), 1.42 (s, 3H, H$_{Art}$), 1.40–1.36 (m, 1H, H$_{Art}$), 1.31–1.26 (m, 1H, H$_{Art}$), 1.18 (sl, 2H, H$_{Art}$), 1.16, (sl, 1H, H$_{Art}$), 1.10–1.01 (m, 1H, H$_{Art}$), 1.00–0.94 (m, 3H, H$_{Art}$), 0.93–0.87 (m, 1H, H$_{Art}$). ^{13}C NMR (101 MHz, CDCl$_3$): δ 139.1 (1C, C$_{Mes}$), 138.9 (1C, C$_2$), 136.7 (2C, C$_{Mes}$), 129.3 (2C, C$_{Mes}$), 127.5 (1C, C$_{Mes}$), 123.0 (1C, C$_4$), 120.6 (1C, C$_5$), 104.1 (1C, C$_{Art}$), 102.2 (1C, C$_{Art}$), 87.9 (1C, C$_{Art}$), 81.1 (1C, C$_{Art}$), 67.7 (1C, C$_{CH2}$), 52.5 (1C, C$_{Art}$), 50.3 (1C, C$_{CH2}$), 44.4 (1C, C$_{Art}$), 37.5 (1C, C$_{Art}$), 36.4 (1C, C$_{Art}$), 34.5 (1C, C$_{Art}$), 30.9 (1C, C$_{Art}$), 27.4 (1C, C$_{CH2}$), 26.2 (1C, C$_{Art}$), 25.0 (1C, C$_{Art}$), 24.5 (1C, C$_{Art}$), 21.2 (1C, C$_{CH2}$), 20.4 (1C, C$_{Art}$), 17.6 (2C, C$_{Mes}$), 17.3 (1C, C$_{Mes}$), 13.2 (1C, C$_{Art}$). HRMS (ESI$^+$): calcd. for C$_{31}$H$_{45}$N$_2$O$_5$ m/z = 525.3328, found 525.3353.

3'-Quinolin-2-yl-1'-[10β-(21-butoxy)dihydroartemisinin]1H-imidazol-3-ium bromide (**L4-Quin** (**9**)). To a stirred solution of **DHA-C4** (128 mg, 0.31 mmol) in CH$_3$CN (3 mL) heated at 70 °C, 1-(quinolin-2-yl)-imidazole (78 mg, 0.40 mmol) was added and the reaction mixture was stirred for 3 days. Then, the solvent was removed under reduced pressure and the crude product was dissolved in CH_2Cl_2 and precipitated with Et_2O. This treatment was repeated three times to afford a white solid (111 mg, 58% yield). Anal. Calcd. for $C_{31}H_{40}BrN_3O_5$: C, 60.58; H, 6.56; N, 6.84. Found C, 60.45; H, 6.72; N, 6.75. ^{1}H-NMR (300 MHz, $CDCl_3$): δ 12.03 (s, 1H, H_2), 8.69–8.63 (m, 1H, H_{Quin}), 8.58–8.50 (m, 2H, H_{Quin}, H_4), 8.04 (d, J = 8.7 Hz, 1H, H_{Quin}), 7.88–7.74 (m, 2H, H_{Quin}, H_5), 7.70–7.57 (m, 1H, H_{Quin}), 7.57 (sl, 1H, H_{Quin}), 5.38 (s, 1H, H_{Art}), 4.78 (d, J = 3.7 Hz, 1H, H_{Art}), 4.70 (t, J = 7.3 Hz, 2H, H_{CH2}), 3.97–3.85 (m, 1H, H_{CH2}), 3.49–3.47 (m, 1H, H_{CH2}), 2.66–2.58 (m, 1H, H_{Art}), 2.44–2.30 (m, 1H, H_{Art}), 2.20–2.11 (m, 2H, H_{Art}), 2.02–1.96 (m, 1H, H_{Art}), 1.88–1.82 (m, 1H, H_{Art}), 1.81–1.64 (m, 4H, H_{CH2}), 1.42 (s, 2H, H_{Art}), 1.38 (s, 3H, H_{Art}), 1.28–1.25 (m, 1H, H_{Art}), 1.21–1.20 (m, 1H, H_{Art}), 0.97 (d, J = 6.4 Hz, 3H, H_{Art}), 0.96–0.93 (m, 1H, H_{Art}), 0.90 (d, J = 7.0, 3H, H_{Art}). ^{13}C NMR (101 MHz, $CDCl_3$): δ 146.1 (1C, C_{Quin}), 144.5 (1C, C_{Quin}), 141.7 (1C, C_{Quin}), 140.3 (1C, C_{Quin}), 137.0 (1C, C_2), 131.5 (1C, C_{Quin}), 128.8 (1C, C_{Quin}), 128.2 (1C, C_4), 127.8 (1C, C_{Quin}), 121.6 (1C, C_5), 119.0 (1C, C_{Quin}), 112.9 (1C, C_{Quin}), 104.2 (1C, C_{Art}), 102.3 (1C, C_{Art}), 88.0 (1C, C_{Art}), 81.1 (1C, C_{Art}), 65.9 (1C, C_{CH2}), 52.5 (1C, C_{Art}), 50.4 (1C, C_{Art}), 44.3 (1C, C_{Art}), 37.5 (1C, C_{Art}), 36.4 (1C, C_{Art}), 34.5 (1C, C_{Art}), 30.9 (1C, C_{Art}), 27.3 (1C, C_{CH2}), 26.5 (1C, C_{CH2}), 26.2 (1C, C_{Art}), 24.7 (1C, C_{Art}), 20.3 (1C, C_{Art}), 15.3 (1C, C_{CH2}), 13.1 (1C, C_{Art}). HRMS (ESI^+): calcd. for $C_{31}H_{40}N_3O_5$ m/z = 534.2962, found 534.2976.

Complex **Aubis(4-Bn)** **(20)**. Under a nitrogen atmosphere, K_2CO_3 (36 mg, 0.26 mmol) was added to **L4-Bn** (108 mg, 0.19 mmol) in dry CH_3CN (4 mL) and heated at 60 °C under stirring. Then, **Au(SMe$_2$)Cl** (25 mg, 0.09 mmol) was added and the mixture was stirred for 10 h. After cooling to room temperature, the solution was filtered through a pad of celite and the solvent removed under reduced pressure. The complex was purified by flash chromatography on silica with CH_2Cl_2-MeOH as eluent (100/0 to 100/10) to give a white solid (100 mg, 98% yield). Anal. Calcd. for $C_{58}H_{80}AuClN_4O_{10}$: C, 56.84; H, 6.58; N, 4.57. Found C, 56.75; H, 6.46; N, 4.51. ^{1}H-NMR (300 MHz, $CDCl_3$): δ 7.35–7.31 (m, 5H, H_{Bn}), 7.26 (sl, 2H, H_4, H_5), 5.45 (sl, 2H, H_{Bn}), 5.36 (s, 1H, H_{Art}), 5.32 (s, 1H, H_{CH2}), 4.77–4.71 (m, 1H, H_{Art}), 4.26 (t, J = 7.1 Hz, 2H, H_{CH2}), 3.81 (dt, J = 9.9, 6.3 Hz, 1H, H_{CH2}), 3.37 (dt, J = 9.9, 6.3 Hz, 2H, H_{CH2}), 2.66–2.58 (m, 1H, H_{Art}), 2.45–2.32 (m, 1H, H_{Art}), 2.16–2.11 (m, 1H, H_{Art}), 2.10–2.00 (m, 1H, H_{Art}), 1.97–1.86 (m, 3H, H_{CH2}, H_{Art}), 1.78–1.68 (m, 2H, H_{Art}), 1.65–1.54 (m, 2H, H_{Art}), 1.44 (s, 3H, H_{Art}), 1.34–1.24 (m, 2H, H_{Art}), 0.96 (d, J = 5.8 Hz, 3H, H_{Art}), 0.90 (d, J = 2.2 Hz, 1H, H_{Art}), 0.87 (d, J = 2.5 Hz, 3H, H_{Art}). ^{13}C NMR (75 MHz, $CDCl_3$): δ 183.6 (1C, C_2), 135.7 (1C, C_{Bn}), 129.1 (2C, C_{Bn}), 128.6 (1C, C_{Bn}), 127.4 (2C, C_{Bn}), 122.4 (1C, C_4), 121.8 (1C, C_5), 104.2 (1C, C_{Art}), 102.0 (1C, C_{Art}), 87.9 (1C, C_{Art}), 81.0 (1C, C_{Art}), 67.5 (1C, C_{Art}), 54.8 (1C, C_{Bn}), 52.5 (1C, C_{Art}), 51.3 (1C, C_{CH2}), 44.3 (1C, C_{Art}), 37.5 (1C, C_{Art}), 36.4 (1C, C_{Art}), 34.6 (1C, C_{Art}), 30.8 (1C, C_{Art}), 29.7 (1C, C_{CH2}), 28.2 (1C, C_{CH2}), 26.2 (1C, C_{Art}), 24.7 (1C, C_{Art}), 24.5 (1C, C_{Art}), 22.3 (1C, C_{CH2}), 13.1 (1C, C_{Art}). HRMS (ESI^+): calcd. for $C_{58}H_{80}AuN_4O_{10}$ m/z = 1189.5534, found 1189.5468.

Complex **Aubis(4-Mes)** **(21)**. Under a nitrogen atmosphere, K_2CO_3 (17 mg, 0.13 mmol) was added to **L4-Mes** (55 mg, 0.09 mmol) in dry CH_3CN (4 mL). The mixture was then heated at 60 °C. After, **Au(SMe$_2$)Cl** (15 mg, 0.05 mmol) was added and the mixture was stirred for 10 h. After cooling to room temperature, the solution was filtered through a pad of celite and the solvent removed under reduced pressure. The complex was purified by flash chromatography on silica with CH_2Cl_2-MeOH as eluent (100/0 to 100/10) to give a white solid (55 mg, 99% yield). Anal. Calcd. for $C_{62}H_{88}AuClN_4O_{10}$: C, 58.10; H, 6.92; N, 4.37. Found C, 58.19; H, 6.90; N, 4.37. ^{1}H-NMR (300 MHz, $CDCl_3$): δ 7.68 (t, J = 1.7 Hz, 1H, H_4), 6.97–6.94 (m, 3H, H_5, H_{Mes}), 5.36 (s, 1H, H_{Art}), 5.29 (s, 1H, H_{Art}), 4.75 (d, J = 3.5 Hz, 1H, H_{Art}), 4.10 (t, J = 6.9 Hz, 2H, H_{CH2}), 3.79 (dt, J = 9.8, 6.3 Hz, 1H, H_{CH2}), 3.34 (dt, J = 9.8, 6.4 Hz, 1H, H_{CH2}), 2.67–2.60 (m, 1H, H_{Art}), 2.38 (s, 6H, H_{Mes}), 2.09–1.99 (m, 2H, H_{Art}), 1.87 (d, J = 2.3 Hz, 9H, H_{CH2}, H_{Art}), 1.75 (sl, 3H, H_{Mes}), 1.68–1.61 (m, 2H, H_{CH2}), 1.43 (s, 3H, H_{Art}), 0.97 (d, J = 5.8 Hz, 3H, H_{Art}), 0.90 (d, J = 7.3 Hz, 4H, H_{Art}). ^{13}C NMR (101 MHz, $CDCl_3$): δ 183.9 (1C, C_2), 139.6 (1C, C_{Mes}), 134.9 (2C, C_{Mes}), 134.8 (1C, C_{Mes}), 129.2 (2C, C_{Mes}), 122.6 (1C, C_4), 122.5 (1C, C_5), 102.9 (1C, C_{Art}), 102.7 (1C, C_{Art}), 89.4 (1C, C_{Art}), 81.8 (1C, C_{Art}), 68.1 (1C, C_{CH2}), 51.7 (1C, C_{Art}), 46.7 (1C, C_{CH2}), 40.2 (1C, C_{Art}), 37.3 (1C, C_{Art}), 36.5 (1C, C_{Art}), 34.3 (1C, C_{Art}), 31.7 (1C, C_{Art}), 28.3 (1C, C_{CH2}), 26.6 (1C, C_{Art}), 26.0 (1C, C_{Art}),

24.7 (1C, C$_{Art}$), 21.2 (1C, C$_{CH2}$), 20.0 (1C, C$_{Mes}$), 19.4 (1C, C$_{Art}$), 17.6 (2C, C$_{Mes}$), 15.3 (1C, C$_{Art}$). HRMS (ESI$^+$): calcd. for C$_{62}$H$_{88}$AuN$_4$O$_{10}$ m/z = 1245.6166, found 1245.6188.

Complex **Aubis(4-Quin)** (**22**). Under a nitrogen atmosphere, K$_2$CO$_3$ (28 mg, 0.20 mmol) was added to **L4-Quin** (89 mg, 0.14 mmol) in dry CH$_3$CN (4 mL). The stirred mixture was then heated at 60 °C. Then, **Au(SMe$_2$)Cl** (30 mg, 0.10 mmol) was added and the mixture was stirred for 10 h. After cooling to room temperature, the solution was filtered through a pad of celite and the solvent removed under reduced pressure to give a white solid (84 mg, 92% yield). Anal. Calcd. For C$_{62}$H$_{78}$AuClN$_6$O$_{10}$: C, 57.29; H, 6.05; N, 6.47. Found C, 57.35; H, 6.01; N, 6.57. ^{1}H-NMR (400 MHz, CDCl$_3$): δ 8.41–8.29 (m, 1H, H$_{Quin}$), 8.20–8.14 (m, 1H, H$_{Quin}$), 8.09–8.05 (m, 1H, H$_4$), 7.90–7.85 (m, 1H, H$_{Quin}$), 7.79–7.73 (m, 1H, H$_{Quin}$), 7.71–7.64 (m, 1H, H$_{Quin}$), 7.57–7.47 (m, 2H, H$_5$, H$_{Quin}$), 5.35–5.32 (m, 1H, H$_{Art}$), 4.77–4.65 (m, 1H, H$_{Art}$), 4.46–4.45 (m, 2H, H$_{CH2}$), 3.93–3.91 (m, 1H, H$_{CH2}$), 3.81–3.74 (m, 1H, H$_{CH2}$), 3.29–3.35 (m, 2H, H$_{CH2}$), 2.63–2.62 (m, 1H, H$_{Art}$), 2.42–2.32 (m, 1H, H$_{Art}$), 2.15–2.11 (m, 2H, H$_{CH2}$), 2.07–1.96 (m, 1H, H$_{Art}$), 1.91–1.82 (m, 1H, H$_{Art}$), 1.74–1.66 (m, 2H, H$_{Art}$), 1.64–1.55 (m, 1H, H$_{Art}$), 1.43 (s, 1H, H$_{Art}$), 1.34–1.25 (m, 1H, H$_{Art}$), 1.25–1.21 (m, 3H, H$_{Art}$), 1.20–1.98 (m, 1H, H$_{Art}$), 1.22–1.16 (m, 1H, H$_{Art}$), 0.95 (d, *J* = 6.2 Hz, 3H, H$_{Art}$), 0.87–0.85 (m, 4H, H$_{Art}$). ^{13}C NMR (126 MHz, CDCl$_3$): δ 181.9 (1C, C$_2$), 149.2 (1C, C$_{Quin}$), 146.3 (1C, C$_{Quin}$), 139.8 (1C, C$_{Quin}$), 131.0 (1C, C$_{Quin}$), 128.5 (1C, C$_{Quin}$), 127.9 (1C, C$_{Quin}$), 127.7 (1C, C$_{Quin}$), 127.5 (1C, C$_{Quin}$), 122.4 (1C, C$_4$), 121.6 (1C, C$_5$), 116.1 (1C, C$_{Quin}$), 104.1 (1C, C$_{Art}$), 102.0 (1C, C$_{Art}$), 87.9 (1C, C$_{Art}$), 81.0 (1C, C$_{Art}$), 67.8 (1C, C$_{CH2}$), 65.9 (1C, C$_{CH2}$), 52.5 (C1, C$_{Art}$), 52.3 (1C, C$_{Art}$), 44.3 (1C, C$_{Art}$), 37.5 (1C, C$_{Art}$), 36.4 (1C, C$_{Art}$), 34.5 (1C, C$_{Art}$), 30.8 (1C, C$_{Art}$), 28.2 (1C, C$_{CH2}$), 26.2 (1C, C$_{Art}$), 24.7 (1C, C$_{Art}$), 20.3 (1C, C$_{Art}$), 15.3 (1C, C$_{CH2}$), 13.1 (1C, C$_{Art}$). HRMS (ESI$^+$): calcd. for C$_{62}$H$_{78}$AuN$_6$O$_{10}$ m/z = 1263.5439, found 1263.5468.

3′-Benzyl-1′-[10β-(22-pentoxy)dihydroartemisinin]1H-imidazol-3-ium bromide (**L5-Bn** (**10**)). To a stirred solution of **DHA-C5** (103 mg, 0.24 mmol) in CH$_3$CN (4 mL) heated at 70 °C, 1-benzylimidazole (34 mg, 0.21 mmol) was added and the reaction mixture was stirred 3 days. Then, the solvent was removed under reduced pressure and the crude product was dissolved in CH$_2$Cl$_2$ and precipitated with Et$_2$O. This treatment was repeated three times to afford a white solid (64 mg, 52% yield). Anal. Calcd. for C$_{30}$H$_{43}$BrN$_2$O$_5$: C, 60.91; H, 7.33; N, 4.74. Found C, 60.91; H, 7.45; N, 4.68. ^{1}H-NMR (300 MHz, CDCl$_3$): δ 10.73 (t, *J* = 1.6 Hz, 1H, H$_2$), 7.54–7.46 (m, 2H, H$_{Bn}$, H$_4$/H$_5$), 7.41–7.35 (m, 5H, H$_{Bn}$, H$_4$/H$_5$), 5.63 (s, 2H, H$_{Bn}$), 5.35 (s, 1H, H$_{Art}$), 4.75–4.71 (m, 1H, H$_{Art}$), 4.32–4.28 (m, 2H, H$_{CH2}$), 3.85–3.76 (m, 1H, H$_{CH2}$), 3.38–3.30 (m, 1H, H$_{CH2}$), 2.65–2.53 (m, 1H, H$_{Art}$), 2.41–2.30 (m, 1H, H$_{Art}$), 2.07–1.90 (m, 3H, H$_{Art}$), 1.89–1.82 (m, 1H, H$_{CH2}$), 1.78–1.68 (m, 3H, H$_{CH2}$, H$_{Art}$), 1.66–1.57 (m, 4H, H$_{CH2}$, H$_{Art}$), 1.41 (s, 3H, H$_{Art}$), 1.35–1.10 (m, 3H, H$_{Art}$), 0.95 (d, *J* = 6.1 Hz, 4H, H$_{Art}$), 0.85 (d, *J* = 7.3 Hz, 3H, H$_{Art}$). ^{13}C NMR (101 MHz, CDCl$_3$): δ 137.9 (1C, C$_2$), 135.0 (1C, C$_{Bn}$), 129.6 (1C, C$_{Bn}$), 129.5 (2C, C$_{Bn}$), 129.1 (2C, C$_{Bn}$), 121.4 (1C, C$_4$), 121.3 (1C, C$_5$), 104.1 (1C, C$_{Art}$), 102.1 (1C, C$_{Art}$), 89.7 (1C, C$_{Art}$), 81.1 (1C, C$_{Art}$), 67.9 (1C, C$_{CH2}$), 53.6 (1C, C$_{Bn}$), 52.6 (1C, C$_{Art}$), 50.0 (1C, C$_{Art}$), 44.4 (1C, C$_{Art}$), 37.5 (1C, C$_{Art}$), 36.4 (1C, C$_{Art}$), 34.6 (1C, C$_{Art}$), 30.9 (1C, C$_{CH2}$), 30.0 (1C, C$_{Art}$), 29.3 (1C, C$_{CH2}$), 29.0 (1C, C$_{CH2}$), 26.2 (1C, C$_{Art}$), 24.7 (1C, C$_{Art}$), 22.2 (1C, C$_{CH2}$), 20.4 (1C, C$_{Art}$), 13.1 (1C, C$_{Art}$). HRMS (ESI$^+$): calcd. for C$_{30}$H$_{43}$N$_2$O$_5$ m/z = 511,3172, found 511.3171.

3′-Mesityl-1′-[10β-(22-pentoxy)dihydroartemisinin]1H-imidazol-3-ium bromide (**L5-Mes** (**11**)). To a stirred solution of **DHA-C5** (160 mg, 0.37 mmol) in CH$_3$CN (4 mL) heated at 70 °C, 1-mesitylimidazole (51 mg, 0.27 mmol) was added and the reaction mixture was stirred for 3 days. The solvent was removed under reduced pressure and the crude product was dissolved in CH$_2$Cl$_2$ and precipitated with Et$_2$O. This treatment was repeated three times to afford a white solid (101 mg, 60% yield). Anal. Calcd. for C$_{32}$H$_{47}$BrN$_2$O$_5$: C, 62.03; H, 7.65; N, 4.52. Found C, 62.15; H, 7.75; N, 4.62. ^{1}H-NMR (400 MHz, CDCl$_3$): δ 10.64 (t, *J* = 1.5 Hz, 1H, H$_2$), 7.58 (t, *J* = 1.7 Hz, 1H, H$_4$), 7.16 (t, *J* = 1.8 Hz, 1H, H$_5$), 7.03 (sl, 2H, H$_{Mes}$), 5.40 (s, 1H, H$_{Art}$), 4.87–4.71 (m, 3H, H$_{Art}$, H$_{CH2}$), 3.85 (dt, *J* = 9.8, 6.4 Hz, 1H, H$_{CH2}$), 3.41 (dt, *J* = 9.8, 6.4 Hz, 1H, H$_{CH2}$), 2.69–2.59 (m, 1H, H$_{Art}$), 2.44–2.34 (m, 4H, H$_{Mes}$, H$_{Art}$), 2.11 (s, 6H, H$_{Mes}$), 2.10–2.01 (m, 3H, H$_{Art}$), 1.94–1.87 (m, 1H, H$_{Art}$), 1.76–1.74 (m, 2H, H$_{CH2}$, H$_{Art}$), 1.72–1.66 (m, 2H, H$_{CH2}$), 1.64 (s, 2H, H$_{CH2}$), 1.55–1.47 (m, 3H, H$_{Art}$), 1.45 (s, 3H, H$_{Art}$), 1.41–1.31 (m, 1H, H$_{Art}$), 1.30–1.23 (m, 1H, H$_{Art}$),

0.98 (d, J = 6.2 Hz, 3H, H$_{Art}$), 0.94–0.92 (m, 1H, H$_{Art}$), 0.90 (d, J = 7.4 Hz, 3H, H$_{Art}$). ^{13}C NMR (101 MHz, CDCl$_3$): δ 141.5 (1C, C$_{Mes}$), 138.7 (1C, C$_2$), 134.2 (2C, C$_{Mes}$), 130.6 (1C, C$_{Mes}$), 130.0 (2C, C$_{Mes}$), 122.9 (1C, C$_4$), 122.0 (1C, C$_5$), 104.1 (1C, C$_{Art}$), 102.1 (1C, C$_{Art}$), 88.0 (1C, C$_{Art}$), 81.1 (1C, C$_{Art}$), 68.0 (1C, C$_{CH2}$), 52.6 (1C, C$_{Art}$), 50.5 (1C, C$_{CH2}$), 44.4 (1C, C$_{Art}$), 37.5 (1C, C$_{Art}$), 36.4 (1C, C$_{Art}$), 34.6 (1C, C$_{Art}$), 30.9 (1C, C$_{Art}$), 30.4 (1C, C$_{CH2}$), 29.1 (1C, C$_{CH2}$), 26.2 (1C, C$_{Art}$), 24.7 (1C, C$_{Art}$), 24.5 (1C, C$_{Art}$), 23.0 (1C, C$_{CH2}$), 21.1 (1C, C$_{Art}$), 20.4 (1C, C$_{Mes}$), 17.7 (2C, C$_{Mes}$), 13.1 (1C, C$_{Art}$). HRMS (ESI$^+$): calcd. for C$_{32}$H$_{47}$N$_2$O$_5$ m/z = 539.3485, found 539.3490.

3′-Quinolin-2-yl-1′-[10β-(22-pentoxy)dihydroartemisinin]1H-imidazol-3-ium bromide (**L5-Quin** (12)). To a stirred solution of **DHA-C5** (142 mg, 0.33 mmol) in CH$_3$CN (3 mL) heated at 70 °C, 1-(quinolin-2-yl)-imidazole (84 mg, 0.43 mmol) was added and the reaction mixture was stirred for 3 days. Then, the solvent was removed under reduced pressure and the crude product was dissolved in CH$_2$Cl$_2$ and precipitated with Et$_2$O. This treatment was repeated three times to afford a white solid (136 mg, 66% yield). Anal. Calcd. for C$_{32}$H$_{42}$BrN$_3$O$_5$: C, 61.14; H, 6.73; N, 6.68. Found C, 61.18; H, 6.67; N, 6.69. ^{1}H-NMR (300 MHz, CDCl$_3$): δ 11.99 (s, 1H, H$_2$), 8.67–8.64 (m, 1H, H$_{Quin}$), 8.55–8.52 (m, 1H, H$_{Quin}$), 8.34–8.31 (m, 1H, H$_4$), 8.05–8.02 (m, 1H, H$_{Quin}$), 7.95–7.90 (m, 1H, H$_{Quin}$), 7.88–7.83 (m, 1H, H$_{Quin}$), 7.84–7.77 (m, 1H, H$_{Quin}$), 7.59–7.53 (m, 1H, H$_5$), 5.39–5.36 (m, 1H, H$_{Art}$), 4.78–4.75 (m, 1H, H$_{Art}$), 4.66–4.61 (m, 2H, H$_{CH2}$, H$_{Art}$), 3.84–3.80 (m, 1H, H$_{CH2}$), 3.69–3.65 (m, 1H, H$_{CH2}$), 3.46–3.31 (m, 3H, H$_{CH2}$), 2.69–2.52 (m, 1H, H$_{Art}$), 2.44–2.29 (m, 2H, H$_{Art}$), 2.19–2.08 (m, 2H, H$_{Art}$), 1.93–1.78 (m, 2H, H$_{Art}$), 1.75–1.67 (m, 4H, H$_{CH2}$), 1.58–1.47 (m, 4H, H$_{Art}$), 1.28–1.25 (m, 2H, H$_{Art}$), 0.96 (d, J = 6.4 Hz, 3H, H$_{Art}$), 0.95 (m, 1H, H$_{Art}$), 0.93 (d, J = 7.4 Hz, 3H, H$_{Art}$). ^{13}C NMR (101 MHz, CDCl$_3$): δ 146.1 (1C, C$_{Quin}$), 144.5 (1C, C$_{Quin}$), 141.6 (1C, C$_{Quin}$), 136.8 (1C, C$_2$), 131.5 (1C, C$_{Quin}$), 129.0 (1C, C$_{Quin}$), 128.8 (1C, C$_{Quin}$), 128.3 (1C, C$_{Quin}$), 128.1 (1C, C$_{Quin}$), 122.2 (1C, C$_4$), 119.0 (1C, C$_5$), 112.8 (1C, C$_{Quin}$), 104.3 (1C, C$_{Art}$), 102.1 (1C, C$_{Art}$), 87.9 (1C, C$_{Art}$), 81.1 (1C, C$_{Art}$), 67.9 (1C, C$_{CH2}$), 51.0 (1C, C$_{Art}$), 50.4 (1C, C$_{Art}$), 44.4 (1C, C$_{Art}$), 37.5 (1C, C$_{Art}$), 36.4 (1C, C$_{Art}$), 34.4 (1C, C$_{Art}$), 31.1 (1C, C$_{CH2}$), 30.0 (1C, C$_{Art}$), 29.5 (1C, C$_{CH2}$), 26.2 (1C, C$_{Art}$), 26.2 (1C, C$_{CH2}$), 23.1 (1C, C$_{Art}$), 22.2 (1C, C$_{CH2}$), 20.5 (1C, C$_{Art}$), 13.1 (1C, C$_{Art}$). HRMS (ESI$^+$): calcd. for C$_{32}$H$_{42}$N$_3$O$_5$ m/z = 548.3119, found 548.3118.

Complex **Aubis(5-Bn)** (24). Under a nitrogen atmosphere, K$_2$CO$_3$ (20 mg, 0.14 mmol) was added to **L5-Bn** (60 mg, 0.10 mmol) in dry CH$_3$CN (4 mL) and heated at 60 °C under stirring. Then, **Au(SMe$_2$)Cl** (15 mg, 0.05 mmol) was added and the mixture was stirred for 10 h. After cooling to room temperature, the solution was filtered through a pad of celite and the solvent removed under reduced pressure. The complex was purified by flash chromatography on silica with CH$_2$Cl$_2$-MeOH as eluent (100/0 to 100/10) to give a white solid (28 mg, 45% yield). Anal. Calcd. for C$_{60}$H$_{84}$AuClN$_4$O$_{10}$: C, 57.48; H, 6.75; N, 4.47. Found C, 57.58; H, 6.89; N, 4.32. ^{1}H-NMR (300 MHz, CDCl$_3$): δ 7.34–7.32 (m, 4H, H$_{Bn}$), 7.26–7.25 (m, 3H, H$_4$, H$_5$), 5.42 (s, 2H, H$_{Bn}$), 5.34 (s, 1H, H$_{Art}$), 4.74 (m, 1H, H$_{Art}$), 4.22–4.17 (m, 2H, H$_{CH2}$), 3.81–3.74 (m, 1H, H$_{CH2}$), 3.36–3.28 (m, 1H, H$_{CH2}$), 2.66–2.56 (m, 1H, H$_{Art}$), 2.42–2.32 (m, 1H, H$_{Art}$), 2.10–2.00 (m, 1H, H$_{Art}$), 1.96–1.82 (m, 3H, H$_{CH2}$), 1.76–1.68 (m, 3H, H$_{Art}$), 1.66–1.53 (m, 3H, H$_{CH2}$), 1.50–1.45 (s, 1H, H$_{Art}$), 1.40–1.18 (m, 6H, H$_{Art}$), 0.96–0.94 (m, 3H, H$_{Art}$), 0.91 (d, J = 7.4 Hz, 2H, H$_{Art}$), 0.86 (d, J = 7.3 Hz, 3H, H$_{Art}$). ^{13}C NMR (101 MHz, CDCl$_3$): δ 183.8 (1C, C$_2$), 135.7 (1C, C$_{Bn}$), 129.1 (2C, C$_{Bn}$), 128.6 (1C, C$_{Bn}$), 127.4 (2C, C$_{Bn}$), 122.3 (1C, C$_4$), 122.1 (1C, C$_5$), 104.1 (1C, C$_{Art}$), 101.9 (1C, C$_{Art}$), 87.9 (1C, C$_{Art}$), 81.1 (1C, C$_{Art}$), 67.9 (1C, C$_{CH2}$), 54.8 (1C, C$_{Bn}$), 52.5 (1C, C$_{Art}$), 51.5 (1C, C$_{CH2}$), 44.4 (1C, C$_{Art}$), 37.5 (1C, C$_{Art}$), 36.4 (1C, C$_{Art}$), 34.6 (1C, C$_{Art}$), 31.2 (1C, C$_{CH2}$), 30.9 (1C, C$_{Art}$), 29.2 (1C, C$_{CH2}$), 26.2 (1C, C$_{Art}$), 24.7 (1C, C$_{Art}$), 24.5 (1C, C$_{Art}$), 23.3 (1C, C$_{CH2}$), 20.4 (1C, C$_{Art}$), 13.1 (1C, C$_{Art}$). HRMS (ESI$^+$): calcd. for C$_{60}$H$_{84}$AuN$_4$O$_{10}$ m/z = 1217.5847, found 1217.5889.

Complex **Aubis(5-Mes)** (25). Under a nitrogen atmosphere, K$_2$CO$_3$ (36 mg, 0.26 mmol) was added to **L5-Mes** (101 mg, 0.16 mmol) in dry CH$_3$CN (4 mL). The mixture was then heated at 60 °C. After, **Au(SMe$_2$)Cl** (27 mg, 0.09 mmol) was added and the mixture was stirred for 10 h. After cooling to room temperature, the solution was filtered through a pad of celite and the solvent removed under reduced pressure. The complex was purified by flash chromatography on silica with CH$_2$Cl$_2$-MeOH as eluent (100/0 to 100/10) to give a white solid (78 mg, 74% yield). Anal. Calcd. for C$_{64}$H$_{92}$AuClN$_4$O$_{10}$:

C, 58.69; H, 7.08; N, 4.28. Found C, 58.78; H, 7.02; N, 4.31. ^{1}H-NMR (300 MHz, CDCl$_3$): δ 7.66 (d, J = 1.8 Hz, 1H, H$_4$), 6.97 (s, 2H, H$_{Mes}$), 6.93 (d, J = 1.8 Hz, 1H, H$_5$), 5.40 (s, 1H, H$_{Art}$), 4.78 (d, J = 3.3 Hz, 1H, H$_{Art}$), 4.11 (t, J = 6.9 Hz, 2H, H$_{CH2}$), 3.80 (dt, J = 9.7, 6.9 Hz, 1H, H$_{CH2}$), 3.34 (dt, J = 9.7, 6.9 Hz, 1H, H$_{CH2}$), 2.65–2.63 (m, 1H, H$_{Art}$), 2.40 (s, 3H, H$_{Mes}$), 2.35 (m, 1H, H$_{Art}$), 2.10–2.00 (m, 2H, H$_{Art}$), 1.96–1.90 (m, 1H, H$_{Art}$), 1.87 (d, J = 3.0 Hz, 6H, H$_{Mes}$), 1.82–1.73 (m, 6H, H$_{CH2}$), 1.72–1.60 (m, 3H, H$_{Art}$), 1.56–1.49 (m, 1H, H$_{Art}$), 1.45 (s, 4H, H$_{Art}$), 1.33–1.26 (m, 1H, H$_{Art}$), 0.98 (d, J = 6.0 Hz, 3H, H$_{Art}$), 0.95–0.92 (m, 1H, H$_{Art}$), 0.90 (d, J = 7.4 Hz, 3H, H$_{Art}$). ^{13}C NMR (101 MHz, CDCl$_3$): δ 183.8 (1C, C$_2$), 139.6 (1C, C$_{Mes}$), 134.8 (2C, C$_{Mes}$), 129.4 (1C, C$_{Mes}$), 129.2 (2C, C$_{Mes}$), 122.7 (1C, C$_4$), 122.5 (1C, C$_5$), 104.1 (1C, C$_{Art}$), 102.0 (1C, C$_{Art}$), 87.9 (1C, C$_{Art}$), 81.1 (1C, C$_{Art}$), 68.1 (1C, C$_{CH2}$), 52.5 (1C, C$_{Art}$), 51.1 (1C, C$_{CH2}$), 44.4 (1C, C$_{Art}$), 37.5 (1C, C$_{Art}$), 36.4 (1C, C$_{Art}$), 34.6 (1C, C$_{Art}$), 31.1 (1C, C$_{CH2}$), 30.9 (1C, C$_{Art}$), 29.3 (1C, C$_{CH2}$), 26.2 (1C, C$_{Art}$), 24.7 (1C, C$_{Art}$), 24.5 (1C, C$_{Art}$), 23.0 (1C, C$_{CH2}$), 21.2 (1C, C$_{Art}$), 20.4 (2C, C$_{Mes}$), 17.7 (1C, C$_{Mes}$), 13.1 (1C, C$_{Art}$). HRMS (ESI$^+$): calcd. for C$_{64}$H$_{92}$AuN$_4$O$_{10}$ m/z = 1273.6473, found 1273.6495.

Complex **Aubis(5-Quin)** (**26**). Under a nitrogen atmosphere, K$_2$CO$_3$ (37 mg, 0.27 mmol) was added to **L5-Quin** (121 mg, 0.19 mmol) in dry CH$_3$CN (4 mL). The stirred mixture was then heated at 60 °C. Then, **Au(SMe$_2$)Cl** (34 mg, 0.12 mmol) was added and the mixture was stirred for 10 h. After cooling to room temperature, the solution was filtered through a pad of celite and the solvent removed under reduced pressure to give a white solid (59 mg, 47% yield). Anal. Calcd. For C$_{64}$H$_{82}$AuClN$_6$O$_{10}$: C, 59.48; H, 6.40; N, 6.50. Found C, 59.45; H, 6.53; N, 6.45. ^{1}H-NMR (300 MHz, CDCl$_3$): δ 8.36 (m, 1H, H$_{Quin}$), 8.18 (m, 1H, H$_{Quin}$), 8.04 (m, 1H, H$_4$), 7.89 (m, 1H, H$_{Quin}$), 7.77 (m, 1H, H$_{Quin}$), 7.71–7.65 (m, 1H, H$_{Quin}$), 7.54 (m, 1H, H$_5$), 7.51–7.48 (m, 1H, H$_{Quin}$), 5.35–5.32 (m, 1H, H$_{Art}$), 4.71 (m, 1H, H$_{Art}$), 4.49–4.45 (m, 2H, H$_{Art}$), 3.73–3.70 (m, 1H, H$_{CH2}$), 3.53–3.46 (m, 3H, H$_{CH2}$), 3.30–3.22 (m, 1H, H$_{CH2}$), 2.63–2.57 (m, 1H, H$_{Art}$), 2.42–2.32 (m, 1H, H$_{Art}$), 2.13 (s, 1H, H$_{Art}$), 2.02 (sl, 2H, H$_{Art}$), 1.97–1.92 (m, 2H, H$_{Art}$), 1.75–1.69 (m, 1H, H$_{CH2}$), 1.61–1.59 (m, 1H, H$_{CH2}$), 1.54–1.49 (m, 2H, H$_{CH2}$), 1.44 (s, 3H, H$_{Art}$), 1.34–1.27 (m, 3H, H$_{Art}$), 0.94 (d, J = 5.9 Hz, 3H, H$_{Art}$), 0.87 (m, 1H, H$_{Art}$), 0.85 (d, J = 7.4 Hz, 3H, H$_{Art}$). ^{13}C NMR (75 MHz, CDCl$_3$): δ 181.8 (1C, C$_2$), 149.2 (1C, C$_{Quin}$), 146.3 (1C, C$_{Quin}$), 139.8 (1C, C$_{Quin}$), 130.9 (1C, C$_{Quin}$), 128.5 (1C, C$_{Quin}$), 127.9 (1C, C$_{Quin}$), 127.7 (1C, C$_{Quin}$), 127.5 (1C, C$_{Quin}$), 122.5 (1C, C$_4$), 121.5 (1C, C$_5$), 116.1 (1C, C$_{Quin}$), 104.1 (1C, C$_{Art}$), 101.9 (1C, C$_{Art}$), 88.0 (1C, C$_{Art}$), 81.0 (1C, C$_{Art}$), 67.9 (1C, C$_{CH2}$), 52.5 (C1, C$_{CH2}$), 52.5 (1C, C$_{Art}$), 50.6 (1C, C$_{CH2}$), 44.4 (1C, C$_{Art}$), 37.5 (1C, C$_{Art}$), 36.4 (1C, C$_{Art}$), 34.6 (1C, C$_{Art}$), 31.0 (1C, C$_{CH2}$), 30.8 (1C, C$_{Art}$), 29.1 (1C, C$_{CH2}$), 26.2 (1C, C$_{Art}$), 24.7 (1C, C$_{Art}$), 24.5 (1C, C$_{Art}$), 20.4 (1C, C$_{Art}$), 13.1 (1C, C$_{Art}$). HRMS (ESI$^+$): calcd. for C$_{64}$H$_{82}$AuN$_6$O$_{10}$ m/z = 1291.5758, found 1291.5785.

3.2. Biology

3.2.1. Parasite Cultures

The *Plasmodium falciparum* F32-ART and F32-TEM parasite lines, resistant and sensitive to artemisinins respectively [9,15], were cultured in vitro in type O human erythrocytes (Etablissement Français du sang (EFS), Toulouse, France), diluted to 2% hematocrit, in RPMI-1640 medium (GIBCO, Illkirch, France) and supplemented with 5% Human Serum AB (EFS, Toulouse, France) at 37 °C and 5% CO$_2$ [33]. Every other day and before each experiment, *P. falciparum* F32-ART and F32-TEM parasites were synchronized at ring stage using 5% D-sorbitol solution [34].

3.2.2. Evaluation of Antiplasmodial Activity

In vitro antiplasmodial activities of the synthesized hybrid molecules were evaluated against the *P. falciparum* strain F32-TEM (corresponding to the parental strain F32-Tanzania). Each molecule was tested at least in three independent experiments (except **Aubis(5-Bn)**, tested twice) by a SYBR Green Fluorescence assay [33] but also at least once with the standard chemosensitivity assay recommended by the WHO and based on the incorporation of [^{3}H] hypoxanthine [33].

For the SYBR Green Fluorescence assay, ring stage parasites were treated with the drugs for 48 h. Then, the pellets were washed twice with PBS and frozen at −20 °C. Thawed plates were incubated for

2 h at room temperature with the SYBR Green (Thermo-Fisher, Illkirch, France) lysis buffer (20 mm Tris base pH 7.5, 5 mm EDTA, 0.008% *w/v* saponin, 0.08% *w/v* Triton X-100). The plates were then read using a fluorescence plate reader (FLx800, BioTek, Illkirch, France) at an excitation wavelength of 485 nm and 535 nm for the emission wavelength. The IC_{50} values (concentration inhibiting 50% of the parasite's growth) were determined using GraphPad Prism software 7 (GraphPad Software, San Diego, CA, USA).

For [^{3}H] hypoxanthine assay, ring stage parasites were incubated with the drug dilutions for 24 h, then, [^{3}H] hypoxanthine (50 µL/0.25 µCi; Perkin-Elmer, Courtaboeuf, France) was added for another 24 h period. After that, plates were frozen at −20 °C. The next step is to thaw the plates and to collect the nucleic acids. Tritium incorporation was then determined thanks to a β-counter (Perkin-Elmer, Courtaboeuf, France).

The antiplasmodial activities reported in Table 1 correspond thus to the mean of IC_{50} values from at least 4 independent experiments acquired by the two methods, SYBR Green and radioactivity.

3.2.3. Evaluation of the Cytotoxicity

The most active compounds were tested for their cytotoxicity using the Vero cell line (monkey epithelial cell line), according to a previously described method [35] with some modifications. The cells were cultured in MEM medium (Dutscher, Brumath, France) supplemented with 10% fetal bovine serum (Dutscher), 0.7 mM glutamine and 100 µg/mL gentamicin.

The cells were seeded at 10^4 cells per well in a 96-well plates and incubated during 24 h. Then, cells were incubated for additional 48 h with the drugs. Cell proliferation was measured with MTT (1-(4,5-dimethylthiazol-2-yl)-3,5-diphenylformazan, Sigma, Saint-Quentin Fallavier, France) which is added to each well for 1 h at 37° C and 5% CO_2. Subsequently, DMSO was added to the wells containing the cells and MTT to dissolve the formed crystals. The plates were then read to determine the absorbance at wavelength of 540 nm (µQuant, BioTek, Illkirch, France). Cell proliferation was calculated from at least three independent experiments using GraphPad Prism software 7 (GraphPad Software, San Diego, CA, USA). The cytotoxic/antiplasmodial activity ratio corresponds to the selectivity index.

3.2.4. Recrudescence Assay

P. falciparum strains F32-ART and F32-TEM, synchronized at ring stage parasites at 3% parasitemia and 2% hematocrit have undergone a 48 h-treatment with the drugs to be tested. The parasites were then washed with RPMI-1640 medium and re-cultivated in drug-free culture conditions with 10% human serum. The parasitemia was then monitored daily to determine the time required for each parasite culture to recover the initial parasitemia of 3%. If no parasites were seen up to 30 days, the parasites were considered as "not recrudescent" [9,15]. The drug doses were chosen in order to discriminate the phenotype response between the artemisinin-resistant and the -sensitive strains. A range from 1-fold to >100-fold the antiplasmodial IC_{50} value previously found has been tested to determine the most appropriate drug dose to use in this recrudescence assay.

4. Conclusions

Three original families of gold(I) NHCs complexes incorporating a covalently attached DHA derivative were synthetized and fully characterized. All the proligands and complexes were tested for their antiplasmodial potency on the *P. falciparum* strains, F32-TEM artemisinin-sensitive and F32-ART artemisinin-resistant. Among the 29 compounds tested, ten gold(I) complexes have shown high antiplasmodial activities, with IC_{50} values less than 50 nM and very low cytotoxicity, with selectivity indexes up to 294. However, even though a simple gold(I) bis(NHC) had shown in a previous work [20] no cross-resistance with artemisinins, the presence of this metal could not prevent cross-resistance in the hybrid gold(I)-DHA complexes **Aubis(3-Me)**, **Aubis(4-Me)** and **Aubis(5-Me)** tested. These data confirm that the presence of an endoperoxide moiety whatever the structure and the other parts of the hybrid molecules tested leads to artemisinins cross-resistance. Therefore, these findings raise concerns about the potential development of new artemisinin derivatives and more broadly endoperoxide-based antiplasmodial drugs even if they include a moiety metabolically active on biochemical pathways involved in the quiescence state.

Author Contributions: Conceptualization, C.H. and H.G.; methodology, C.H.; synthesis, purification and characterization of the hybrid molecules, G.B. and Á.F.Á.; in vitro antimalarial and cytotoxic activities experiments, M.O.; in vitro cross-resistance assays, M.O.; writing-review and editing, C.H., H.G., M.O., F.B.-V. and J.-M.A.; supervision, C.H., H.G., F.B.-V. and J.-M.A.; funding acquisition, F.B.-V. All authors have read and agreed to the published version of the manuscript.

Funding: This study was supported in part by the French "Agence Nationale de la Recherche" (ANR grant INMAR ANR16 CE35 0003) and the "Centre National de la Recherche Scientifique".

Conflicts of Interest: The authors declare no conflict of interest. The founding sponsors had no role in the design of the study, analyses or interpretation of data, in the writing of the manuscript, and in the decision to publish the results.

References

1. World Health Organisation. *World Malaria Report*; WHO: Geneva, Suisse, 2018; ISBN 9789241565653.
2. Wongsrichanalai, C.; Meshnick, S.R. Declining Artesunate-Mefloquine Efficacy against Falciparum Malaria on the Cambodia–Thailand Border. *Emerg. Infect. Dis. J.* **2008**, *14*, 716. [CrossRef] [PubMed]
3. Amato, R.; Lim, P.; Miotto, O.; Amaratunga, C.; Dek, D.; Pearson, R.D.; Almagro-Garcia, J.; Neal, A.T.; Sreng, S.; Suon, S.; et al. Genetic markers associated with dihydroartemisinin–piperaquine failure in *Plasmodium falciparum* malaria in Cambodia: A genotype–phenotype association study. *Lancet Infect. Dis.* **2017**, *17*, 164–173. [CrossRef]
4. Witkowski, B.; Duru, V.; Khim, N.; Ross, L.S.; Saintpierre, B.; Beghain, J.; Chy, S.; Kim, S.; Ke, S.; Kloeung, N.; et al. A surrogate marker of piperaquine-resistant *Plasmodium falciparum* malaria: A phenotype–genotype association study. *Lancet Infect. Dis.* **2017**, *17*, 174–183. [CrossRef]
5. Ouji, M.; Augereau, J.M.; Paloque, L.; Benoit-Vical, F. *Plasmodium falciparum* resistance to artemisinin-based combination therapies: A sword of Damocles in the path toward malaria elimination. *Parasite* **2018**, *25*, 1–12. [CrossRef] [PubMed]
6. Walsh, J.J.; Coughlan, D.; Heneghan, N.; Gaynor, C.; Angus, B. A novel artemisinin-quinine hybrid with potent antimalarial activity. *Bioorg. Med. Chem. Lett.* **2007**, *17*, 3599–3602. [CrossRef]
7. Fröhlich, T.; Karagöz, A.Ç.; Reiter, C.; Tsogoeva, S.B. Artemisinin-derived dimers: Potent antimalarial and anticancer agents. *J. Med. Chem.* **2006**, *59*, 7360–7388. [CrossRef]
8. Elsohly, M.A.; Gul, W.; Khan, S.L.; Tekwani, B.L. New orally active artemisinin dimer antimalarials. *World J. Tradit. Chin. Med.* **2017**, *3*, 3. [CrossRef]
9. Witkowski, B.; Lelièvre, J.; Barragán, M.J.L.; Laurent, V.; Su, X.Z.; Berry, A.; Benoit-Vical, F. Increased tolerance to artemisinin in plasmodium *falciparum* is mediated by a quiescence mechanism. *Antimicrob. Agents Chemother.* **2010**, *54*, 1872–1877. [CrossRef]
10. Ariey, F.; Witkowski, B.; Amaratunga, C.; Beghain, J.; Langlois, A.C.; Khim, N.; Kim, S.; Duru, V.; Bouchier, C.; Ma, L.; et al. A molecular marker of artemisinin-resistant *Plasmodium falciparum* malaria. *Nature* **2014**, *505*, 50–55. [CrossRef]
11. Teuscher, F.; Gatton, M.L.; Chen, N.; Peters, J.; Kyle, D.E.; Cheng, Q. Artemisinin-Induced Dormancy in *Plasmodium falciparum*: Duration, Recovery Rates, and Implications in Treatment Failure. *J. Infect. Dis.* **2010**, *202*, 1362–1368. [CrossRef]
12. Intharabut, B.; Kingston, H.W.; Srinamon, K.; Ashley, E.A.; Imwong, M.; Dhorda, M.; Woodrow, C.; Stepniewska, K.; Silamut, K.; Day, N.P.J.; et al. Artemisinin Resistance and Stage Dependency of Parasite Clearance in Falciparum Malaria. *J. Infect. Dis.* **2019**, *219*, 1483–1489. [CrossRef] [PubMed]
13. Paloque, L.; Ramadani, A.P.; Mercereau-Puijalon, O.; Augereau, J.M.; Benoit-Vical, F. *Plasmodium falciparum*: Multifaceted resistance to artemisinins. *Malar. J.* **2016**, *15*, 149. [CrossRef] [PubMed]
14. Chen, N.; LaCrue, A.N.; Teuscher, F.; Waters, N.C.; Gatton, M.L.; Kyle, D.E.; Cheng, Q. Fatty acid synthesis and pyruvate metabolism pathways remain active in dihydroartemisinin-induced dormant ring stages of plasmodium *falciparum*. *Antimicrob. Agents Chemother.* **2014**, *58*, 4773–4781. [CrossRef] [PubMed]

15. Ménard, S.; Haddou, T.B.; Ramadani, A.P.; Ariey, F.; Iriart, X.; Beghain, J.; Bouchier, C.; Witkowski, B.; Berry, A.; Mercereau-Puijalon, O.; et al. Induction of multidrug tolerance in *Plasmodium falciparum* by extended artemisinin pressure. *Emerg. Infect. Dis.* **2015**, *21*, 1733–1741. [CrossRef] [PubMed]
16. Peatey, C.L.; Chavchich, M.; Chen, N.; Gresty, K.J.; Gray, K.A.; Gatton, M.L.; Waters, N.C.; Cheng, Q. Mitochondrial Membrane Potential in a Small Subset of Artemisinin-Induced Dormant *Plasmodium falciparum* Parasites in vitro. *J. Infect. Dis.* **2015**, *212*, 426–434. [CrossRef]
17. Krnajski, Z.; Gilberger, T.W.; Walter, R.D.; Cowman, A.F.; Müller, S. Thioredoxin reductase is essential for the survival of *Plasmodium falciparum* erythrocytic stages. *J. Biol. Chem.* **2002**, *277*, 25970–25975. [CrossRef] [PubMed]
18. Hemmert, C.; Fabié, A.; Fabre, A.; Benoit-Vical, F.; Gornitzka, H. Synthesis, structures, and antimalarial activities of some silver(I), gold(I) and gold(III) complexes involving N-heterocyclic carbene ligands. *Eur. J. Med. Chem.* **2013**, *60*, 64–75. [CrossRef]
19. Hemmert, C.; Ramadani, A.P.; Boselli, L.; Fernández Álvarez, Á.; Paloque, L.; Augereau, J.-M.; Gornitzka, H.; Benoit-Vical, F. Antiplasmodial activities of gold(I) complexes involving functionalized N-heterocyclic carbenes. *Bioorg. Med. Chem.* **2016**, *24*, 3075–3082. [CrossRef]
20. Ouji, M.; Delmas, S.B.; Álvarez, Á.F.; Augereau, J.-M.; Valentin, A.; Hemmert, C.; Gornitzka, H.; Benoit-Vical, F. Design, Synthesis and Efficacy of Hybrid Triclosan-gold Based Molecules on Artemisinin-resistant *Plasmodium falciparum* and *Leishmania infantum* Parasites. *ChemistrySelect* **2020**, *5*, 619–625. [CrossRef]
21. Paloque, L.; Hemmert, C.; Valentin, A.; Gornitzka, H. Synthesis, characterization, and antileishmanial activities of gold(I) complexes involving quinoline functionalized N-heterocyclic carbenes. *Eur. J. Med. Chem.* **2015**, *94*, 22–29. [CrossRef]
22. Zhang, C.; Bourgeade Delmas, S.; Fernández Álvarez, Á.; Valentin, A.; Hemmert, C.; Gornitzka, H. Synthesis, characterization, and antileishmanial activity of neutral N-heterocyclic carbenes gold(I) complexes. *Eur. J. Med. Chem.* **2018**, *143*, 1635–1643. [CrossRef] [PubMed]
23. Boselli, L.; Ader, I.; Carraz, M.; Hemmert, C.; Cuvillier, O.; Gornitzka, H. Synthesis, structures, and selective toxicity to cancer cells of gold(I) complexes involving N-heterocyclic carbene ligands. *Eur. J. Med. Chem.* **2014**, *85*, 87–94. [CrossRef] [PubMed]
24. Zhang, C.; Hemmert, C.; Gornitzka, H.; Cuvillier, O.; Zhang, M.; Sun, R.W.-Y. Cationic and Neutral N-Heterocyclic Carbene Gold(I) Complexes: Cytotoxicity, NCI-60 Screening, Cellular Uptake, Inhibition of Mammalian Thioredoxin Reductase, and Reactive Oxygen Species Formation. *ChemMedChem* **2018**, *13*, 1218–1229. [CrossRef] [PubMed]
25. Zhang, C.; Maddelein, M.L.; Wai-Yin Sun, R.; Gornitzka, H.; Cuvillier, O.; Hemmert, C. Pharmacomodulation on Gold-NHC complexes for anticancer applications—Is lipophilicity the key point? *Eur. J. Med. Chem.* **2018**, *157*, 320–332. [CrossRef] [PubMed]
26. Bindoli, A.; Rigobello, M.P.; Scutari, G.; Gabbiani, C.; Casini, A.; Messori, L. Thioredoxin reductase: A target for gold compounds acting as potential anticancer drugs. *Coord. Chem. Rev.* **2009**, *253*, 1692–1707. [CrossRef]
27. Haynes, R.K.; Chan, H.-W.; Ho, W.-Y.; Ko, C.K.-F.; Gerena, L.; Kyle, D.E.; Peters, W.; Robinson, B.L. Convenient Access Both to Highly Antimalaria-Active 10-Arylaminoartemisinins, and to 10-Alkyl Ethers Including Artemether, Arteether, and Artelinate. *ChemBioChem* **2005**, *6*, 659–667. [CrossRef] [PubMed]
28. Zhang, C.; Fortin, P.-Y.; Barnoin, G.; Qin, X.; Wang, X.; Fernandez Alvarez, A.; Bijani, C.; Maddelein, M.-L.; Hemmert, C.; Cuvillier, O.; et al. Artemisinin-Derivative-NHC-gold(I)-Hybrid with Enhanced Cytotoxic Activity Through Inhibiting NRF2 Transcriptional Activity. *Angew. Chem. Int. Ed.* **2020**. [CrossRef]
29. Strassner, T.; Unger, Y.; Zeller, A. Use of Pt- and Pd-bis- and tetracarbon complexes with bridged carbon ligands in OLEDs. 20090326237, 31 December 2009.
30. Witkowski, B.; Khim, N.; Chim, P.; Kim, S.; Ke, S.; Kloeung, N.; Chy, S.; Duong, S.; Leang, R.; Ringwald, P.; et al. Reduced artemisinin susceptibility of *Plasmodium falciparum* ring stages in western Cambodia. *Antimicrob. Agents Chemother.* **2013**, *57*, 914–923. [CrossRef] [PubMed]
31. Paloque, L.; Witkowski, B.; Lelièvre, J.; Ouji, M.; Ben Haddou, T.; Ariey, F.; Robert, A.; Augereau, J.M.; Ménard, D.; Meunier, B.; et al. Endoperoxide-based compounds: Cross-resistance with artemisinins and selection of a *Plasmodium falciparum* lineage with a K13 non-synonymous polymorphism. *J. Antimicrob. Chemother.* **2018**, *73*, 395–403. [CrossRef] [PubMed]

32. Straimer, J.; Gnädig, N.F.; Stokes, B.H.; Ehrenberger, M.; Crane, A.A.; Fidock, D.A. *Plasmodium falciparum* K13 mutations differentially impact ozonide susceptibility and parasite fitness in vitro. *MBio* **2017**, *8*, e00172-17. [CrossRef] [PubMed]
33. Desjardins, R.E.; Canfield, C.J.; Haynes, J.D.; Chulay, J.D. Quantitative assessment of antimalarial activity in vitro by a semiautomated microdilution technique. *Antimicrob. Agents Chemother.* **1979**, *16*, 710–718. [CrossRef] [PubMed]
34. Lambros, C.; Vanderberg, J.P. Synchronization of *Plasmodium falciparum* Erythrocytic Stages in Culture. *J. Parasitol.* **1979**, *65*, 418. [CrossRef] [PubMed]

35. Tengchaisri, T.; Chawengkirttikul, R.; Rachaphaew, N.; Reutrakul, V.; Sangsuwan, R.; Sirisinha, S. Antitumor activity of triptolide against cholangiocarcinoma growth in vitro and in hamsters. *Cancer Lett.* **1998**, *133*, 169–175. [CrossRef]

Sample Availability: Samples of the compounds are available from the authors.

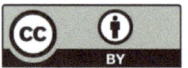

© 2020 by the authors. Licensee MDPI, Basel, Switzerland. This article is an open access article distributed under the terms and conditions of the Creative Commons Attribution (CC BY) license (http://creativecommons.org/licenses/by/4.0/).

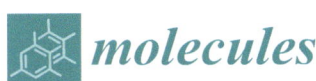

Article

A Self-Assembling NHC-Pd-Loaded Calixarene as a Potent Catalyst for the Suzuki-Miyaura Cross-Coupling Reaction in Water

Arnaud Peramo [1], Ibrahim Abdellah [2], Shannon Pecnard [1], Julie Mougin [1], Cyril Martini [2,3], Patrick Couvreur [1], Vincent Huc [2,*] and Didier Desmaële [1,*]

[1] Institut Galien Paris-Sud, CNRS UMR 8612, Université Paris-Saclay, Faculté de Pharmacie, 5 rue JB Clément, 92296 Châtenay-Malabry, France; arnaud.peramo@gmail.com (A.P.); shannon.pecnard@u-psud.fr (S.P.); julie.mougin@u-psud.fr (J.M.); patrick.couvreur@u-psud.fr (P.C.)

[2] Institut de Chimie Moléculaire et des Matériaux d'Orsay, CNRS UMR 8182, Université Paris Saclay, Bâtiment 420, 91405 Orsay, France; ibrahim_abdellah@hotmail.com (I.A.); cyril.martini@novecal.com (C.M.)

[3] NOVECAL, 86 rue de Paris, 91400 Orsay, France

* Correspondence: vincent.huc@u-psud.fr (V.H.); didier.desmaele@u-psud.fr (D.D.); Tel.: +33-(0)-1-6915-7436 (V.H.); +33-(0)-1-4683-5753 (D.D.)

Academic Editor: Yves Canac
Received: 9 March 2020; Accepted: 22 March 2020; Published: 24 March 2020

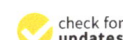

Abstract: Nanoformulated calix[8]arenes functionalized with N-heterocyclic carbene (NHC)-palladium complexes were found to be efficient nano-reactors for Suzuki-Miyaura cross-coupling reactions of water soluble iodo- and bromoaryl compounds with cyclic triol arylborates at low temperature in water without any organic co-solvent. Combined with an improved one-step synthesis of triol arylborates from boronic acid, this remarkably efficient new tool provided a variety of 4′-arylated phenylalanines and tyrosines in good yields at low catalyst loading with a wide functional group tolerance.

Keywords: NHC; nanoparticle; calixarene; palladium catalyst; Suzuki-Miyaura reaction; amino-acids; water

1. Introduction

The Suzuki-Miyaura reaction has emerged as one of the most powerful tool for C–C bond formation because of its compatibility with a broad range of functional groups giving rise to numerous applications throughout organic chemistry, synthesis of pharmaceutical compounds [1–3] and materials science [4,5]. Aqueous Suzuki-Miyaura cross-coupling reactions are particularly promising due to the water tolerance of boronic acids compared with the organometallic reagents required for other cross-coupling protocols. As a consequence, the Suzuki-Miyaura reaction has been widely developed under homogenous or heterogenous catalytic conditions in water media and a large array of different ligands and palladium complexes including micellar catalysis conditions nanoparticulate formulations have been designed to increase efficiency under aqueous conditions [6–16]. The water and functional group tolerance of the Suzuki-Miyaura reaction culminated in the cross-coupling of iodoarylated proteins under physiological conditions opening the way to a realm of chemical-biology applications [17–20]. Reactions in water are not restricted to those with biomolecules: due to water's ideal proprieties (abundance, environmental compatibility, non-toxicity and nonflammability) a wide range of catalytic and organic reactions have been developed in water as solvent [21]. In this context, calixarene macromolecules have been used for Suzuki-Miyaura cross-coupling reactions as supports for palladium catalyst. In particular, calix[4]arenes bearing phosphine or N-heterocyclic carbene (NHC) ligands have demonstrated good catalytic efficiencies in this reaction [22–26]. There are a few examples of the use of calix[4]arenes as catalyst supports in mixtures of water and dioxane [22], however, to our knowledge no reactions in pure water have been reported using unsupported calixarene. Recently, the synthesis of a large-cavity calix[8]arene anchoring eight NHC-palladium catalytic heads (Pd-Calix, Figure 1) was reported [27]. This catalyst demonstrated good catalytic properties and low metal leaching for Suzuki-Miyaura cross-coupling reactions with bromoarenes in green solvent such as ethanol, but the Pd-Calix was also tested in water/organic mixtures giving promising results. On the other hand this catalyst was found much less efficient in pure water [27]. Assuming that nanoparticles (NPs) embedding the Pd-Calix would show improved catalytic efficiency over the bulk material, a nanoformulation of this Pd-Calix was realized. Herein we describe the use of Pd-Calix nanosuspension (Pd-Calix-NS) as an efficient catalyst for the Suzuki-Miyaura reaction in aqueous solution at 37 °C. A variety of water-soluble cyclic triolborates were obtained in a one-step process from boronic acids, and their reactions with different haloarenes under Suzuki-Miyaura cross-coupling conditions using the Pd-Calix-NS are described.

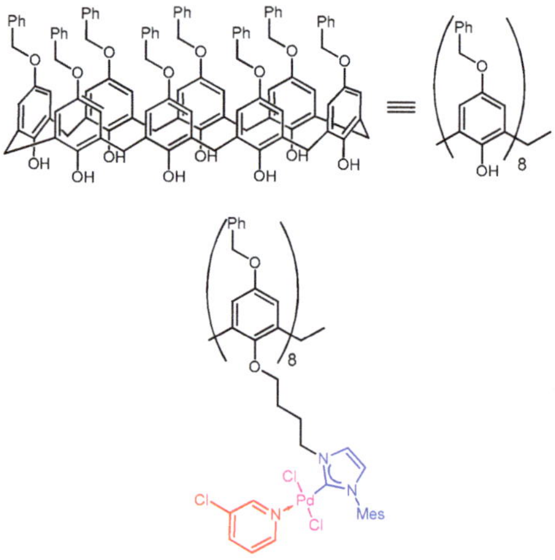

Figure 1. General structure of calix [8]arenes (top) and structure of the calix[8]arene bearing eight NHC-palladium units (Pd-Calix) (bottom). Mes = Mesityl.

2. Results and Discussion

The calix [8] arene-NHC-Pd catalyst was synthesized according to the method previously reported [27]. Briefly, chlorobutyl appendages were first bound to the eight free phenol groups of benzyloxycalix[8]arene and the chlorides then displaced with 3-(mesityl)-2,3-dihydro-1*H*-imidazole. The palladium carbene complexes were next generated with palladium chloride in the presence of potassium carbonate and 3-chloropyridine as extra ligand.

Formulation of Pd-Calix was first performed using the nanoprecipitation/solvent evaporation method using THF as organic solvent [28]. Nanoparticles with a 116 nm average hydrodynamic diameter were obtained as revealed by dynamic light scattering (DLS) (Table 1). Unfortunately, this formulation was found quite unstable after few days. To address this problem, the emulsion-solvent evaporation method was attempted using CH_2Cl_2 to solubilize the catalyst [29]. The organic phase was poured into an aqueous solution containing sodium cholate (1.5%) as surfactant, the two phases were emulsified by sonication and the solvent was evaporated.

Monodisperse NPs with a mean diameter of 112 nm (Z average determined by DLS) and a polydispersity index (PdI) of 0.2 were thus obtained. The formulation was found stable upon 30-day storage thanks to their quite negative zeta potential (Table 1). CryoTEM imaging revealed spherical NPs in line with DLS measurements (Figure 2).

Table 1. Size, polydispersity index (PDI) and ζ-Potential of the Pd-Calix-NPs as measured by dynamic light scattering according to the method of preparation.

Method of Formulation	Size (nm)	PDI	ζ-Potential (mV)
Nanoprecipitation	116	0.18	−3.14
Emulsion evaporation	112	0.21	−16.8

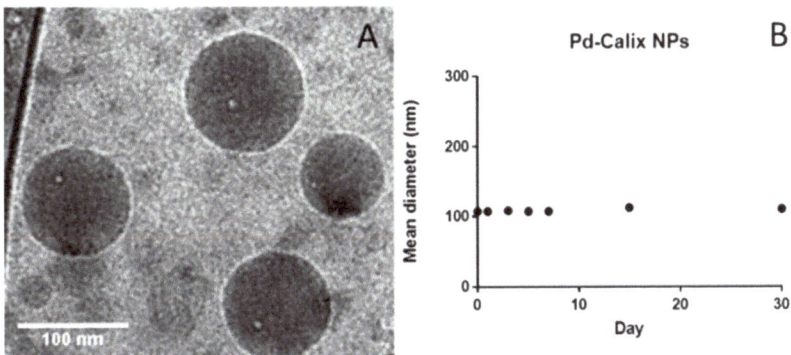

Figure 2. (**A**): Cryo-TEM images of the nanoparticles of the Pd-Calix-NS prepared by emulsion-solvent evaporation; (**B**): Evolution of the mean diameter of the nanoparticles of the Pd-Calix-NS upon incubation at 25 °C in water over one-month.

Following our early finding that palladium stabilized PLGA-PEG NPs were an efficient catalyst for the Suzuki-Miyaura couplings of 4-iodophenylalanine with phenylboronic acid derivatives, we chose to evaluate the present catalyst in the same model reaction [30]. Thus, reaction of N-Boc-4-iodo-L-phenylalanine (**1a**) with phenylboronic acid in the presence of 0.005 mol% of Pd-Calix-NS (0.04 mol% of Pd per mol of substrate) in pH 8.0 phosphate buffer at 37 °C reached 40% conversion into diphenylalanine **3a** after 3 h (Table 2, entry 1).

Although boronic acids are the originally used organoboron derivative for Suzuki-Miyaura reaction, they suffered from some drawbacks such as protodeboronation and oxidation. More nucleophilic organoboron reagents were thus developed with an improved stability and reactivity profile [31]. Among them, potassium phenylfluoroborate [32] and N-methyliminodiacetic acid phenylboronates (MIDA) [33] provided very low conversion rate or no reaction. On the other hand, cyclic triol phenylborate [34] turned out to give a full conversion in 3 h using 0.005 mol% of catalyst (0.04 mol% of palladium) per mol of substrate (Table 2, entry 4). Such a superior reactivity of borate salts squared with our previous results with Pd NPs stabilized by PLGA-PEG in water [30]. The hydrolytic stability of the cyclic triol borate derivatives in the reaction conditions (checked by NMR in D_2O-PBS) must be emphasized and clearly accounted for the efficiency of the process. Interestingly, there was no need of added base to carry out the reaction and the control of the pH was simply achieved using PBS buffer. This feature is of crucial interest to enlarge the process to biomolecules.

To evaluate the influence of the nanoformulation, the bulk catalyst without sodium cholate was used at the same concentration on the same benchmark reaction (Table 2, entry 4). However, less than 5% of conversion was observed highlighting the tremendous impact of the nano-reactor design on the catalysis efficiency. Interestingly, the amount of catalyst can be further diminished to 0.001 mol% on small scale reactions (3–4 mg) without reducing the overall conversion rate, highlighting the remarkable catalytic efficiency of the present nanosuspension. Although similar full conversion was achieved with the Pd-PLGA-PEG NPs catalyst (Entry 6), this formulation suffered of long-term stability issue. On the other hand, the water-soluble Davis catalyst (Entry 7) is very easy to handle but required much higher amount of palladium.

Table 2. Influence of the organoboron derivative on the cross-coupling reaction of N-Boc-4-iodo-L-phenylalanine.

Entry	Pd Catalyst	X	Conv (%) [a]
1	Pd-Calix-NS	B(OH)$_2$	40
2	Pd-Calix-NS	BF$_3$-K$^+$	10
3	Pd-Calix-NS	N-methyl-boronic acid MIDA ester	0
4	Pd-Calix-NS	cyclic triol borate K$^+$	98
5	Bulk Pd-Calix	cyclic triol borate K$^+$	<5
6	Pd-PLGA-PEG NPs	cyclic triol borate K$^+$	97[b]
7	[NaO-pyrimidine-NH$_2$]$_2$ Pd(OAc)$_2$	B(OH)$_2$	95[c]

[a] N-Boc-4-iodo-L-phenylalanine (1 equiv.), boronic acid derivatives (3 equiv.), Pd-Calix-NS (0.005 mol%), phosphate buffer (20 mM, pH = 8), 37 °C for 3 h. Conversion determined by ^{1}H NMR analysis of the C-3 methylene signal. [b] 0.01% Pd, according to reference [30]. [c] 1 mol% Pd, according to reference [18].

Having identified the best organoboron partner we turned our efforts to expand the scope of the process to other water-soluble aryl halides. The results obtained using various halides with cyclic triol phenylborate **2a** and 0.005 mol% of Pd-Calix-NS as catalyst are summarized in Figure 3. The influence of the halide was briefly investigated. 4-Iodo- and 4-bromophenylalanine underwent reaction with similar high yield. By contrast the chloride derivative **1c** was found completely unreactive. In addition to amino acid derivatives, we investigated several water soluble simple aromatic halides. The presence of carboxylic acid, phenol or amino groups on the arene ring did not affect the reaction, the main limitation being the solubility of the starting material in water. Even 2-iodoaniline underwent the desired coupling albeit at lower rate.

The influence of the structure of the cyclic triol borate was next explored. Synthesis of cyclic triol borates from boronic acids usually involved initial ester formation with 1,1,1-tris (hydroxymethyl) ethane in toluene with azeotropic removal of water followed by cyclization upon treatment with KOH in the same conditions. We found that the requisite cyclic triol borates can more easily be obtained in a one-step process from boronic acids by a simple stirring with the triol in the presence of 1 equiv. of KOH in dioxane at 30 °C.

The desired compounds were then isolated by simple filtration. This new method was found more convenient that the original procedure and was amenable to large laboratory scale preparation [34]. The bench-stable borate salts were thus obtained in good yields with a variety of aryl and heteroaryl compounds (Table 3). Hindered or electron poor boronic acids required longer reaction time (compounds **2g**, **2h**). Replacement of KOH base by another alkaline earth metal afforded the corresponding metal borate salt in similar yield (compounds **2b–d**). On the other hand, the poorly crystallizing tetrabutylammonium cyclic triol borate (**2e**) was obtained in only 20% yield.

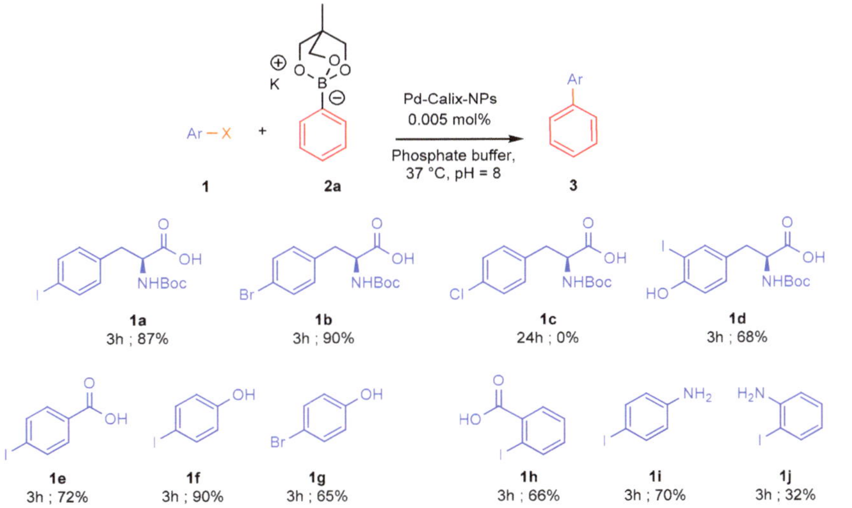

Figure 3. Reactivity of cyclic phenyltriolborate with selected water-soluble aryl halides. Aryl halide (1 equiv.), cyclic triol phenylborate (3 equiv.), Pd-Calix-NS (0.005 mol%), phosphate buffer (20 mM, pH = 8), 37 °C 3 h. Isolated yield after chromatographic purification.

Table 3. Synthesis of cyclic triolborates from boronic acids.

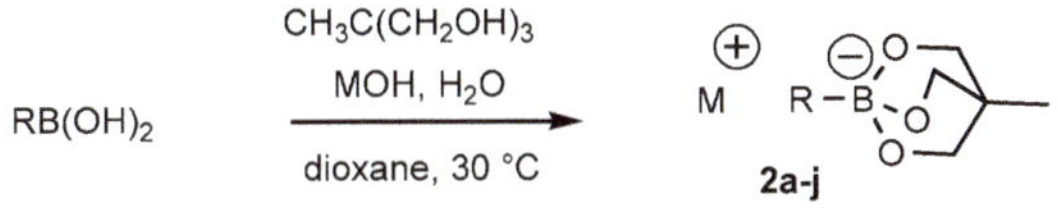

Compound	R	M	Time (h)	Yield (%)
2a	Ph	K	3	80
2b	Ph	Li	3	46
2c	Ph	Na	3	87
2d	Ph	Cs	3	67
2e	Ph	n-Bu$_4$N	3	20
2f	p-MeOPh	K	3	69
2g	o-Tol	K	16	59[a]
2h	m-NO$_2$Ph	K	16	72
2i	2-furanyl	K	3	67
2j	3-thiophenyl	K	3	65

[a] The reaction was conducted at 60 °C.

With the small library of cyclic triol borate salts in hand, their reaction with N-Boc-4-iodo-L-phenylalanine (**1a**) was next examined (Table 4). The screenings of the influence of the counter anion clearly established that potassium and at a lesser extend sodium salts were the most effective. On the other hand the NBu$_4$ counter ion was found detrimental to the efficiency of the coupling. It appears that electron withdrawing group on the aromatic ring or steric hindrance made the reaction slower. Nevertheless both, 3′-nitrodiphenylalanine (**3ah**) and [(2′-methylphenyl) phenyl] alanine (**3ag**) were isolated in good yields by prolonging the reaction time to 16 h. Moreover, when the pH was reduced to 7 and 6 the coupling still took place with only a small reduction of yield (Entries **2** and **3**). The latter result may be useful for substrates poorly soluble at basic pH and to conduct reaction with biomolecules at physiological pH [35]. Heterocyclic triolborates, including furan and thiophene rings could also be used affording **3ai**, **3aj** in satisfactory yields. Possibility to recycle the catalyst was briefly investigated. Unfortunately attempts to resuspend the catalyst pellet obtained by centrifugation after the first reaction cycle failed, presumably because it was not possible to adjust the require amount of sodium cholate.

Table 4. Reactivity of aryl and heteroaryl cyclic triolborates with *N*-Boc-4-iodophenylalanine.

Entry	Cyclic borate	R	Metal	pH	Product	Yield(%) [a]
1	2a	Ph	K	8.0	3a	98
2	2a	Ph	K	7.0	3a	67
3	2a	Ph	K	6.0	3a	56
4	2b	Ph	Li	8.0	3a	30
5	2c	Ph	Na	8.0	3a	90
6	2d	Ph	Cs	8.0	3a	47
7	2e	Ph	TBA	8.0	3a	22
8	2f	*p*-MeOPh	K	8.0	3af	98
9	2g	*o*-Tol	K	8.0	3ag	79 [b]
10	2h	*m*-NO$_2$Ph	K	8.0	3ah	72 [b]
11	2i	2-furanyl	K	8.0	3ai	87
12	2j	3-thiophenyl	K	8.0	3aj	63

[a] The reaction was conducted at 60 °C.

3. Experimental

3.1. General Information

Infrared (IR) spectra were obtained using a Fourier Transform Bruker Vector 22 spectrometer. Only significant absorptions are listed. The ^{1}H and ^{13}C NMR were recorded using a Bruker Advance 300 (300 and 75 MHz, respectively) spectrometer. Recognition of methyl, methylene, methine and quaternary carbon nuclei in ^{13}C NMR spectra rests on the J-modulated spin-echo sequence. All chemical shifts are quoted on the δ scale in ppm using residual solvent as the internal standard (^{1}H NMR: CDCl$_3$ = 7.26; D$_2$O = 4.79; DMSO-d_6 = 2.50; D$_3$COD = 3.33 and ^{13}C NMR: DMSO-d_6 = 39.5). Coupling constants (J) are reported in Hz with the following splitting abbreviations: s = singlet, d = doublet, t = triplet, q = quartet, quint = quintet and m = multiplet. ^{1}H and ^{13}C NMR spectra of compounds **2a, 2e-j, 3a, 3d, 3e-f, 3h-j, 3af, 3ag, 3ah, 3ai, 3aj** are provided in Supplementary Materials. Mass spectra were recorded using an LTQ-Velos Pro Thermofisher Scientific spectrometer. The sizes of the obtained Pd nanoformulations were measured using a Malvern particle size analyzer [nano ZS (173° scattering angle)]. The morphology of the different palladium nanoformulations was examined by transmission electron microscope (TEM) using a JEOL JEM 100CXII transmission electron microscope at an accelerating voltage of 100 kV and for high resolution image using a JEOL JEM 2010 instrument at 200 kV. Deionized water was used for chemical reactions and Milli-Q purified water for nanoparticle preparation. Bidistilled MilliQ water was produced using a water purification system (Millipore). Chemicals were obtained from Carbosynth Limited (UK), Sigma Aldrich Chemical Co (France), Fluorochem and Alfa Aesar (France) and were used without further purification. Solvents of analytical grade were obtained from VWR. Phosphate buffer saline (PBS) pH 7.4 was obtained from Sigma Aldrich. Anhydrous DMF and dioxane were obtained from Sigma Aldrich. Tetrahydrofuran (THF) was distilled from sodium/benzophenone ketyl and CH$_2$Cl$_2$ from CaH$_2$. The calix [8]arene-NHC-Pd catalyst was synthesized according to the method previously reported [27]. All reactions involving air- or water-sensitive compounds were routinely conducted in glassware, which was flame-dried under a positive pressure of nitrogen or argon. Analytical thin-layer chromatography was performed on Merck silica gel 60F254 glass precoated plates (0.25 mm layer). Column chromatography was performed on Merck silica gel 60 (230–400 mesh ASTM (American Standard Test Sieve Series). Diaryl and heteroaryl compounds were chromatographed eluting with AcOEt/cyclohexane mixture 1:4 to 1:1. The 4-substituded phenylalanine derivatives were chromatographed eluting with CH_2Cl_2/MeOH 98:2 to 95:15.

3.2. Nanoformulation of the Calix [8]arene-NHC-Pd Catalyst

Pd-Calix-NS were prepared by the emulsion-evaporation technique. Practically, the calix [8] arene-NHC-Pd catalyst (29.74 mg, 0.005 mmol) was dissolved into CH_2Cl_2 (5 mL). The organic phase was emulsified into 10 mL of 1.5% sodium cholate (w/w) aqueous solution using a vortex for 1 min and then a vibrating metallic tip at 30% amplitude for 1 min at 0 °C. The organic solvent was evaporated by magnetic stirring overnight in an open flask under a laminar flow hood and readjusted to 10 mL to provide a stock suspension of Pd-Calix-NS at 2.97 mg/mL.

3.3. Nanoparticles Characterization by DLS

Mean hydrodynamic diameters of the nanoassemblies and polydispersity index were measured at 25 °C by quasi-elastic light scattering with a Nano ZS (Malvern Instrument, 173 scattering angle). The NPs surface charge was investigated by ζ-potential measurement at 25 °C after dilution with 1 mM NaCl solution, applying the Smoluchowski equation. Measurements were carried out in triplicate. Colloidal stability in MilliQ water at 20 °C and 4 °C was investigated by measuring the Pd NPs mean diameter over a period of 30 days.

3.4. Cryogenic Transmission Electron Microscopy (CryoTEM) of Pd-Calix-NS

Morphology of the NPs of Pd-Calix-NS was observed by CryoTEM. Few drops of the nanosuspension (2.97 mg/mL) were deposited on EM grids covered with a holey carbon film (Quantifoil R2/2) previously treated with a plasma glow discharge. Observations were conducted at low temperature (−180 °C) on a JEOL 2010 FEG microscope operated at 200 kV. Images were recorded with a Gatan camera.

3.5. General Method for the Synthesis of Potassium Aren-2,6,7-trioxa-1-borate-bicyclo[2.2.2]octane Salts

To a solution of the given boronic acid (1.64 mmol) and 1,1,1-tris(hydroxymethyl)ethane (197 mg, 1.65 mmol) in dioxane (10 mL) was added ground KOH (92 mg, 1.64 mmol). The mixture was flushed with argon and water (29 µL, 1.65 mmol) was added. The resulting mixture was stirred at 30 °C for 3 h. Cyclohexane (5 mL) was then added and the precipitated potassium triolborate salt was filtered on a sintered glass funnel and washed twice with acetone. The solid was dried under vacuum to afford the potassium borate salts as amorphous solids.

Potassium 4-methyl-1-phenyl-2,6,7-trioxa-1-borabicyclo-[2.2.2]octan-1-uide (**2a**), The general method using phenyl boronic acid gave the title compound 14 in 87% yield. ^{1}H NMR (300 MHz, DMSO-d_6): δ = 7.30 ppm (d, J = 7.2 Hz, 2H, H-2, H-6), 6.98–6.88 (m, 3H, H-3, H-4, H-5), 3.57 (s, 6H, CH_2OB), 0.47 (s, 3H, CH_3) ppm; ^{13}C NMR (75 MHz, DMSO-d6): δ = 132.1 (2CH, C-2, C-6), 125.5 (2CH, C-3, C-5), 124.0 (CH, C-4), 73.6 (3CH2, B(OCH$_2$)$_3$), 34.4 (C, CCH_3), 16.2 (CH_3, CCH_3) ppm. The C-B was not observed; IR (neat, cm^{-1}): 3064, 2958, 2843, 1613, 1351, 1207, 1093, 1042, 914, 878, 850, 714; MS (ESI$^-$): m/z (%) = 205.1 (100) [M − K]$^-$, 204.1 (20).

Tetra-n-butylammonium 4-methyl-1-phenyl-2,6,7-trioxa-1-borabicyclo-[2.2.2]octan-1-uide (**2e**), The general method using 1 equivalent of n-Bu$_4$NOH as base provided the tetra-n-butylammonium borate salt **2e** [36] in 20% yield as an off-white amorphous solid. ^{1}H NMR (300 MHz, DMSO-d_6): δ, =; 733

(d, J = 6.6 Hz, 2H, H-2,H-6), 7.02–6.85 (m, 3H, H-3,H-4, H-5), 3.58 (s, 6H, CH$_2$OB), 3.20–3.10 (m, 8H, CH$_2$N), 1.62–1.42 (m, 8H, CH$_2$CH$_2$N); 1.30 (hex, J = 7.3 Hz, 8H, CH$_2$CH$_2$CH$_2$N), 0.93 (t, 7.3 Hz, 12H, CH$_3$CH$_2$CH$_2$CH$_2$N), 0.48 (s, 3H, CH$_3$) ppm; ^{13}C NMR (75 MHz, DMSO-d_6): δ = 132.2 (2CH, C-2, C-6), 125.4 (2CH, C-3, C-5), 123.9 (CH, C-4), 73.5 (3CH$_2$, B(OCH$_2$)$_3$), 57.5 (4CH$_2$, CH$_3$CH$_2$CH$_2$CH$_2$N), 34.4 (C, CCH$_3$), 23.0 (4CH$_2$, CH$_3$CH$_2$CH$_2$CH$_2$N), 19.1 (4CH$_2$, CH$_3$CH$_2$CH$_2$CH$_2$N), 16.2 (CH$_3$, CCH$_3$), 13.4 (4CH$_3$, CH$_3$CH$_2$CH$_2$CH$_2$N) ppm. The C-B was not observed.

Potassium 1-(4-methoxyphenyl)-4-methyl-2,6,7-trioxa-1-borabicyclo-[2.2.2]octan-1-uide (**2f**), The general method using 4-methoxyphenyl boronic acid give the title compound [34] as a white powder in 69% yield; ^{1}H NMR (300 MHz, DMSO-d_6): δ = 7.22 (d, J = 8.1 Hz, 2H, H-2, H-6), 6.57 (d, J = 8.1 Hz, 2H, H-3, H-5), 3.63 (s, 3H, OCH$_3$), 3.57 (s, 6H, CH$_2$OB), 0.48 (s, 3H, CH$_3$) ppm; ^{13}C NMR (75 MHz, DMSO-d_6): δ = 157.2 (C, C-4), 133.5 (2CH, C-2, C-6), 111.7 (2CH, C-3, C-5), 74.0 (3CH$_2$, B(OCH$_2$)$_3$), 54.9 (CH3, OCH$_3$), 34.9 (C, CCH$_3$), 16.8 (CH$_3$) ppm, the C-B was not observed; IR (neat, cm^{-1}): 3230, 2863, 2841, 1598, 1510, 1451, 1399, 1283, 1214, 1178, 1078, 1045, 1024, 933, 854, 815,729, 697, 608; MS (ESI$^-$): *m/z* (%) = 235.1 (100) [M-K]$^-$, 234.1 (20).

Potassium 4-methyl-1-(3-nitrophenyl)-2,6,7-trioxa-1-borabicyclo-[2.2.2] octan-1-uide (**2h**), The general method using 3-nitrophenyl boronic acid gave the title compound [37] in 72% yield, ^{1}H NMR (300 MHz, DMSO-d_6): δ = 8.17 (d, J = 1.5 Hz, 1H, H-2), 7.83 (dd, J = 8.1, 1.5 Hz, 1H, H-4), 7.75 (d, 1H, J = 6.9 Hz, H-6), 7.29 (t, 1H, J = 7.6 Hz, H-5), 3.62 (s, 6H, CH$_2$OB), 0.51 (s, 3H, CH$_3$) ppm; ^{13}C NMR (75 MHz, DMSO-d_6): δ = 146.48 (C, C-3), 138.98 (CH, C-6), 126.90 (CH, C-2 or C-5), 126.30 (CH, C-2 or C-5), 119.26 (CH, C-4), 73.52 (3CH2, B(OCH$_2$)$_3$), 34.56 (C, CCH$_3$), 15.97 (CH$_3$) ppm, the C-B was not observed; IR (neat, cm^{-1}): 3015, 2948, 2850, 1606, 1519, 1458, 1402, 1342, 1278, 1238, 1216, 1083, 1054, 885, 863; MS (ESI$^-$): m/z (%) = 250.0 (100) [M − K]$^-$, 249 (20).

Potassium 4-methyl-1-(o-tolyl)-2,6,7-trioxa-1-borabicyclo-[2.2.2]octan-1-uide (**2g**), The general method using *o*-tolylboronic acid gave the title compound [37] in 59% yield, ^{1}H NMR (300 MHz, DMSO-d_6): δ = 7.38 (d, J = 6.0 Hz, 1H, H-6), 6.90–6.75 (m, 3H, H-3,H-4,H-5), 3.61 (s, 6H, CH$_2$OB), 2.37 (s, 3H, ArCH$_3$), 0.52 (s, 3H, CH$_3$) ppm; ^{13}C NMR (75 MHz, DMSO-d_6): δ = 141.6 (C, C-2), 132.4 (CH, C-6), 128.0 (CH), 124.5 (CH), 122.8 (CH), 73.0 (3CH$_2$, B(OCH$_2$)$_3$), 34.5 (C, CCH$_3$), 22.2 (CH$_3$, ArCH3), 16.3 (CH$_3$) ppm, the C-B was not observed; IR (neat, cm^{-1}): 3158, 2855, 1396, 1210, 1178, 1066, 1035, 970, 945, 928, 891, 829, 750, 689; MS (ESI$^-$): *m/z* (%) = 219.1 (100) [M-K]$^-$, 218 (20).

Potassium 1-(furan-2-yl)-4-methyl-2,6,7-trioxa-1-borabicyclo-[2.2.2]octan-1-uide (**2i**), The general method using 2-furylboronic acid gave the title compound [38] in yield 67%; ^{1}H NMR (300 MHz, DMSO-D$_6$): δ = 7.31 (s, 1H, H-5), 6.10 (m, 1H, H-3), 5.94 (d, J = 3.0 Hz, 1H, H-4), 3.54 (s, 6H, CH$_2$OB), 0.48 (s, 3H, CH$_3$) ppm; ^{13}C NMR (75 MHz, DMSO-d_6): δ = 140.6 (CH, C-5), 110.3 (CH, C-3 or C-4), 108.4 (CH, C-3 or C-4), 72.9 (3CH$_2$, B(OCH$_2$)$_3$), 34.4 (C, CCH$_3$), 16.1 (CH$_3$) ppm, the C-B was not observed; MS (APCI$^-$): m/z (%) = 195.1 (100) [M$^-$], 194.1 (20).

Potassium 4-methyl-1-(thiophen-3-yl)-2,6,7-trioxa-1-borabicyclo-[2.2.2]octan-1-uide (**2j**), The general method using 3-thienylboronic acid gave the title compound [39] in yield 65%; ^{1}H NMR (300 MHz, DMSO-d_6): δ = 7.01 (dd, J = 4.5 Hz, J = 2.7 Hz, 1H, H-5), 6.93 (d, J = 4.5 Hz 1H, H-4), 6.85 (d, J = 1.8 Hz, 1H, H-2), 3.54 (s, 6H, CH$_2$OB), 0.46 (s, 3H, CH$_3$) ppm; ^{13}C NMR (75 MHz, DMSO-d_6): δ = 132.9 (CH, C-4), 123.7 (CH, C-2), 120.9 (CH, C-5), 73.6 (3CH$_2$, B(OCH$_2$)$_3$), 34.4 (C, CCH$_3$), 16.2 (CH$_3$) ppm, the C-B was not observed; IR (neat, cm^{-1}): 2948, 2847, 1630, 1468, 1421, 1400, 1351, 1215, 1172, 1071, 1000, 926, 869, 839, 774, 599, 622; MS (ESI$^-$): *m/z* (%) = 211.2 (5) [M − H]$^-$, 195.1 (100).

3.6. General Method for the Small-Scale Suzuki-Miyaura Coupling with Pd-Calix-NS

In an Eppendorf tube, the arylhalide (0.008 mmol, 1 equiv.) and the boronic acid/cyclic-triolborate salt (0.024 mmol, 3 equiv.) were suspended in phosphate buffer pH 8.0–6.0 (200 mM, 50 µL) and MilliQ Water (370 µL). The suspension of Pd-Calix-NS was added (3.2·10^{-6} mmol; 0.00004 equiv.; 80 µL) and the reaction was mixed and shaken on a thermostated shaker (Biosan TS-100) at 800 rpm at 37 °C. After

3 h, the reaction was frozen in liquid nitrogen and the solution lyophilized. The crude product was taken up in CD$_3$OD and analyzed by ^{1}H-NMR.

3.7. General Method for the Preparative Suzuki-Miyaura Coupling with Pd-Calix-NS

The arylhalide (0.25 mmol, 1 equiv.) and the boronic acid (0.75 mmol, 3 equiv.) were suspended in phosphate buffer pH 8.0 (200 mM, 5 mL) and water (The stock solution of Pd-Calix-NS (0.025 mmol Pd, 0.01 equiv.) was added and the reaction was stirred at 37 °C. After 3/16 h, the reaction was frozen in liquid nitrogen and the solution was lyophilized. The crude product was purified by flash chromatography on silica gels to afford the expected cross-coupling product.

4-Phenylbenzoic Acid (**3e**), The general method using 4-iodobenzoic acid and potassium phenyltriolborate gave 4-phenylbenzoic acid [40] (Yield = 72%); ^{1}H NMR (300 MHz, CDCl$_3$): δ = 8.19 (d, *J* = 8.2 Hz, 2H, H-2′, H-6′), 7.71 (d, *J* = 8.2 Hz, 2H, H-3′, H-5′), 7.64 (d, *J* = 7.8 Hz, 2H, H-2″, H-6″), 7.55–7.38 (m, 3H, H3″, H-4″, H-5″) ppm; ^{13}C NMR (75 MHz, DMSO-d$_6$): δ = 167.2 (C, CO$_2$H), 144.3 (C), 139.1 (C), 130.0 (2CH), 129.7 (C), 129.1 (2CH), 128.3 (CH), 127.0 (2CH), 126.8 (2CH), ppm; MS (ESI$^-$) m/z = 197.1 (100) [M − H]$^-$.

4-Phenylphenol (**3f**), The general method using 4-iodophenol and potassium phenyltriolborate gave 4-phenylphenol [41] (Yield = 90%); ^{1}H NMR (300 MHz, CD$_3$OD): δ = 10.38 (1H, br s, OH), 8.37 (d, *J* = 8.1 Hz, 2H, H-2′, H-6′), 8.28 (d, *J* = 8.7 Hz, 2H, H-3, H-5), 8.21 (t, *J* = 7.5 Hz, 2H, H-3′, H-5′), 8.07 (td, *J* = 7.2, 0.9 Hz, 1H, H-4′), 7.66 (d, *J* = 8.4 Hz, 2H, H-2, H-6) ppm; ^{13}C NMR (75 MHz, CD$_3$OD): δ = 160.6 (C, C-1), 149.7 (C, C-1′), 140.5 (C, C-4), 138.3 (2CH, C-3, C-5), 137.3 (2CH, C-3′, C-5′), 135.9 (CH, C-4′), 135.5 (2CH, C-2′, C-6′), 125.3 (2CH, C-2, C-6) ppm; MS (ESI$^-$) m/z (%) = 169.1 (100) [M − H]$^-$.

2-Phenylbenzoic Acid (**3h**), The general method using 2-iodobenzoic acid and potassium phenyltriolborate gave 2-phenylbenzoic acid [42] (Yield = 66%) ^{1}H NMR (300 MHz, DMSO-d$_6$): δ = 12.70 (s, 1H, OH), 7.72 (d, *J* = 7.5 Hz, 1H, H-6, 1H), 7.57 (t, *J* = 7.5 Hz, 1H, H-4, 1H), 7.45 (t, *J* = 7.3 Hz, 1H, H-5, 1H), 7.45–7.30 (m, 6H) ppm; ^{13}C NMR (75 MHz, CDCl$_3$): δ = 173.6 (C, CO$_2$H), 143.5 (C, C-2), 141.1 (C, C-1′), 132.2 (CH), 131.3 (CH), 130.8 (CH), 129.4 (C, C-1), 128.6 (2CH), 128.2 (2CH), 127.5 (CH), 127.3 (CH) ppm.

4-Phenylaniline (**3i**), The general method using 4-iodooaniline and potassium phenyltriolborate gave 4-phenylaniline [43] (Yield = 70%) ^{1}H NMR (300 MHz, DMSO-d$_6$): δ = 7.52 (d, *J* = 8.2 Hz, 2H, H-2, H-5, 2H), 7.42–7.32 (m, 4H, H-2′, H-3′, H-5′, H-6′), 7.20 (t, *J* = 7.3 Hz, 1H, H-4′), 6.67 (d, *J* = 8.2 Hz, 2H, H-2, H-6), 5.19 (br s, 2H, NH$_2$) ppm; ^{13}C NMR (75 MHz, DMSO-d$_6$): δ = 148.3 (C), 140.7(C), 128.7 (2CH), 127.5 (C), 127.1 (2CH), 125.6 (CH), 125.3 (2CH), 114.3 (2CH) ppm; MS (ESI$^+$) m/z (%) = 170.1 (100) [M + H]$^+$.

2-Phenylaniline (**3j**), The general method using 2-iodooaniline and potassium phenyltriolborate gave 2-phenylaniline [44] (Yield = 32%) ^{1}H NMR (300 MHz, CD$_3$OD): δ = 7.50–7.25(m, 5H), 7.09 (dt, *J* = 8.1 Hz, 1.5 Hz, 1H, H-5), 7.02 (d, *J* = 7.8 Hz, 1H, H-3), 6.81 (d, *J* = 7.8 Hz, 1H, H-6), 6.75 (t, *J* = 7.3 Hz, 1H, H-4) ppm; ^{13}C NMR (75 MHz, CD$_3$OD): δ = 144.85 (C, C-2), 139.7 (C, C-1′), 130.0 (CH), 128.7 (2CH, C-3′, C-5′), 128.6 (2CH, C-2′, C-6′), 128.2 (CH), 126.7 (CH), 125.9 (C, C-1), 116.8 (CH, C-5), 115.3 (CH, C-3) ppm; MS (ESI$^+$) *m/z* (%) = 170.1 (100) [M + H]$^+$.

N-boc-4-phenyl-L-phenylalanine (**3a**), The general method using *N*-Boc-4-iodo-L-phenylalanine and potassium phenyltriolborate (2a) gave the title compound [45] in 87% yield: ^{1}H NMR (300 MHz, CD$_3$OD) δ 7.62–7.48 (m, 4H), 7.40 (t, *J* = 7.5 Hz, 2H), 7.35–7.27 (m, 3H), 4.46–4.30 (m, 1H, H-2), 3.20 (dd, *J* = 13.8, 5.1 Hz, 1H, H-3), 2.95 (dd, *J* = 13.8, 8.7 Hz, 1H, H-3), 1.40 (s, 9H, NCO2C(CH$_3$)$_3$) ppm; ^{13}C NMR (75 MHz, CD$_3$OD): δ = 175.4 (C, CO$_2$H), 157.8 (C, CO$_2$*t*-Bu), 142.3 (C), 141.0 (C), 137.8 (C), 130.8 (2CH), 129.8 (2CH), 128.2 (CH), 128.0 (2CH), 127.9 (2CH), 80.5 (C, NCO$_2$C(CH$_3$)$_3$)), 56.3 (CH, C-2), 38.4 (CH2, C-3), 28.7 (3CH3, NCO$_2$C(CH$_3$)$_3$) ppm; MS (ESI-) *m/z* (%): 340.17 (100) [M − H]$^-$, 266.2 (80) [M-t-BuOH-H]$^-$.

N-boc-3-phenyltyrosine (**3d**), The general method using *N*-Boc-4-iodo-L-tyrosine and potassium phenyltriolborate (2a) gave the title compound [46] in 68% yield; ^{1}H NMR (300 MHz, CD$_3$OD): δ = 7.55 (d, *J* = 7.3 Hz, 2H, H-2″, H-6″), 7.36 (t, *J* = 7.3 Hz, 2H, H-3″, H-5″), 7.26 (t, *J* = 7.3 Hz, 1H, H-4″), 7.12 (s, 1H, H-2′), 7.02 (d, *J* = 8.2 Hz, 1H, H-6′), 6.82 (d, *J* = 8.2 Hz, 1H, H-5′), 4.45–4.25 (m, 1H, H-3), 3.10 (dd, *J* = 13.1, 1.8 Hz, 1H, H-3), 2.89 (dd, *J* = 13.1, 7.7 Hz, 1H, H-3), 1.37 (s, 9H, NCO2C(CH$_3$)$_3$) ppm; ^{13}C NMR (75 MHz, CD$_3$OD): δ = 175.4 (C, CO$_2$H), 157.8 (C, CO$_2$*t*-Bu), 154.1 (C, C-4′), 140.2 (C, C-1′), 132.7 (C), 130.4 (2CH), 130.2 (CH), 129.6 (C), 129.5 (C), 128.9 (2CH), 127.6 (CH), 117.0 (CH), 80.5 (C, NCO$_2$C(CH$_3$)), 56.4 (CH, C-2), 37.9 (CH2, C-3), 28.7 (3CH3, NCO$_2$C(CH$_3$)$_3$) ppm; MS m/z (%) (ESI$^-$): 356.2 (100) [M − H]$^-$, 282.2 (65) [M-t-BuOH-H]$^-$.

N-Boc-4-(4-methoxyphenyl)-L-phenylalanine (**3af**), The general method using *N*-Boc-4-iodo-L-phenyl alanine and potassium 4-methoxy-1-phenyl-2,6,7-trioxa-1-borabicyclo[2.2.2]octan-1-uide (2f) gave the title compound [47] in 98% yield; ^{1}H NMR (300 MHz, CD$_3$OD): δ = 7.49 (t, *J* = 8.4 Hz, 4H, H-2′, H-6′, H-2″, H-6″), 7.27 (d, *J* = 7.8 Hz, 2H, H-2′, H-6′), 6.97 (d, *J* = 8.7 Hz, 2H, H-3″, H-5″), 4.45–4.30 (m, 1H, H-2), 3.82 (s, 3H, OMe), 3.18 (dd, *J* = 13.8, 4.8 Hz, 1H, H-3), 2.95 (dd, *J* = 13.8, 9.3 Hz, 1H, H-3), 1.38 (s, 9H, NCO2C(CH$_3$)$_3$) ppm; ^{13}C NMR (75 MHz, CD$_3$OD): δ = 175.4 (C, CO2H), 160.7 (C-4″), 157.7 (C, CO2t-Bu), 140.6 (C, C-1′), 137.0 (C), 134.7 (C), 130.8 (2CH), 128.8 (2CH), 127.5 (2CH), 115.2 (2CH, C-3″, C-5″), 80.5 (C, NCO$_2$C(CH$_3$)), 56.4 (CH, C-2), 55.7 (CH$_3$, OCH$_3$), 38.4 (CH$_2$, C-3), 28.7 (3CH$_3$, NCO$_2$C(CH$_3$)$_3$) ppm.

N-boc-4-(2-methylphenyl)-L-phenylalanine (**3ag**), The general method using *N*-Boc-4-iodo-L-phenylalanine and potassium 2-methyl-1-phenyl-2,6,7-trioxa-1-borabicyclo[2.2.2]octan-1-uide (2g) gave the title compound [46] in 79% yield after 16 h reaction time. ^{1}H NMR (300 MHz, CD$_3$OD): δ = 7.30 (d, *J* = 8.7 Hz, 2H), 7.28–7.10 (m, 6H), 4.45–4.30 (m, 1H, H-2), 3.21 (dd, *J* = 13.8, 4.5 Hz, 1H, H-3), 2.95 (dd, *J* = 13.8, 9.3 Hz, 1H, H-3), 2.21 (s, 3H, ArCH$_3$), 1.39 (s, 9H, NCO2C(CH$_3$)$_3$) ppm; ^{13}C NMR (75 MHz, CD$_3$OD): δ = 175.4 (C, CO$_2$H), 157.8 (C, CO$_2$*t*-Bu), 143.0 (C, C-1′), 141.8 (C), 137.2 (C), 136.2 (C), 131.2 (CH), 130.6 (CH), 130.1 (4CH), 128.2 (CH), 126.7 (CH), 80.5 (C, NCO$_2$C(CH$_3$)), 56.3 (CH, C-2), 38.5 (CH$_2$, C-3), 28.7 (3CH$_3$, NCO$_2$C(CH$_3$)$_3$), 20.6 (CH$_3$, ArCH$_3$) ppm; MS m/z (%) (ESI$^-$): 354.2 (100) [M − H]$^-$, 280.2 (85) [M-t-BuOH-H]$^-$.

N-boc-4-(3-nitrophenyl) phenylalanine (**3ah**), The general method using *N*-Boc-4-iodo-L-phenylalanine and potassium 3-nitro-1-phenyl-2,6,7-trioxa-1-borabicyclo[2.2.2]octan-1-uide (2h) gave the title compound [47] in 72% yield after 16 h reaction time; 1H NMR (300 MHz, CD$_3$OD): δ = 8.45 (s, 1H, H-2″), 8.19 (d, *J* = 8.0 Hz, 1H, H-4″), 8.02 (d, *J* = 7.9 Hz, 1H, H-6″), 7.68 (t, *J* = 7.9 Hz, 1H, H-5″), 7.63 (d, *J* = 8.1 Hz, 2H, H-3′, H-5′), 7.39 (d, *J* = 8.1 Hz, 2H, H-2′, H-6′), 4.45–4.30 (m, 1H, H-2), 3.24 (dd, *J* = 13.8, 4.8 Hz, 1H, H-3), 2.98 (dd, *J* = 13.8, 8.4 Hz, 1H, H-3), 1.39 (s, 9H, NCO$_2$C(CH$_3$)$_3$) ppm; ^{13}C NMR (75 MHz, CD$_3$OD): δ = 175.2 (C, CO$_2$H), 157.8 (C, CO$_2$*t*-Bu), 150.2 (C, C-3″), 144.0 (C), 139.4 (C), 138.4 (C), 134.0 (CH), 131.3 (2CH), 131.2 (CH), 128.4 (2CH), 122.9 (CH), 122.4 (CH), 80.6 (C, NCO$_2$C(CH$_3$)), 56.2 (CH, C-2), 38.4 (CH$_2$, C-3), 28.7 (3CH$_3$, NCO$_2$C(CH$_3$)$_3$), MS m/z (%) (ESI$^-$): 385.2 (100) [M − H]$^-$, 311.2 (65) [M-*t*-BuOH-H]$^-$.

N-boc-4-(2-furanyl) phenylalanine (**3ai**), The general method using *N*-Boc-4-iodo-L-phenylalanine and potassium 4-methyl-1-(furan-2-yl)-2,6,7-trioxa-1-borabicyclo[2.2.2]octan-1-uide (2i) gave the title compound in 87% yield ^{1}H NMR (300 MHz, CD$_3$OD): δ = 7.60 (d, *J* = 8.0 Hz, 2H, H-3′, H-5′), 7.51 (s, 1H, H-4″), 7.25 (d, *J* = 8.0 Hz, 2H, H-2′, H-6′), 6.70 (d, *J* = 2.8 Hz, 1H, H-3″), 6.50 (br s 1H, H-4″), 4.45–4.25 (m, 1H, H-2), 3.16 (dd, *J* = 13.8, 4.5, Hz, 1H, H-3), 2.92 (dd, *J* = 13.8, 9.3 Hz, 1H, H-3), 1.39 (s, 9H, NCO$_2$C(CH$_3$)$_3$); ^{13}C NMR (75 MHz, CD$_3$OD): δ = 175.3 (C, CO$_2$H), 157.7 (C, CO$_2$*t*-Bu), 155.2 (C, C-2″), 143.2 (CH), 137.8 (C), 130.7 (2CH, C-2′, C-6′), 129.8 (C), 124.7 (2CH, C-3′, C-5′), 112.6 (CH, C-3″), 105.7 (CH, C-4″), 80.5 (C, NCO$_2$C(CH$_3$)), 56.2 (CH, C-2), 38.5 (CH2, C-3), 28.6 (3CH$_3$, NHCO$_2$C(CH$_3$)$_3$); MS m/z (%) (ESI$^-$): 330.2 (100) [M − H]$^-$, 256.2 (85) [M-tBuOH-H]$^-$.

N-boc-4-(4-thienyl) phenylalanine (**3aj**), The general method using *N*-Boc-4-iodo-L-phenylalanine and potassium 4-methyl-1-(thiophen-3-yl)-2,6,7-trioxa-1-borabicyclo[2.2.2]octan-1-uide (2j) gave the title compound [48] in 63% yield ^{1}H NMR (300 MHz, CD$_3$OD): δ = 7.58–7.49 (m, 3H, H-2″, H-3′, H-5′), 7.45–7.38 (m, 2H, H-4″, H-5″), 7.25 (d, J = 7.8 Hz, 2H, H-2′, H-6′), 4.35–4.20 (m, 1H, H-2), 3.18 (dd, J = 13.5, 4.5, Hz, 1H, H-3), 2.94 (dd, J = 13.5, 7.2 Hz, 1H, H-3), 1.38 (s, 9H, NCO$_2$C(CH$_3$)$_3$); ^{13}C NMR (75 MHz, CD$_3$OD): δ = 175.4 (C, CO$_2$H), 157.8 (C, CO$_2$$t$-Bu), 143.3 (C, C-3″), 137.5 (C), 135.7 (C), 130.8 (2CH, C-2′, C-6′), 127.9 (2CH, C-3′, C-5′), 127.2 (CH, C-3″ or C-4″), 127.1 (CH, C-3″ or C-4″), 120.9 (CH, C-2″), 80.5 (C, NCO$_2$C(CH$_3$)), 56.3 (CH, C-2), 38.4 (CH2, C-3), 28.7 (3CH3, NHCO$_2$C(CH$_3$)$_3$); MS (ESI$^-$): m/z (%) 346.2 (100) [M − H]$^-$, 272.1 (50) [M-t-BuOH-H]$^-$.

4. Conclusions

To conclude, we have shown that the nanoformulation of benzyloxycalix [8] arene supported NHC-palladium complexes gave highly stable nanosuspension endowed with high catalytic activity for the Suzuki–Miyaura couplings in pure water. In combination with cyclic triol boronates as nucleophilic partner, this nanoformulation was successfully engaged in coupling reactions with water-soluble substrates bearing a wide range of functional groups using a low catalyst loading.

The high catalytic activity of the Pd-Calix-NS can be attributed to the specific characteristics of the nanostructure exalting the high catalytic power the NHC-Pd structure previously observed in organic solvents [27,49]. The exact origin of the increase reactivity of the nanoparticulate formulation remain to be addressed, nevertheless it may be hypothesis that the self-assembling of the calix molecules driven by hydrophobic interaction would give NPs embedding the lipophilic crown of benzyl groups into the core of the particles, while the more polar palladium NHC appendages would be disposed on the surface. Such an arrangement would favorably influence the oxidative addition step with water soluble aryl halides and hence increase the rate of the overall process.

Supplementary Materials: Copies of ^{1}H NMR and ^{13}C NMR spectra of the compound are available in the online supplementary materials.

Author Contributions: V.H., D.D. and P.C. conceived and designed the experiments; A.P. and I.A. performed the experiments; S.P. synthetized the arylborate salts; C.M. Design and synthesis the Pd-Calix complex; J.M. performed the TEM imaging of the nanoparticles. All authors have read and agreed to the published version of the manuscript.

Funding: The authors thank the Ministère de la Recherche et de la Technologie (Fellowship to A.P.) and the Fondation pour la Recherche Médicale (FRM 2018 Fellowship to A.P.).

Conflicts of Interest: The authors declare no conflict of interest.

References

1. Torborg, C.; Beller, M. Recent Applications of Palladium-Catalyzed Coupling Reactions in the Pharmaceutical, Agrochemical, and Fine Chemical Industries. *Adv. Synth. Catal.* **2009**, *351*, 3027–3043. [CrossRef]
2. Magano, J.; Dunetz, J.R. Large-Scale Applications of Transition Metal-Catalyzed Couplings for the Synthesis of Pharmaceuticals. *Chem. Rev.* **2011**, *111*, 2177–2250. [CrossRef] [PubMed]
3. Hayler, D.; Leahy, K.D.; Simmons, E.M. A Pharmaceutical Industry Perspective on Sustainable Metal Catalysis. *Organometallics* **2019**, *38*, 36–46. [CrossRef]
4. Cheng, F.; Adronov, A. Suzuki Coupling Reactions for the Surface Functionalization of Single-Walled Carbon Nanotubes. *Chem. Mater.* **2006**, *18*, 5389–5391. [CrossRef]
5. Fei, Z.; Soo Kim, J.; Smith, J.; Buchaca Domingo, E.; Anthopoulos, T.D.; Stingelin, N.; Watkins, S.E.; Kim, J.S.; Heeney, M. A low band gap co-polymer of dithienogermole and 2,1,3-benzothiadiazole by Suzuki polycondensation and its application in transistor and photovoltaic cells. *J. Mater. Chem.* **2011**, *21*, 16257–16263. [CrossRef]
6. Polshettiwar, V.; Decottignies, A.; Len, C.; Fihri, A. Suzuki–Miyaura Cross-Coupling Reactions in Aqueous Media: Green and Sustainable Syntheses of Biaryls. *ChemSusChem* **2010**, *3*, 502–522. [CrossRef]
7. Levin, E.; Ivry, E.; Diesendruck, C.E.; Lemcoff, N.G. Water in N-Heterocyclic Carbene-Assisted Catalysis. *Chem. Rev.* **2015**, *115*, 4607–4692. [CrossRef]

8. Chatterjee, A.; Ward, T.R. Recent Advances in the Palladium Catalyzed Suzuki–Miyaura Cross-Coupling Reaction in Water. *Catal. Lett.* **2016**, *146*, 820–840. [CrossRef]
9. Handa, S.; Andersson, M.P.; Gallou, F.; Reilly, J.; Lipshutz, B.H. HandaPhos: A General Ligand Enabling Sustainable ppm Levels of Palladium-Catalyzed Cross-Couplings in Water at Room Temperature. *Angew. Chem. Int. Ed.* **2016**, *55*, 4914–4918. [CrossRef]
10. Giacalone, F.; Campisciano, V.; Calabrese, C.; La Parola, V.; Syrgiannis, Z.; Prato, M.; Gruttadauria, M. Single-Walled Carbon Nanotube–Polyamidoamine Dendrimer Hybrids for Heterogeneous Catalysis. *ACS Nano* **2016**, *10*, 4627–4636. [CrossRef]
11. Isley, N.A.; Wang, Y.; Gallou, F.; Handa, S.; Aue, D.H.; Lipshutz, B.H. A Micellar Catalysis Strategy for Suzuki–Miyaura Cross-Couplings of 2-Pyridyl MIDA Boronates: No Copper, in Water, Very Mild Conditions. *ACS Catal.* **2017**, *7*, 8331–8337. [CrossRef]
12. Patel, N.D.; Rivalti, D.; Buono, F.G.; Chatterjee, A.; Qu, B.; Braith, S.; Desrosiers, J.-N.; Rodriguez, S.; Sieber, J.D.; Haddad, N.; et al. Effective BI-DIME Ligand for Suzuki–Miyaura Cross-Coupling Reactions in Water with 500 ppm Palladium Loading and Triton X. *Asian J. Org. Chem.* **2017**, *6*, 1285–1291. [CrossRef]
13. Takale, B.S.; Thakore, R.R.; Handa, S.; Gallou, F.; Reilly, J.; Lipshutz, B.H. A new, substituted palladacycle for ppm level Pd-catalyzed Suzuki–Miyaura cross couplings in water. *Chem. Sci.* **2019**, *10*, 8825–8831. [CrossRef] [PubMed]
14. Thakore, R.R.; Takale, B.S.; Gallou, F.; Reilly, J.; Lipshutz, B.H. N,C-Disubstituted Biarylpalladacycles as Precatalysts for ppm Pd-Catalyzed Cross Couplings in Water under Mild Conditions. *ACS Catal.* **2019**, *9*, 11647–11657. [CrossRef]
15. Veisi, H.; Mirzaei, A.; Mohammadi, P. Palladium nanoparticles decorated into a biguanidine modified-KIT-5 mesoporous structure: A recoverable nanocatalyst for ultrasound-assisted Suzuki–Miyaura cross-coupling. *RSC Adv.* **2019**, *9*, 41581–41590. [CrossRef]
16. Sharma, P.; Arora, A.; Oswal, P.; Rao, G.K.; Kaushal, J.; Kumar, S.; Kumar, S.; Singh, M.P.; Singh, A.J.; Kumar, A. Bidentate organochalcogen ligands (N., E.; E = S/Se) as stabilizers for recyclable palladium nanoparticles and their application in Suzuki–Miyaura coupling reactions. *Polyhedron* **2019**, *171*, 120–127. [CrossRef]
17. Ojida, A.; Tsutsumi, H.; Kasagi, N.; Hamachi, I. Suzuki coupling for protein modification. *Tetrahedron Lett.* **2005**, *46*, 3301–3305. [CrossRef]
18. Chalker, J.M.; Wood, C.S.C.; Davis, B.G. A Convenient Catalyst for Aqueous and Protein Suzuki−Miyaura Cross-Coupling. *J. Am. Chem. Soc.* **2009**, *131*, 16346–16347. [CrossRef]
19. Jbara, M.; Maity, S.D.; Brik, A. Palladium in the Chemical Synthesis and Modification of Proteins. *Angew. Chem. Int. Ed.* **2017**, *56*, 10644–10655. [CrossRef]
20. Isengger, P.G.; Davis, B.G. Concepts of Catalysis in Site-Selective Protein Modifications. *J. Am. Chem. Soc.* **2019**, *141*, 8005–8013. [CrossRef]
21. Kitanosono, T.; Masuda, K.; Xu, P.; Kobayashi, S. Catalytic Organic Reactions in Water toward Sustainable Society. *Chem. Rev.* **2018**, *118*, 679–746. [CrossRef] [PubMed]
22. Frank, M.; Maas, G.; Schatz, J. Calix[4]arene-Supported *N*-Heterocyclic Carbene Ligands as Catalysts for Suzuki Cross-Coupling Reactions of Chlorotoluene. *Eur. J. Org. Chem.* **2004**, 607–613. [CrossRef]
23. Brendgen, T.; Frank, M.J.; Schatz, J. The Suzuki Coupling of Aryl Chlorides in Aqueous Media Catalyzed by in situ Generated Calix[4]arene-Based N-Heterocyclic Carbene Ligands. *Eur. J. Org. Chem.* **2006**, 2378–2383. [CrossRef]
24. Monnereau, L.; Sémeril, D.; Matt, D.; Toupet, L. Cavity-Shaped Ligands: Calix[4]arene-Based Monophosphanes for Fast Suzuki–Miyaura Cross-Coupling. *Chem. Eur. J.* **2010**, *16*, 9237–9247. [CrossRef]
25. Brenner, E.; Matt, D.; Henrion, M.; Teci, M.; Toupet, L. Calix[4]arenes with one and two *N*-linked imidazolium units as precursors of *N*-heterocyclic carbene complexes. Coordination chemistry and use in Suzuki–Miyaura cross-coupling. *Dalton Trans.* **2011**, *40*, 9889–9898. [CrossRef]
26. Narkhede, N.; Uttam, B.; Pulla Rao, C. Calixarene-Assisted Pd Nanoparticles in Organic Transformations: Synthesis, Characterization, and Catalytic Applications in Water for C–C Coupling and for the Reduction of Nitroaromatics and Organic Dyes. *ACS Omega* **2019**, *4*, 4908–4917. [CrossRef]
27. Abdellah, I.; Kasongo, P.; Labattut, A.; Guillot, R.; Schulz, E.; Martini, C.; Huc, V. Benzyloxycalix[8]arene: A new valuable support for NHC palladium complexes in C–C Suzuki–Miyaura couplings. *Dalton Trans.* **2018**, *47*, 13843–13848. [CrossRef]

28. Fessi, H.; Puisieux, F.; Devissaguet, J.P.; Ammoury, N.; Benita, S. Nanocapsule formation by interfacial polymer deposition following solvent displacement. *Int. J. Pharm.* **1989**, *55*, R1–R4. [CrossRef]

29. Pisani, E.; Fattal, E.; Paris, J.; Ringard, C.; Rosilio, V.; Tsapis, N. Surfactant dependent morphology of polymeric capsules of perfluorooctyl bromide: Influence of polymer adsorption at the dichloromethane–water interface. *J. Colloid Interface Sci.* **2008**, *326*, 66–71. [CrossRef]

30. Dumas, A.; Peramo, A.; Desmaële, D.; Couvreur, P. PLGA-PEG-supported Pd Nanoparticles as Efficient Catalysts for Suzuki-Miyaura Coupling Reactions in Water. *Chimia* **2016**, *70*, 252–257. [CrossRef]

31. Lennox, A.J.J.; Lloyd-Jones, G.C. Selection of boron reagents for Suzuki–Miyaura coupling. *Chem. Soc. Rev.* **2014**, *43*, 412–443. [CrossRef] [PubMed]

32. Molander, G.A.; Canturk, B. Organotrifluoroborates and Monocoordinated Palladium Complexes as Catalysts—A Perfect Combination for Suzuki–Miyaura Coupling. *Angew. Chem. Int. Ed.* **2009**, *48*, 9240–9261. [CrossRef]

33. Lee, S.J.; Gray, K.C.; Paek, J.S.; Burke, M.D. Simple, Efficient, and Modular Syntheses of Polyene Natural Products via Iterative Cross-Coupling. *J. Am. Chem. Soc.* **2008**, *130*, 466–468. [CrossRef]

34. Yamamoto, Y.; Takizawa, M.; Yu, X.-Q.; Miyaura, N. Cyclic Triolborates: Air- and Water-Stable Ate Complexes of Organoboronic Acids. *Angew. Chem. Int. Ed.* **2008**, *47*, 928–931. [CrossRef] [PubMed]

35. Peramo, A.; Dumas, A.; Remita, H.; Benoît, M.; Yen-Nicolay, S.; Corre, R.; Louzada, A.; Dupuy, C.; Pecnard, S.; Lambert, B.; et al. Selective modification of a native protein in a patient tissue homogenate using palladium nanoparticles. *Chem. Commun.* **2019**, *55*, 15121–15124. [CrossRef] [PubMed]

36. Sakashita, S.; Takizawa, M.; Sugai, J.; Ito, H.; Yamamoto, Y. Tetrabutylammonium 2-Pyridyltriolborate Salts for Suzuki–Miyaura Cross-Coupling Reactions with Aryl Chlorides. *Org. Lett.* **2013**, *15*, 4308–4311. [CrossRef]

37. Akula, M.R.; Yao, M.-L.; Kabalka, G.W. Triolborates: Water-soluble complexes of arylboronic acids as precursors to iodoarenes. *Tetrahedron Lett.* **2010**, *51*, 1170–1171. [CrossRef]

38. Chen, Y.J.; Cui, Z.; Feng, C.-G.; Lin, G.-Q. nantioselective Addition of Heteroarylboronates to Arylimines Catalyzed by a Rhodium-Diene Complex. *Adv. Synth. Catal.* **2015**, *357*, 2815–2820. [CrossRef]

39. Yu, X.-Q.; Yamamoto, Y.; Miyaura, N. Rhodium-Catalyzed Asymmetric 1,4-Addition of Heteroaryl Cyclic Triolborate to α,β-Unsaturated Carbonyl Compounds. *Synlett* **2009**, 994–998. [CrossRef]

40. Schulman, E.M.; Christensen, K.A.; Grant, D.M.; Walling, C. Substituent effects on carbon-13 chemical shifts in 4-substituted biphenyls and benzenes. Substituent effect transmitted through eight covalent bonds. *J. Org. Chem.* **1974**, *39*, 2686–2690. [CrossRef]

41. Paterson, W.G.; Tipman, N.R. The nuclear magnetic resonance spectra of para-substituted phenols. *Can. J. Chem.* **1962**, *40*, 2122–2125. [CrossRef]

42. Wu, Z.-C.; Lu, Y.-N.; Ren, Y.-M.; Chen, Z.-M.; Tao, T.-X. Suzuki Cross-Coupling of Aryl Halides with Phenylboronic Acid Catalysed by an Amidoxime Fibres-Nickel(0) Complex. *J. Chem. Res.* **2013**, *37*, 451–454. [CrossRef]

43. Lynch, B.M.; Macdonald, B.C.; Webb, J.G.K. NMR spectra of aromatic amines and amides-I Correlations of amino proton shifts with Hammett substituents constants with Hückel electron densities. *Tetrahedron* **1968**, *24*, 3595–3605. [CrossRef]

44. Appleton, J.M.; Andrews, B.D.; Rae, I.D.; Reichert, B.E. Aromatic amides V. Intramolecular hydrogen bonding in ortho-substituted anilides. *Aust. J. Chem.* **1970**, *23*, 1667–1677.

45. Ksander, G.M.; Ghai, R.D.; deJesus, R.; Diefenbacher, C.G.; Yuan, A.; Berry, C.; Sakane, Y.; Trapani, A. Dicarboxylic Acid Dipeptide Neutral Endopeptidase Inhibitors. *J. Med. Chem.* **1995**, *38*, 1689–1700. [CrossRef]

46. Knör, S.; Laufer, B.; Kessler, H. Efficient Enantioselective Synthesis of Condensed and Aromatic-Ring-Substituted Tyrosine Derivatives. *J. Org. Chem.* **2006**, *71*, 5625–5630. [CrossRef]

47. De Vasher, R.B.; Moore, L.R.; Shaughnessy, K.H. Aqueous-Phase, Palladium-Catalyzed Cross-Coupling of Aryl Bromides under Mild Conditions, Using Water-Soluble, Sterically Demanding Alkylphosphines. *J. Org. Chem.* **2004**, *69*, 7919–7927. [CrossRef]

48. Willemse, T.; Van Imp, K.; Goss, R.J.M.; van Vlijmen, H.W.T.; Schepens, W.; Maes, B.U.W.; Ballet, S. Suzuki–Miyaura Diversification of Amino Acids and Dipeptides in Aqueous Media. *ChemCatChem* **2015**, *7*, 2055–2070. [CrossRef]

49. Zhou, X.-X.; Shao, L.-X. N-Heterocyclic Carbene/Pd(II)/1-Methylimidazole Complex Catalyzed Suzuki-Miyaura Coupling Reaction of Aryl Chlorides in Water. *Synthesis* **2011**, 3138–3142. [CrossRef]

Sample Availability: Samples of the compounds **2a-j, 3a_j, 3af, 3ag, 3ah, 3ai and 3aj** are available from the authors.

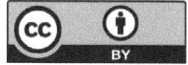 © 2020 by the authors. Licensee MDPI, Basel, Switzerland. This article is an open access article distributed under the terms and conditions of the Creative Commons Attribution (CC BY) license (http://creativecommons.org/licenses/by/4.0/).

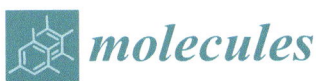

Article

The Influence of Various *N*-Heterocyclic Carbene Ligands on Activity of Nitro-Activated Olefin Metathesis Catalysts

Michał Pieczykolan [1,2], Justyna Czaban-Jóźwiak [1], Maura Malinska [2], Krzysztof Woźniak [2], Reto Dorta [3], Anna Rybicka [2], Anna Kajetanowicz [2,*] and Karol Grela [1,2,*]

1. Institute of Organic Chemistry Polish Academy of Sciences, Kasprzaka 44/52, 01-224 Warsaw, Poland; michalpieczykolan@gmail.com (M.P.); czaban.justyna@gmail.com (J.C.-J.)
2. Faculty of Chemistry, Biological and Chemical Research Centre, University of Warsaw, Żwirki i Wigury 101, 02-089 Warsaw, Poland; mmalinska@chem.uw.edu.pl (M.M.); kwozniak@chem.uw.edu.pl (K.W.); annamariarybicka@gmail.com (A.R.)
3. Department of Chemistry, School of Molecular Sciences, University of Western Australia, 35 Stirling Highway, Perth 6009, Australia; reto.dorta@uwa.edu.au
* Correspondence: a.kajetanowicz@uw.edu.pl (A.K.); prof.grela@gmail.com (K.G.)

Academic Editor: Yves Canac
Received: 16 April 2020; Accepted: 8 May 2020; Published: 12 May 2020

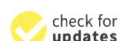

Abstract: A set of nitro-activated ruthenium-based Hoveyda-Grubbs type olefin metathesis catalysts bearing sterically modified *N*-hetero-cyclic carbene (NHC) ligands have been obtained, characterised and studied in a set of model metathesis reactions. It was found that catalysts bearing standard SIMes and SIPr ligands (**4a** and **4b**) gave the best results in metathesis of substrates with more accessible C–C double bonds. At the same time, catalysts bearing engineered naphthyl-substituted NHC ligands (**4d–e**) exhibited high activity towards formation of tetrasubstituted C–C double bonds, the reaction which was traditionally Achilles' heel of the nitro-activated Hoveyda–Grubbs catalyst.

Keywords: metathesis; ruthenium; nitro catalysts; NHC ligands; olefins

1. Introduction

Although first transition metal complexes bearing *N*-heterocyclic carbene (NHC) ligands were studied independently by Wanzlick [1] and Öfele [2] in the late 1960s, these intriguing species remained unexplored for many years. They re-entered the stage in 1991 when Arduengo and co-workers prepared the first stable and crystalline *N*-heterocyclic carbene (IAd) [3]. Since then, because of easy fine-tuning of the steric and electronic properties of these compounds [4], NHCs have been widely used both as organocatalysts and as ligands for numerous transition metals catalysed reactions [5].

Olefin metathesis is a useful methodology enabling formation of multiple carbon–carbon double bonds [6–8]. Pioneering studies on this reaction were undertaken by scientists working in industry and in academia, where one might mention milestone contributions by Anderson and Merckling (Du Pont–norbornene polymerization) [9], Banks and Bailey (Philips Petroleum—so-called the three-olefin process) [10], and Natta (linear and cyclic olefin polymerization) [11]. In these early contributions, undefined catalytic systems and harsh conditions were usually applied, which limited the applicability of this transformation to rather simple systems. The discovery of Schrock's molybdenum [12] and Grubbs' first-generation ruthenium [13] complexes in the 1990s significantly enhanced pertinence of this methodology, but the real avalanche of olefin metathesis applications happened only after the introduction of the so-called second-generation Ru catalysts, i.e., Ru-complexes bearing at least one NHC ligand [14–16]. Currently, a number of complexes are commercially available, inter alia, general-use catalysts like Umicore Grubbs Catalyst M2a (**1a**) [17] introduced in 1999 [18] and its SIPr variant (**1b**), Umicore M2 (**2a**) [19], Hoveyda–Grubbs' catalyst (**3a**) [20] and SIPr analogue (**3b**), and nitro-catalysts **4a,b** (Figure 1) [21–23].

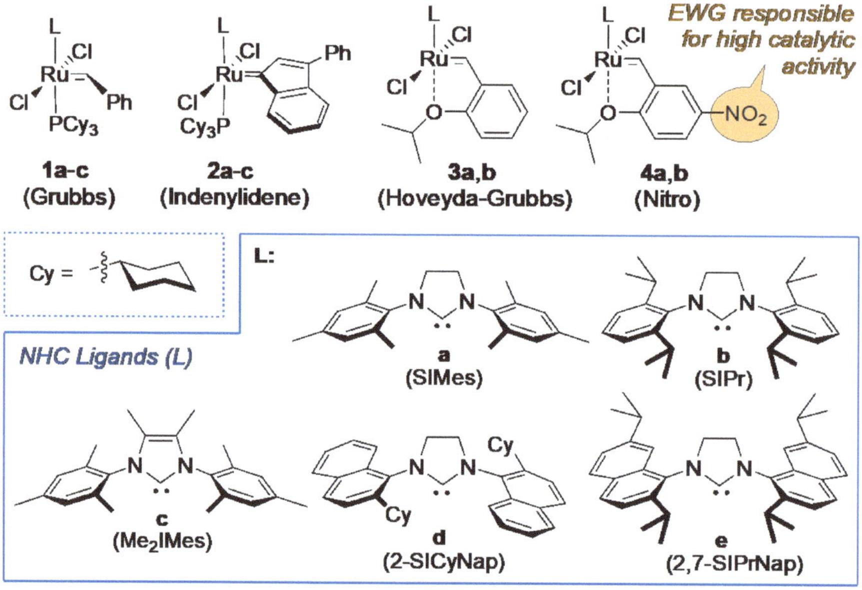

Figure 1. Examples of commercial Ru-based olefin metathesis catalysts and *N*-heterocyclic carbene (NHC) ligands (**a**–**e**).

Given the importance of the NHC ligand in ruthenium olefin metathesis catalysts, these ligands (L) have been optimised over the years. It was found that modification of the central five-membered *N*-heterocycle leads to decreasing activity or faster decomposition of the corresponding complex [24,25]. Similar results were obtained when replacing the aromatic side chain substituents with aliphatic ones [26–30]. However, unsymmetrically substituted NHC ligands, bearing one aromatic and one aliphatic *N*-substituent, have found their important niche as specialised catalysts [31–33]. On the other hand, introducing slightly bulkier aryl substituents compared to SIMes [34–37] or modifications of the 4 and 5 position in the imidazolium ring [26,38–40] cause usually an opposite effect resulting in an increase of the catalysts' activity.

Besides varying the NHC ligand, benzylidene ligands offer a broad testing ground for modifications of the catalytic properties of these ruthenium complexes [41]. Our group has developed a nitro-activated version of the Hoveyda complex **4a** [42–45]. The presence of an electron-withdrawing group (EWG) [43,46] in *para* position results in weakening of Ru-O bond, therefore accelerating the initiation rate of the resulting catalyst. As a consequence, **4a** has been utilised as a successful metathesis catalyst in natural products and target-oriented syntheses [47,48], as well as the industrial context, such as in the ring-closing metathesis (RCM) at scale up to 7 kg leading to the antiviral BILN 2061 agent precursor at Boehringer–Ingelheim plant [49,50], anticancer agent Largazole at decagrams scale at Oceanyx Pharmaceuticals, Inc. [51], and in continuous flow using a scalable membrane pervaporation device at Snapdragon Chemistry, Inc. [52]. Interestingly, the iodide-containing analogue of **4a** gave very good results in a number of challenging CM and RCM reactions [53]. Importantly, increased stability towards ethylene makes this diiodo derivative especially suitable for macrocyclization RCM of unbiased dienes [53]. Based on the excellent results reported by Bertrand and Grubbs on cyclic-alkyl-amino carbene (CAAC) ligands [54], Skowerski et al. obtained a CAAC analogue of **4a** that promoted difficult RCM macrocyclization at 30 ppm, and cross metathesis of acrylonitrile at 300 ppm Ru loading and lower [55]. In addition, the successful nitro-catalyst design has provided an impetus for developing a number of derivative catalysts utilising the same EWG-activation concept [46,56–58]. On the other hand, replacement of the chelating oxygen atom by groups containing sulphur [59–61] or nitrogen [61–63] results in so-called latent complexes [64,65]. These catalysts exhibit increased stability, but have to be activated thermally, chemically or photochemically.

Herein, we describe the synthesis of a small set of nitro-activated catalysts bearing NHC ligands (L) of different steric properties (Figure 1 and Scheme 1). Catalyst **4a** bearing a well-known SIMes ligand (Figure 1, NHC structures: **a**) was chosen as the benchmark, while the less known SIPr (Figure 1, **4b**) [53] and the new complexes with Me$_2$IMes [40] and with two naphthalene based ligands (Figure 1, NHC structures: **c–e**) developed by Dorta, were studied in detail [66–69]. These five complexes were characterised structurally and then tested in model olefin metathesis reactions [70] to check how steric properties of the different NHC ligands influence structural and catalytic properties of the resulting Ru complexes.

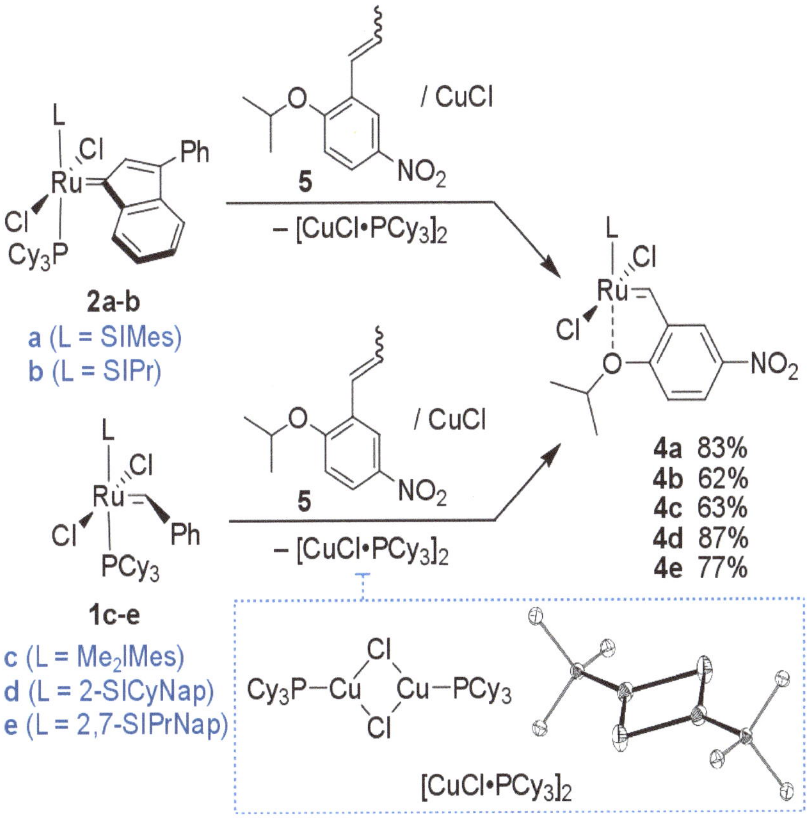

Scheme 1. Synthesis of complexes **4a–e**.

2. Results and Discussion

2.1. Synthesis of the Ruthenium Complexes

All complexes were synthesised via the stoichiometric metathesis-ligand exchange reaction according to a procedure initially disclosed by Hoveyda [71] and illustrated on Scheme 1. Depending on the NHC precursor, the reactions were performed either in toluene or in DCM, in the presence of copper(I) chloride—a commonly used phosphine scavenger [71]. Complexes **4a** and **4b** were obtained from commercially available second-generation indenylidene complexes **2a** and **2b** in 83% and 62% yield, respectively. Interestingly, during these syntheses, we were able to isolate the putative CuCl•PCy$_3$ complex in pure form and solve its crystallographic structure. It is stated that despite the fact that CuCl is being used as a phosphine scavenger in the preparation of various Hoveyda complexes for almost 20 years [71], according to our knowledge the product of this reaction has not yet been unambiguously characterised [72]. The synthesis of complexes **4c–e** was carried out using appropriate Grubbs second generation complexes **1c–e** as the source of ruthenium [40,66,68,73].

Complex **4c** was obtained in the reaction of **1c** with propenylbenzene derivative **5** in the presence of CuCl as a microcrystalline brownish solid with a moderate yield of 63%. Complexes **4d** and **4e** were obtained in a similar way from **5** and corresponding Grubbs-type catalysts [66,68,73] **1d** or **1e** as greenish microcrystalline solids in good yields, 87% and 77% respectively. General conditions for the synthesis of complexes **4a–e** are shown in Table 1. As solids, all new Ru-compounds were stable when under an inert atmosphere and were stored for weeks without any sign of decomposition (acc. to TLC and NMR). Having these catalysts in hand, we were ready to study how different NHC arrangements [74] present in **4a–e** influence the resulted complex structures and activity.

Table 1. Detailed conditions used in synthesis of **4a–e**.

Catalyst	Solvent	Time (min)	Temp. (°C)	Yield (%)
4a	Toluene	60	80	83
4b	Toluene	60	80	60
4c	Toluene	60	60	63
4d	DCM	20	40	87
4e	DCM	10	40	77

2.2. Structure Analysis

The crystal structures of **4b–e** have been determined by applying single crystal X-ray diffraction (Figure 2). It allows for investigation of structural conformations and steric subtleties of the studied compounds. The structure of **4a** has been previously reported [75] and another related molecule—a catalyst **4f** (Figure 3) developed by Buchmeiser [24] that contains saturated 1,3-*bis*(2,4,6-trimethylphenyl) 3,4,5,6-tetrahydropyrimidin-2-ylidene ligand—was included in Table 2 for comparison purposes [24] (while selected bond lengths and angles are given in Table 2, the full set of X-ray data is provided in Table S1 in Supplementary Materials).

All ruthenium complexes adopt a distorted square bi-pyramid coordination mode around the central ruthenium atom. The top of these pyramids are the O(1) oxygen of the benzylidene chelate and the C(1) carbon atoms of the NHC ligand. The average distance for the Ru-Cl bond amounts to 2.33 Å with a small variation from this value and the chloride atoms are in the trans configuration.

Most of the geometrical parameters do not differ much as they stay in the range of the 3σ threshold, however some interesting trends can be observed. The substitution of various NHC ligands strongly influences the Ru-O(1) bond. The bond is shortened in comparison to the parent SIMes-bearing (**4a**) compound (2.287(1) Å) with the exception of the NHC ring modification to the 6-member one in the **4f** moiety (2.310(2) Å).

An opposite trend was found for the Ru-C(1) bond, which is elongated except for the **4d** molecule. The Ru-C(2) bond changes within a smaller range with the shortest distance for the **4a** and **4c** (1.825(2)Å and 1.821(3) Å, respectively), whereas the longest bond distance is recorded for the **4e** structure 1.836(9) Å and 1.838(9) Å).

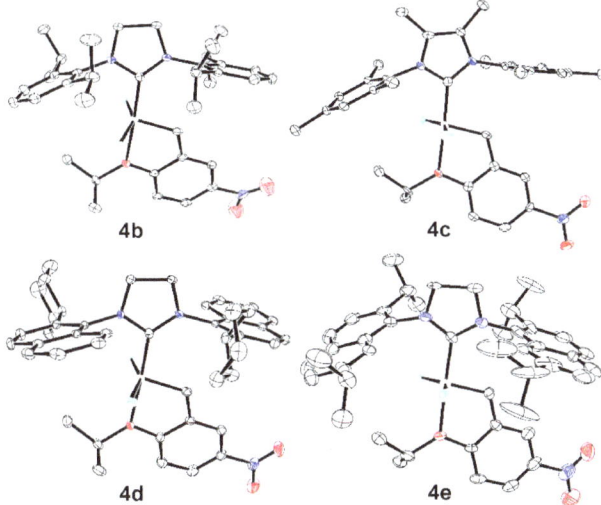

Figure 2. Solid state crystallographic structures of **4a**, **4b**, **4c** and **4e** complexes. Colour codes: blue—nitrogen, red—oxygen, green—chlorine.

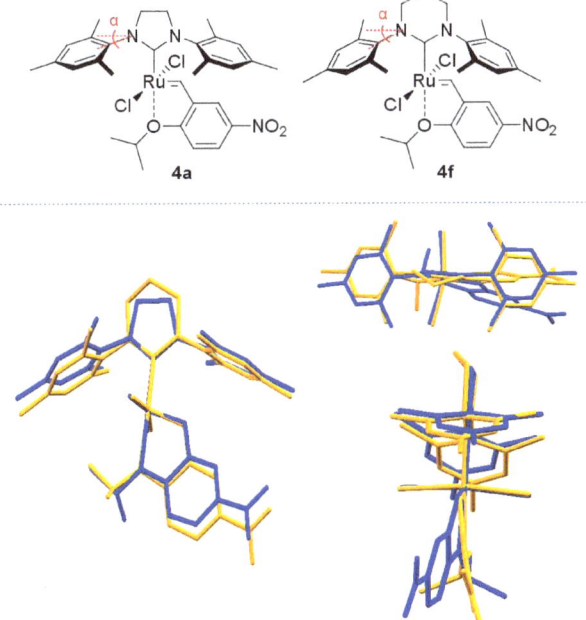

Figure 3. Molecular structures of **4a** and **4f**. Front, top, and side view of molecule overlay of **4a** (blue), **4f** (orange). For angle α values see Table 2.

Table 2. Selected bond lengths (Å) and angles (deg) in complexes **4a–e**. The **4e** structure contains two molecules in the asymmetric unit.

	4a [75]	4b	4c	4d	4e [a]	4f [24]
Ru-C(1)	1.979(3)	1.985(4)	1.990(4)	1.970(3)	2.002(9) 2.012(9)	2.013(2)
Ru-O(1)	2.287(1)	2.244(2)	2.232(2)	2.254(2)	2.285(5) 2.252(5)	2.310(2)
Ru-C(2)	1.825(2)	1.829(4)	1.821(3)	1.827(3)	1.836(9) 1.838(9)	1.825(3)
Ru-Cl(1)	2.333(1)	2.324(1)	2.335(1)	2.328(1)	2.328(2) 2.328(2)	2.343(1)
Ru-Cl(2)	2.330(1)	2.333(1)	2.339(1)	2.331(1)	2.328(2) 2.324(2)	2.343(1)
C(1)-Ru-O(1)	178.45(6)	172.5(1)	175.6(1)	175.4(1)	176.8(3) 177.8(3)	175.93(8)
C(1)-Ru-C(2)	101.36(8)	102.1(1)	103.0(1)	102.4(1)	99.9(4) 101.6(4)	105.1(1)
Ru-C(2)-C(3)-C(4)	8.6(2)	−8.9(5)	5.9(4)	−5.4(3)	−2(1) 2(1)	−4.5(3)
C(2)-Ru-C(1)-N(1)	7.6(2)	14.2(4)	5.5(4)	13.0(3)	−31.8(9) 27(1)	0.8(2)
α	19.8(1)	20.8(3)	20.1(2)	19.0(2)	19.4(7) 12.4(7)	25.4(2)
V_{Bur} (%)	35.4	36.5	34.7	34.6	34.8 36.1	38.0

[a] The **4e** structure contains two molecules in the asymmetric unit.

The torsion angles are the most sensitive parameters in the crystal studies, and they differ in all studied complexes, although not that significantly. The Ru-C(2)-C(3)-C(4)-O(1) ring in the Hoveyda pre-catalyst is almost planar. The Ru-C(2)-C(3)-C(4) torsion angle, which defines the mutual orientation of the carbene bond and the NHC ligand is more flexible (Figure 4). Yet again, similar values were found for complexes **4a** and **4c** that form negative torsion angles, whereas one can see positive values of this angle for the **4b** and **4d** complexes, with the **4e** precatalyst in the middle of the range. The ligands with more bulky character demand a bigger rotation of the C(2)-Ru-C(1)-N(1) torsion angle (**4b**, **4d** and **4e**).

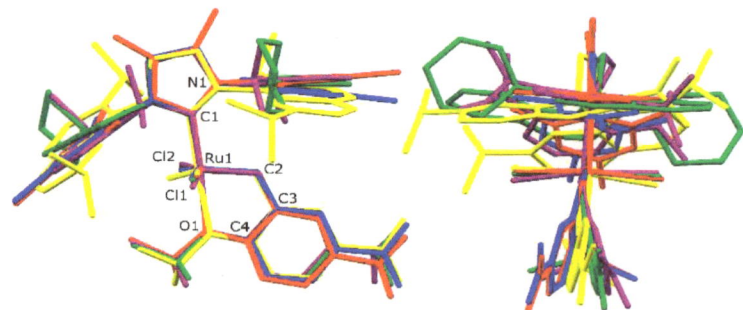

Figure 4. Front and side view of molecule overlay of **4a** (blue), **4b** (purple), **4c** (red), **4d** (green) and **4e** (yellow) complexes with label used to define selected geometrical parameters.

The angle α (Figure 3) represents visually how much the *N*-aryl 'wings' of the NHC ligands are lowered towards the metal centre. For (S)IMes-decorated complexes (**4a**, **4c**) this angle measures 19.8 and 20.1°, and is only slightly larger (20.8°) in the case of SIPr bearing **4b**. Importantly, the naphthyl members of the series have the N-substituents more 'up' (19.0° for **4d**), being in strong contrast to complex **4f** where the NHC wings are visibly lowered (25.4°) thus shielding the Ru centre more. However, some individual geometrical parameters can mislead the overall comparison. The root means square (RMS) analysis, taking into account the following six atoms: Ru, C(1), C(2), O(1), Cl(1) and Cl(2), has revealed similarity of the studied structures to the initial **4a** compound. The RMS values are 0.090, 0.053, 0.057, 0.049, 0.062 Å and 0.104 Å for **4b**, **4c**, **4d**, **4e'**, **4e''** and **4f**, respectively. The structures **4c**, **4d** and **4e'** revealed a bigger similarity to the **4a** complex, and this finding agrees with the $V_{bur\%}$ values.

Using the data obtained from diffraction studies, we also calculated the buried volume ($V_{bur\%}$) parameters [76] for the studied series of nitro-catalysts bearing NHC ligands (Figure 5). As expected, $V_{bur\%}$ value of SIPr in **4b** (36.5%) was bigger than the one of SIMes in **4a** (35.4%) and Me$_2$IMes in **4c** (34.7%). The value obtained for Dorta's 2-SICyNap, present in catalyst **4d** (34.6%) was similar to the one obtained for Me$_2$IMes in **4c** (34.7%), even though the (cyclohexyl)naphthyl groups in **4d** can be considered as relatively bulkier in comparison with smaller Mes N-substituents in **4c**. Therefore it seems that they have similar steric demand of ligand (at least in the proximity of Ru).

Because crystals of catalyst **4e** that were measured by us contained two molecules in the asymmetric unit (**4e'** and **4e''**), the $V_{bur\%}$ values were calculated for each of them (Table 2). The relatively big difference between them was probably caused by various spatial arrangements of the naphthyl groups in both of these molecules. **4a** and **4c** had the smallest NHC, while the **4d** and **4e''** the largest. In the case of compounds **4b** and **4e''** the greater steric hindrance around the Ru atom is visible on the V_{bur} maps, which directly influenced the increased calculated V_{bur} value. The least protected Ru centre in this series is visible for complexes **4c** and **4d** and corresponds to the lowest V_{bur} values. Buchmeiser's catalyst **4f** has the highest V_{bur} value, which is probably correlated to the presence of the pyrimidine ring and different electron density than for the other NHCs. The difference between **4f** and other catalysts is marginal and is best visible for 10 Å radii (Figure 5f), where below the central atom some negative electron density is visible.

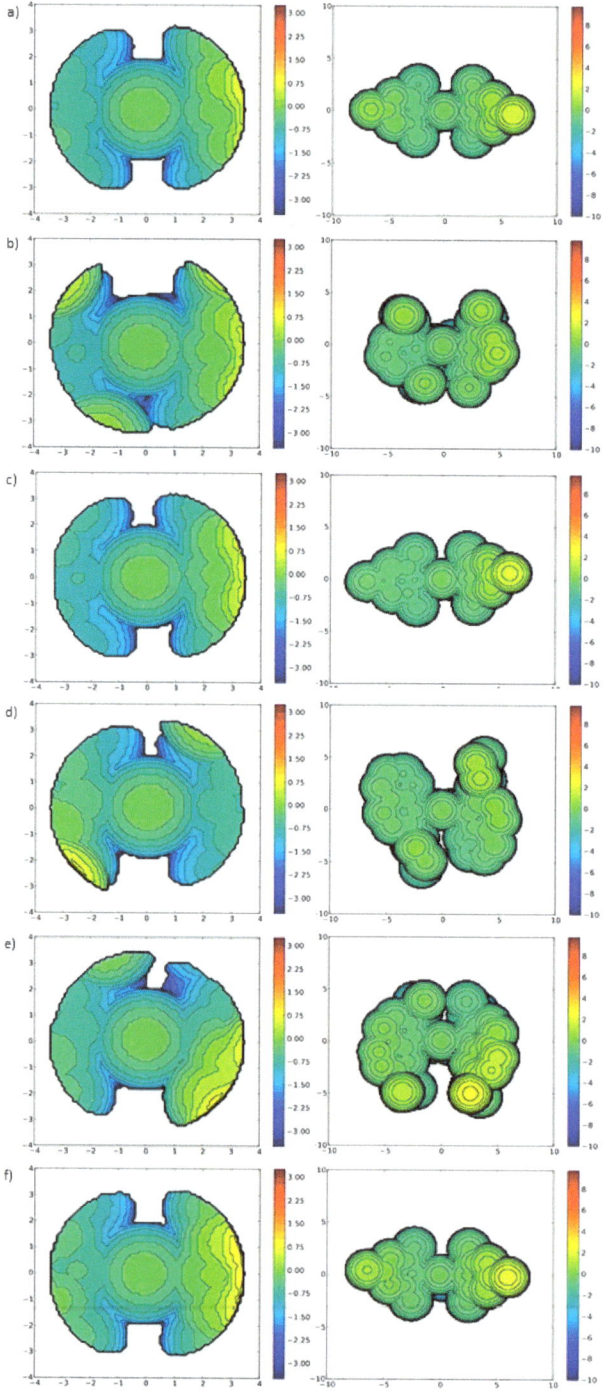

Figure 5. Steric maps calculated in SambVca software for complexes **4a** to **4f**. Standard (3.5 Å) and enlarged (10 Å) radii were used. (**a**) Catalyst **4a**, (**b**) Catalyst **4b**, (**c**) Catalyst **4c**, (**d**) Catalyst **4d**, (**e**) Catalyst **4e**, (**f**) Catalyst **4f**.

2.3. Comparative Catalytic Activity Studies of Nitro-Catalysts 4a–e

The performance of the nitro-catalysts **4a–e** was evaluated in the ring-closing and ene-yne metathesis of six model substrates: diethyl 2,2-diallylmalonate (**6**), diethyl 2-allyl-2-(2-methylallyl)malonate (**8**), 2,2-di(2-methylallyl)tosylate (**10**), diethyl 2,2-di(2-methylallyl)malonate (**12**), allyl 1,1-diphenylpropargyl ether (**14**), and (1-(prop-1-en-2-yl-methoxy)prop-2-yne-1,1-diyl)dibenzene (**16**). In the first stage of this research the RCM reaction of 2,2-diallylmalonate (**6**), the most commonly used model substrate [77] was examined in the presence of 1 mol% of nitro-catalysts **4a–e** (Scheme 2). Reactions were performed in NMR tubes at ambient temperature.

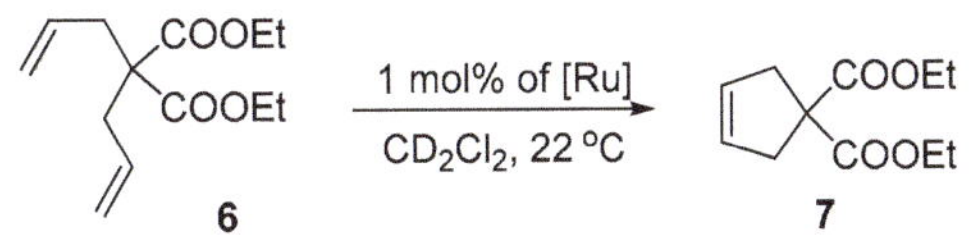

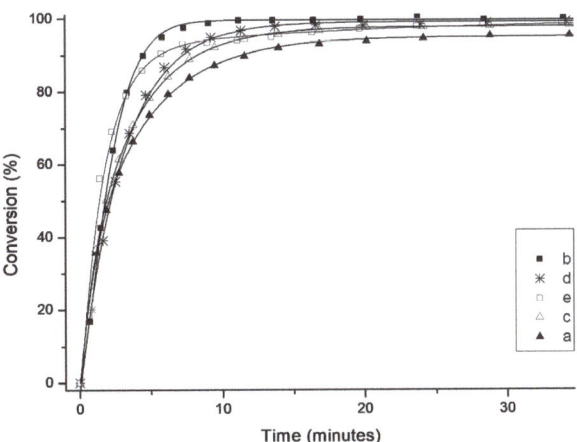

Scheme 2. Ring-closing metathesis (RCM) of diethyl 2,2-diallylmalonate (**6**).

As expected for the EWG-activated family of catalysts, all tested complexes showed high activity and almost quantitative conversion was achieved after only 10–15 min (Figure 6).

Figure 6. Time/conversion curves for the RCM reaction of diethyl 2,2-diallylmalonate (**6**) with 1 mol% of **4a–e** at 23 °C (monitored by ^{1}H-NMR). Lines are visual aids only.

Interestingly, the least active complex was the SIMes-containing **4a**. Complex **4c** with an unsaturated Me$_2$IMes ligand initiated slightly faster and provided maximal conversion after approximately 15 minutes. Both catalysts containing naphthyl substituents in their NHC ligands **4d** and **4e** exhibited even higher activity, with a slightly better result obtained for cyclohexyl-substituted catalyst **4d**. The most active complex in the series was **4b** bearing the SIPr ligand, which gave full conversion in less than 10 min.

Diethyl 2,2-diallylmalonate (**6**) is a rather simple substrate to ring-close and is used more to examine whether a newly obtained complex exhibits any catalytic metathesis activity than to show in detail the subtle differences between similarly active catalysts. To determine how the activity of the new Ru-complexes compare, a more difficult substrate containing substituted double bonds, diethyl 2-allyl-2-(2-methyllyl)malonate (**8**) was studied next (Scheme 3, Figure 7).

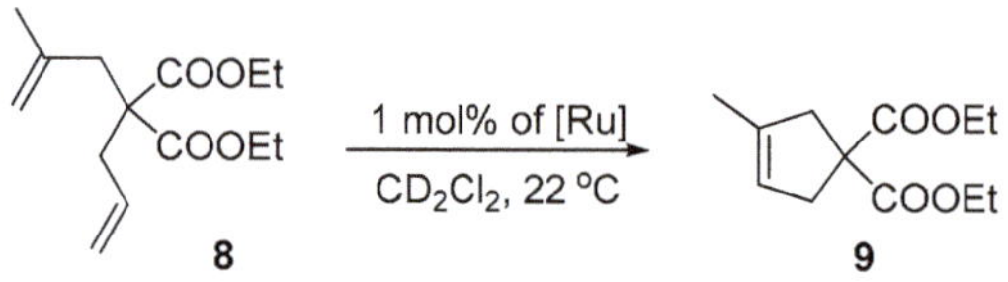

Scheme 3. RCM reaction of diethyl 2-allyl-2-(2-methylallyl)malonate (8).

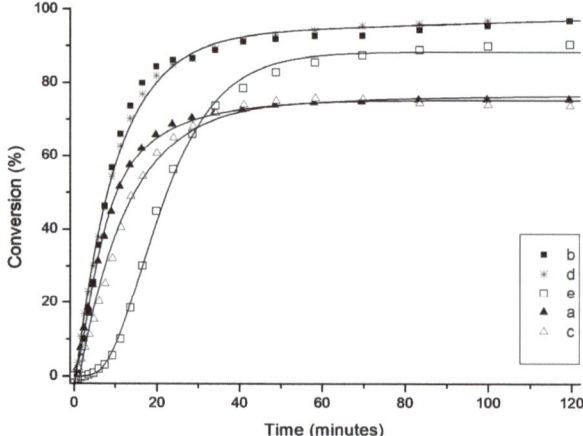

Figure 7. Time/conversion curves for the RCM reaction of diethyl 2-allyl-2-(2-methylallyl)malonate (8) with 1 mol% of 4a–e at 23 °C (monitored by ^{1}H-NMR). Lines are visual aids only.

In this case, under similarly mild conditions as used for the RCM of 6, namely in the presence of 1 mol% catalyst and at room temperature, the general trend was maintained, although higher diversity between the tested catalysts was found (Figure 7). The highest activity was observed for 4b (SIPr) and 4d, (2-SICyNap) complexes containing relatively large aryl substituents in the NHC ligand. After 20 minutes they reached 84 and 81% yield, respectively, reaching in both cases 97% of RCM product 9 within 2 h.

An interesting S-shaped curve was observed for the second complex bearing bulky naphthyl-substituted NHC (4e). The latter admittedly initialised slower than the other counterparts, as after 20 min it reached only 45% conversion. Interestingly, after this initial latency period 4e initiated in a fast rate giving after 100 min 90% conversion of 8. As observed previously for the conversion of 6 to 7, the least reactive complexes in this model reaction were 4a and 4c, which initiated quicker than 4e but after two hours provided the product with only 75 and 73% yield, respectively.

Next, we examined the activity of the nitro-catalysts in the RCM formation of tetrasubstituted olefins. Dienes 2,2-di(2-methyl allyl)tosylate (10) and diethyl 2,2-di(2-methyl allyl)malonate (12) are known to be more demanding and usually require the use of harsh conditions and specifically designed catalysts in order to achieve high yields [78]. Here, the reactions were performed in the presence of 5 mol% of complexes 4a–e at 80 °C (Scheme 4).

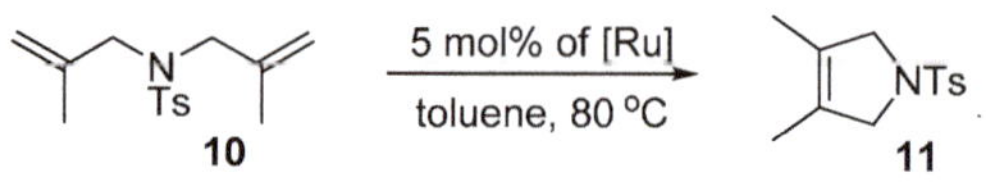

Scheme 4. RCM reaction of 2,2-di(2-methylallyl)tosylate (10).

When tosylate **10** was used (Scheme 4), good to very good yields were achieved, however a significant difference between complexes bearing bulky naphthyl substituted NHCs (**4d** and **4e**) and the more standard ones (**4a–c**) was observed (Figure 8). Despite the forcing conditions such as high catalyst loading and elevated temperature, the SIMes, SIPr and Me$_2$IMes-bearing catalysts produced **10** in 76–83% yield after one hour. In contrast, bulkier Dorta-type complexes **4d** and **4e** reached almost quantitative conversion, 90 and 91% respectively, after only 20 min. Interestingly, when the reaction time was extended to 24 h also complex with SIPr ligand (**4b**) achieved a similar conversion of 91%, while **4a** and **4c** died reaching 80–82% only (Table 3).

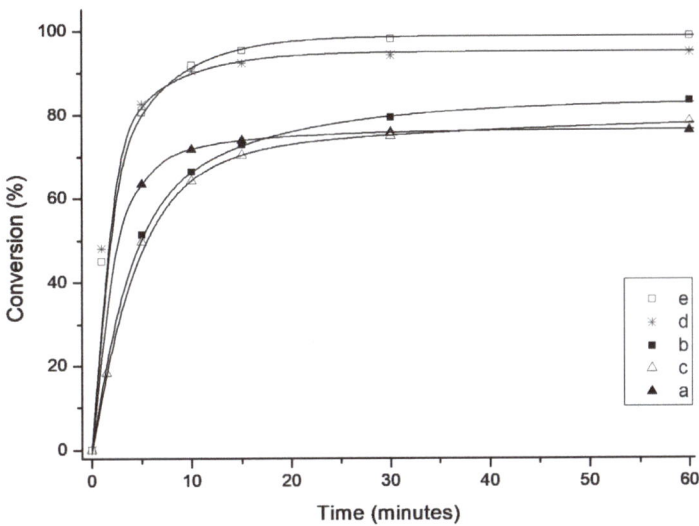

Figure 8. Time/conversion curves for the RCM reaction of 2,2-di(2-methylallyl)tosylate (**10**) with 5 mol% of **4a–e** at 80 °C (monitored by GC). Lines are visual aids only.

Table 3. RCM reaction of 2,2-di(2-methylallyl)tosylate (**10**) with 5 mol% of **4a–e** at 80 °C (monitored by GC) after 1 and 24 h.

Catalyst	Conversion (%)	
	After 1 h	After 24 h
4a	76	82
4b	83	91
4c	78	80
4d	98	99
4e	95	97

When even more challenging diethyl 2,2-di(2-methylallyl)malonate (**12**) was used instead of 2,2-di(2-methylallyl)tosylate (**10**) in the presence of 5 mol% of Ru at 80 °C (Scheme 5, Table 4), only the most bulky Dorta complex **4e** provided a relatively satisfactory result of 62% yield in 6 h. The other complexes (**4a–d**) were less active, leading to 9–21% of the desired product **13**.

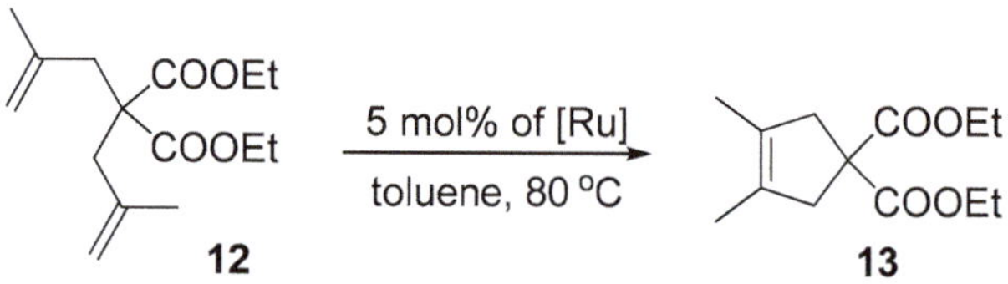

Scheme 5. RCM reaction of diethyl 2,2-di(2-methylallyl)malonate (**12**).

Table 4. RCM reaction of diethyl 2,2-di(2-methylallyl)malonate (**12**) with 5 mol% of **4a–e** at 80 °C (monitored by GC) after 6 and 24 h.

Catalyst	Conversion (%)	
	After 6 h	After 24 h
4a	16	18
4b	9	63
4c	21	21
4d	14	66
4e	62	84

After extending the reaction time to 24 h, virtually no changes in conversion were observed in the case of complexes with mesitylene-based NHC ligands (**4a** and **4c**). Pleasurably, we noticed a huge improvement in yield of the desired product when the reaction was conducted in the presence of Dorta-type (**4e** and **4d**) and SIPr-based (**4b**) catalysts (Table 4). Especially in the case of the latter two, changes were significant (from 14% to 66% for **4d** and from 9% to 63% for **4b**).

Ene-yne metathesis is a highly selective and atom-economical methodology for the synthesis of 1,3 dienes, which are valuable building blocks in organic synthesis [79]. To picture the application profile of the studied catalysts, two members of the ene-yne class of compounds were investigated with catalysts **4a–e**. Reactivity profiles for the metathesis of allyl 1,1-diphenylpropargyl ether (**14**) were established first (Scheme 6).

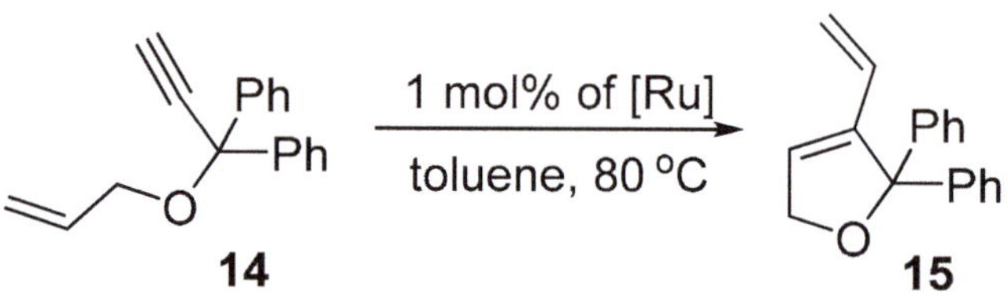

Scheme 6. Ene-yne reaction of allyl 1,1-diphenylpropargyl ether (**14**).

In the ene-yne cycloisomerisation of easy to react **14** [80] the most active were catalysts containing the smallest substituents (**4a–c**), while those with more bulky side chain groups (**4d–e**) showed diminished conversions (Figure 9). Nevertheless, all catalysts, but one, **4d** contain a large cyclohexyl substituent in the *ortho* position of the aryl ring, provided the desired product with yields above 80% during the first 6 h of the reaction. Further extension of the reaction time to 24 h resulted in slight improvement of the results leading to essentially quantitative conversions (over 90%) for **4a** and **4c** (Table 5).

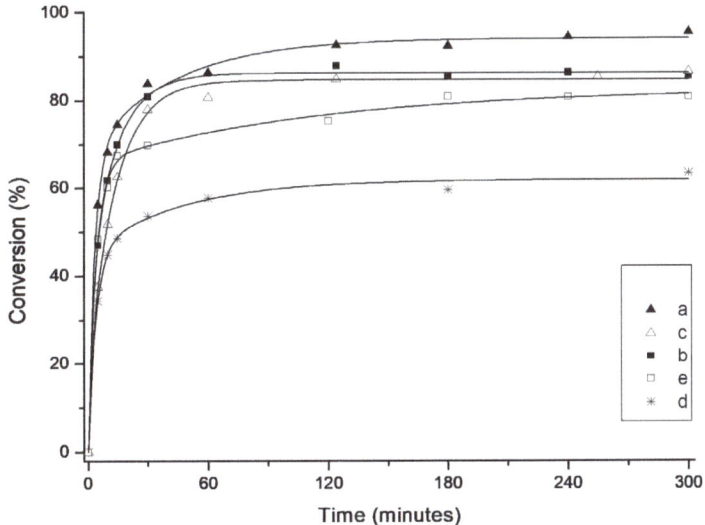

Figure 9. Time/conversion curves for the ene-yne reaction of allyl 1,1-diphenylpropargyl ether (**14**) with 1 mol% of **4a–e** at 80 °C (monitored by GC). Lines are visual aids only.

Table 5. Ene-yne reaction of allyl 1,1-diphenylpropargyl ether (**14**) with 1 mol% of **4a–e** at 80 °C (monitored by GC) after 6 and 24 h.

Catalyst	Conversion (%)	
	After 6 h	After 24 h
4a	93	99
4b	87	87
4c	90	93
4d	60	73
4e	81	88

Next, the more challenging cycloisomerisation substrate (1-(prop-1-en-2-yl-methoxy)prop-2-yne-1,1-diyl)dibenzene (**16**) [81–83] was utilised (Scheme 7). As for substrate **12**, also in this case the loading of the catalysts was increased from 1 to 5 mol% in order to obtain near-quantitative conversions.

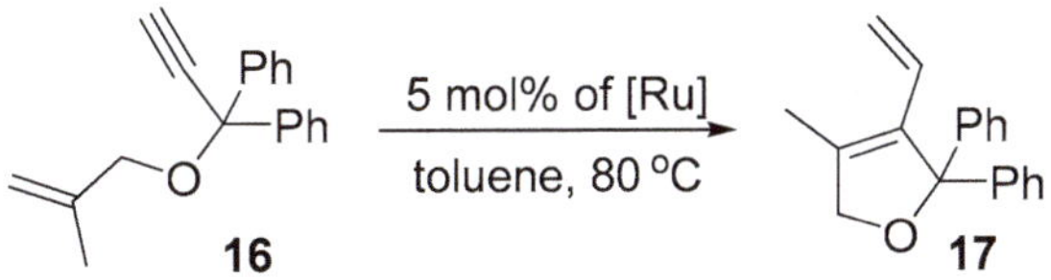

Scheme 7. Ene-yne reaction of (1-(prop-1-en-2-yl-methoxy)prop-2-yne-1,1-diyl)dibenzene (**16**).

Indeed, most of the complexes used gave the expected product with a yield of 90–100% in less than 6 hours, with **4d** being the most active, and after extension of the reaction time to 24 h 100% of yield was reached (Table 6). The only exception was the complex **4b** containing simple SIPr-ligand, which under these conditions gave only 25 and 41% conversion, after 6 and 24 h respectively.

Table 6. Ene-yne reaction of (1-(prop-1-en-2-yl-methoxy)prop-2-yne-1,1-diyl)dibenzene (16) with 5 mol% of 4a–e at 80 °C (monitored by GC) after 6 and 24 h.

Catalyst	Conversion (%)	
	After 6 h	After 24 h
4a	88	99
4b	15	42
4c	94	97
4d	94	98
4e	74	98

3. Experimental Section

3.1. General

All reactions were carried out under argon flow in pre-dried glassware using Schlenk techniques. Reaction profiles performed in NMR tube were carried out in degassed CD_2Cl_2. CH_2Cl_2 (Sigma-Aldrich Sp. z o.o., Poznan, Poland) was dried by distillation with CaH_2 under argon and was stored under argon. THF, toluene, n-hexane and xylene were dried by distillation with Na/K alloy. Flash chromatography was performed using Merck KGaA (Darmstadt, Germany) silica gel 60 (230–400 mesh). NMR spectra were recorded in $CDCl_3$ or CD_2Cl_2 with Varian Mercury 400 MHz and Varian VNMRS 500 MHz spectrometers. MS (FD/FAB) was recorded with a GCT Premier spectrometer from Waters Corporation (Milford, MA, USA). MS (EI) spectra were recorded with an AMD 604 Intectra GmbH (Harpstedt, Germany) spectrometer. Other commercially available chemicals were used as received.

3.2. Synthesis of Complexes

Synthesis of 4a: Complex (2a) (220 mg, 0.232 mmol) was dissolved in toluene (7 mL), and 1-isopropoxy-4-nitro-2-(prop-1-en-1-yl)benzene (5) (61.6 mg, 0.278 mmol) was added. The mixture was stirred for 5 min, CuCl (45.9 mg, 0.474 mmol) was added, and the mixture was heated at 80 °C for 30 min. The reaction mixture was cooled to room temperature and concentrated in vacuo. From this point, all manipulations were carried out in air with reagent grade solvents. The product was purified by silica gel chromatography (AcOEt/c-hexane = 1:4 v/v). The solvent was evaporated under vacuum, and the residue was dissolved in CH_2Cl_2 (2 mL). MeOH (5 mL) was added and CH_2Cl_2 was slowly removed under vacuum. The precipitated was filtered, washed with MeOH (5 mL), and dried in vacuo to afford **4a** as a green microcrystalline solid (130 mg, 83%). ^{1}H-NMR (CD_2Cl_2, 500 MHz,): δ = 16.42 (s, 1H), 8.46 (dd, J = 9.1, 2.5 Hz, 1H), 7.80 (d, J = 2.5 Hz, 1H), 7.10 (s, 4H), 6.94 (d, J = 9.1 Hz, 1H), 5.01 (sept, J = 6.1 Hz, 1H), 4.22 (s, 4H), 2.46–2.48 (m, 18H), 1.30 (d, J = 6.1 Hz, 6H); ^{13}C-NMR (125 MHz, CD_2Cl_2): δ = 289.1, 208.2, 156.8, 150.3, 145.0, 143.5, 139.6, 139.3, 129.8, 124.5, 117.2, 113.3, 78.2, 52.0, 21.3, 21.2, 19.4; IR (KBr): $\tilde{v}$ = 2924, 2850, 1606, 1521, 1480, 1262, 1093, 918, 745 cm^{-1}; FDMS m/z [M$^+$] 671.1.

Synthesis of 4b: Similar to the preparation of **4a**, **5** (150 mg, 0.68 mmol) was added to the solution of complex **2b** (690 mg, 0.68 mmol) in toluene (15 mL). The mixture was stirred for 5 min, and CuCl (135 mg, 1.36 mmol) was added. **4b** was obtained as green microcrystalline solid (380 mg, 62%). ^{1}H-NMR (500 MHz, CD_2Cl_2): δ = 16.33 (s, 1H), 8.38 (dd, J = 9.0, 2.7 Hz, 1H), 7.69 (d, J = 2.7 Hz, 1H), 7.58 (t, J = 7.7 Hz, 4H), 7.39 (d, J = 7.7 Hz, 4H), 6.90 (d, J = 9.0 Hz, 1H), 4.99 (m, 1H), 4.20 (s, 4H), 3.56 (m, 4H), 1.40 (d, J = 6.1 Hz, 6H), 1.24 (d, J = 6.7 Hz, 12H); ^{13}C-NMR (125 MHz, CD_2Cl_2): δ = 283.7, 210.3, 156.6, 149.0, 143.6, 143.0, 136.2, 130.0, 124.4, 124.0, 116.7, 112.8, 77.7, 77.2, 77.0, 76.7, 54.5, 28.8, 26.5, 23.3, 21.7; IR (KBr):$\tilde{v}$ = 3096, 3069, 2970, 2951, 2927, 2868, 1527, 1341, 1270, 1095, 914, 742 cm^{-1}; FDMS m/z [M$^+$] 755.10.

Synthesis 4c: Complex **2c** (500 mg, 0.571 mmol) was dissolved in toluene (11 mL), and 1-isopropoxy-4-nitro-2-(prop-1-en-1-yl)benzene (5) (190 mg, 0.856 mmol) was added. The mixture was stirred for 5 min, CuCl (113 mg, 1.14 mmol) was added, and the mixture was stirred at 70 °C for 40 min.

The reaction mixture was cooled to room temperature and concentrated in vacuo. From this point, all manipulations were carried out in air with reagent grade solvents. The product was purified by silica gel chromatography (AcOEt/c-hexane = 1:5 v/v). The solvent was evaporated under vacuum, and the residue was dissolved in CH_2Cl_2 (2 mL). MeOH (5 mL) was added and CH_2Cl_2 was slowly removed under vacuum. The precipitated was filtered, washed with MeOH (5 mL) and dried in vacuo to afford **4c** as a brownish microcrystalline solid (250 mg, 63%). ^{1}H-NMR (500 MHz, CD_2Cl_2): δ = 16.57 (s, 1H), 8.42 (dd, J = 9.0, 2.7 Hz, 1H), 7.92 (d, J = 2.5 Hz, 1H), 7.14 (s, 4H), 6.89 (d, J = 9.0 Hz, 1H), 4.98 (m, 1H), 2.48 (s, 6H), 2.18 (s, 12H), 1.97 (s, 6H), 1.35 (d, J = 6.1 Hz, 6H); ^{13}C-NMR (125 MHz, CD_2Cl_2): δ = 287.0, 167.0, 156.4, 145.0, 143.2, 139.7, 138.4, 129.2, 127.8, 123.3, 116.7, 112.7, 77.5, 77.3, 77.0, 76.8, 21.8, 21.1, 21.1, 19.1, 19.1; IR (KBr): $\tilde{v}$ = 3103, 3084, 2986, 2969, 2921, 1604, 1571, 1520, 1384, 1337, 1320, 1095, 746, 660 cm^{-1}; FDMS m/z [M$^+$] 697.1.

Synthesis of 4d: Similar to the preparation of **4c**, **5** (86 mg, 0.389 mmol) was added to the solution of complex **1d** (250 mg, 0.243 mmol) in CH_2Cl_2 (15 mL). The mixture was stirred for 5 min, and CuCl (48 mg, 0.486 mmol) was added. **4d** was obtained as green microcrystalline solid (180 mg, 87 %). ^{1}H-NMR (500 MHz, CD_2Cl_2): δ = 16.04 (s, 1H), 8.30 (d, J = 8.1 Hz, 2H), 8.23 (dd, J = 9.0, 2.7 Hz, 1H), 8.08 (d J = 8.6 Hz, 2H), 7.95 (d, J = 7.9 Hz, 2H), 7.68 (d, J = 8.6 Hz, 2H), 7.60 (td, J = 6.9, 1.0 Hz, 2H), 7.52 (td, J = 6.9, 1.0 Hz, 2H), 7.33 (d J = 2.5, 1H), 6.71 (d, J = 9.0 Hz, 1H), 4.77 (m, 1H), 4.48–4.34 (m, 4H), 4.12 (q, J = 14.2, 7.1 Hz, 1H), 3.11 (s, 2H), 2.16 (s, 1H), 2.04 (s, 2H), 1.98–1.96 (m, 12H), 1.74–1.55 (m, 10H), 1.48–1.37 (m, 4H), 1.25 (t, J = 7.1 Hz, 4H), 1.09 (d, J = 6.1 Hz, 2H), 1.01 (d, J = 6.1 Hz, 2H); ^{13}C-NMR (125 MHz, CD_2Cl_2): δ = 211.5, 156.5, 145.1, 143.7, 142.8, 133.0, 131.6, 129.8, 127.9, 127.0, 126.2, 125.2, 123.9, 116.6, 112.4, 77.5, 77.2, 77.0, 76.7, 60.3, 54.5, 53.4, 39.8, 36.2, 32.5, 31.5, 30.9, 28.2, 27.5, 26.6, 26.3, 25.8, 21.1; IR (KBr): $\tilde{v}$ = 3067, 2925, 2849, 1735, 1523, 1441, 1340, 1267, 1091, 914, 818, 747 cm^{-1}; FDMS m/z [M$^+$] 851.2.

Synthesis of 4e: Similar to the preparation of **4c**, **5** (64.4 mg, 0.291 mmol) was added to the solution of complex **1e** (200 mg, 0.194 mmol) in CH_2Cl_2 (10 mL). The mixture was stirred for 5 min, and CuCl (38.4 mg, 0.388 mmol) was added. **4e** was obtained as green microcrystalline solid (128 mg, 77 %). ^{1}H-NMR (500 MHz, CD_2Cl_2): δ = 16.39 (s, 1H), 16.21 (s, 1H), 8.21 (dq, J = 8.9, 2.5 Hz, 1H), 8.05 (d, J = 8.9 Hz, 2H), 7.95 (s, 1H), 7.86 (dd J = 8.3, 3.2, 2H), 7.63 (t, J = 8.9 Hz, 2H), 7.50 (d, J = 2.5 Hz, 1H), 7.47–7.40 (m, 2H), 6.69 (t, J = 8.3 Hz, 1H), 4.80–4.70 (m 1H), 4.60 (s, 1H), 4.47 (t, J = 5.8 Hz, 2H), 3.65 (quint, J = 13.1, 6.7 Hz, 1H), 3.22 (quint, J = 13.5, 6.7 Hz, 1H), 3.11 (quint, J = 13.5, 6.8 Hz, 1H), 1.44–1.36 (m, 25H), 1.13 (d, J = 5.9 2H), 1.04 (d, J = 6.0 Hz, 2H), 0.93 (d, J = 6.0 Hz, 2H); ^{13}C-NMR (125 MHz, CD_2Cl_2): δ = 286.9, 286.6, 211.2, 210.7, 156.5, 147.0, 146.1, 143.9, 143.8, 142.9, 131.7, 131.0, 129.8, 129.7, 127.7, 126.3, 125.5, 123.7, 123.3, 123.2, 122.4, 116.6, 112.5, 112.4, 77.4, 77.2, 77.0, 76.7, 54.0, 34.7, 34.4, 29.2, 29.1, 25.8, 24.0, 23.5, 23.5, 23.3, 22.8, 22.6, 21.1, 21.0, 20.7; IR (KBr): $\tilde{v}$ = 3090, 3058, 2960, 2870, 1604, 1525, 1473, 1340, 1256, 1092, 845 cm^{-1}; FDMS m/z [M$^+$] 855.3.

4. Conclusions

The family of nitro-complexes containing NHC ligands with different steric properties was synthesised, characterised and investigated in terms of activity. Analysis of the solid-state geometrical parameters manifested some interesting relationships. Intuitively, the most important difference in geometry was expressed by angle α, representing visually how the *N*-aryl 'wings' of the NHC ligand are lowered towards the metal centre (Figure 4, Table 2). In the case of the SIPr-bearing **4b** the *N*-aryl 'flaps' are slightly lowered compared to (S)IMes-decorated **4a,c**. Interestingly, the naphthyl members of this series (**4d–e**) have the *N*-substituents even slightly more 'elevated' compared to their (S)IMes and SIPr counterparts (**4a–b**). This is in strong contrast to complex **4f** where the NHC wings are visibly lowered, thus shielding much more the Ru centre. Interestingly, the latter complex, although very useful in cyclopolymerization of diynes, in model RCM reactions was found to be less reactive than the analogue SIMes Hoveyda-Grubbs complex [24]. The $V_{bur\%}$ values and steric maps calculated for the studied complexes illustrated the same picture, rendering the naphthyl-containing complexes

4d–e being the least crowded and **4f** having the highest $V_{bur\%}$ value. The model reactions also sorted the tested complexes into two groups. While in the reaction of a simple model diene (**6**) all catalysts exhibited similarly high activity, in the case of a still rather straightforward cycloisomerisation of ene-yne **14**, the less bulky NHC containing complexes **4a–c** were more active. At the same time, with more demanding sterically crowded substrates, a significant advantage of complexes with bulkier NHC ligands (**4b**, **4d–e**) was evident. Importantly, complexes **4d–e** demonstrated high activity in formation of tetra-substituted C–C double bonds [78,84], the reaction which was traditionally Achilles' heel of the nitro-catalyst [42–45]. It is stressed that in all cases the studied model reactions were very clean and no side-products were observed.

Overall, the comparative study here suggests that the elaborated naphthyl-based catalysts (**4d–e**) may be better for challenging, sterically crowded substrates, while the 'easy' substrates can be transformed more readily in the presence of catalysts with standard NHC ligands (**4a–b**). Interestingly, catalysts **4c** bearing Me$_2$IMes ligand seemed the least utile.

These results show again [85] that different catalysts can be optimal for different applications, and that even small, sometimes incremental, variations can result in substantial changes in reactivity.

Supplementary Materials: The following are available online. Figure S1: Atomic Displacement Parameters (ADPs) and the labeling of atoms in **4b** and **4c**; Figure S2: Atomic Displacement Parameters (ADPs) and the labeling of atoms in **4d**; Figure S3: Atomic Displacement Parameters (ADPs) and the labeling of atoms in 4e for two molecules in asymmetric unit (**4e′** and **4e″**); Figure S4: Overlay of molecules from the **4a** structure (black) with the **4b** (magenta), **4c** structure (blue), **4d** structure (green), **4f** structure (grey), **4e′** structure (red) and **4e″** (yellow) and **4g** (grey); Figure S5: Atomic Displacement Parameters; Table S1: Experimental details for **4b–4e** structures; Table S2: Experimental details for the CuClPCy3 measurement.

Author Contributions: Experiments and data analysis, M.P. and J.C.-J.; naphthyl ligands synthesis, R.D.; X-Ray measurements, M.M. and K.W. V_{bur} calculation, A.R.; writing—original draft preparation, A.K. and K.G.; writing—review and editing, A.K., R.D. and K.G.; supervision, A.K. and K.G. All authors have read and agreed to the published version of the manuscript.

Funding: This research was funded by the OPUS project financed by the National Science Centre, Poland on the basis of a decision DEC-2014/15/B/ST5/02156.

Conflicts of Interest: The authors declare no conflict of interest. K.G. is an advisory board member of the Apeiron Synthesis company, the producer of catalyst **4a–b**.

References

1. Wanzlick, H.-W.; Schönherr, H.-J. Direct Synthesis of a Mercury Salt-Carbene Complex. *Angew. Chem. Int. Ed.* **1968**, *7*, 141–142. [CrossRef]
2. Öfele, K. 1,3-Dimethyl-4-imidazolinyliden-(2)-pentacarbonylchrom ein neuer übergangsmetall-carben-komplex. *J. Organomet. Chem.* **1968**, *12*, P42–P43. [CrossRef]
3. Arduengo, A.J.; Harlow, R.L.; Kline, M. A stable crystalline carbene. *J. Am. Chem. Soc.* **1991**, *113*, 361–363. [CrossRef]
4. Gómez-Suárez, A.; Nelson, D.J.; Nolan, S.P. Quantifying and understanding the steric properties of N-heterocyclic carbenes. *Chem. Commun.* **2017**, *53*, 2650–2660. [CrossRef]
5. Cazin, C. (Ed.) *N-Heterocyclic Carbenes in Transition Metal Catalysis and Organocatalysis*; Springer: Dordrecht, The Netherlands, 2011; Volume 32, pp. 1–336.
6. Grubbs, R.H.; Wenzel, A.G.; O'Leary, D.J.; Khosravi, E. *Handbook of Metathesis*; Wiley-VCH: Weinheim, Germany, 2015.
7. Grela, K. *Olefin Metathesis: Theory and Practice*; John Wiley & Sons, Inc.: Hoboken, NJ, USA, 2014.
8. Michrowska, A.; Grela, K. Quest for the ideal olefin metathesis catalyst. *Pure Appl. Chem.* **2008**, *80*, 31–43. [CrossRef]
9. Anderson, A.W.; Merckling, N.G. Polymeric Bicyclo-(2, 2, 1)-2-Heptene. U.S. Patent 2,721,189, 18 October 1955.
10. Banks, R.L.; Bailey, G.C. Olefin Disproportionation. A New Catalytic Process. *Ind. Eng. Chem. Prod. Res. Dev.* **1964**, *3*, 170–173. [CrossRef]
11. Natta, G.; Dall'Asta, G.; Mazzanti, G. Stereospecific Homopolymerization of Cyclopentene. *Angew. Chem. Int. Ed.* **1964**, *3*, 723–729. [CrossRef]

12. Schrock, R.R.; Murdzek, J.S.; Bazan, G.C.; Robbins, J.; Dimare, M.; O'Regan, M. Synthesis of molybdenum imido alkylidene complexes and some reactions involving acyclic olefins. *J. Am. Chem. Soc.* **1990**, *112*, 3875–3886. [CrossRef]
13. Schwab, P.; Grubbs, R.H.; Ziller, J.W. Synthesis and Applications of RuCl2(CHR')(PR3)2: The Influence of the Alkylidene Moiety on Metathesis Activity. *J. Am. Chem. Soc.* **1996**, *118*, 100–110. [CrossRef]
14. Ackermann, L.; Fürstner, A.; Weskamp, T.; Kohl, F.J.; Herrmann, W.A. Ruthenium carbene complexes with imidazolin-2-ylidene ligands allow the formation of tetrasubstituted cycloalkenes by RCM. *Tetrahedron Lett.* **1999**, *40*, 4787–4790. [CrossRef]
15. Huang, J.; Stevens, E.D.; Nolan, S.P.; Petersen, J.L. Olefin Metathesis-Active Ruthenium Complexes Bearing a Nucleophilic Carbene Ligand. *J. Am. Chem. Soc.* **1999**, *121*, 2674–2678. [CrossRef]
16. Scholl, M.; Trnka, T.M.; Morgan, J.P.; Grubbs, R.H. Increased ring closing metathesis activity of ruthenium-based olefin metathesis catalysts coordinated with imidazolin-2-ylidene ligands. *Tetrahedron Lett.* **1999**, *40*, 2247–2250. [CrossRef]
17. Available online: https://pmc.umicore.com/en/products/umicore-grubbs-catalyst-m2a-c848/ (accessed on 15 April 2020).
18. Scholl, M.; Ding, S.; Lee, C.W.; Grubbs, R.H. Synthesis and activity of a new generation of ruthenium-based olefin metathesis catalysts coordinated with 1,3-dimesityl-4,5-dihydroimidazol-2-ylidene ligands. *Org. Lett.* **1999**, *1*, 953–956. [CrossRef] [PubMed]
19. Available online: https://catalysts.evonik.com/product/catalysts/downloads/homogeneous_catalysts_evonik.pdf (accessed on 15 April 2020).
20. Available online: https://pmc.umicore.com/en/products/umicore-grubbs-catalyst-m2/ (accessed on 15 April 2020).
21. Available online: https://www.sigmaaldrich.com/catalog/product/sial/901755?lang=pl&region=PL (accessed on 15 April 2020).
22. Available online: https://www.strem.com/catalog/v/44-0758/59/ruthenium_502964-52-5 (accessed on 15 April 2020).
23. Available online: https://www.strem.com/catalog/v/44-0770/59/ruthenium_928795-51-1 (accessed on 15 April 2020).
24. Yang, L.; Mayr, M.; Wurst, K.; Buchmeiser, M.R. Novel metathesis catalysts based on ruthenium 1,3-dimesityl-3,4,5,6-tetrahydropyrimidin-2-ylidenes: Synthesis, structure, immobilization, and catalytic activity. *Chem. Eur. J.* **2004**, *10*, 5761–5770. [CrossRef]
25. Despagnet-Ayoub, E.; Grubbs, R.H. A ruthenium olefin metathesis catalyst with a four-membered N-heterocyclic carbene ligand. *Organometallics* **2005**, *24*, 338. [CrossRef]
26. Fürstner, A.; Ackermann, L.; Gabor, B.; Goddard, R.; Lehmann, C.W.; Mynott, R.; Stelzer, F.; Thiel, O.R. Comparative investigation of ruthenium-based metathesis catalysts bearing N-heterocyclic carbene (NHC) ligands. *Chem.-A Eur. J.* **2001**, *7*, 3236–3253. [CrossRef]
27. Dinger, M.B.; Nieczypor, P.; Mol, J.C. Adamantyl-Substituted N-Heterocyclic Carbene Ligands in Second-Generation Grubbs-Type Metathesis Catalysts. *Organometallics* **2003**, *22*, 5291. [CrossRef]
28. Yun, J.; Marinez, E.R.; Grubbs, R.H. A new ruthenium-based olefin metathesis catalyst coordinated with 1,3-dimesityl-1,4,5,6-tetrahydropyrimidin-2-ylidene: synthesis, X-ray structure, and reactivity. *Organometallics* **2004**, *23*, 4172. [CrossRef]
29. Vehlow, K.; Maechling, S.; Blechert, S. Ruthenium metathesis catalysts with saturated unsymmetrical N-heterocyclic carbene ligands. *Organometallics* **2006**, *25*, 25. [CrossRef]
30. Ledoux, N.; Allaert, B.; Pattyn, S.; Vander Mierde, H.; Vercaemst, C.; Verpoort, F. *N,N*′-Dialkyl- and *N*-Alkyl-*N*-mesityl-Substituted *N*-Heterocyclic Carbenes as Ligands in Grubbs Catalysts. *Chem. Eur. J.* **2006**, *12*, 4654. [CrossRef]
31. Tornatzky, J.; Kannenberg, A.; Blechert, S. New catalysts with unsymmetrical N-heterocyclic carbene ligands. *Dalton Trans.* **2012**, *41*, 8215. [CrossRef] [PubMed]
32. Hamad, F.B.; Sun, T.; Xiao, S.; Verpoort, F. Olefin metathesis ruthenium catalysts bearing unsymmetrical heterocyclic carbenes. *Coord. Chem. Rev.* **2013**, *257*, 2274–2292. [CrossRef]
33. Paradiso, V.; Costabile, C.; Grisi, F. Ruthenium-based olefin metathesis catalysts with monodentate unsymmetrical NHC ligands. *Beilstein J. Org. Chem.* **2018**, *14*, 3122–3149. [CrossRef] [PubMed]
34. Dinger, M.B.; Mol, J.C. High turnover numbers with ruthenium-based metathesis catalysts. *Adv. Synth. Catal.* **2002**, *344*, 671–677. [CrossRef]
35. Banti, D.; Mol, J.C. Degradation of the ruthenium-based metathesis catalyst [RuCl2(CHPh)(H2IPr)(PCy3)] with primary alcohols. *J. Organomet. Chem.* **2004**, *689*, 3113. [CrossRef]

36. Clavier, H.; Urbina-Blanco, C.A.; Nolan, S.P. Indenylidene Ruthenium Complex Bearing a Sterically Demanding NHC Ligand: An Efficient Catalyst for Olefin Metathesis at Room Temperature. *Organometallics* **2009**, *28*, 2848–2854. [CrossRef]
37. Gallenkamp, D.; Fürstner, A. Stereoselective Synthesis ofE,Z-Configured 1,3-Dienes by Ring-Closing Metathesis. Application to the Total Synthesis of Lactimidomycin. *J. Am. Chem. Soc.* **2011**, *133*, 9232–9235. [CrossRef]
38. Bieniek, M.; Bujok, R.; Stepowska, H.; Jacobi, A.; Hagenkötter, R.; Arlt, D.; Jarzembska, K.N.; Makal, A.; Woźniak, K.; Grela, K. New air-stable ruthenium olefin metathesis precatalysts derived from bisphenol S. *J. Organomet. Chem.* **2006**, *691*, 5289–5297. [CrossRef]
39. Arduengo, A.J.; Davidson, F.; Dias, H.V.R.; Goerlich, J.R.; Khasnis, D.; Marshall, W.J.; Prakasha, T.K. An Air Stable Carbene and Mixed Carbene "Dimers. " *J. Am. Chem. Soc.* **1997**, *119*, 12742–12749. [CrossRef]
40. Kadyrov, R.; Rosiak, A.; Tarabocchia, J.; Szadkowska, A.; Bieniek, M.; Grela, K. New concepts in designing ruthenium-based second generation olefin metathesis catalysts and their application. In *Catalysis of Organic Reactions*; CRC Press: Boca Raton, FL, USA, 2008; pp. 217–222.
41. Ginzburg, Y.; Lemcoff, N. Hoveyda-Type Olefin Metathesis Complexes. In *Olefin Metathesis*; Wiley: Hoboken, NJ, USA, 2014; pp. 437–451.
42. Grela, K.; Harutyunyan, S.; Michrowska, A. A Highly Efficient Ruthenium Catalyst for Metathesis Reactions. *Angew. Chem. Int. Ed.* **2002**, *41*, 4038–4040. [CrossRef]
43. Michrowska, A.; Bujok, R.; Harutyunyan, S.; Sashuk, V.; Dolgonos, G.; Grela, K.; Dolgonos, G.A. Nitro-Substituted Hoveyda–Grubbs Ruthenium Carbenes: Enhancement of Catalyst Activity through Electronic Activation. *J. Am. Chem. Soc.* **2004**, *126*, 9318–9325. [CrossRef] [PubMed]
44. Grela, K. Ruthenium Complexes as (Pre)catalysts for Metathesis Reactions. U.S. Patent 6,867,303, 15 March 2005.
45. Bieniek, M.; Michrowska, A.; Gułajski, Ł.; Grela, K. A Practical Larger Scale Preparation of Second-Generation Hoveyda-Type Catalysts. *Organometallics* **2007**, *26*, 1096–1099. [CrossRef]
46. Zhan, Z.-Y.J. Recyclable Ruthenium Catalysts for Metathesis Reactions. U.S. Patent 7,632,772, 15 December 2009.
47. Lindner, F.; Friedrich, S.; Hahn, F. Total Synthesis of Complex Biosynthetic Late-Stage Intermediates and Bioconversion by a Tailoring Enzyme from Jerangolid Biosynthesis. *J. Org. Chem.* **2018**, *83*, 14091–14101. [CrossRef] [PubMed]
48. Stellfeld, T.; Bhatt, U.; Kalesse, M. Synthesis of the A,B,C-Ring System of Hexacyclinic Acid. *Org. Lett.* **2004**, *6*, 3889–3892. [CrossRef] [PubMed]
49. Shu, C.; Zeng, X.; Hao, M.-H.; Wei, X.; Yee, N.K.; Busacca, C.A.; Han, Z.; Farina, V.; Senanayake, C.H. RCM Macrocyclization Made Practical: An Efficient Synthesis of HCV Protease Inhibitor BILN. *Org. Lett.* **2008**, *10*, 1303–1306. [CrossRef] [PubMed]
50. Farina, V.; Shu, C.; Zeng, X.; Wei, X.; Han, Z.; Yee, N.K.; Senanayake, C.H. Second-Generation Process for the HCV Protease Inhibitor BILN 2061: A Greener Approach to Ru-Catalyzed Ring-Closing Metathesis†. *Org. Process Res. Dev.* **2009**, *13*, 250–254. [CrossRef]
51. Chen, Q.-Y.; Chaturvedi, P.R.; Luesch, H. Process development and scale-up total synthesis of largazole, a potent class i histone deacetylase inhibitor. *Org. Process Res. Dev.* **2018**, *22*, 190–199. [CrossRef]
52. Breen, C.P.; Parrish, C.; Shangguan, N.; Majumdar, S.; Murnen, H.; Jamison, T.F.; Bio, M.M. A scalable membrane pervaporation approach for continuous flow olefin metathesis. *Org. Process Res. Dev.* **2020**. [CrossRef]
53. Tracz, A.; Matczak, M.; Urbaniak, K.; Skowerski, K. Nitro-grela-type complexes containing iodides–robust and selective catalysts for olefin metathesis under challenging conditions. *Beilstein J. Org. Chem.* **2015**, *11*, 1823–1832. [CrossRef]
54. Marx, V.M.; Sullivan, A.H.; Melaimi, M.; Virgil, S.C.; Keitz, B.K.; Weinberger, D.S.; Bertrand, G.; Grubbs, R.H. Cyclic alkyl amino carbene (caac) ruthenium complexes as remarkably active catalysts for ethenolysis. *Angew. Chem. Int. Ed.* **2015**, *54*, 1919–1923. [CrossRef]
55. Gawin, R.; Tracz, A.; Chwalba, M.; Kozakiewicz, A.; Trzaskowski, B.; Skowerski, K. Cyclic Alkyl Amino Ruthenium Complexes—Efficient Catalysts for Macrocyclization and Acrylonitrile Cross Metathesis. *ACS Catal.* **2017**, *7*, 5443–5449. [CrossRef]
56. Schmid, T.E.; Dumas, A.; Colombel-Rouen, S.; Crévisy, C.; Baslé, O.; Mauduit, M. From environmentally friendly reusable ionic-tagged ruthenium-based complexes to industrially relevant homogeneous catalysts: Toward a sustainable olefin metathesis. *Synlett* **2017**, *28*, 773–798.

57. Bieniek, M.; Bujok, R.; Milewski, M.; Arlt, D.; Kajetanowicz, A.; Grela, K. Making the family portrait complete: Synthesis of electron withdrawing group activated Hoveyda-Grubbs catalysts bearing sulfone and ketone functionalities. *J. Organomet. Chem.* **2020**, *918*, 121276. [CrossRef]
58. Bieniek, M.; Samojłowicz, C.; Sashuk, V.; Bujok, R.; Śledź, P.; Lugan, N.; Lavigne, G.; Arlt, D.; Grela, K. Rational design and evaluation of upgraded Grubbs/Hoveyda olefin metathesis catalysts: Polyfunctional benzylidene ethers on the test bench. *Organometallics* **2011**, *30*, 4144–4158. [CrossRef]
59. Eivgi, O.; Sutar, R.L.; Reany, O.; Lemcoff, N.G. Bichromatic photosynthesis of coumarins by UV filter-enabled olefin metathesis. *Adv. Synth. Catal.* **2017**, *359*, 2352–2357. [CrossRef]
60. Ivry, E.; Frenklah, A.; Ginzburg, Y.; Levin, E.; Goldberg, I.; Kozuch, S.; Lemcoff, N.G.; Tzur, E. Light- and thermal-activated olefin metathesis of hindered substrates. *Organometallics* **2018**, *37*, 176–181. [CrossRef]
61. Tzur, E.; Szadkowska, A.; Ben-Asuly, A.; Makal, A.; Goldberg, I.; Woźniak, K.; Grela, K.; Lemcoff, N.G. Studies on electronic effects in *O*-, *N*- and *S*-chelated ruthenium olefin-metathesis catalysts. *Chem.-A Eur. J.* **2010**, *16*, 8726–8737. [CrossRef]
62. Żukowska, K.; Szadkowska, A.; Pazio, A.E.; Woźniak, K.; Grela, K. Thermal switchability of *N*-chelating Hoveyda-type catalyst containing a secondary amine ligand. *Organometallics* **2012**, *31*, 462–469. [CrossRef]
63. Gawin, A.; Pump, E.; Slugovc, C.; Kajetanowicz, A.; Grela, K. Ruthenium amide complexes—Synthesis and catalytic activity in olefin metathesis and in ring-opening polymerisation. *Eur. J. Inorg. Chem.* **2018**, *2018*, 1766–1774. [CrossRef]
64. Monsaert, S.; Lozano Vila, A.; Drozdzak, R.; Van Der Voort, P.; Verpoort, F. Latent olefin metathesis catalysts. *Chem. Soc. Rev.* **2009**, *38*, 3360–3372. [CrossRef]
65. Eivgi, O.; Lemcoff, N.G. Turning the light on: Recent developments in photoinduced olefin metathesis. *Synthesis* **2018**, *50*, 49–63.
66. Luan, X.; Mariz, R.; Gatti, M.; Costabile, C.; Poater, A.; Cavallo, L.; Linden, A.; Dorta, R. Identification and characterization of a new family of catalytically highly active imidazolin-2-ylidenes. *J. Am. Chem. Soc.* **2008**, *130*, 6848–6858. [CrossRef] [PubMed]
67. Vieille-Petit, L.; Luan, X.; Mariz, R.; Blumentritt, S.; Linden, A.; Dorta, R. A new class of stable, saturated *N*-heterocyclic carbenes with *N*-naphthyl substituents: Synthesis, dynamic behavior, and catalytic potential. *Eur. J. Inorg. Chem.* **2009**, *2009*, 1861–1870. [CrossRef]
68. Vieille-Petit, L.; Clavier, H.; Linden, A.; Blumentritt, S.; Nolan, S.P.; Dorta, R. Ruthenium olefin metathesis catalysts with *N*-heterocyclic carbene ligands bearing *N*-naphthyl side chains. *Organometallics* **2010**, *29*, 775–788. [CrossRef]
69. Winter, P.; Hiller, W.; Christmann, M. Access to Skipped Polyene Macrolides through Ring-Closing Metathesis: Total Synthesis of the RNA Polymerase Inhibitor Ripostatin B. *Angew. Chem. Int. Ed.* **2012**, *51*, 3396–3400. [CrossRef]
70. Ritter, T.; Hejl, A.; Wenzel, A.G.; Funk, T.W.; Grubbs, R.H. A standard system of characterization for olefin metathesis catalysts. *Organometallics* **2006**, *25*, 5740–5745. [CrossRef]
71. Garber, S.B.; Kingsbury, J.S.; Gray, B.L.; Hoveyda, A.H. Efficient and Recyclable Monomeric and Dendritic Ru-Based Metathesis Catalysts. *J. Am. Chem. Soc.* **2000**, *122*, 8168–8179. [CrossRef]
72. Rivard, M.; Blechert, S. Effective and Inexpensive Acrylonitrile Cross-Metathesis: Utilisation of Grubbs II Precatalyst in the Presence of Copper(I) Chloride. *Eur. J. Org. Chem.* **2003**, *2003*, 2225–2228. [CrossRef]
73. Vieille-Petit, L.; Luan, X.; Gatti, M.; Blumentritt, S.; Linden, A.; Clavier, H.; Nolan, S.P.; Dorta, R. Improving Grubbs' II type ruthenium catalysts by appropriately modifying the N-heterocyclic carbene ligand. *Chem. Commun.* **2009**, *25*, 3783–3785. [CrossRef]
74. Samojłowicz, C.; Bieniek, M.; Grela, K. Ruthenium-based olefin metathesis catalysts bearing *N*-heterocyclic carbene ligands. *Chem. Rev.* **2009**, *109*, 3708–3742. [CrossRef]
75. Barbasiewicz, M.; Szadkowska, A.; Makal, A.; Jarzembska, K.N.; Grela, K.; Woźniak, K. Is the Hoveyda-Grubbs Complex a Vinylogous Fischer-Type Carbene? Aromaticity-Controlled Activity of Ruthenium Metathesis Catalysts. *Chem.-A Eur. J.* **2008**, *14*, 9330–9337. [CrossRef] [PubMed]
76. Falivene, L.; Credendino, R.; Poater, A.; Petta, A.; Serra, L.; Oliva, R.; Scarano, V.; Cavallo, L. SambVca A Web Tool for Analyzing Catalytic Pockets with Topographic Steric Maps. *Organometallics* **2016**, *35*, 2286–2293. [CrossRef]
77. Chatterjee, A.K.; Choi, T.-L.; Sanders, D.P.; Grubbs, R.H. A general model for selectivity in olefin cross metathesis. *J. Am. Chem. Soc.* **2003**, *125*, 11360–11370. [CrossRef] [PubMed]

78. Mukherjee, N.; Planer, S.; Grela, K. Formation of tetrasubstituted C–C double bonds via olefin metathesis: Challenges, catalysts, and applications in natural product synthesis. *Org. Chem. Front.* **2018**, *5*, 494–516. [CrossRef]
79. Diver, S.T.; Griffiths, J.R. Ene-yne metathesis. In *Olefin Metathesis: Theory and Practice*; Grela, K., Ed.; John Wiley & Sons: Hoboken, NJ, USA, 2014; pp. 153–185.
80. Grotevendt, A.G.D.; Lummiss, J.A.M.; Mastronardi, M.L.; Fogg, D.E. Ethylene-Promoted versus Ethylene-Free Enyne Metathesis. *J. Am. Chem. Soc.* **2011**, *133*, 15918–15921. [CrossRef]
81. Schmid, T.E.; Bantreil, X.; Citadelle, C.A.; Slawin, A.; Cazin, C.S.J. Phosphites as ligands in ruthenium-benzylidene catalysts for olefin metathesis. *Chem. Commun.* **2011**, *47*, 7060–7062. [CrossRef]
82. Guidone, S.; Blondiaux, E.; Samojłowicz, C.; Gułajski, Ł.; Kędziorek, M.; Malinska, M.; Pazio, A.; Wozniak, K.; Grela, K.; Doppiu, A.; et al. Catalytic and Structural Studies of Hoveyda-Grubbs Type Pre-Catalysts Bearing Modified Ether Ligands. *Adv. Synth. Catal.* **2012**, *354*, 2734–2742. [CrossRef]
83. Broggi, J.; Urbina-Blanco, C.A.; Clavier, H.; Leitgeb, A.; Slugovc, C.; Slawin, A.; Nolan, S.P. The Influence of Phosphane Ligands on the Versatility of Ruthenium-Indenylidene Complexes in Metathesis. *Chem.-A Eur. J.* **2010**, *16*, 9215–9345. [CrossRef]
84. Lecourt, C.; Dhambri, S.; Allievi, L.; Sanogo, Y.; Zeghbib, N.; Ben Othman, R.; Lannou, M.-I.; Sorin, G.; Ardisson, J. Natural products and ring-closing metathesis: synthesis of sterically congested olefins. *Nat. Prod. Rep.* **2018**, *35*, 105–124. [CrossRef]
85. Bieniek, M.; Michrowska, A.; Usanov, D.L.; Grela, K. In an attempt to provide a user's guide to the galaxy of benzylidene, alkoxybenzylidene, and indenylidene ruthenium olefin metathesiss catalysts. *Chem. A Eur. J.* **2008**, *14*, 806–818. [CrossRef]

Sample Availability: Samples of the compounds are not available from the authors.

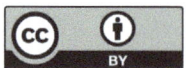

© 2020 by the authors. Licensee MDPI, Basel, Switzerland. This article is an open access article distributed under the terms and conditions of the Creative Commons Attribution (CC BY) license (http://creativecommons.org/licenses/by/4.0/).

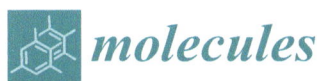

Review

NHC Core Pincer Ligands Exhibiting Two Anionic Coordinating Extremities

Rachid Taakili and Yves Canac *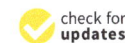

LCC–CNRS, Université de Toulouse, CNRS, 31077 Toulouse, France; rachid.taakili@lcc-toulouse.fr
* Correspondence: yves.canac@lcc-toulouse.fr

Academic Editor: Vito Lippolis
Received: 20 April 2020; Accepted: 6 May 2020; Published: 9 May 2020

Abstract: The chemistry of NHC core pincer ligands of LX$_2$ type bearing two pending arms, identical or not, whose coordinating center is anionic in nature, is here reviewed. In this family, the negative charge of the coordinating atoms can be brought either by a carbon atom via a phosphonium ylide (R$_3$P$^+$–CR$_2^-$) or by a heteroatom through amide (R$_2$N$^-$), oxide (RO$^-$), or thio(seleno)oxide (RS$^-$, RSe$^-$) donor functionalities. Through selected examples, the synthetic methods, coordination properties, and applications of such tridentate systems are described. Particular emphasis is placed on the role of the donor ends in the chemical behavior of these species.

Keywords: carbon ligand; amide; negative charge; NHC; phosphonium ylide; oxide; pincer

---

1. Introduction

The term 'pincer' was introduced in 1989 by van Koten to refer to a tridentate ligand featuring a central anionic carbon atom coordinated through a covalent σ bond and associated with two flanking arms that donate their electron lone pairs and force the metal center to adopt a meridional geometry [1]. This geometry has the main advantage of leaving an open coordination shell for any incoming molecule and of preventing undesired ligand redistribution processes [2–6]. The high stability, variability and activity of pincer ligands have made these species essential today in modern organometallic chemistry and homogeneous catalysis [7–9]. The first pincer system prepared by Shaw et al. in the late 1970s was based on an anionic carbon atom belonging to a central phenyl ring and bearing two neutral pendant phosphine donors, the so-called PCP pincer ligands [10]. This pioneering report was followed shortly after by the preparation of the NCN analogues by van Koten and Noltes [11]. From there, a wide variety of chemical motifs were designed, and the term 'pincer' was generally extended to any metallic complex adopting a meridional geometry whatever the bonding mode of the coordinating ends, as opposed to the facial coordination mode found in tripodal systems [12–14]. According to the Green formalism [15], although mono-anionic pincers (L$_2$X-type) remain the most exemplified, other systems containing neutral (L$_3$-type), di- (LX$_2$-type), or tri-anionic (X$_3$-type) pincer frameworks were also developed allowing an efficient control of the metal coordination sphere and the stabilization of a broad range of metal centers with different oxidation states [16–22]. Among all pincer-type ligands, di-anionic representatives (LX$_2$-type) have been relatively little explored, and considering only the cases where the central donor moiety is neutral [23], three main sub-structures of this family have been reported over the years featuring either a pyridine [24–29], a carbodiphosphorane [30–32], or a N-heterocyclic carbene (NHC) [33,34]. The latter architecture **B** built from a neutral NHC core (2-e$^-$ donor (L-type)) and two anionic peripheral groups (1-e$^-$ donor (X-type)) is formally characterized by an opposite bonding mode to that encountered in the Shaw's prototype **A** derived from a central anionic aryl group (1-e$^-$ donor (X-type)) and two neutral donor moieties (2-e$^-$ donor (L-type)) (Scheme 1). In both structures, in addition to the thermodynamically favored chelate effect, the association of coordinating extremities of different nature extends naturally the scope of accessible metal fragments, but more generally of all centers having a Lewis acidic character. According to HSAB theory (hard soft acid base) [35,36], combining a soft NHC with two harder anionic groups must inevitably afford metallic complexes with unique properties, as is the case with systems **B**. For instance, a different bonding mode is anticipated with a high degree of covalency in the NHC-metal bond and a more marked ionic character between the negatively charged atoms and the metal center. It follows that anionic functionalized NHC ligands generally prefer to coordinate with electropositive metals, the anionic arms acting as a real anchor counterbalancing the natural tendency of the NHC to dissociate from the metal [37–41]. With late transition metals, an opposite behavior is expected with a possible lability of the anionic donor extremities [42–44]. All of these electronic criteria, combined with geometric parameters, govern the reactivity vs stability of these pincers, thus making each of them a unique system.

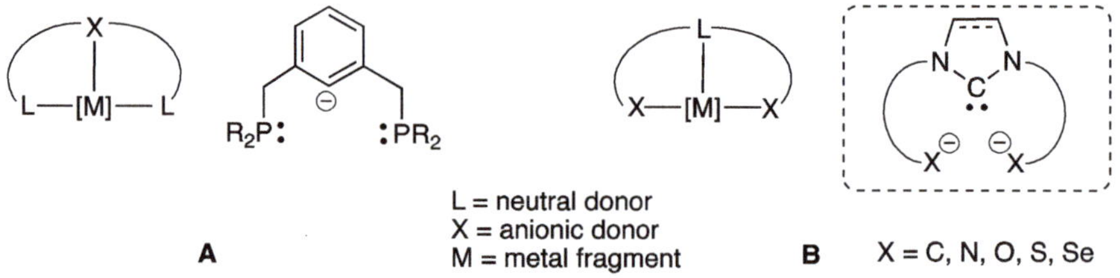

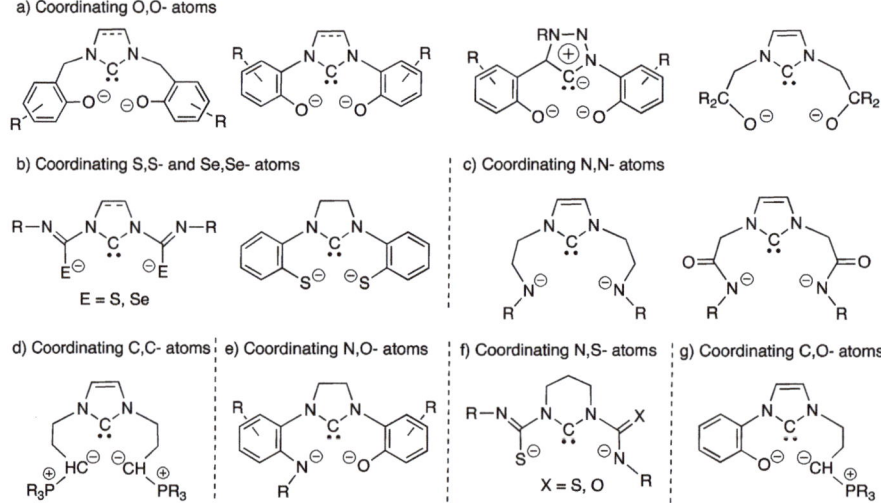

Scheme 1. Representation of the XL$_2$ prototype pincer **A** and LX$_2$ pincers **B** of interest.

This review aims to account for this class of LX$_2$-type pincer ligands **B** where the central NHC is N-substituted by two side arms bearing identical or different anionic coordinating atoms, and which remains to this day underdeveloped compared to other families of pincer ligands. Through selected examples, the preparation methods, coordination properties, and applications of NHC core pincers exhibiting amide, oxide, thio(seleno)oxide, and phosphonium ylide donor extremities, which belong to this class of ligands, will be thus presented (Scheme 2).

Scheme 2. Representation of the general structure of known pincer structures of type **B** based on a central N-heterocyclic carbene (NHC) and two peripheral anionic coordinating atoms being identical or not.

2. NHC Core Pincer Ligands of LX$_2$-Type

2.1. Based on Two Identical Side Arms

2.1.1. With Two Coordinating O- Atoms

The first representatives of the family were reported by Kawaguchi et al. from the 1,3-bis(4,6-di-*tert*-butyl-2-hydroxybenzyl) imidazolium bromide **1** prepared in 60% yield via sequential N-alkylation of imidazole with 2-bromomethyl-4,6-di-*tert*-butylphenol. By reacting the imidazolium salt **1** with TiCl$_4$(THF)$_2$ in the presence of NaN(SiMe$_3$)$_2$, the bis(aryloxide) NHC Ti(IV) pincer complex **2** was formed in 74% yield (Scheme 3) [45]. An X-ray diffraction analysis confirms the meridional coordination mode of the NHC where the pseudo-octahedral geometry adopted by the Ti(IV) center is completed by a THF molecule and two chlorine atoms in mutual *cis* position. Using the same protocol, the Zr(IV) analogue **3** was prepared but with a lower yield (20%) since it was obtained as a mixture with the corresponding homoleptic bis(NHC) Zr complex isolated in 38% yield [46]. It should be mentioned that although the latter complex could be synthetized in 84% yield by the reaction of ZrCl$_4$(THF)$_2$ with two equivalents of ligand, attempts to prepare complex **3** in a better yield failed. The larger ionic radius of Zr with respect to Ti was proposed to explain the more favorable formation of the bis(NHC) complex in the case of Zr. Both pincer complexes **2** and **3** could be converted to their alkyl derivatives via chloride displacement upon addition of Grignard reagents. For example, the chloro ligands in complexes **2–3** could be substituted using 2 equivalents of PhCH$_2$MgCl to form the corresponding dialkyl pincer complexes. Whatever the series, the benzyl complexes display a distorted trigonal bipyramidal geometry with a meridional coordination of the NHC.

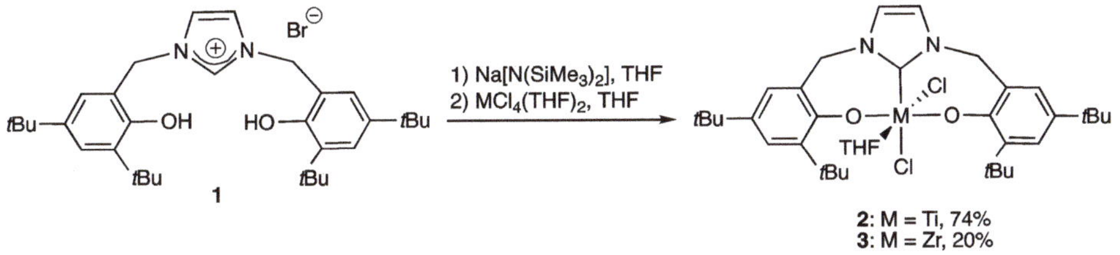

Scheme 3. Preparation of group 4 pincer complexes **2–3** (M = Ti, Zr) featuring a bis(aryloxide) NHC ligand from the imidazolium salt **1** [45,46].

Another striking fact concerns the dibromide analogue of complex **2**, which, upon reduction with an equivalent of LiBEt$_3$H, led to the formation of a rare Ti(III) complex exhibiting a distorted octahedral geometry and where the coordination sphere around the metal is completed by the pincer ligand occupying meridional positions, two THF molecules in mutual *trans* position and a bromide co-ligand [47]. Following this, dinuclear complexes [48] and macrocyclic structures of the same tridentate ligand with group 4 metals were also reported by the same authors [49]. These metallic systems as well as the Ti(IV) pincer complex **2** showed significant catalytic activity for the polymerization of ethylene.

Based on the same flanking donor arms but with a central saturated six-membered NHC, rare earth pincer complexes (Nd, Y, Sm) were prepared, fully characterized, and applied in the polymerization of *n*-hexyl isocyanate [50]. The polymer formed showed very high molecular weight and narrow molecular weight distribution. It was also demonstrated that the catalytic activity depends on the radius of rare earth metal, solvent, polymerization temperature, and the ligand structure. The saturated NHC moiety was in particular found to play a critical role in the initiation step of the polymerization process.

More rigid representatives of the same family were prepared via a different route, which consists of the elimination of alcohols from imidazolium salts. For instance, Ti(IV) complexes **5** and **6** were quantitatively formed by the reaction of the imidazolium salt **4** with TiCl(O*i*Pr)$_3$ and Ti(O*i*Pr)$_4$

precursors, respectively (Scheme 4) [51]. Deduced from a solid state analysis, complexes **5** and **6** exhibit a slightly distorted octahedral geometry with the bis(aryloxide) NHC ligand coordinated in a meridional manner. The NHC Ti(IV) complex **6** was shown to readily initiate the ring-opening polymerization of *rac*-lactide in a controlled fashion without the NHC a priori playing any role in the catalytic transformation. Related pincer complexes were obtained using the same protocol in the Zr(IV) and Hf(IV) series [52]. Despite lower yields, amine elimination was also found to be a possible route to afford such pincer complexes. The reaction of salt **4** with M(NMe$_2$)$_4$ (M = Ti, Zr) thus afforded the corresponding bis(phenoxy) NHC amido complexes.

Homoleptic bis-ligated NHC complexes could be also synthetized in high yields by reacting the imidazolium salt **4** with half of an equivalent of MCl$_4$ complexes (M = Ti, Zr, Hf) in the presence of Et$_3$N [53]. In all complexes, the metal atom adopts a distorted octahedral geometry with the two NHCs located in *trans* position one from each other. These three NHC pincer complexes were described to be redox-active and, in the case of Zr and Hf derivatives, to present luminescent properties, constituting the first examples of emissive non-metallocene group 4 metal complexes. It must be mentioned that tetravalent Ti(IV) complexes bearing the same pincer ligand were found to be active and selective for the copolymerization of cyclohexene oxide with CO$_2$ [54].

In the Zr series, toluene elimination was observed from the imidazolium salt **4** by using Zr(CH$_2$Ph)$_4$ as a metal precursor leading to the corresponding chlorobenzyl NHC pincer complex **7** in quantitative yield (Scheme 4) [55]. However, while this complex is stable in non-coordinating solvents, in the presence of THF the quantitative formation of the unexpected Zr-THF adduct **8** as a single isomer was observed. The complex **8** is characterized by the presence of a heptacoordinate Zr center featuring an *O,N,C,N,O*-pentadentate trianionic ligand. The formation of **8** was rationalized through a Lewis base assisted benzyl migration from the Zr atom to the carbenic center. This unusual benzyl migration was also observed with other group 4 metals (Ti, Hf) [56]. More recently, the reversibility of this benzyl migration was demonstrated by the addition of PMe$_3$ to a bis(phenolate) benzylimidazolylidene(dibenzyl)zirconium complex and then abstraction of the coordinated PMe$_3$ on the Zr complex formed with a Ni(0) complex [57].

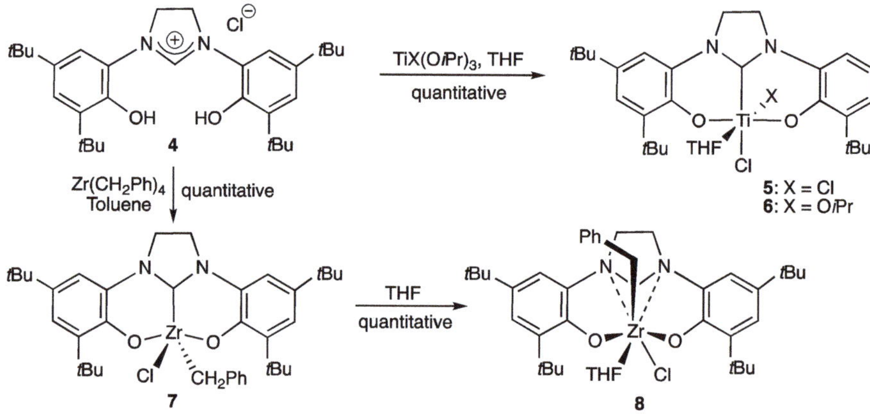

Scheme 4. Preparation of Ti(IV) and Zr(IV) pincer complexes **5–7** featuring a more rigid bis(aryloxide) NHC ligand from the imidazolium salt **4**, and unexpected rearrangement to the benzyl complex **8** [51,52,55].

Bis(aryloxide) NHC pincer ligands were successfully coordinated to a wide variety of metal centers, such as metals of groups 5 (V) [58], 6 (Mo) [59], 7 (Mn) [58], 9 (Ir [60], Co [61,62]), 10 (Ni, Pd, Pt) [63], and 13 (Al) [64]. More precisely from the imidazolium salt **4**, high oxidation sate V(V) and Mn(III) metal complexes were readily prepared using triisopropoxyvanadium(V) oxide [(*i*PrO)$_3$V=O] and manganese(III) acetylacetonate [Mn(aca)$_3$] precursors, respectively [58]. Al(III) complexes supported by such a dianionic NHC pincer ligand were obtained via various synthetic methods [64]. A possible route involved first, via alcohol elimination, the formation of the zwitterionic bis(phenolate) imidazolinium complex **9** featuring a four-coordinate tetrahedral Al(III) center *O,O*- chelated by the two phenolate extremities (Scheme 5). The latter was then readily converted to the pincer NHC Al(III) complex **10** upon reaction with an equivalent of LDA. The dimeric nature of **10** is indicated by an X-ray diffraction analysis where the two Al centers are supported by a *O,C,O*- coordinated NHC bis(phenolate) ligand and connected to one another via *µ*-O bridging Al-O*i*Pr groups. Both Al centers display a slightly distorted trigonal bipyramidal geometry with a meridional coordination of the bis(phenolate) NHC ligand. Moreover, the pincer Al complex **10** was reported to efficiently polymerize *rac*-lactive and trimethylene carbonate in a highly controlled fashion for the production of narrow disperse materials with catalytic performance in the range of conventional group 13 based ROP catalysts.

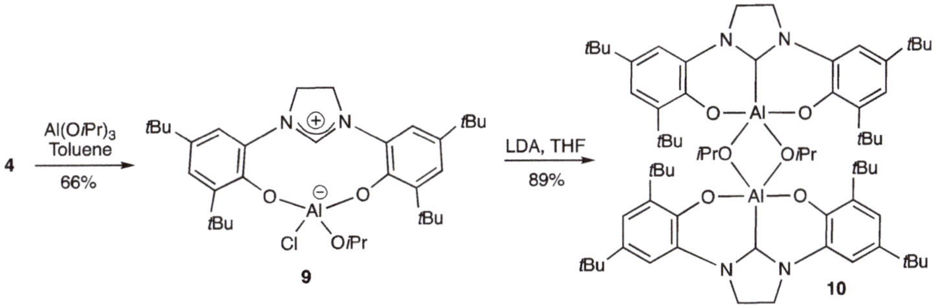

Scheme 5. Preparation of the dimeric Al(III) complex **10** featuring a more rigid bis(aryloxide) NHC ligand from the imidazolium salt **4** [64].

To accommodate heavy metal centers, the introduction of a benzimidazol-2-ylidene core was also considered, on the assumption that the presence of a π-conjugated system over the three six-membered aromatic rings should provide additional stabilization to the metal center. High-valent NHC Mo(VI) complexes featuring a *O,C,O*- benzimidazolylidene pincer ligand were prepared, as illustrated with the complex **12** isolated in 75% yield by addition of (DME)MoO$_2$Cl$_2$ in THF to the benzimidazolium precursor **11** in the presence of Et$_3$N (Scheme 6, top) [59]. In the solid state, the dioxo complex **12** was found to crystallize following two different arrangements, namely a dimeric structure with two six-coordinate Mo(VI) atoms in a strongly distorted octahedral environment and a monomeric form with the five-coordinate Mo(VI) center lying in between a square pyramidal and a trigonal bipyramidal geometry. The dioxo complex **12**, which represents a rare example of five-coordinated Mo(VI) complex, was found to be stable toward air and moisture in the solid state and in solution. The pre-ligand **11** was also reported to stabilize oxo-imido and bis(imido) Mo(VI) pincer complexes.

A series of group 10 metal complexes, **13**–**15**, was prepared in good yield (66–79%) when the same precursor **11** was treated with one equivalent of MCl$_2$ (M = Ni, Pd, Pt) in the presence of an excess of potassium carbonate in pyridine at 100 °C (Scheme 6, bottom) [63]. This one-pot procedure was also successfully applied in the imidazolylidene series. Imposed by the tridentate NHC, these complexes adopt a distorted square-planar geometry. DFT studies performed on Pd and Pt representatives indicated that the HOMO is centered on the metal and the aryloxide fragment while the LUMO involves mainly the pyridine co-ligand. Based on these findings, optical properties were studied evidencing the absence of luminescence at room temperature but in the case of Pt complexes the presence of an emission band in the green region of the visible spectrum at 77 K, which was attributed to a long-lived triplet-manifold excited state featuring MLLCT character [63].

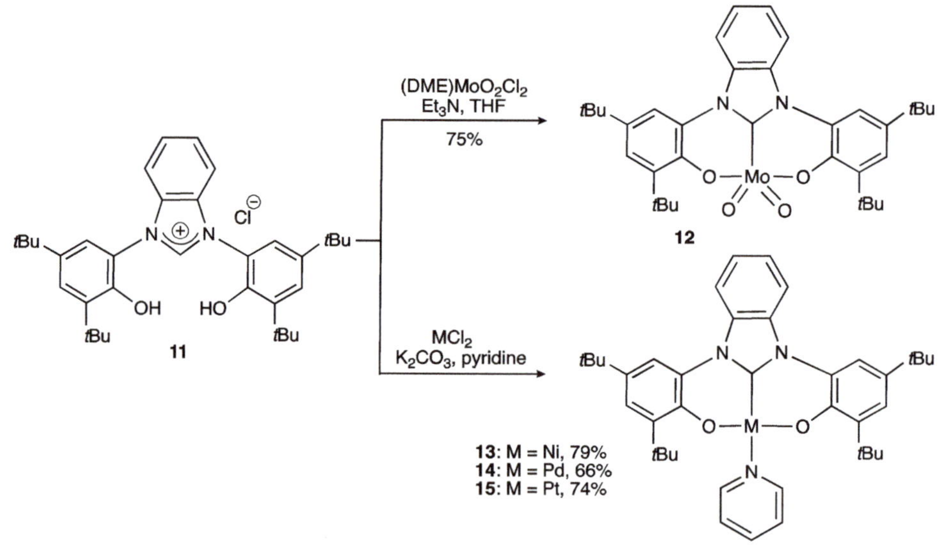

Scheme 6. Preparation of metal complexes **12–15** (M = Mo, Ni, Pd, Pt) from the benzimidazolium salt **11** [59,63].

In the Co series, the trifluoromethylation of (hetero)arenes was reported, thanks to the thermally stable pincer Co(III) complex **16**, which is able under light exposure to release a CF_3 radical (Scheme 7) [62]. This result represents an elegant strategy to activate strong M-CF_3 bonds for the functionalization of small molecules. From a synthetic point of view, the Co(III) complex **16** was formed by oxidation of the corresponding four-coordinate Co(II) complex using AgCF_3 in MeCN. An X-ray diffraction analysis of **16** indicates that the CF_3 group is orthogonal to the O,C,O- Co plane with a short Co-CF_3 bond in favor of a high degree of covalency. The complex **16** appeared to be diamagnetic well described as a low-spin Co(III) center stabilized by a closed-shell dianionic bis(phenolate) NHC core pincer ligand.

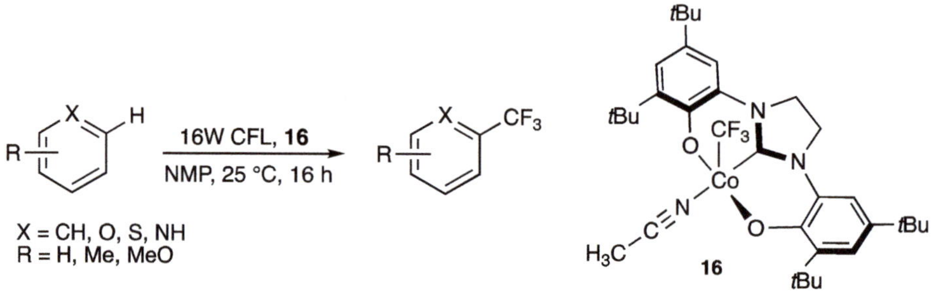

Scheme 7. Photoinduced trifluoromethylation of (hetero)arenes by the pincer Co(III) complex **16** [62].

Very recently, the first bis(phenolate) mesoionic carbene was reported by Hohloch et al. following a ten-step procedure and was shown to be a valuable ligand for the preparation of various heteroleptic early transition metal pincer complexes (group 4 to group 6) (Scheme 8) [65]. The triazolium salt **17**, which can be prepared on a multi-gram scale, was obtained by reacting phenyl substrates bearing alkyne and azide functionalities under classical click conditions. Prior to N-methylation, the two alcohol functions were protected in the presence of bis(trimethylsilyl)acetamide (BSA). Treatment with MeOH followed by salt metathesis with tetraethylammonium chloride afforded finally the pre-ligand **17** in 51% overall yield. From the latter, rare examples of Ti, Mo, and Nb imido complexes were prepared, as illustrated with the Nb complex **18** isolated in 62% yield. The Nb atom in **18** resides in a distorted octahedral environment where the coordination sphere is completed by the *O,C,O*- pincer ligand and imido, chloro, and pyridine co-ligands. Comparison of the electrochemical properties of these carbenic complexes with more classical bis(phenolate) NHC complexes conclude that, as expected, triazolylidenes are more difficult to oxidize than imidazolinylidene-based systems.

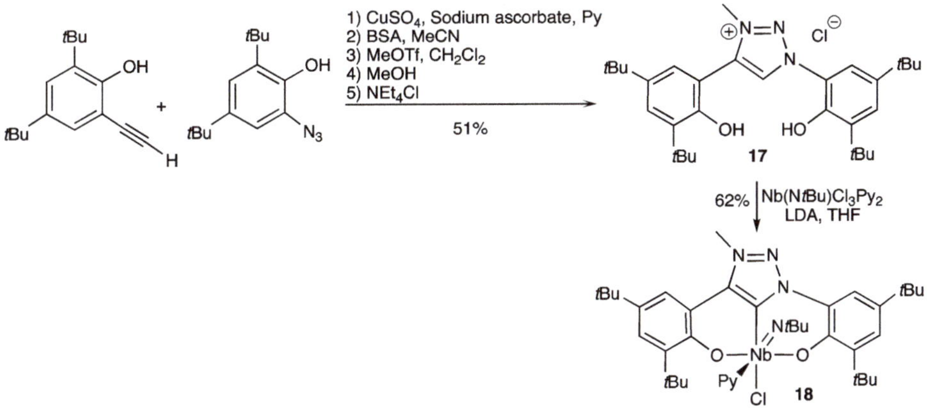

Scheme 8. Preparation of the Nb complex **18** featuring a bis(phenolate) mesoionic carbene ligand [65].

After the development of various bis(aryloxy) NHC core systems, bis(alkoxy) analogues were naturally considered. For such purpose and based on preliminary studies on bidentate systems [66,67], the introduction of electron-withdrawing CF$_3$ groups was envisaged to decrease the acidity of the alcohol hydrogen atoms. Indeed, the stability of fluoroalkoxy carbenes has been reported, in particular the reluctance of the alkoxy fragment not to react with the electrophilic imidazolium center as may be the case with more basic alkoxides [68]. Under phase-transfer catalysis, the imidazolium salt **19** as a stable zwitterion was thus prepared through a sequential method by reacting 1*H*-imidazole with hexafluoroisobutylene oxide (Scheme 9) [69]. It is noteworthy that the salt **19** could be obtained in excellent yield (94%) via a one-pot procedure without isolating the imidazole intermediate. This methodology was extended to 3,4-disubstituted imidazole and triazole derivatives. Treatment of **19** with two equivalents of *t*BuOK generated the corresponding free carbene, which was observed to be relatively stable in solution. Addition of [NiCl$_2$(PPh$_3$)$_2$] to this carbene resulted in the formation of the NHC pincer **20** and the bis(NHC) complex **21** in a 2/1 ratio. While an X-ray diffraction analysis of **20** confirmed the square-planar geometry around the Ni(II) center with the meridional coordination of the bis(alkoxy) NHC that of **21** indicated that two alkoxy groups of the same NHC are bound to Ni and the two hydroxyl groups from the other NHC are hydrogen-bonded to the adjacent oxygen atoms.

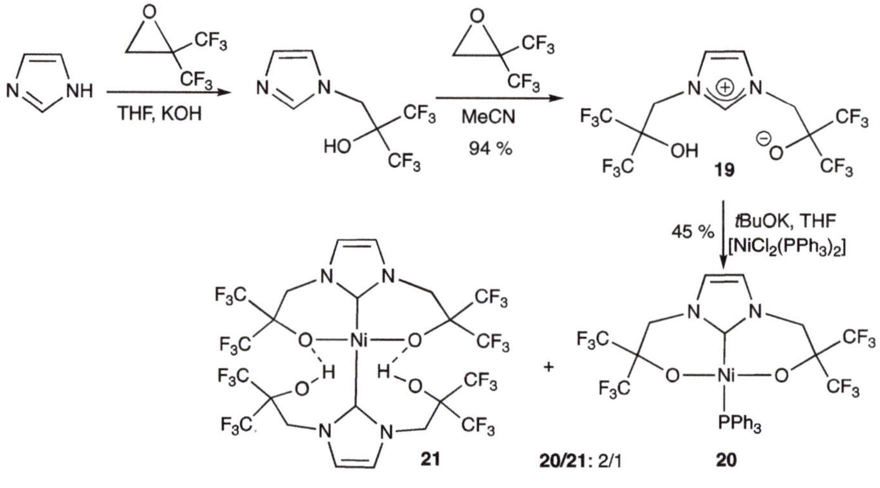

Scheme 9. Preparation of bis(alkoxy) NHC Ni(II) complexes 20 and 21 from 1*H*-imidazole [69].

2.1.2. With Two Coordinating S- (or Se) Atoms

Bis(thiolate) NHC core complexes were actually reported before their oxygenated analogues. The first complexes were obtained by reacting Pd(PPh$_3$)$_4$ and RhCl(PPh$_3$)$_3$ with tetraazapentalene derivatives 22, the latter exhibiting unique reactivity due to the presence of hypervalent sulfur (Scheme 10) [70]. In both cases, the formation of Pd(II) and Rh(III) complexes 23 and 24 was accompanied by the release of triphenylphosphine sulfide. It is noteworthy that, depending on the nature of the amine substituents (R), the bis(thiolate) NHC complexes were isolated as a mixture with their isostructural complexes containing an unsymmetrical amido, NHC, thiolate pincer ligand, knowing that more hindered R substituents, disadvantage a priori the latter form. The best ratios in favor of the *S,C,S*- pincer complexes 23 and 24 were observed with small *p*-Cl- and *p*-MeOC$_6$H$_4$ amine substituents with yields between 86% and 99%. The complexes based on a *N,C,S*- ligand were generally found to be less stable than their analogues exhibiting the symmetrical *S,C,S*- ligand. In a Pd complex of type 23 bearing N-Me groups, an X-ray diffraction analysis was performed confirming the square planar geometry around the Pd(II) center surrounded by two sulfur, one phosphorus, and a carbenic carbon atom. This Pd complex was found to be very stable in organic solvents under air. For Rh(III) complexes of type 24, the octahedral geometry of the metal center with two phosphine ligands located in *trans* position was deduced on the basis of a solid state analysis performed in the case of a Rh complex featuring the hybrid *SCN*- pincer ligand. Following the same strategy, a diselenato version of 22 based on a five-membered saturated NHC was prepared by the same authors and coordinated with different metal centers such as Pd(PPh$_3$)$_4$, Pt(PPh$_3$)$_4$, and RhCl(PPh$_3$)$_3$, affording corresponding *Se,C,Se*- pincer complexes. [71,72]

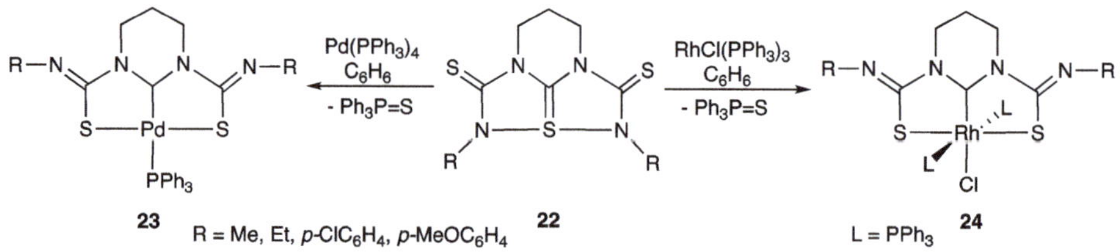

Scheme 10. Preparation of tridentate bis(thiolate) NHC Pd(II) and Rh(III) complexes 23 and 24 from tetraazapentalene derivatives 22 [70].

Another representative of the family was described by Sellmann et al. who observed the unexpected formation of bis(thiolate) NHC Ni(II) pincer complexes **27** upon dissociation of the dimeric complex **26** by addition of different metallic salts (KCN, LiMe, NaSPh) (Scheme 11) [73]. X-ray structure determinations confirmed the square planar geometry around the metal center with a characteristic propeller-like twist resulting from positioning the phenyl rings above and below the coordination plane. If the pincer complexes **27** exhibit remarkable thermal stability, in the presence of Brönsted acids, the regeneration of dimer **26** was noticed.

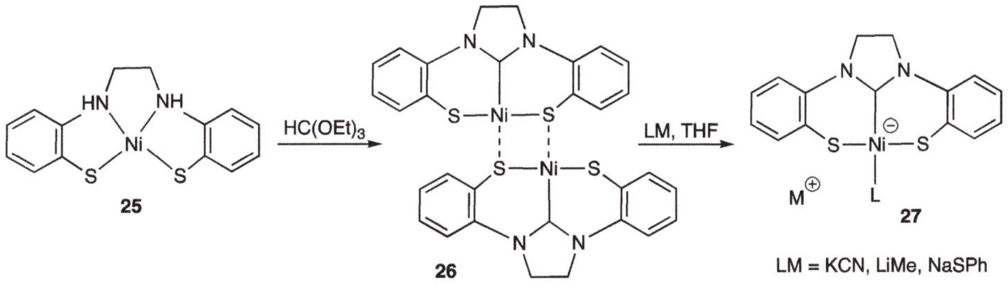

Scheme 11. Preparation of bis(thiolate) NHC Ni(II) pincer complexes **27** through dissociation of the dimeric precursor **26** [73].

2.1.3. With Two Coordinating N- Atoms

The first bis(amido) NHC pincer complex was described by Fryzuk et al. in 2004 in the Zr(IV) series [74]. The corresponding pre-ligand, namely the bis(amine) imidazolium salt **28** (Ar = Tol) was synthetized by the reduction of a bis(amide) imidazolium salt using borane-dimethylsulfide. Later, in order to introduce larger N-aryl groups (Ar = Mes, Xy), an alternative route was developed consisting of melting the appropriate N-substituted imidazole with a β-chloroethylarylamine [75]. Whatever the preparation method, imidazolium salts **28** were treated with $KN(SiMe_3)_2$ to give in good yield the stable free NHCs substituted by two amine donor arms. The latter reacted cleanly with $M(NMe_2)_4$ complexes (M = Zr, Hf), providing a convenient entry to N,C,N- group 4 pincer complexes (Scheme 12). The dimethylamido co-ligands could be readily removed by adding an excess of chlorotrimethylsilane, affording the corresponding dichloride adducts which were then converted into dialkyl complexes by treatment with Grignard reagents. In the case of a Hf complex of type **30** bearing two isobutyl groups, an X-ray diffraction analysis evidences a distorted trigonal bipyramidal geometry around the metal atom with the two amido moieties in pseudo-*trans* position [75]. It should be noted that Hf dialkyl complexes are more thermally stable than Zr representatives, with the exception of the Hf diethyl complex which undergoes β-hydrogen transfer and subsequent C-H bond activation with the neighboring N-Mes substituent to afford a cyclometalled complex [75]. The Hf dialkyl complexes were also shown to insert carbon monoxide and isocyanides to give the related η^2- acyl and η^2- iminoacyl derivatives. After activation with $[Ph_3C, B(C_6F_5)_4]$, the Zr dimethyl complex showed moderate catalytic activity for ethylene polymerization.

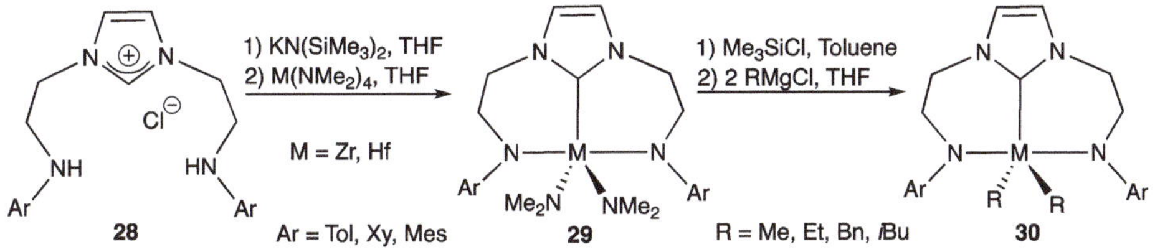

Scheme 12. Preparation of bis(amido) NHC pincer complexes (M = Zr, Hf) **29** and **30** from the imidazolium salt **28** [74,75].

From the same pre-ligand, bis(amido) NHC tantalum pincer complexes were also reported [76]. However, to reach such systems, the formation of the dilithiated diamido NHC ligand **32** prepared by addition of 2 equivalents of BuLi to the free carbene **31** was a prerequisite. Indeed, from the free carbene **31**, only the formation of bidentate amido NHC Ta complexes were observed, the remaining amine arm being reluctant to coordinate the metal center. By contrast, the metathesis reaction of **32** in the presence of various $TaCl_x(NMe_2)_{5-x}$ precursors proceeded under mild conditions and in good yield to afford the desired pincer complexes, as illustrated with complex **33** (Scheme 13, top). However, attempts to synthesize trialkyl derivatives following this methodology were not successful, yielding instead metallaziridines, as demonstrated with the formation of N,C,C,N- NHC Ta(V) complexes **34** (Scheme 13, bottom). An X-ray diffraction analysis of one of these representatives (with R = Np) emphasizes the facial orientation of the activated C-H bond and the distorted pseudo trigonal bipyramidal geometry around the Ta center. DFT calculations confirm that such cyclometallated species formed by the endocyclic C-H activation of one of the amido arms are thermodynamically favored over the targeted trialkyl derivatives.

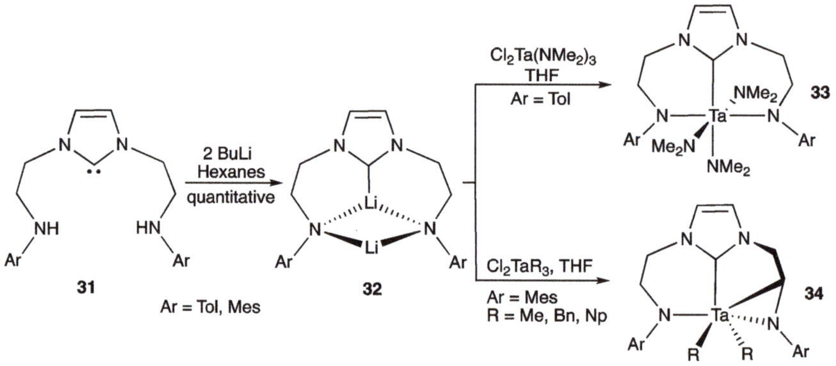

Scheme 13. Preparation of bis(amido) NHC Ta(V) complexes **33** and **34** from the free NHC **31** [76].

Bis(amido) NHC ligands were also coordinated to group 10 metal centers. The Pd(II) complex **36** was prepared from the tridentate imidazolium salt **35** exhibiting two side amide arms and $PdCl_2$ in the presence of the K_2CO_3/pyridine system (Scheme 14) [77]. This square planar pincer Pd complex isolated in 77% yield showed significant catalytic activity in Suzuki coupling reactions of aryl bromides with phenylboronic acid, although less than corresponding monodentate NHC Pd complexes bearing a pendant neutral amine arm. This difference was attributed to the too strongly anionic amido coordinating ends, which do not allow in the case of **36** the release of vacant sites during the catalytic process. The dissociation of the neutral NHC moiety is expected to be more favorable with electropositive early transition metal centers.

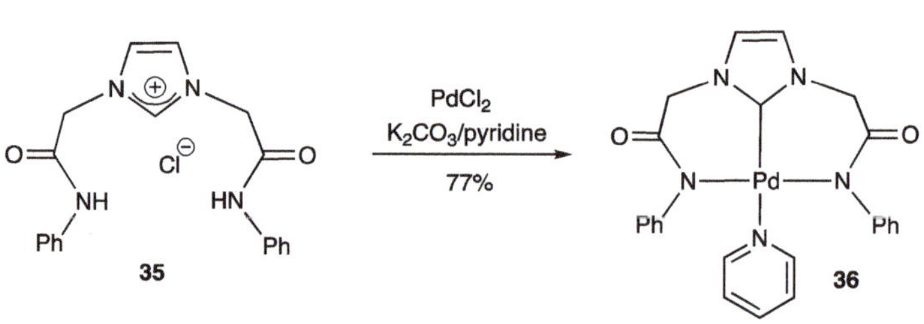

Scheme 14. Preparation of the bis(amido) NHC Pd(II) pincer complex **36** from the imidazolium salt **35** [77].

2.1.4. With Two Coordinating C- Atoms

Phosphonium ylides are globally neutral in their free state, characterized by an almost planar carbanion stabilized by an adjacent tetrahedral phosphonium center. In their coordination state, phosphonium ylides act exclusively as η^1- carbon centered ligands, rather than as η^2- C=P ligands [78], and can therefore be considered locally as anionic carbon ligands [79]. This chemical description means that phosphonium ylides like NHCs behave as strong σ-donor carbon ligands while differing in their bonding mode (NHC, 2e$^-$ donor (L type); P$^+$-ylide, 1e$^-$ donor (X type)) [80,81]. Following preliminary reports in the field aimed at developing ylide-based metal complexes [82–85], NHC and phosphonium ylide donor moieties were recently associated by a C$_3$-propyl bridge in the bi- [86], tetradente [87], and in the pincer series forming very electron-rich complexes [88], thanks to the design of a general synthetic strategy [89].

A new family of pincer Pd(II) complexes bearing an electron-rich *C,C,C*- NHC, diphosphonium bis(ylide) ligand was indeed prepared from the imidazolium salt **37** featuring two phosphonium side chains obtained through the dual N-functionalization of 1*H*-imidazole by (3-bromopropyl)triphenylphosphonium bromide (Scheme 15) [88]. Due to a difference in acidity between the cationic moieties, the imidazolium salt **37** was sequentially coordinated to Pd(II) centers leading first to the NHC Pd complex **38** and then to the *ortho*-metallated Pd complex **39**. Protonation of the latter afforded the NHC, diphosphonium bis(ylide) pincer Pd(II) complex **40** as a mixture of *meso*- and *dl*-diastereomers (de = 50%). The pincer complex **40** isolated in 94% yield appeared to be perfectly stable in air both in the solid state and in solution. The selectivity of C-coordination was rationalized on the basis of DFT calculations, indicating the quasi-degeneracy of the two diastereomeric forms. Thanks to its electronic properties, this NHC core pincer was shown to efficiently stabilize Pd(II) complexes bearing isocyanide **41** and carbonyl co-ligands **42**, whose examples of this latter type remain rare due to easy Pd–CO dissociation (Scheme 15). In the isocyanide case, an X-ray diffraction analysis of both isomers was achieved showing that the Pd(II) atom is an integral part of two strongly distorted fused six-membered metallacycles and resides in a quasi-square planar environment with the two phosphonium ylides occupying mutually *trans* positions [88].

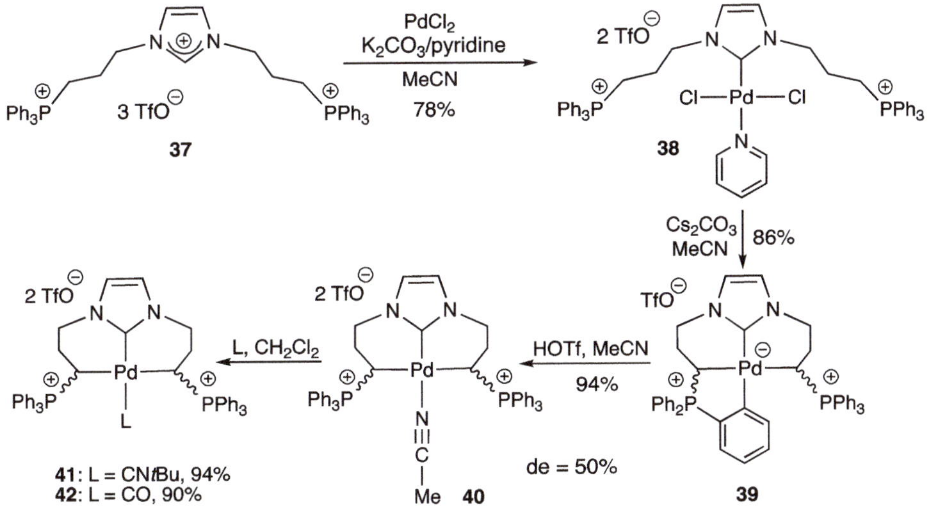

Scheme 15. Preparation of NHC, diphosphonium bis(ylide) Pd(II) pincer complexes **40–42** from the imidazolium salt **37** [88].

NHC core diphosphonium bis(ylide) Pd complexes **40–42** represent the sole examples of LX$_2$-type pincer complexes where the metal center is bonded only with carbon atoms, in the present case being of different nature: one carbenic (sp^2) and two ylidic (sp^3) carbon atoms. Their availability combined with their stability should benefit catalytic processes requiring extremely electron-rich ligands.

2.2. Based on Two Different Side Arms

The interest in unsymmetrical pincer ligands has considerably increased in recent years since they can provide significantly different chemical donor extremities with a more or less pronounced hard/soft character, thus affording metal complexes with unprecedented properties. This may lead in particular to catalysts exhibiting unique reactivity and selectivity profiles. In this direction, NHC core pincers of LX$_2$-type bearing two different side arms are rare and their synthesis represent an additional synthetic challenge because their formation requires the coordination of three different donors having their own chemical features at the same metallic center. For instance, the coordination of neutral and/or anionic donor ends possessing a wide range of basicity will have to take into account the relative acidity of each H-atom in the corresponding conjugated acid precursors.

2.2.1. With N,O- Coordinating Atoms

In the last decade, the preparation of the imidazolium salt **43** bearing pending amine and phenol arms was reported in four steps in 52% overall yield from 2-(*N*-mesitylamino) aniline [90]. However, while this cation appeared to be stable in the solid state, it was observed to quantitatively rearrange in solution to form the thermodynamically favored benzimidazolium salt **44** (Scheme 16) [91]. DFT calculations were performed to rationalize the mechanism of this unprecedented rearrangement. Despite its instability, various attempts to coordinate the pre-ligand **43** were carried out with group 4 metals, all leading to unexpected species but not to the desired pincer complexes. It is worth mentioning the formation of the Zr(IV) complex **45**, which was obtained when the precursor **43** was reacted with ZrBn$_4$ and BnMgCl in toluene. The formation of **45** results formally from the migration of a benzyl group and a proton to the carbenic center, converting the heterocycle to an imidazolidine. The latter stands as a Zr(IV) complex where the metallic center interacts with a tetradentate *N,N,N,O*-dianionic ligand featuring two X-type (amide and phenoxide) and two L-type (amine) donor moieties. Similar benzyl migration was already evidenced in Zr(IV) complexes supported by bis(phenoxy) NHC pincer ligands [55]. These surprising results tend to illustrate the difficulty of access to unsymmetrical pincer systems containing different coordinating ends.

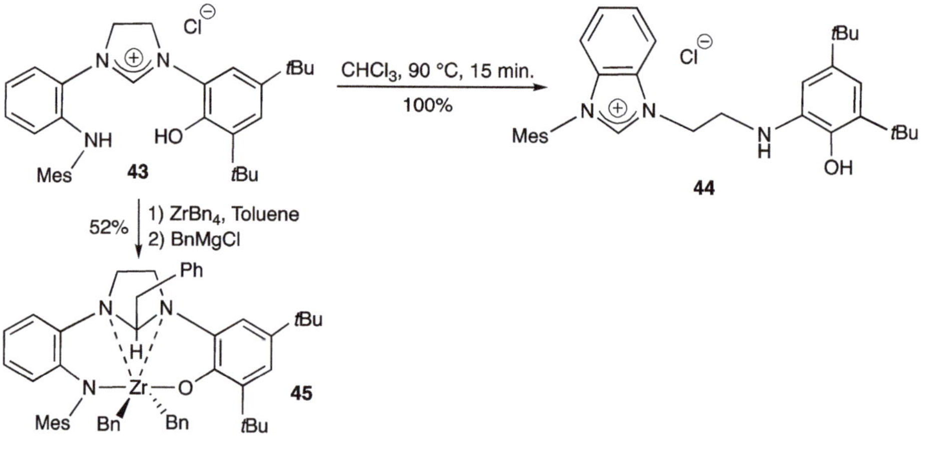

Scheme 16. Preparation of the tridentate *N,C,O*- imidazolium salt **43** with corresponding thermal rearrangement to the benzimidazolium salt **44** and coordination to the Zr(IV) complex **45** [90,91].

2.2.2. With N,S- Coordinating Atoms

The method developed to prepare S,C,S- pincer complexes (see Scheme 10) also enabled the synthesis of unsymmetrical pincer complexes as illustrated with the formation of the S,C,N- Pt(II) **47** and Rh(III) **48** complexes. The difference lies in the nature of the tetraazapentalene substrates **46** where a thiocarbonyl function is replaced by a carbonyl group (Scheme 17) [92]. As demonstrated in the Rh(III) series, the substitution of both thiocarbonyls by two carbonyl groups does not lead, as one might have expected, to the formation of N,C,N- pincers but to a bidentate N,S- Rh complex [92].

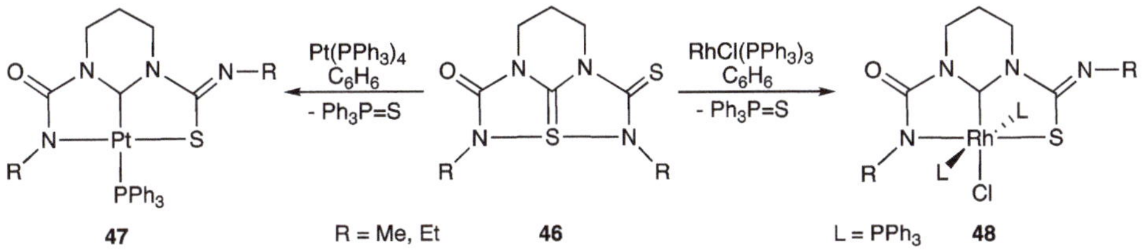

Scheme 17. Preparation of S,C,N- pincer complexes **47** (M = Pt) and **48** (M = Rh) from unsymmetrical tetraazapentalenes **46** [92].

2.2.3. With C,O- Coordinating Atoms

With the previous cases **47–48**, the Pd(II) complex **52** constitutes one of the very rare examples of NHC core pincer complex of LX$_2$-type exhibiting two different peripheral coordinating extremities reported to date [93]. The latter, featuring pending phenolate and phosphonium ylide moieties, was readily obtained from the *ortho*-metallated Pd complex **51** in 94% yield, thanks to the selective acid cleavage of a C$_{ar}$-Pd bond using HOTf in MeCN (Scheme 18). The highly strained zwitterionic C,C,C,O- Pd complex **51** was prepared through two distinct routes, either directly from the tridentate imidazolium salt **49** by adding PdCl$_2$ in the presence of Cs$_2$CO$_3$ in 84% yield or in a two-step procedure via the NHC Pd pyridine adduct **50** in 64% overall yield. The pincer complex **52** was readily converted to its isocyanide analogue **53** by an exchange reaction at the Pd center. In this case, the formation of a Pd–CO adduct was not experimentally observed, due probably to the too weak donor character of the C,C,O- pincer ligand.

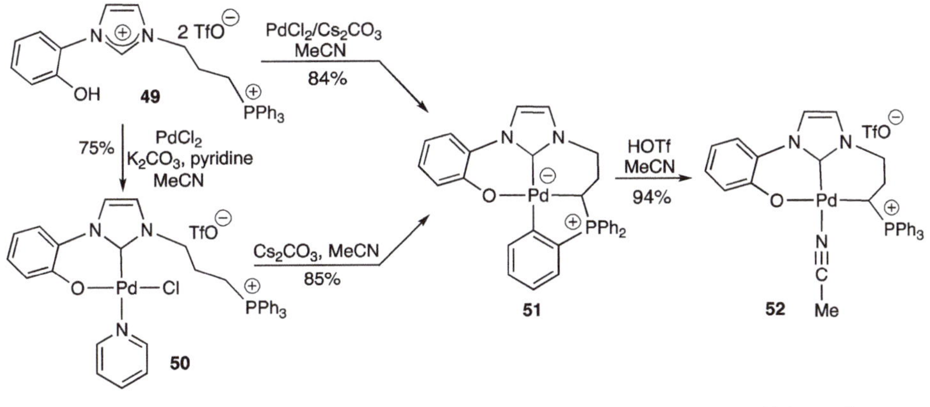

Scheme 18. Preparation of the C,C,O- phenolate, NHC, phosphonium ylide pincer Pd(II) complex **52** from the imidazolium salt **49** following two different routes [93].

The overall donating character of the C,C,O- ligand of complex **52** was further analyzed on the basis of IR ν_{CO} and ν_{CN} stretching frequencies, oxidation potentials, and DFT calculations by comparison with isostructural phosphonium ylide-based pincer Pd complexes. Notably, the IR ν_{CN} frequency values of Pd complexes **53** (2207 cm^{-1}) and **55** (2206 cm^{-1}) indicate that the *C,C,O-* NHC, phenolate, phosphonium ylide, and the *C,C,C-* bis(NHC) phosphonium ylide have similar electronic properties. These IR values, which appear at higher frequency than that of the Pd-CN*t*Bu complex **41** (2194 cm^{-1}), bearing the *C,C,C-* bis(ylide) NHC ligand lead to the conclusion that the substitution of a NHC or a phenolate for a phosphonium ylide increases significantly the donor character of corresponding pincer ligands (Scheme 19) [93]. The Pd–CO complex **42** only experimentally observed in the case of the bis(ylide) ligand is in perfect agreement with these findings. This trend was also found to be in line with previous studies performed on an isoelectronic series of *C,C-* chelating NHC, phosphonium ylide $Rh(CO)_2$ complexes. [94,95]

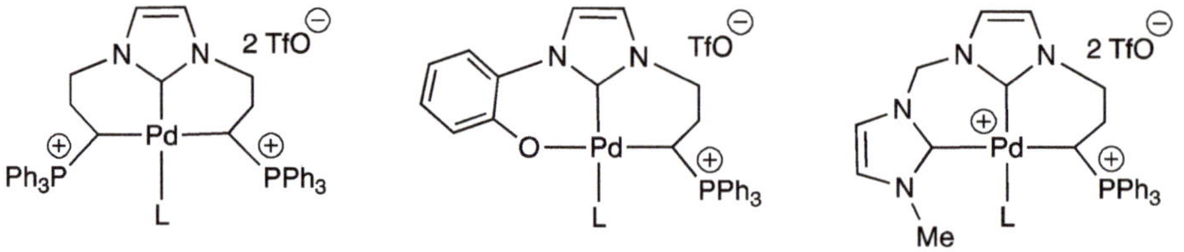

41: L = CN*t*Bu, ν_{CN} = 2194
42: L = CO, ν_{CO} = 2114

53: L = CN*t*Bu, ν_{CN} = 2207
54: L = CO, not formed

55: L = CN*t*Bu, ν_{CN} = 2206
56: L = CO, not formed

Scheme 19. Experimental IR ν_{CO} and ν_{CN} stretching frequencies (cm^{-1}) for NHC core phosphonium ylide-based pincer Pd(II) complexes (L = CN*t*Bu or CO) [93].

The electronic properties of these phosphonium ylide-based pincer Pd(II) complexes were exploited in homogeneous catalysis for the Pd-catalyzed allylation of aldehydes. It was in particular observed that the Pd complex bearing the most donor pincer ligand, namely the NHC, bis(ylide), was the most active in this catalytic process [93].

3. Conclusions and Perspectives

In perpetual search for new ligands, those based on pincer architecture have a promising future, not only because of a structural diversity, which remains to be discovered, but also because of their many potential applications, especially in the fields of organometallic chemistry, homogeneous catalysis, and materials. In this large family, pincer ligands of LX_2-type which position two anionic donor units on either side of a neutral central donor are less common and undoubtedly deserve to be more considered. Combining neutral with anionic donor extremities indeed offers several advantages such as the efficient coordination of a wide range of metal centers and the access to unusual oxidation states. For instance, anionic donors are more likely to bind early transition metals, while neutral ones generally prefer to coordinate late transition metals. In this category of pincer ligands, NHCs substituted by two anionic arms represent a promising family. The association of NHCs with anionic donors indeed makes it possible to stabilize but also to modulate the reactivity of various metal complexes across the periodic table. Independently of the two anionic arms, the nature of the central donor allows a fine adjustment of the electronic properties of the pincer structure since saturated, unsaturated, five- or six-membered NHCs, as well as mesoionic carbenes can be introduced. However, the preparation of such chelating systems generally represents a synthetic challenge in terms of coordination selectivity and choice of metal center in order to reach a good compromise between stability and reactivity. As pointed out in this review, the nature of the donors used in this family of pincer ligand remains very limited to date, and there is no doubt that the introduction of other donor functionalities should allow the development of new properties in the area of redox and photo-active systems but would also be beneficial for the activation of small molecules and for homogeneous catalysis.

Author Contributions: R.T.: literature survey; Y.C.: conceptualization, writing, editing. All authors have read and agreed to the published version of the manuscript.

Funding: This research received no external funding.

Acknowledgments: The authors thank the Centre National de la Recherche Scientifique (CNRS) for financial support. R.T. is grateful to French MENESR for a PhD fellowship.

Conflicts of Interest: The authors declare no conflict of interest.

References

1. Van Koten, G. Tuning the reactivity of metals held in a rigid ligand environment. *Pure Appl. Chem.* **1989**, *61*, 1681–1694. [CrossRef]
2. Morales-Morales, D.; Jensen, C.G.M. *The Chemistry of Pincer Compounds*, 1st ed.; Elsevier Science: Amsterdam, The Netherlands, 2011.
3. Van Koten, G.; Milstein, D. *Organometallic Pincer Chemistry*; Van Koten, G., Milstein, D., Eds.; Springer: Berlin/Heidelberg, Germany, 2013; Volume 40, pp. 1–356.
4. Adams, G.M.; Weller, A.S. POP-type ligands: Variable coordination and hemilabile behaviour. *Coord. Chem. Rev.* **2018**, *355*, 150–172. [CrossRef]
5. Benito-Garagorri, D.; Kirchner, K. Modularly designed transition metal PNP and PCP pincer complexes based on aminophosphines: Synthesis and catalytic applications. *Acc. Chem. Res.* **2008**, *41*, 201–213. [CrossRef] [PubMed]
6. Roddick, D.M.; Zargarian, D. Pentacoordination for pincer and related tertendate coordination compounds: Revisiting structural properties and trends for d^8 transition metal systems. *Inorg. Chim. Acta* **2014**, *422*, 251–264. [CrossRef]
7. Szabó, K.J.; Wendt, O.F. (Eds.) *Pincer and Pincer-Type Complexes: Applications in Organic Synthesis and Catalysis*; Willey-VCH: Weinheim, Germany, 2014.
8. Gunanathan, G.; Milstein, D. Bond activation and catalysis by ruthenium pincer complexes. *Chem. Rev.* **2014**, *114*, 12024–12087. [CrossRef]
9. Maser, L.; Vondung, L.; Langer, R. The ABC in pincer chemistry–from amine to borylene and carbon-based pincer ligands. *Polyhedron* **2018**, *143*, 28–42. [CrossRef]
10. Moulton, C.J.; Shaw, B.L. Transition metal-carbon bonds. Part XLII. Complexes of nickel, palladium, platinum, rhodium and iridium with the tridentate ligand 2,6-bis[(di-t-butylphosphino)methyl]phenyl. *J. Chem. Soc. Dalton Trans.* **1976**, *11*, 1020–1024. [CrossRef]
11. Van Koten, G.; Timmer, K.; Noltes, J.G.; Spek, A.L. A novel type of Pt–C interaction and a model for the final stage in reductive elimination processes involving C–C coupling at Pt; synthesis and molecular geometry of [1,N,N'-η-2,6-bis{(dimethylamino)methyl}toluene]iodoplatinum(II) tetrafluoroborate. *J. Chem. Soc. Chem. Commun.* **1978**, *6*, 250–252. [CrossRef]
12. Parkin, G. The bioinorganic chemistry of zinc: Synthetic analogues of zinc enzymes that feature tripodal ligands. *Chem. Commun.* **2000**, *20*, 1971–1985. [CrossRef]
13. Blackman, A.G. Tripodal tetraamine ligands containing three pyridine units: The other polypyridyl ligands. *Eur. J. Inorg. Chem.* **2008**, *2008*, 2633–2647. [CrossRef]
14. Gamble, A.J.; Lynam, J.M.; Thatcher, R.J.; Walton, P.H.; Whitwood, A.C. Cis-1,3,5-triaminocyclohexane as a facially cappind ligand for ruthenium(II). *Inorg. Chem.* **2013**, *52*, 4517–4527. [CrossRef] [PubMed]
15. Green, M.L.H. A new approach for the formal classification of covalents compounds of the elements. *J. Organomet. Chem.* **1995**, *500*, 127–148. [CrossRef]
16. Pugh, D.; Danapoulos, A.A. Metal complexes with 'pincer'-type ligands incorporating N-heterocyclic carbene functionalities. *Coord. Chem. Rev.* **2007**, *251*, 610–641. [CrossRef]
17. Niu, J.L.; Hao, X.Q.; Gong, J.F.; Song, M.P. Symmetrical and unsymmetrical pincer complexes with group 10 metals: Synthesis *via* aryl C–H activation and some catalytic applications. *Dalton Trans.* **2011**, *40*, 5135–5150. [CrossRef] [PubMed]
18. O'Reilly, M.E.; Veige, A.S. Trianionic pincer and pincer-type metal complexes and catalysts. *Chem. Soc. Rev.* **2014**, *43*, 6325–6369. [CrossRef]
19. Deng, Q.H.; Melen, R.L.; Gade, L.H. Anionic chiral tridentate N-donor pincer ligands in asymmetric catalysis. *Acc. Chem. Res.* **2014**, *47*, 3162–3173. [CrossRef]

20. Murugesan, S.; Kirchner, K. Non-precious metal complexes with an anionic PCP pincer architecture. *Dalton Trans.* **2016**, *45*, 416–439. [CrossRef]
21. Peris, E.; Crabtree, R.H. Key factors in pincer ligand design. *Chem. Soc. Rev.* **2018**, *27*, 1959–1968. [CrossRef]
22. Liu, J.K.; Gong, J.F.; Song, M.P. Chiral palladium pincer complexes for asymmetric catalytic reactions. *Org. Biomol. Chem.* **2019**, *17*, 6069–6098. [CrossRef]
23. Luconi, L.; Rossin, A.; Motta, A.; Tuci, G.; Giambastiani, G. Group IV organometallic compounds based on dianionic pincer ligands: Synthesis, characterization, and catalytic activity in intramolecular hydroamination reactions. *Chem. Eur. J.* **2013**, *19*, 4906–4921. [CrossRef]
24. Agapie, T.; Day, M.W.; Bercaw, J.E. Synthesis and reactivity of tantalum complexes supported by bidentate X_2 and tridentate LX_2 ligand with two phenolates linked to pyridine, thiophene, furan, and benzene connectors: Mechanistic studies of the formation of a tantalum benzylidene and insertion chemistry for tantalum−carbon bonds. *Organometallics* **2008**, *27*, 6123–6142.
25. Winston, M.S.; Bercaw, J.E. A novel bis(phosphido)pyridine [PNP]$^{2-}$ pincer ligand and its potassium and bis(dimethylamido)zirconium(IV) complexes. *Organometallics* **2010**, *29*, 6408–6416. [CrossRef]
26. Lenton, T.N.; VanderVelde, D.G.; Bercaw, J.E. Synthesis of a bis(thiophenolate)pyridine ligand and its titanium, zirconium, and tantalum complexes. *Organometallics* **2012**, *31*, 7492–7499. [CrossRef]
27. Komiyama, Y.; Kuwabara, J.; Kanbara, T. Deprotonation-induced structural changes in SNS-pincer ruthenium complexes with secondary thioamide groups. *Organometallics* **2014**, *33*, 885–891. [CrossRef]
28. Suzuki, T.; Kajita, Y.; Masuda, H. Deprotonation/protonation-driven change of the σ-donor ability of a sulfur atom in iron(II) complexes with a thioamide SNS pincer type ligand. *Dalton Trans.* **2014**, *43*, 9732–9739. [CrossRef] [PubMed]
29. Islam, M.J.; Smith, M.D.; Peryshkov, D.V. Sterically encumbered dianionic dicarboranyl pincer ligand $(C_5H_3N)(C_2B_{10}H_{11})_2$ and its CNC nickel(II) complex. *J. Organomet. Chem.* **2018**, *867*, 208–2013. [CrossRef]
30. Kubo, K.; Jones, N.D.; Ferguson, M.J.; McDonald, R.; Cavell, R.G. Chelate and pincer carbene complexes of rhodium and platinum derived from hexaphenylcarbodiphosphorane, Ph_3=C=PPh_3. *J. Am. Chem. Soc.* **2005**, *127*, 5314–5315. [CrossRef]
31. Petz, W.; Neumüller, B. New platinum complexes with carbodiphosphorane as pincer ligand via ortho phenyl metallation. *Polyhedron* **2011**, *30*, 1779–1784. [CrossRef]
32. Kubo, K.; Okitsu, H.; Miwa, H.; Kume, S.; Cavell, R.G. Carbon(0)-bridged Pt/Ag dinuclear and tetranuclear complexes based on a cyclometalated pincer carbodiphosphorane platform. *Organometallics* **2017**, *36*, 266–274. [CrossRef]
33. Liddle, S.T.; Edworthy, I.S.; Arnold, P.L. Anionic tethered N-heterocyclic carbene chemistry. *Chem. Soc. Rev.* **2007**, *36*, 1732–1744. [CrossRef]
34. Zhang, D.; Zi, G. N-heterocyclic carbene (NHC) complexes of group 4 transition metals. *Chem. Soc. Rev.* **2015**, *44*, 1898–1921. [CrossRef] [PubMed]
35. Pearson, R.G. Antisymbiosis and the trans effect. *Inorg. Chem.* **1973**, *12*, 712–713. [CrossRef]
36. Pearson, R.G. Absolute electronegativity and hardness: Application to inorganic chemistry. *Inorg. Chem.* **1988**, *27*, 734–740. [CrossRef]
37. Arnold, P.L.; Liddle, S.T. F-block N-heterocyclic carbenes. *Chem. Commun.* **2006**, *38*, 3959–3971. [CrossRef] [PubMed]
38. Fliedel, C.; Schnee, G.; Avilés, T.; Dagorne, S. Group 13 metal (Al, Ga, In, Tl) complexes supported by heteroatom-bonded carbene ligands. *Coord. Chem. Rev.* **2014**, *275*, 63–86. [CrossRef]
39. Bellemin-Laponnaz, S.; Dagorne, S. Group 1 and 2 and early transition metal complexes bearing N-heterocyclic carbene ligands: Coordination chemistry, reactivity and applications. *Chem. Rev.* **2014**, *114*, 8747–8774. [CrossRef]
40. Hameury, S.; de Frémont, P.; Braunstein, P. Metal complexes with oxygen-functionalized NHC ligands: Synthesis and applications. *Chem. Soc. Rev.* **2017**, *46*, 632–733. [CrossRef]
41. Guérin, V.; Ménard, A.; Guernon, H.; Moutounet, O.; Legault, C.Y. From chelating to bridging ligands: N-sulfonyliminoimidazolium ylides as precursors to anionic N-heterocyclic carbene ligands. *Organometallics* **2019**, *38*, 409–416. [CrossRef]
42. Bartoszewicz, A.; Marcos, R.; Sahoo, S.; Inge, A.K.; Zou, X.; Martin-Matute, B. A highly active bifunctional iridium complex with an alcohol/alkoxide-tethered N-heterocyclic carbene for alkylation of amines with alcohols. *Chem. Eur. J.* **2012**, *18*, 14510–14519. [CrossRef]

43. Pape, F.; Teichert, J.F. Dealing at arm's length: Catalysis with N-Heterocyclic carbene ligands bearing anionic tethers. *Eur. J. Org. Chem.* **2017**, *2017*, 4206–4229. [CrossRef]
44. Evans, K.J.; Campbell, C.L.; Haddow, M.F.; Luz, C.; Morton, P.A.; Mansell, S.M. Lithium complexes with bridging and terminal NHC ligands: The decisive influence of an anionic tether. *Eur. J. Inorg. Chem.* **2019**, *2019*, 4894–4901. [CrossRef]
45. Aihara, H.; Matsuo, T.; Kawaguchi, H. Titanium N-heterocyclic carbene complexes incorporating an imidazolium-linked bis(phenol). *Chem. Commun.* **2003**, *17*, 2204–2205. [CrossRef] [PubMed]
46. Zhang, D.; Aihara, H.; Watanabe, T.; Matsuo, T.; Kawaguchi, H. Zirconium complexes of the tridentate bis(aryloxide)-N-heterocyclic-carbene ligand: Chloride and alkyl functionalized derivatives. *J. Organomet. Chem.* **2007**, *692*, 234–242. [CrossRef]
47. Zhang, D.; Liu, N. Titanium complexes bearing bisaryloxy-N-heterocyclic carbenes: Synthesis, reactivity, and ethylene polymerization study. *Organometallics* **2009**, *28*, 499–505. [CrossRef]
48. Zhang, D. Dinuclear titanium(IV) complexes bearing phenoxide-tethered N-heterocyclic carbene ligands with *cisoid* conformation through control of hydrolysis. *Eur. J. Inorg. Chem.* **2007**, *2007*, 4839–4845. [CrossRef]
49. Zhang, D.; GengShi, G.; Wang, J.; Yue, Q.; Zheng, W.; Weng, L. Macrocyclic hexanuclear zirconium(IV) complex bearing a bisaryloxyl N-heterocyclic-carbene ligand: Synthesis, structure, and catalytic properties. *Inorg. Chem. Commun.* **2010**, *13*, 433–435. [CrossRef]
50. Zhang, M.; Zhang, J.; Ni, X.; Shen, Z. Bis(phenolate) N-heterocyclic carbene rare earth metal complexes: Synthesis, characterization and applications in the polymerization of *n*-hexyl isocyanate. *RSC Adv.* **2015**, *5*, 83295–83303. [CrossRef]
51. Romain, C.; Brelot, L.; Bellemin-Laponnaz, S.; Dagorne, S. Synthesis and structural characterization of a novel family of titanium complexes bearing a tridentate bis-phenolate-N-heterocyclic carbene dianionic ligand and their use in the controlled ROP of *rac*-lactide. *Organometallics* **2010**, *29*, 1191–1198. [CrossRef]
52. Dagorne, S.; Bellemin-Laponnaz, S.; Romain, C. Neutral and cationic N-heterocyclic carbene zirconium and hafnium benzyl complexes: Highly regioselective oligomerization of 1-hexene with a preference for trimer formation. *Organometallics* **2013**, *32*, 2736–2743. [CrossRef]
53. Romain, C.; Choua, S.; Collin, J.P.; Heinrich, M.; Bailly, C.; Karmazin-Brelot, L.; Bellemin-Laponnaz, S.; Dagorne, S. Redox and luminescent properties of robust and air-stable N-heterocyclic carbene group 4 metal complexes. *Inorg. Chem.* **2014**, *53*, 7371–7376. [CrossRef]
54. Quadri, C.C.; Le Roux, E. Copolymerization of cyclohexene oxide with CO_2 catalyzed by tridentate N-heterocyclic carbene titanium(IV) complexes. *Dalton Trans.* **2014**, *43*, 4242–4246. [CrossRef] [PubMed]
55. Romain, C.; Miqueu, K.; Sotiropoulos, J.M.; Bellemin-Laponnaz, S.; Dagorne, S. Non-innocent behavior of a tridentate NHC chelating ligand coordinated onto a zirconium(IV) center. *Angew. Chem. Int. Ed.* **2010**, *49*, 2198–2201. [CrossRef] [PubMed]
56. Romain, C.; Specklin, D.; Miqueu, K.; Sotiropoulos, J.M.; Fliedel, C.; Bellemin-Laponnaz, S.; Dagorne, S. Unusual benzyl migration reactivity in NHC-bearing group 4 metal chelates: Synthesis, characterization, and mechanistic investigations. *Organometallics* **2015**, *34*, 4854–4863. [CrossRef]
57. Despagnet-Ayoub, E.; Takase, M.K.; Labinger, J.A.; Bercaw, J.E. Reversible 1,2-alkyl migration to carbene and ammonia activation in an N-heterocyclic carbene–zirconium complex. *J. Am. Chem. Soc.* **2015**, *137*, 10500–10503. [CrossRef] [PubMed]
58. Bellemin-Laponnaz, S.; Welter, R.; Brelot, L.; Dagorne, S. Synthesis and structure of V(V) and Mn(III) NHC complexes supported by a tridentate bis-aryloxide-N-heterocyclic carbene ligand. *J. Organomet. Chem.* **2009**, *694*, 604–606. [CrossRef]
59. Baltrun, M.; Watt, F.A.; Schoch, R.; Hohloch, S. Dioxo-, oxo-imido-, and bis-imido-molybdenum(VI) complexes with a bis-phenolate-NHC ligand. *Organometallics* **2019**, *38*, 3719–3729. [CrossRef]
60. Weinberg, D.R.; Hazari, N.; Labinger, J.A.; Bercaw, J.E. Iridium(I) and iridium(III) complexes supported by a diphenolate imidazolyl-carbene ligand. *Organometallics* **2010**, *29*, 89–100. [CrossRef]
61. Harris, C.F.; Bayless, M.B.; van Leest, N.P.; Bruch, Q.J.; Livesay, B.N.; Basca, J.; Hardcastle, K.I.; Shores, M.P.; de Bruin, B.; Soper, J.D. Redox-active bis(phenolate) N-heterocyclic carbene [OCO] pincer ligands support cobalt electron transfer series spannning four oxidation states. *Inorg. Chem.* **2017**, *56*, 12421–12435. [CrossRef]
62. Harris, C.F.; Kuehner, C.S.; Basca, J.; Soper, J.D. Photoinduced cobalt(III)–trifluoromethyl bond activation enables arene C–H trifluoromethylation. *Angew. Chem. Int. Ed.* **2018**, *57*, 1311–1315. [CrossRef]

63. Borré, E.; Dahm, G.; Aliprandi, A.; Mauro, M.; Dagorne, S.; Bellemin-Laponnaz, S. Tridentate complexes of group 10 bearing bis-aryloxide N-heterocyclic carbene ligands: Synthesis, structural, spectroscopic, and computational characterization. *Organometallics* **2014**, *33*, 4374–4384. [CrossRef]
64. Romain, C.; Fliedel, C.; Bellemin-Laponnaz, S.; Dagorne, S. NHC bis-phenolate aluminium chelates: Synthesis, structure, and use in lactide and trimethylene carbonate polymerization. *Organometallics* **2014**, *33*, 5370–5379. [CrossRef]
65. Baltrun, M.; Watt, F.A.; Schoch, R.; Wölper, C.; Neuba, A.G.; Hohloch, S. A new bis-phenolate mesoionic carbene ligand for early transition metal chemistry. *Dalton Trans.* **2019**, *48*, 14611–14625. [CrossRef] [PubMed]
66. Arnold, P.L.; Rodden, M.; Davis, K.M.; Scarisbrick, A.C.; Blake, A.J.; Wilson, C. Asymmetric lithium(I) and copper(II) alkoxy-N-heterocyclic carbene complexes; crystallographic characterization and Lewis acid catalysis. *Chem. Commun.* **2004**, *14*, 1612–1613. [CrossRef] [PubMed]
67. Arnold, P.L.; Wilson, C. Sterically demanding bi- and tridentate alkoxy-N-heterocyclic carbenes. *Inorg. Chim. Acta* **2007**, *360*, 190–196. [CrossRef]
68. Arnold, P.L.; Casely, I.J.; Turner, Z.R.; Carmichael, C.D. Functionalized saturated-backbone carbene ligands: Yttrium and uranyl alkoxy-carbene complexes and bicyclic carbene-alcohol adducts. *Chem. Eur. J.* **2008**, *14*, 10415–10422. [CrossRef]
69. Arduengo, A.J., III; Dolpin, J.S.; Gurau, G.; Marshall, W.J.; Nelson, J.C.; Petrov, V.A.; Runyon, J.W. Synthesis and complexes of fluoroalkoxy carbenes. *Angew. Chem. Int. Ed.* **2013**, *52*, 5110–5114. [CrossRef]
70. Matsumura, N.; Kawano, J.I.; Fukunishi, N.; Inoue, H. Synthesis of new transition metal carbene complexes from π-sulfurane compounds: Reaction of 10-S-3 tetraazapentalene derivatives with Pd(PPh$_3$)$_4$ and RhCl(PPh$_3$)$_3$. *J. Am. Chem. Soc.* **1995**, *117*, 3623–3624. [CrossRef]
71. Iwasaki, F.; Manabe, N.; Nishiyama, H.; Takada, K.; Yasui, M.; Kusamiya, M.; Matsumura, N. Crystal and molecular structures of hypervalent thia/selena pentalenes. *Bull. Chem. Soc. Jpn.* **1997**, *70*, 1267–1275. [CrossRef]
72. Iwasaki, F.; Nishiyama, H.; Yasui, M.; Kusamiya, M.; Matsumura, N. Structures and formation mechanism of novel metal-carbene complexes derived from hypervalent thiadiselenadiazapentalenes. *Bull. Chem. Soc. Jpn.* **1997**, *70*, 1277–1287. [CrossRef]
73. Sellmann, D.; Allmann, C.; Heinemann, F.; Knoch, F.; Sutter, J. Ubergangsmetallkomplexe mit schwefelliganden CXXIV. *J. Organomet. Chem.* **1997**, *541*, 291–305. [CrossRef]
74. Spencer, L.P.; Winston, S.; Fryzuk, M.D. Tridentate amido carbene ligands in early-transition-metal coordination chemistry. *Organometallics* **2004**, *23*, 3372–3374. [CrossRef]
75. Spencer, L.P.; Fryzuk, M.D. Synthesis and reactivity of zirconium and hafnium complexes incorporating chelating diamido-N-heterocyclic-carbene ligands. *J. Organomet. Chem.* **2005**, *690*, 5788–5803. [CrossRef]
76. Spencer, L.P.; Beddie, C.; Hall, M.B.; Fryzuk, M.D. Synthesis, reactivity, and DFT studies of tantalum complexes incorporating diamido-N-heterocyclic carbene ligands. Facile endocyclic C–H bond activation. *J. Am. Chem. Soc.* **2006**, *128*, 12531–12543. [CrossRef] [PubMed]
77. Liao, C.Y.; Chan, K.T.; Zeng, J.Y.; Hu, C.H.; Tu, C.Y.; Lee, H.M. Nonchelate and chelate complexes of palladium(II) with N-heterocyclic carbene ligands of amido functionality. *Organometallics* **2007**, *26*, 1692–1702. [CrossRef]
78. IUPAC. *Compendium of Chemical Terminoly*, 2nd ed.; (The Gold Book) Online Corrected Version **2006** η (eta or hapto) in Inorganic Nomenclature; McNaught, A.D., Wilkinson, A., Eds.; RSC: Cambridge, UK, 1997.
79. Schmidbaur, H. Phosphorus ylides in the coordination sphere of transition metals: An inventory. *Angew. Chem. Int. Ed.* **1983**, *22*, 907–927. [CrossRef]
80. Chauvin, R.; Canac, Y. *Late Transition Metals of Neutral η^1-Carbon Ligands*; Springer: Berlin/Heidelberg, Germany, 2010; Volume 30, pp. 1–252.
81. Abdalilah, M.; Canac, Y.; Lepetit, C.; Chauvin, R. Towards the stability limit of cyclic diphosphonium bis-ylides. *C. R. Chimie* **2010**, *3*, 1091–1098. [CrossRef]
82. Canac, Y.; Duhayon, C.; Chauvin, R. A diaminocarbene-phosphonium ylide: Direct access to C,C-chelating ligands. *Angew. Chem. Int. Ed.* **2007**, *46*, 6313–6315. [CrossRef]
83. Abdellah, I.; Debono, N.; Canac, Y.; Duhayon, C.; Chauvin, R. Atropochiral (C,C)-chelating NHC-ylide ligands: Synthesis and resolution of palladium(II) complexes thereof. *Dalton Trans.* **2009**, *35*, 7196–7202. [CrossRef]

84. Canac, Y.; Chauvin, R. Atropochiral C,X- and C,C-chelating carbon ligands. *Eur. J. Inorg. Chem.* **2010**, *16*, 2325–2335. [CrossRef]
85. Maaliki, C.; Abdalilah, M.; Barthes, C.; Duhayon, C.; Canac, Y.; Chauvin, R. Bis-ylide ligands from acyclic proximal diphosphonium precursors. *Eur. J. Inorg. Chem.* **2012**, *2012*, 4057–4064. [CrossRef]
86. Benaissa, I.; Taakili, R.; Lugan, N.; Canac, Y. A convenient access to N-phosphonio-substituted NHC metal complexes [M = Ag(I), Rh(I), Pd(II)]. *Dalton Trans.* **2017**, *46*, 12293–12305. [CrossRef] [PubMed]
87. Barthes, C.; Bijani, C.; Lugan, N.; Canac, Y. A palladium(II) complex of a C_4 chelating bis(NHC) diphosphonium bis(ylide) ligand. *Organometallics* **2018**, *37*, 673–678. [CrossRef]
88. Taakili, R.; Lepetit, C.; Duhayon, C.; Valyaev, D.A.; Lugan, N.; Canac, Y. Palladium(II) pincer complexes of a C,C,C-NHC, diphosphonium bis(ylide) ligand. *Dalton Trans.* **2019**, *48*, 1709–1721. [CrossRef] [PubMed]
89. Canac, Y. Carbeniophosphines versus phosphoniocarbenes: The role of the positive charge. *Chem. Asian. J.* **2018**, *13*, 1872–1887. [CrossRef]
90. Despagnet-Ayoub, E.; Miqueu, K.; Sotiropoulos, J.M.; Henling, L.M.; Day, M.W.; Labinger, J.A.; Bercaw, J.E. Unexpected rearrangements in the synthesis of an unsymmetrical tridentate dianionic N-heterocyclic carbene. *Chem. Sci.* **2013**, *4*, 2117–2121. [CrossRef]
91. Despagnet-Ayoub, E.; Henling, L.M.; Labinger, J.A.; Bercaw, J.E. Group 4 transition-metal complexes of an aniline-carbene-phenol ligand. *Organometallics* **2013**, *32*, 2934–2938. [CrossRef]
92. Manabe, N.; Yasui, M.; Nishiyama, H.; Shimamoto, S.; Matsumura, N.; Iwasaki, F. Crystal and molecular structures of novel metal–carbene complexes IV. Effect of carbonyl groups and formation mechanism. *Bull. Chem. Soc. Jpn.* **1996**, *69*, 2771–2780. [CrossRef]
93. Taakili, R.; Barthes, C.; Goëffon, A.; Lepetit, C.; Duhayon, C.; Valyaev, D.A.; Canac, Y. NHC Core Phosphonium Ylide-based Palladium(II) Pincer Complexes: The Second Ylide Extremity Makes the Difference. *Inorg. Chem.* **2020**. [CrossRef]
94. Canac, Y.; Lepetit, C.; Abdalilah, M.; Duhayon, C.; Chauvin, R. Diaminocarbene and phosphonium ylide ligands: A systematic comparison of their donor character. *J. Am. Chem. Soc.* **2008**, *130*, 8406–8413. [CrossRef]
95. Canac, Y.; Lepetit, C. Classification of the electronic properties of chelating ligands in *cis*-[LL'Rh(CO)$_2$] complexes. *Inorg. Chem.* **2017**, *56*, 667–675. [CrossRef]

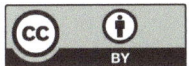

© 2020 by the authors. Licensee MDPI, Basel, Switzerland. This article is an open access article distributed under the terms and conditions of the Creative Commons Attribution (CC BY) license (http://creativecommons.org/licenses/by/4.0/).

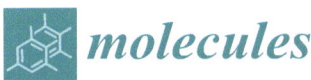 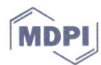

Article

Towards the Preparation of Stable Cyclic Amino(ylide)Carbenes

Henning Steinert, Christopher Schwarz, Alexander Kroll and Viktoria H. Gessner *

Faculty of Chemistry and Biochemistry, Chair of Inorganic Chemistry II, Ruhr University Bochum, Universitätsstr. 150, 44801 Bochum, Germany; henning.steinert@rub.de (H.S.); christopher.m.schwarz@rub.de (C.S.); Alexander.kroll@rub.de (A.K.)
* Correspondence: viktoria.gessner@rub.de; Tel.: +49-(0)234/32-24174

Academic Editor: Yves Canac
Received: 25 January 2020; Accepted: 11 February 2020; Published: 12 February 2020

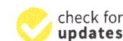

Abstract: Cyclic amino(ylide)carbenes (CAYCs) are the ylide-substituted analogues of N-heterocyclic Carbenes (NHCs). Due to the stronger π donation of the ylide compared to an amino moiety they are stronger donors and thus are desirable ligands for catalysis. However, no stable CAYC has been reported until today. Here, we describe experimental and computational studies on the synthesis and stability of CAYCs based on pyrroles with trialkyl onium groups. Attempts to isolate two CAYCs with trialkyl phosphonium and sulfonium ylides resulted in the deprotonation of the alkyl groups instead of the formation of the desired CAYCs. In case of the PCy$_3$-substituted system, the corresponding ylide was isolated, while deprotonation of the SMe$_2$-functionalized compound led to the formation of ethene and the thioether. Detailed computational studies on various trialkyl onium groups showed that both the α- and β-deprotonated compounds were energetically favored over the free carbene. The most stable candidates were revealed to be α-hydrogen-free adamantyl-substituted onium groups, for which β-deprotonation is less favorable at the bridgehead position. Overall, the calculations showed that the isolation of CAYCs should be possible, but careful design is required to exclude decomposition pathways such as deprotonations at the onium group.

Keywords: carbenes; ylides; DFT calculations; electronic structure; catalysis; ligands; structure–activity relationship

1. Introduction

Since the isolation of the first stable singlet carbenes by Bertrand and Arduengo [1] 30 years ago, these divalent carbon ligands have led to a revolution in coordination chemistry and produced most remarkable developments in various fields of chemistry. Owing to their high donor strength, they are applied as potent ligands in transition metal catalysis [2–5] (e.g., in the second generation Grubbs catalyst [6]), in organo catalysis [2,7–10], or main group chemistry [2,11,12], such as for the stabilization of reactive [2,12], electron-deficient [2,12], or low-valent species [2,12]. The success of carbenes is mostly based on their thermal stability and high donor capacity, which usually surpasses that of phosphines or amines. Furthermore, detailed studies by various research groups over the world have demonstrated the straightforward tunability of the electronic structure, particularly the HOMO–LUMO gap, thus allowing for the adjustment of the donor and acceptor properties for the desired application. While the first years of the "carbene revolution" were defined by the Arduengo-type N-heterocyclic carbenes (NHC) **A** (Figure 1), the past years have seen a huge expansion of the carbene portfolio by variation of the substituents [13–18] or the geometry (cyclic versus acyclic) [18] at the carbenic carbon atom. This has led to drastic changes in the carbene properties and hence to a myriad of new fields of applications. For example, in a landmark report, Bertrand and coworkers demonstrated that the replacement of one nitrogen substituent in an NHC by a sp^3-carbon substituent to form acyclic and cyclic alkyl(amino)carbenes (CAAC, **B**) significantly increases the donor and acceptor properties of these compounds [18]. This results in a sufficiently small HOMO–LUMO (highest molecular orbital, lowest molecular orbital, respectively) gap to allow for straightforward dihydrogen activation [19].

In recent years, many different types of carbenes with different donor/acceptor properties have been reported, many of which, however, suffer from insufficient stability for broad applications. One particularly interesting class of singlet carbenes is the amino(ylide)carbenes (CAYCs, **C**). Here, one of the nitrogen substituents of an NHC was replaced by an ylide group. Due to the lower electronegativity of carbon compared to nitrogen, such an ylide-substitution should result in increased HOMO and LUMO levels, thus making CAYCs particularly strong donors with interesting electronic properties [20–24].

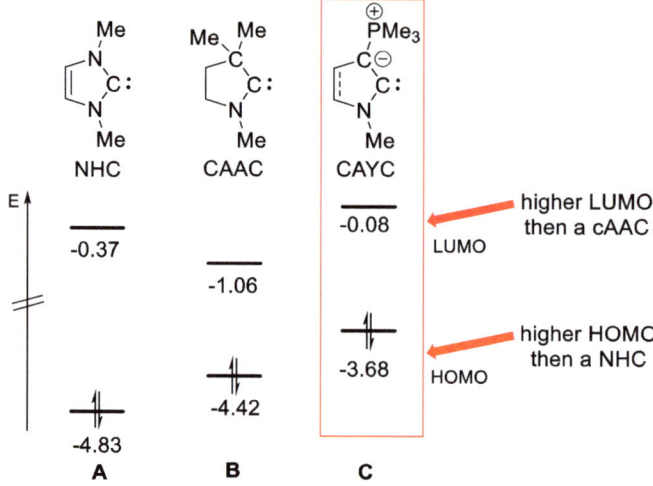

Figure 1. Schematic representation of the HOMO and LUMO properties of different singlet carbenes. Eigenvalues of the frontier orbitals were taken from Reference [21].

Initial attempts to isolate CAYCs were reported in 2008. Kawashima and Fürstner targeted the isolation of **1** and **2**, respectively (Figure 2) [25,26]. However, both compounds were found to decompose at low temperatures, and no room temperature stable CAYC has been reported until today. Nonetheless, the successful synthesis of the CAYCs could be unambiguously confirmed by trapping the carbenes in the coordination sphere of a metal. Isolation of an anionic CAYC was also reported by Bertand and coworkers. They likewise failed in the isolation of the CAYC **5** by deprotonation of phosphonium salt **4** with different bases (Figure 2). However, employment of two equiv. of methyllithium resulted in the formation of the anionic CAYC **6** via P-C cleavage and elimination of one of the phosphorus-bound phenyl groups [27]. In contrast to carbenes, a couple of ylide-substituted heavier tetrylenes have been isolated in recent years due to the generally higher stability of the heavier carbenes resulting from the increased stability of the +2 oxidation state as a consequence of the larger s,p orbital separation [28–30]. They impressively demonstrated unique reactivities owing to their high donor capacity imparted by the ylide-substituents.

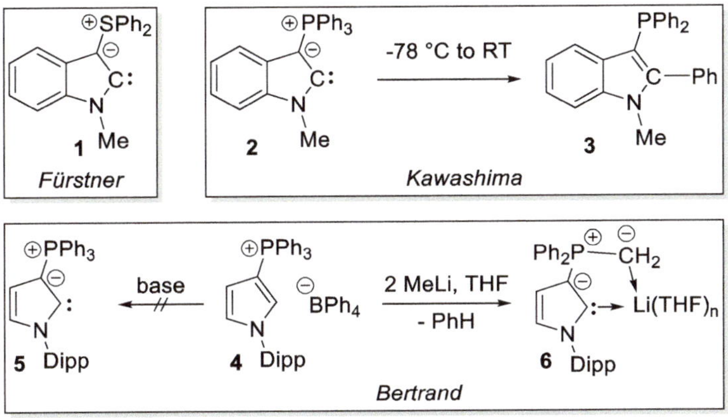

Figure 2. Attempts to isolate CAYCs (Dipp = 2,6-diisopropylphenyl) [25–27].

During their attempts to isolate a CAYC, Kawashima and coworkers uncovered a decomposition reaction pathway of **2** which led to the formation of indole **3** via transfer of an aryl substituent of the onium group to the carbene center [25]. Due to the lower bond strength of a P-C_{sp2} and S-C_{sp2}, respectively, compared to bonds with a sp^3 hybridized carbon atom, such a transfer should be less likely for trialkyl substituted onium moieties. With this in mind, we set out to synthesize CAYCs **7** and **8** with a dialkylsulfonium and trialkylphosphonium group.

2. Results

2.1. Attempted Synthesis of CAYCs with Trialklyl Onium Groups

We started our investigations with the attempt to synthesize the dimethylsulfonium carbene **7**. The sulfonium salt **9** was synthesized according to a literature procedure [26,31,32] via treatment of N-(2,6-diisopropylphenyl)pyrrole [33] with DMSO and trifluoroacetic anhydride, and was isolated in 58% yield as colorless solid. The salt **9** exhibited a pseudo triplet in the ^{1}H NMR spectrum at 7.35 ppm for the NCHCSMe$_2$ moiety. Recently, Szostak and coworkers showed that the σ-donor strengths of carbenes can easily be estimated by measurement of the $^1J_{CH}$ coupling constant in the protonated carbene precursors [34]. Measurement of the $^1J_{CH}$ coupling constant of **9** revealed a value of 194.0 Hz, which suggests that the CAYC **7** is a stronger donor than typical NHCs and of a strength comparable to CAACs. The structure of **9** was unambiguously confirmed by single-crystal X-ray diffraction analysis (Figure 3). Deprotonation was next attempted at low temperatures. Addition of methyllithium (MeLi) or lithium diisopropylamide (LDA) at −78 °C to a solution of **9** in THF led to a color change from colorless to brown and the selective formation of a single new compound, as assessed by NMR spectroscopy (Scheme 1). Isolation revealed the product to be thioether **10**, which could be isolated as colorless oil in 94% yield. Compound **5** is characterized by a signal at 6.69 ppm in the ^{1}H NMR spectrum for the imidazolium hydrogen atom and at 2.22 ppm for the sulfur-bound methyl group. The formation of **10** clearly resulted from the deprotonation of the sulfonium salt at the methyl group and the intermediate generation of yilde **10-Int**. This ylide intermediate presumably reacted in a kind of Corey–Chaykovsky reaction [35,36] with itself to form **8** under concomitant formation of ethene. Indeed, NMR monitoring of the formation of **10** clearly showed the formed ethene by appearance of a signal at 5.35 ppm in the ^{1}H NMR spectrum.

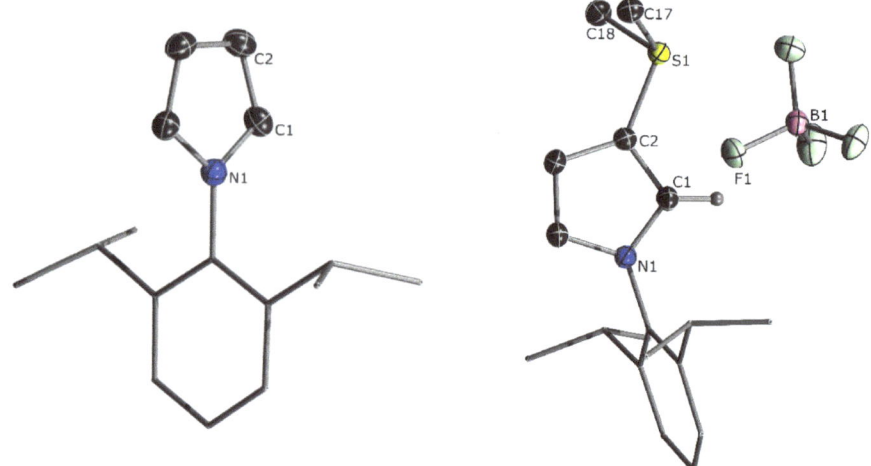

Figure 3. Molecular structure of *N*-(2,6-diisopropylphenyl)pyrrole (left) and **9**. Ellipsoids are drawn at the 50% probability level. Selected bond lengths (Å) and angles (°): N-(1,2-Diisopropylphenyl)pyrrole: N1–C1 1.374(2), N1–C4 1.375(2), C1–C2 1.370(2), C2–C3 1.416(3), C3–C4 1.367(2). **9**: S2–C2 1.748(1), N1–C1 1.362(1), C1–C2 1.376(2), C2–C3 1.412(2).

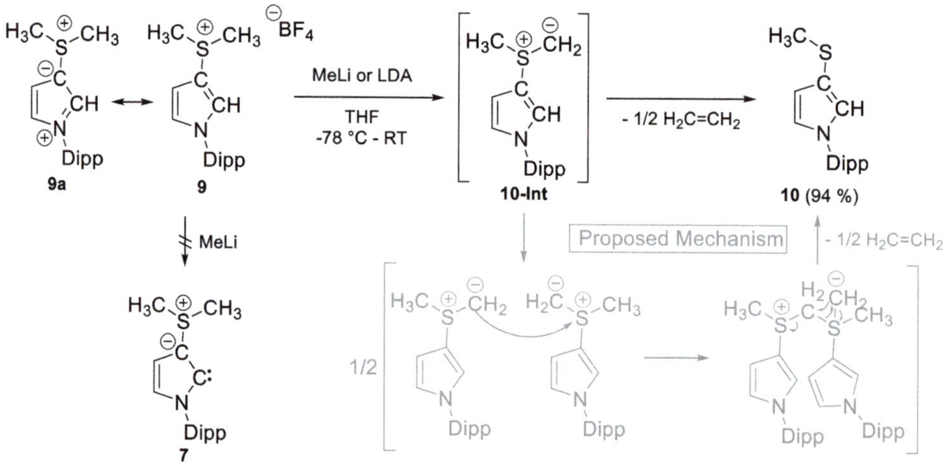

Scheme 1. Deprotonation of the sulfonium salt **9** to form thioether **10** and proposed mechanism.

Comparison of the structure of the sulfonium salt **9** with that of the pyrrole precursor *N*-(2,6-diisopropylphenyl)pyrrole revealed similar structural changes upon introduction of the onium moiety, as previously observed by Fürstner and coworkers. [26] As a result of the delocalization of the charge of the sulfonium moiety into the pyrrole ring of **9** and the thus more pronounced contribution of the ylidic resonance structure **9b** to the overall electronic structure of **9**, the C1–C2 bond in **9** (1.376(2) Å) was elongated compared the one found in *N*-(2,6-diisopropylphenyl)pyrrole (1.370(3) and 1.367(2) Å). Likewise, the C1–N1 bond shortened from approx. 1.374 Å in the unsubstituted pyrrole to 1.362(1) Å in **9**.

Since deprotonation of **9** at the methyl group was clearly kinetically favored over the desired carbene formation, we next turned our attention towards a tricyclohexyl phosphonium salt.

We envisioned that the cyclohexyl group should be less prone to ylide formation (due to electronic and steric reasons) and thus allow for the formation of carbene **8**. The phosphonium precursor **11** was synthesized by treatment of the corresponding iodo compound, obtained similarly to a known procedure [37] with tricyclohexylphosphine in the presence of 5 mol% Ni(cod)$_2$ (cod = 1,5-cyclooctadiene) at elevated temperatures and isolated as colorless solid in 61% yield. Compound **11** was characterized by multi-nuclear NMR spectroscopy, elemental, and single-crystal X-ray diffraction analysis (Figure 4). The phosphonium salt exhibited a signal at 26.1 ppm in the ^{31}P NMR spectrum and a multiplet at 7.23–7.26 ppm in the ^{1}H NMR spectrum for the pyrrole hydrogen atom. The $^1J_{CH}$ coupling constant of 189.2 Hz suggested a slightly stronger σ-donating character of **8** compared to **7** [34]. Treatment of **11** with an equiv. amount of methyllithium or lithium diisopropylamide at low temperatures resulted in the formation of a single new product, as evidenced by a new signal at 6.6 ppm in the ^{31}P NMR spectrum (Scheme 2). Isolation again revealed selective deprotonation at the cyclohexyl group instead of formation of the desired carbene species. Phosphorus ylide **12** could be isolated in 60% yield as colorless solid. It was characterized by a doublet at 12.0 ppm with a coupling constant of 125.0 Hz in the ^{13}C{^{1}H} NMR spectrum corresponding to the ylidic carbon atom.

Table 1. Comparison of the bond lengths in **11** and **12**.

Structural Parameters		11	12
bond length (Å)	C1–C2	1.358(4)	1.379(2)
	C1-N1	1.358(4)	1.364(1)
	C2–P1	1.765(3)	1.790(1)
	P1–C29	1.830(3)	1.679(1)
bond angle (°)	P1–C29–C30	110.9(2)	122.20(10)
	P1–C29–C34	111.1(2)	120.68(10)
	C30–C29–C34	110.0(2)	113.02(11)
	Σ	332.0(6)	355.90(31)

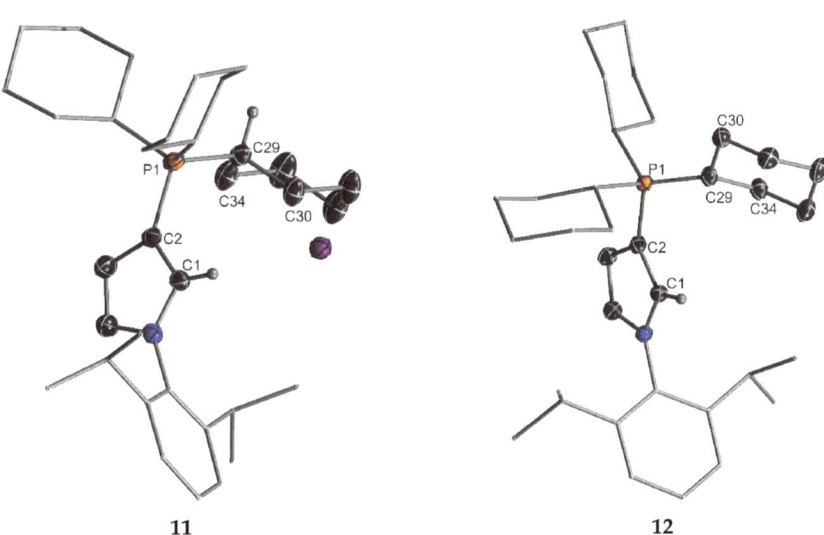

Figure 4. Molecular structures of (left) **11** and (right) **12**. Ellipsoids are drawn at the 50% probability level. Selected bond lengths are provided in Table 1.

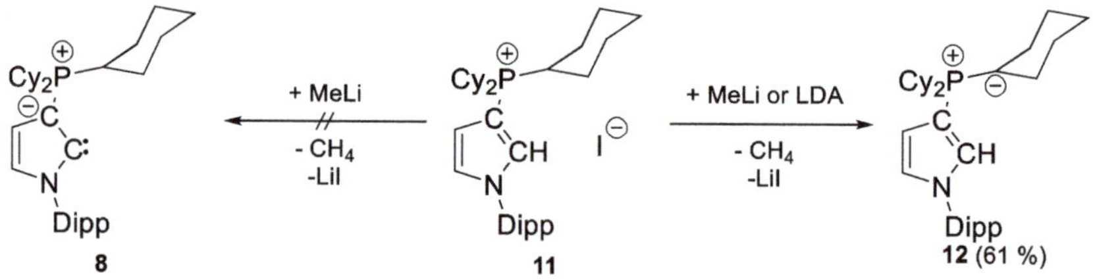

Scheme 2. Deprotonation of the phosphonium salt **11** to form **12**.

Single crystals of **12** were grown by diffusion of *n*-hexanes into a solution of **12** in benzene (Figure 4). The ylide crystallized in the *P*2$_1$/c space group and confirmed the nature of the compound suggested by NMR spectroscopy. The ylidic carbon atom was—as expected for a non-stabilized ylide—pyramidalized, albeit the deviation from planarity was only small, with a sum of angles of 355.9(3)° (Table 1). In comparison to its protonated precursor **11**, **12** exhibited a shortened P-C29 bond due to the ylidic bonding situation, while the P1–C2 bond slightly elongated due to the weaker electrostatic interaction between the onium group and the π-electrons. Despite this weaker ylidic interaction in the P1–C2 linkage of **12**, the C1–C2 bond in **12** was slightly elongated compared to **11**, while the C–N bond changed insignificantly.

2.2. Computational Studies

The unsuccessful formation of the CAYCs **7** and **8** led us to more closely look into the stability of different CAYCs. We particularly wondered whether there are stable CAYCs, or if proton shifts from any moiety in the carbene to the divalent carbon center is always energetically favorable. Thus, the energetics of possible proton transfers in the carbene were examined using computational methods. The calculations were performed on the PBE0-def2svp/PBE0-def2tzvp level of theory, including THF as solvent via the polarizable continuum model. At first, decomposition pathways for carbene **I** (onium group = PCy$_3$ = **8**) were investigated (Figure 5). Besides the proton shift from the α-position of the onium group to the carbene center (via **TS**$_{I→II}$) to form the ylide observed in experiment, we also probed the viability of a deprotonation in β-position (via **TS**$_{I→III}$). For this β-deprotonation, three different pathways were considered: (i) abstraction of a proton in equatorial position and (ii) in axial position of the cyclohexyl ring followed by cyclohexene elimination (**TS**$_{III→IV}$), as well as (iii) a concerted mechanism, in which proton abstraction and cyclohexene elimination occur simultaneously (**TS**$_{I→IV}$). The results showed that from a thermodynamic point of view, both the α- and β-deprotonation (with subsequent cyclohexene elimination) were clearly favored over the free carbene **I**. Thereby, the cyclohexene elimination product was the most favored decomposition product, being 106 kJ/mol favored over the AYC and 46 kJ/mol over ylide **II** (onium group = PCy$_3$ = **11**). This preference was expected, since the β-elimination product **IV** is lacking any reactive carbenic, ylidic or carbanionic site in the molecule and thus should be more stable. However, kinetically the transfer of the proton in α-position to the phosphorus atom was favored over the abstraction of the β-hydrogen atom, so that **II** was the kinetically favored species. With a barrier of only 58 kJ/mol, the required activation energy for TSα was small enough to be easily overcome at temperatures below room temperature, thus explaining the impossible isolation of **8** and the selective formation of **12**.

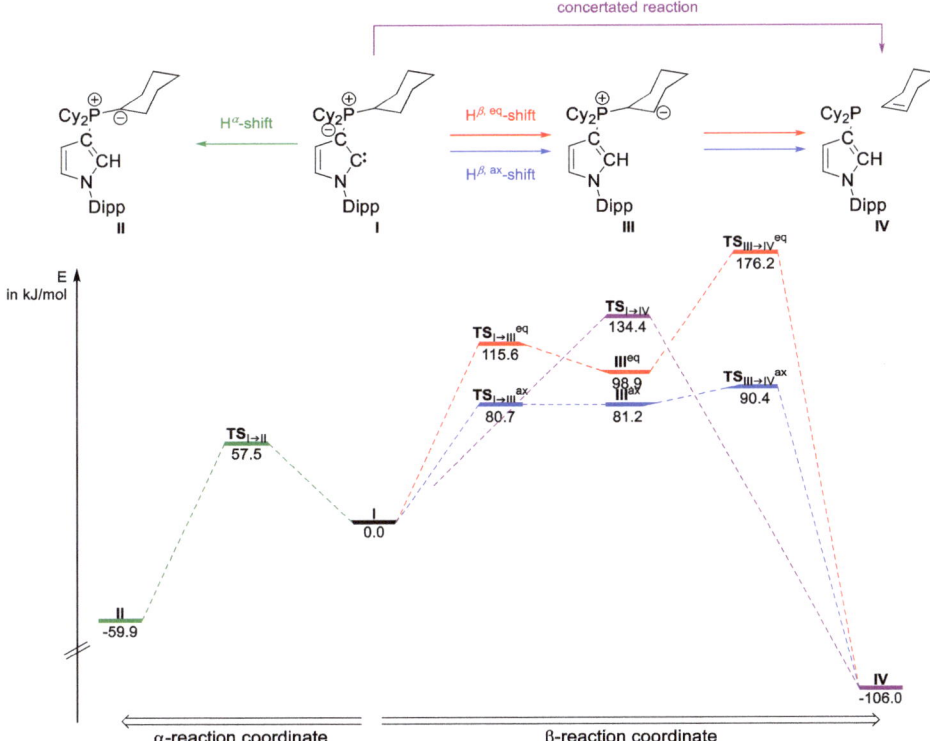

Figure 5. Different pathways for the decomposition of a PCy$_3$-substituted CAYC. Energies are given relative to CAYC **I** (PBE0-def2svp/PBE0-def2tzvp; PCM with THF as solvent).

Next, detailed studies on the decomposition pathways with different onium moieties were performed to unveil molecular structures advantageous for the isolation of stable CAYCs. Besides phosphonium, sulfonium and sulfoxonium units with different alkyl substituents were also considered. The results for the different CAYCs **I** are summarized in Table 2. It should be noted that in some cases, the β-deprotonated species **III** was found to be not stable and decomposed directly under formation of the alkene and the corresponding sulfide, sulfoxide and phosphine, respectively (concerted mechanism). The calculations revealed that in every case, the deprotonation in α-position to the heteroatom was thermodynamically favored over the corresponding CAYC. For example, α-deprotonation at a cyclohexyl group was favored by approx. 60 kJ/mol for phosphonium, sulfonium, and sulfoxonium groups. Furthermore, the activation energy for the H$_\alpha$-shift from the methyl or cyclohexyl group to the carbene center was always low enough to be easily overcome at room temperature. Thus, substituents with α-H atoms seem to be unsuitable for the formation of isolable CAYCs.

Table 2. Comparison of the proton shifts from the α- and β-position of the onium group to the carbene center. Energies are given relative to the corresponding CAYC **I** (PBE0-def2svp/PBE0-def2tzvp; PCM with THF as solvent).

Onium Group	II (kJ/mol)	TS$_{I \to II}$ (kJ/mol)	TS$_{I \to III}$ (kJ/mol)	III (kJ/mol)	TS$_{III \to IV}$ (kJ/mol)	IV (kJ/mol)
	α-deprotonation		β-deprotonation			
SCy$_2$	−61.4	44.1		66.9 (concerted)		−239.9
SOCy$_2$	−61.7	50.6	100.1^{eq}	102.7 (concerted) 107.4^{eq}	119.1^{eq}	−203.5
PCy$_3$	−59.9	57.5	115.6^{eq} 80.7^{ax}	134.4 (concerted) 98.9^{eq} 81.2^{ax}	176.2^{eq} 90.4^{ax}	−106.0
SMe$_2$	−52.2	54.8			−	
SOMe$_2$	−85.0	60.3			−	
PMe$_3$	−53.9	56.5			−	
S^{t}Bu$_2$	−			54.0 (concerted)		−236.3
SO^{t}Bu$_2$	−			35.9 (concerted)		−248.0
P^{t}Bu$_3$	−		71.1	40.9	58.5	−185.5
SAd$_2$	−			123.7		−8.3
SOAd$_2$	−			102.4		7.4
PAd$_3$	−		91.6	91.2	108.4	47.1
S(CH$_2$)$_2$	−		38.0^a	−48.6^a	−40.4^a	−275.0
S(CH$_2$)$_3$	−11.9	65.5	105.0	75.4	83.0	−238.8
S(CH$_2$)$_4$	−33.6	56.7		90.5 (concerted)		−180.0

[a] Note that deprotonation always occurs in the α-position to sulfur. Thus, activation energies are lower than those usually seen for β-deprotonations.

Therefore, we turned our attention toward the α-hydrogen-free substituents, *tert*-butyl and adamantyl, where only deprotonation in β-position to the heteroatom can take place. In case of the *tert*-butyl groups, the β-deprotonated species **IV** were clearly thermodynamically favored over the CAYCs. However, the corresponding shifts of the H$^\beta$-atoms were kinetically less favored then the H$^\alpha$-shifts. This was at least suggested by the results obtained from the cyclohexyl-substituted ylides. However, in the case of the *tert*-butyl substituents, the barriers for the β-deprotonation also appeared to be very low, so any attempt to isolate a *tert*-butyl-substituted CAYC **I** should lead to the formation of isobutene and the corresponding pyrrole. The same holds true for the compounds with cyclic sulfonium groups. The only exceptions are the adamantly-substituted compounds. Here, the products formed after deprotonation and elimination were thermodynamically only slightly downhill (sulfonium ylide) or even uphill. This was due to the required formation of a double bond at the bridgehead of the adamantly substituents (Bredt's rule). Overall, the tris(adamantyl) phosphonium-substituted CAYC is thus the most promising candidate for isolation. It features a rather high barrier for intramolecular proton transfer and β-elimination is clearly disfavored by 47 kJ/mol.

3. Discussion and Conclusions

In conclusion, we reported herein on attempts to synthesize and isolate room-temperature-stable CAYCs. While former studies solely focused on aryl-substituted onium moieties, which partly underwent decomposition by cleavage of one of the aryl groups, we examined the impact of alkyl substituents on stability. The experimental and theoretical results clearly showed that the isolation of trialkyl-onium-substituted CAYCs is also preparatively highly challenging. Simple alkyl groups such as methyl or cyclohexyl are not suitable substituents due to their straightforward deprotonation in the α-position to the heteroatom. Thus, in case of the PCy$_3$-substituted pyrrole, no carbene but ylide formation via deprotonation at the cyclohexyl moiety was observed. Likewise, the dimethylsulfonium compound underwent a kind of Corey–Chaykovsky reaction with formation of ethene and the thioether. The calculations demonstrated that even if accessible at low temperatures, trialkyl onium groups show high tendencies to undergo proton shifts not only from the α-position of the heteroatom, but also from the β-position. This observation is true for phosphonium, sulfonium, and sulfoxonium moieties.

These results, together with the previously observed P-C bond cleavage of aryl-substituted onium groups, clearly show that a careful molecular design must be chosen in order to exclude decomposition pathways of these highly basic carbenes. Our calculations suggest that α-hydrogen-free substituents, particularly adamantyl moieties, might be the substituents of choice in terms of stability. Current experimental studies are now addressing the preparation of CAYCs with a molecular design proposed by our calculations. The steric bulk will presumably require additional structural changes for successful synthesis of the carbene precursors. If these difficulties can be handled, stable CAYCs should become available in the near future.

4. Materials and Methods

Detailed experimental procedures, NMR spectra, and crystallographic and computational data as well as the coordinates and energies of the optimized structures can be found in the Supplementary Information File available online.

4.1. Crystal Structure Determination

All data were collected with an OXFORD *SuperNova*. The structures were resolved using direct methods; the *Shelx* software package [38–40] was used for refinement and expansion was carried out using FOURIER techniques. An inert oil was used to mount the crystals and the crystal structure determination was performed at 100 K using Mo-K$_\alpha$ radiation. The corresponding data have been deposited with the CAMBRIDGE CRYSTALLOGRAPHIC DATA CENTRE as supplementary publication no. 1979639-1979642. Copies of the data can be obtained free of charge on application to CAMBRIDGE CRYSTALLOGRAPHIC DATA CENTRE, 12 Union Road, Cambridge CB2 1EZ; UK [Homepage: https://www.ccdc.cam.ac.uk/].

Diamond 4.0 [41] by CRYSTAL IMPACT and *GIMP* 2.10 [42] were used for graphic representation, Ellipsoids are drawn at the 50% probability level.

The structure of **9** contained a highly disordered solvent molecule that was treated using the PLATON/SQUEZZE routine. [43]

4.2. Computational Studies

All computational studies were carried out without symmetry restrictions. If it was not possible to obtain starting coordinates from crystal structures, either *GaussView 3.0* [44] or *GaussView 6.0* [45] were used. Calculations were done either with the *Gaussian09 Revision E.01* [46], the *Gaussian16 Revision B.01* [47], or the *Gaussian16 Revision C.01* [48] program packages using density-functional theory (DFT) [49,50] with PBE0 [51]/def2svp [52] with GRIMMES D3 dispersion correction with Becke–Johnson damping [53–55]. To determine the nature of the structures, harmonic vibrational frequency analysis was performed on the same level of theory. [56] No imaginary frequencies were observed for the ground states; for transition states, one imaginary frequency corresponding to the translational motion was observed. Single point energies were calculated on PBE0 [51]/def2tzvp [52] level of theory. Additional, single-point energies were calculated on the same level of theory with the polarizable continuum model (PCM) the integral equation formalism variant (IEFPCM) [57], as implemented in Gaussian09 and Gaussian16 with the parameters for tetrahydrofurane. The values in the paper are by 7.925867 kJ/mol for each species to convert them to a 1 M standard state.

Supplementary Materials: The following are available online. Supporting information on experimental procedures, NMR spectra, and crystallographic and computational data as well as the coordinates and energies of the optimized structures.

Author Contributions: Conceptualization, H.S. and V.H.G.; Synthetic and computational investigations, H.S.; Data analysis, H.S.; X-ray crystallography, C.S. and A.K.; supervision, V.H.G; project administration, V.H.G.; funding acquisition, V.H.G. All authors have read and agreed to the published version of the manuscript.

Funding: This research was funded by the European Research Council under the European Union's Horizon 2020 research and innovation program (Project: YlideLigands, No 677749).

Conflicts of Interest: The authors declare no conflict of interest.

References

1. Arduengo, A.J.; Harlow, R.L.; Kline, M. A stable crystalline carbene. *J. Am. Chem. Soc.* **1991**, *113*, 361–363. [CrossRef]
2. Hopkinson, M.N.; Richter, C.; Schedler, M.; Glorius, F. An overview of N-heterocyclic carbenes. *Nature* **2014**, *510*, 485–496. [CrossRef] [PubMed]
3. Zhao, Q.; Meng, G.; Nolan, S.P.; Szostak, M. N-Heterocyclic Carbene Complexes in C–H Activation Reactions. *Chem. Rev.* **2020**. [CrossRef] [PubMed]
4. Díez-González, S.; Marion, N.; Nolan, S.P. N-Heterocyclic Carbenes in Late Transition Metal Catalysis. *Chem. Rev.* **2009**, *109*, 3612–3676. [CrossRef]
5. Janssen-Müller, D.; Schlepphorst, C.; Glorius, F. Privileged chiral N-heterocyclic carbene ligands for asymmetric transition-metal catalysis. *Chem. Soc. Rev.* **2017**, *46*, 4845–4854. [CrossRef]
6. Scholl, M.; Ding, S.; Lee, C.W.; Grubbs, R.H. Synthesis and activity of a new generation of ruthenium-based olefin metathesis catalysts coordinated with 1,3-dimesityl-4,5-dihydroimidazol-2-ylidene ligands. *Org. Lett.* **1999**, *1*, 953–956. [CrossRef]
7. Naumann, S.; Dove, A.P. N-Heterocyclic carbenes for metal-freepolymerization catalysis: An update. *Polym. Int.* **2016**, *65*, 16–27. [CrossRef]
8. Enders, D.; Niemeier, O.; Henseler, A. Organocatalysis by N-Heterocyclic Carbenes. *Chem. Rev.* **2007**, *107*, 5606–5655. [CrossRef]
9. Flanigan, D.M.; Romanov-Michailidis, F.; White, N.A.; Rovis, T. Organocatalytic Reactions Enabled by N-Heterocyclic Carbenes. *Chem. Rev.* **2015**, *115*, 9307–9387. [CrossRef]
10. Marion, N.; Díez-González, S.; Nolan, S.P. N-Heterocyclic Carbenes as Organocatalysts. *Angew. Chem. Int. Ed.* **2007**, *46*, 2988–3000. [CrossRef]
11. Nesterov, V.; Reiter, D.; Bag, P.; Frisch, P.; Holzner, R.; Porzelt, A.; Inoue, S. NHCs in Main Group Chemistry. *Chem. Rev.* **2018**, *118*, 9678–9842. [CrossRef] [PubMed]
12. Martin, C.; Soleilhavoup, M.; Bertrand, G. Carbene-stabilized main group radicals and radical ions. *Chem. Sci.* **2013**, *4*, 3020–3030. [CrossRef] [PubMed]
13. Nakano, R.; Jazzar, R.; Bertrand, G. A crystalline monosubstituted carbene. *Nat. Chem.* **2018**, *10*, 1196–1200. [CrossRef] [PubMed]
14. Arduengo, A.J.; Goerlich, J.R.; Marshall, W.J. A Stable Thiazol-2-ylidene and Its Dimer. *Liebigs Ann. -Recl.* **1997**, *1997*, 365–374. [CrossRef]
15. Martin, D.; Baceiredo, A.; Gornitzka, H.; Schoeller, W.W.; Bertrand, G. A stable P-heterocyclic carbene. *Angew. Chem. Int. Ed. Engl.* **2005**, *44*, 1700–1703. [CrossRef]
16. Alcarazo, M.; Suárez, R.M.; Goddard, R.; Fürstner, A.A. A New Class of Singlet Carbene Ligands. *Chem. Eur. J.* **2010**, *16*, 9746–9749. [CrossRef]
17. Lavallo, V.; Canac, Y.; Präsang, C.; Donnadieu, B.; Bertrand, G. Stable cyclic (alkyl)(amino)carbenes as rigid or flexible, bulky, electron-rich ligands for transition-metal catalysts: A quaternary carbon atom makes the difference. *Angew. Chem. Int. Ed. Engl.* **2005**, *44*, 5705–5709. [CrossRef]
18. Lavallo, V.; Mafhouz, J.; Canac, Y.; Donnadieu, B.; Schoeller, W.W.; Bertrand, G. Synthesis, reactivity, and ligand properties of a stable alkyl carbene. *J. Am. Chem. Soc.* **2004**, *126*, 8670–8671. [CrossRef]
19. Frey, G.D.; Lavallo, V.; Donnadieu, B.; Schoeller, W.W.; Bertrand, G. Facile splitting of hydrogen and ammonia by nucleophilic activation at a single carbon center. *Science* **2007**, *316*, 439–441. [CrossRef]
20. Borthakur, B.; Silvi, B.; Dewhurst, R.D.; Phukan, A.K. Theoretical Strategies Toward Stabilization of SingletRemote N-Heterocyclic Carbenes. *J. Comput. Chem.* **2016**, *37*, 1484–1490. [CrossRef]
21. Andrada, D.M.; Holzmann, N.; Hamadi, T.; Frenking, G. Direct estimate of the internal π-donation to the carbene centre within N-heterocyclic carbenes and related molecules. *Beilstein J. Org. Chem.* **2015**, *11*, 2727–2736. [CrossRef] [PubMed]
22. Borthakur, B.; Phukan, A.K. Moving toward Ylide-Stabilized Carbenes. *Chem. Eur. J.* **2015**, *21*, 11603–11609. [CrossRef] [PubMed]
23. Fekete, Á.; Nyulászi, L. Phosphorus stabilized carbenes: Theoretical predictions. *J. Organomet. Chem.* **2002**, *643–644*, 278–284. [CrossRef]

24. Bharadwaz, P.; Chetia, P.; Phukan, A.K. Electronicand Ligand Properties of Skeletally Substituted Cyclic(Alkyl)(Amino)Carbenes(CAACs) and Their Reactivity towardsSmall Molecule Activation: A Theoretical Study. *Chem. Eur. J.* **2017**, *23*, 9926–9936. [CrossRef]
25. Nakafuji, S.-Y.; Kobayashi, J.; Kawashima, T. Generation and coordinating properties of a carbene bearing a phosphorus ylide: An intensely electron-donating ligand. *Angew. Chem. Int. Ed. Engl.* **2008**, *47*, 1141–1144. [CrossRef]
26. Fürstner, A.; Alcarazo, M.; Radkowski, K.; Lehmann, C.W. Carbenes stabilized by ylides: Pushing the limits. *Angew. Chem. Int. Ed. Engl.* **2008**, *47*, 8302–8306. [CrossRef]
27. Asay, M.; Donnadieu, B.; Baceiredo, A.; Soleilhavoup, M.; Bertrand, G. Cyclic (amino)bis(ylide)carbene as an anionic bidentate ligand for transition-metal complexes. *Inorg. Chem.* **2008**, *47*, 3949–3951. [CrossRef]
28. Asay, M.; Inoue, S.; Driess, M. Aromatic ylide-stabilized carbocyclic silylene. *Angew. Chem. Int. Ed. Engl.* **2011**, *50*, 9589–9592. [CrossRef]
29. Alvarado-Beltran, I.; Baceiredo, A.; Saffon-Merceron, N.; Branchadell, V.; Kato, T. Cyclic Amino(Ylide) Silylene: A Stable Heterocyclic Silylene with Strongly Electron-Donating Character. *Angew. Chem. Int. Ed. Engl.* **2016**, *55*, 16141–16144. [CrossRef]
30. Mohapatra, C.; Scharf, L.; Scherpf, T.; Mallick, B.; Feichtner, K.-S.; Schwarz, C.; Gessner, V.H. Isolation of a Diylide-Stabilized Stannylene and Germylene: Enhanced Donor Strength through Coplanar Lone Pair Alignment. *Angew. Chem. Int. Ed. Engl.* **2019**. [CrossRef]
31. Hartke, K.; Teuber, D.; Gerber, H.-D. Indole- and pyrrole-sulfonium ylides. *Tetrahedron* **1988**, *44*, 3261–3270. [CrossRef]
32. Kobayashi, J.; Nakafuji, S.-Y.; Yatabe, A.; Kawashima, T. A novel ylide-stabilized carbene; formation and electron donating ability of an amino(sulfur-ylide)carbene. *Chem. Commun.* **2008**, 6233–6235. [CrossRef] [PubMed]
33. Sergeev, A.G.; Schulz, T.; Torborg, C.; Spannenberg, A.; Neumann, H.; Beller, M. Palladium-catalyzed hydroxylation of aryl halides under ambient conditions. *Angew. Chem. Int. Ed. Engl.* **2009**, *48*, 7595–7599. [CrossRef]
34. Meng, G.; Kakalis, L.; Nolan, S.P.; Szostak, M. A simple ^{1}H NMR method for determining the σ-donor properties of N-heterocyclic carbenes. *Tetrahedron Lett.* **2019**, *60*, 378–381. [CrossRef]
35. Li, J.J. *Name Reactions*, 4th ed.; Springer: Berlin/Heidelberg, Germany, 2009; pp. 146–147.
36. Li, A.-H.; Dai, L.-X.; Aggarwal, V.K. Asymmetric Ylide Reactions: Epoxidation, Cyclopropanation, Aziridination, Olefination, and Rearrangement. *Chem. Rev.* **1997**, *97*, 2341–2372. [CrossRef]
37. Alvarez, A.; Guzman, A.; Ruiz, A.; Velarde, E.; Muchowski, J.M. Synthesis of 3-arylpyrroles and 3-pyrrolylacetylenes by palladium-catalyzed coupling reactions. *J. Org. Chem.* **1992**, *57*, 1653–1656. [CrossRef]
38. Thorn, A.; Dittrich, B.; Sheldrick, G.M. Enhanced rigid-bond restraints. *Acta Cryst. Sect. A: Fundam. Cryst. Cryst.* **2012**, *68*, 448–451. [CrossRef]
39. Sheldrick, G.M. SHELXT—Integrated space-group and crystal-structure determination. *Acta Cryst. Sect. A Fundam. Cryst.* **2015**, *71*, 3–8. [CrossRef]
40. Sheldrick, G.M. A short history of SHELX. *Acta Cryst. Sect. A: Fundam. Cryst.* **2008**, *64*, 112–122. [CrossRef]
41. Pennington, W.T. DIAMOND – Visual Crystal Structure Information System. *J. Appl. Cryst.* **1999**, *32*, 1028–1029. [CrossRef]
42. The GIMP Team. Available online: https://www.gimp.org/news/2019/04/07/gimp-2-10-10-released/ (accessed on 25 January 2020).
43. Spek, A.L. Structure validation in chemical crystallography. *Acta. Cryst. Sect. D: Biol. Cryst.* **2009**, *65*, 148–155. [CrossRef] [PubMed]
44. Producer. *GaussView, Version 3.0*; Gaussian, Inc.: Pittsburgh, PA, USA, 2000. Available online: https://gaussview.software.informer.com/3.0/ (accessed on 25 January 2020).
45. Dennington, R.; Keith, T.A.; Millam, J.M. *GaussView, Version 6.0*; Semichem Inc.: Shawnee, MO, USA, 2016. Available online: https://gaussian.com/gaussview6/ (accessed on 25 January 2020).
46. Frisch, M.J.; Trucks, G.W.; Schlegel, H.B.; Scuseria, G.E.; Robb, M.A.; Cheeseman, J.R.; Scalmani, G.; Barone, V.; Mennucci, B.; Petersson, G.A.; et al. *Gaussian 09, Revision. E.01*; Gaussian, Inc.: Wallingford, CT, USA, 2009. Available online: https://gaussian.com/glossary/g09/ (accessed on 25 January 2020).

47. Frisch, M.J.; Trucks, G.W.; Schlegel, H.B.; Scuseria, G.E.; Robb, M.A.; Cheeseman, J.R.; Scalmani, G.; Barone, V.; Petersson, G.A.; Nakatsuji, H.; et al. *Gaussian 16, Revision, B.01*; Gaussian, Inc.: Wallingford, CT, USA, 2016. Available online: https://gaussian.com/gaussian16/ (accessed on 25 January 2020).
48. Frisch, M.J.; Trucks, G.W.; Schlegel, H.B.; Scuseria, G.E.; Robb, M.A.; Cheeseman, J.R.; Scalmani, G.; Barone, V.; Petersson, G.A.; Nakatsuji, H.; et al. *Gaussian 16, Revision, C.01*; Gaussian, Inc.: Wallingford, CT, USA, 2016. Available online: https://gaussian.com/gaussian16/ (accessed on 25 January 2020).
49. Hohenberg, P.; Kohn, W. Inhomogeneous Electron Gas. *Phys. Rev.* **1964**, *136*, B864–B871. [CrossRef]
50. Kohn, W.; Sham, L.J. Self-Consistent Equations Including Exchange and Correlation Effects. *Phys. Rev.* **1965**, *140*, A1133–A1138. [CrossRef]
51. Adamo, C.; Barone, V. Toward reliable density functional methods without adjustable parameters: The PBE0 model. *J. Chem. Phys.* **1999**, *110*, 6158–6170. [CrossRef]
52. Weigend, F.; Ahlrichs, R. Balanced basis sets of split valence, triple zeta valence and quadruple zeta valence quality for H to Rn: Design and assessment of accuracy. *Phys. Chem. Chem. Phys.* **2005**, *7*, 3297–3305. [CrossRef]
53. Grimme, S.; Antony, J.; Ehrlich, S.; Krieg, H. A consistent and accurate ab initio parametrization of density functional dispersion correction (DFT-D) for the 94 elements H-Pu. *J. Chem. Phys.* **2010**, *132*, 154104. [CrossRef]
54. Grimme, S.; Ehrlich, S.; Goerigk, L. Effect of the damping function in dispersion corrected density functional theory. *J. Comput. Chem.* **2011**, *32*, 1456–1465. [CrossRef]
55. Smith, D.G.A.; Burns, L.A.; Patkowski, K.; Sherrill, C.D. Revised Damping Parameters for the D3 Dispersion Correction to Density Functional Theory. *J. Phys. Chem. Lett.* **2016**, *7*, 2197–2203. [CrossRef]
56. Deglmann, P.; Furche, F. Efficient characterization of stationary points on potential energy surfaces. *J. Am. Chem. Soc.* **2002**, *117*, 9535–9538. [CrossRef]
57. Tomasi, J.; Mennucci, B.; Cammi, R. Quantum mechanical continuum solvation models. *Chem. Rev.* **2005**, *105*, 2999–3093. [CrossRef]

Sample Availability: Samples of the compounds are not available from the authors.

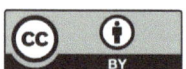

© 2020 by the authors. Licensee MDPI, Basel, Switzerland. This article is an open access article distributed under the terms and conditions of the Creative Commons Attribution (CC BY) license (http://creativecommons.org/licenses/by/4.0/).

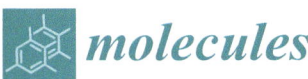

Article

Complexes of Dichlorogermylene with Phosphine/Sulfoxide-Supported Carbone as Ligand [†]

Ugo Authesserre [1], Sophie Hameury [1,2], Aymeric Dajnak [1], Nathalie Saffon-Merceron [3], Antoine Baceiredo [1], David Madec [1,*] and Eddy Maerten [1,*]

1. Université de Toulouse, UPS, and CNRS, LHFA UMR 5069, 118 Route de Narbonne, 31062 Toulouse, France; authesserre@chimie.ups-tlse.fr (U.A.); sophie.hameury@univ-poitiers.fr (S.H.); dajnak@chimie.ups-tlse.fr (A.D.); baceiredo@chimie.ups-tlse.fr (A.B.)
2. Université de Poitiers, IC2MP, UMR CNRS 7285, 1 Rue Marcel Doré, CEDEX 9, 86073 Poitiers, France
3. Université de Toulouse, UPS, and CNRS, ICT UAR2599 118 Route de Narbonne, 31062 Toulouse, France; saffon@chimie.ups-tlse.fr
* Correspondence: madec@chimie.ups-tlse.fr (D.M.); maerten@chimie.ups-tlse.fr (E.M.)
† This paper is dedicated to the memory of Professor André Mortreux.

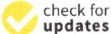

Abstract: Due to their remarkable electronic features, recent years have witnessed the emergence of carbones L_2C, which consist in two donating L ligands coordinating a central carbon atom bearing two lone pairs. In this context, the phosphine/sulfoxide-supported carbone **4** exhibits a strong nucleophilic character, and here, we describe its ability to coordinate dichlorogermylene. Two original stable coordination complexes were obtained and fully characterized in solution and in the solid state by NMR spectroscopy and X-ray diffraction analysis, respectively. At 60 °C, in the presence of **4**, the Ge(II)-complex **5** undergoes a slow isomerization that transforms the bis-ylide ligand into an yldiide.

Keywords: carbone; ligand; germylene; coordination; ylide

1. Introduction

The rapid development of homogeneous catalysis in the last decades is highly related to the intensive research that was accomplished toward ligand design. Due to their lone pair(s) and their related nucleophilic character, oxygen-, nitrogen-, sulfur- and phosphorus-containing ligands have been dominating in the field for several decades [1]. In the late 1980s, the discovery of the first stable carbenes represented the milestone leading to the emergence of carbon-based ligands (**I**, Figure 1) [2,3]. Indeed, the development of these molecules, containing a divalent C(II) atom bearing a vacant orbital and a lone pair, exhibiting a high σ-donation and a strong binding ability toward transition metals, render them essential tools for catalysis. The corresponding organometallic complexes have been proven to be particularly robust and efficient and offering in numerous catalytic processes a larger scope of reaction [4–7]. The related carbon(0) species (**II**), also named carbones, bearing two lone pairs on the central carbon atom are a new emerging class of η^1-carbon ligands. Even though carbodiphosphoranes (**II**, L, L' = PPh$_3$) were discovered in the 1960s by Ramirez [8], these species were at first regarded as two cumulated phosphorus ylide functions on a central carbon atom. It was only in 2006, after the theoretical investigations by Frenking et al. [9–12], that these molecules were considered as a carbon atom in the zero-oxidation state stabilized by two L-phosphine ligands, in agreement with the description initially used by Kaska in 1973 [13]. Since then, this family of ligands has considerably grown, leading to a large structural diversity of carbones **II** and a better understanding of their behavior [14–23]. Naturally, owing to the existence of two lone pairs, they are strong σ- and π-donors (two- or four-electron donating ability); they have been used as original ligands for the preparation of organometallic complexes with interesting applications in catalysis [24–29].

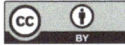

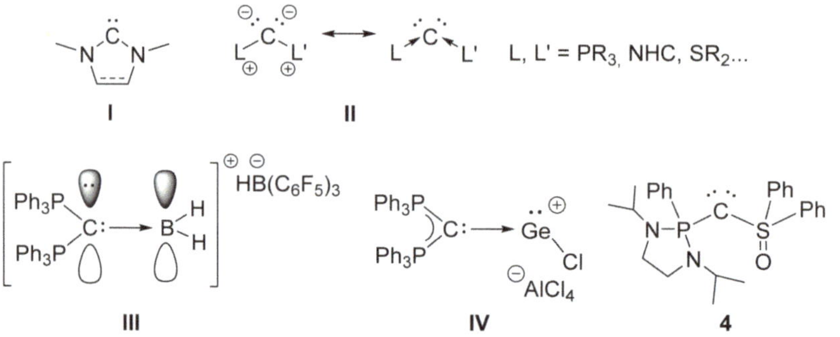

Figure 1. NHC (**I**), carbones (**II**), dihydrido borenium (**III**) and germyliumylidene (**IV**) stabilized by carbodiphosphoranes and phosphine/sulfoxide-supported carbone **4** (for a better readability, formal charges in (**III,IV**) and **4** were omitted).

The strong donor ability of carbones **II** also enables the synthesis of novel reactive species. For example, Alcarazo et al. took advantage of the two available lone pairs of carbodiphosphoranes to stabilize reactive molecules such as dihydrido borenium cation **III** [30]. In the same vein, several groups have used carbones or strong σ-donating ligands to prepare dichlorogermylene adducts giving access to germyliumylidenes (**IV**) or germylones [31–38]. In this context, we report here the coordination ability of a phosphine/sulfoxide-supported carbone **4** [39] towards dichlorogermylene.

2. Results and Discussion

2.1. Synthesis

For the preparation of the phosphine/sulfoxide-supported carbone **4**, we followed the previously described synthesis [39] but several practical aspects were improved. Indeed, after the complete oxidation of methyldiphenylsulfonium, acidification and filtration of the precipitates (carboxylic acids), the expected methyldiphenylsulfoxonium salt **1** was extracted from the aqueous solution by liquid/liquid extraction using dichloromethane as a solvent (Scheme 1). This extraction avoids the possible thermal degradation of the sulfoxonium salt during the evaporation of water under reduced pressure (if prolonged heating above 50 °C is performed). The yield of this step was improved to 53%, after two successive recrystallizations. The coupling reaction between sulfoxonium salt **1** and chlorophosphonium **2** in the presence of two equivalents of lithium di*iso*propylamide (LDA) was also improved in terms of reaction time (Scheme 1). It was found that heating the reaction mixture up to 60 °C considerably sped up the reaction since a full conversion was reached in 24 h instead of 96 h at room temperature. Protonated precursor **3** was obtained as a white powder upon concentration (70% yield). The final deprotonation was performed in THF solution at RT with potassium hydride (KH) leading to the selective formation of **4**, which was isolated in 69% yield.

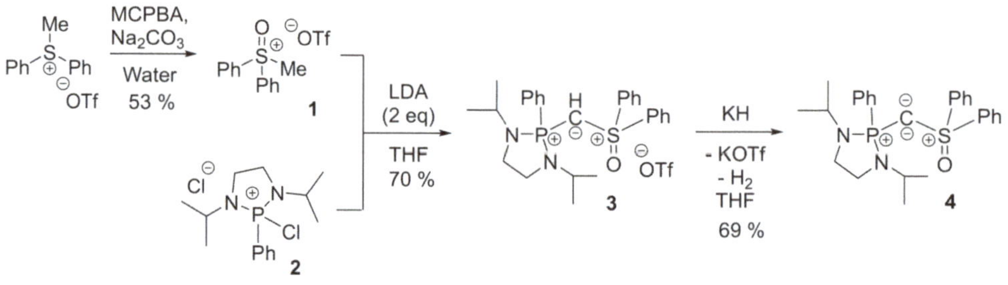

Scheme 1. Synthetic path of phosphine/sulfoxide-supported carbone **4**.

2.2. Dichlorogermylene Coordination

Previous experimental results and DFT calculations have already established that phosphine/sulfoxide-supported carbone **4** exhibits a strong nucleophilic character [39]. The potential usefulness of **4** as a ligand towards transition metals was demonstrated by selective reactions with several organometallic complexes [Au(I), Rh(I)] [39]. Therefore, its coordinating ability toward $GeCl_2$/dioxane should be an interesting approach to access original low-valent germanium derivatives.

Ligand **4** reacts immediately with one equivalent of $GeCl_2$ dioxane leading to the selective formation of complex **5** which has been isolated as colorless crystals from a saturated solution of CH_2Cl_2/pentane (yield 80%, Scheme 2). In comparison with the hexaphenylcarbodiphosphorane analogue [33], complex **5** exhibits a good solubility in common organic solvent and could be fully characterized by NMR spectroscopy. The ^{31}P NMR spectrum displays a signal at lower field (δ = 49.5 ppm) compared to that of free ligand **4** (δ = 29.0 ppm), reminiscent of the protonated precursor **3** (δ = 45.0 ppm). In the ^{13}C NMR spectrum, the central carbon atom appears as a doublet at δ = 47.0 ppm (J_{PC} = 77.3 Hz). The addition of a second equivalent of $GeCl_2$·dioxane to **5**, or the direct use of two equivalents of $GeCl_2$·dioxane with **4**, leads to the quantitative formation of bis-germylene complex **6**, which has been isolated in the crystalline form from C_6D_6 solution (yield 75%). It has been fully characterized by NMR spectroscopy, and particularly, the ^{31}P NMR spectrum indicates a signal at δ = 51.2 ppm and the central carbon atom appears in ^{13}C NMR spectrum as a doublet at δ = 46.6 ppm (J_{PC} = 79.1 Hz).

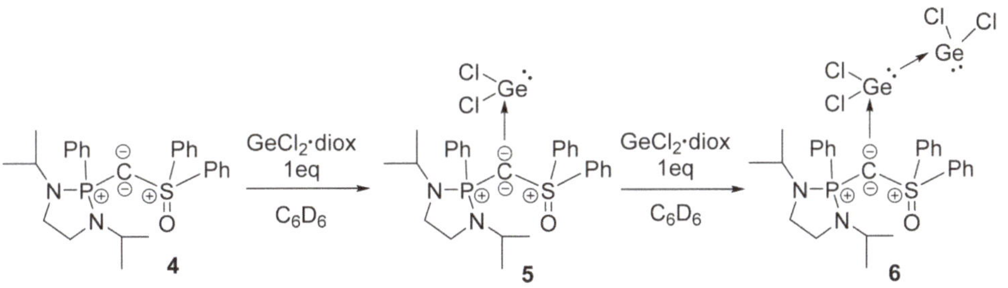

Scheme 2. Coordination of phosphine/sulfoxide-supported carbone **4** with one or two equivalents of germylene dichloride.

Isolated in the crystalline form, the molecular structures of complexes **5** and **6** were confirmed by X-ray diffraction analysis (Figure 2, see Supplementary Materials). The selected geometrical parameters for experimental structures can be found in Table 1.

As expected, the S1-C1 (1.650 Å) and P1-C1 (1.725 Å) bond lengths in **5** are very similar to those observed in the protonated precursor **3** (1.653 Å and 1.719 Å respectively), because of their similar environments. The repulsion between the p_π-lone pair at the carbon and the one at the Ge atom explains the long C1-Ge1 bond length (2.071 Å). It is slightly longer than the one observed by Alcarazo et al. with carbodiphosphoranes (2.063 Å) but much longer than a typical C-Ge bond (1.95 Å) [40]. The P1-C1-S1 angle decreased significantly upon complexation with $GeCl_2$ (from 121° in **3** or **4** to 113.7° in **5**). The introduction of a third heteroatom (Ge) around the carbon, which is less electronegative than P and S, influences the atomic orbital distribution with a pronounced s character toward the C-Ge bond and increased p-character in the C-P and C-S bonds. This phenomenon together with the covalent radius of the germanium atom justify the narrowing of the P1-C1-S1 angle in **5** [41]. Nevertheless, the C1 atom environment remains almost planar ($\sum° $ = 357.5°). In **6**, with the coordination of the second $GeCl_2$ unit, the previously discussed repulsion disappears, leading to a shortening of the C1-Ge1 bond length to 1.980 Å. The other bond lengths and angles (P1-C1, C1-S1, PCS) remain almost unchanged (Table 1). The dative nature of the Ge1-Ge2 bond is confirmed by its length (2.582 Å), way longer than classical Ge-Ge σ-bonds (2.40–2.50 Å) [42]. The same tendency was observed for carbodiphosphoranes [33] or NHC [43].

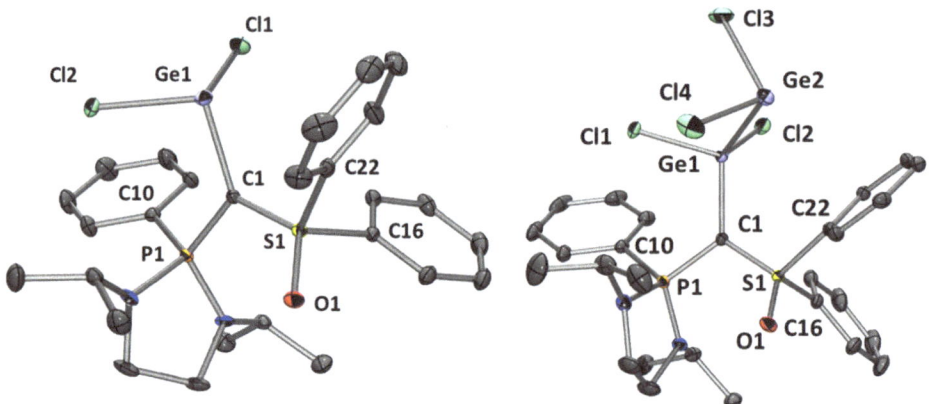

Figure 2. Molecular structures of **5** (left) and **6** (right). Ellipsoids are drawn at the 30% probability level; hydrogen atoms are omitted for clarity. Selected bond lengths (Å) and angles (°): **5**: C1-Ge1 2.071(2), C1-P1 1.725(2), C1-S1 1.650(2), P1-C10 1.802(3), S1-O1 1.457(2), Ge1-Cl2 2.299(1), Ge1-Cl1 2.331(1), S1-C22 1.780(3), S1-C16 1.784(3). P1-C1-S1 113.73(14), P1-C1-Ge1 128.12(13), Ge1-C1-S1 115.65(13), C1-Ge1-Cl2 96.82(7), Cl2-Ge1-Cl1 95.37(3), Cl1-Ge1-C1 98.81(7); **6**: C1-Ge1 1.980(2), C1-P1 1.748(2), C1-S1 1.665(2), Ge1-Ge2 2.582(1), Ge1-Cl1 2.185(1), Ge1-Cl2 2.245(1), Ge2-Cl4 2.267(1), Ge2-Cl3 2.275(1), P1-C10 1.792(2), S1-O1 1.455(1), S1-C22 1.778(2), S1-C16 1.782(2), P1-C1-S1 112.40(10), P1-C1-Ge1 127.01(9), Ge1-C1-S1 117.30(9), C1-Ge1-Cl1 105.44(5), Cl1-Ge1-Cl2 101.33(2), Cl2-Ge1-Ge2 107.25(2), Cl1-Ge1-Ge2 109.25(2), Ge1-Ge2-Cl4 92.09(2), Cl4-Ge2-Cl3 98.84(3), Ge1-Ge2-Cl3 89.41(2).

Table 1. Selected geometrical parameters for **3**, **4**, **5** and **6** [1].

	3	4	5	6
P1-C1	1.719(15)	1.800(1)	1.725(2)	1.748(2)
S1-C1	1.653(13)	1.593(1)	1.650(2)	1.665(2)
P1-C1-S1	120.98(9)	120.74(8)	113.73(14)	112.40(10)
C1-Ge1	-	-	2.071(2)	1.980(2)
Ge1-Ge2	-	-	-	2.582(1)

[1] Bond lengths in Å and angle in deg.

Contrary to the carbodiphosphorane analogues, chloride abstraction from **5** using AlCl$_3$ or KB(C$_6$F$_5$)$_4$ in order to prepare germyliumylidene derivatives only led to complex mixtures. Nevertheless, when **5** is treated in the presence of one equivalent of **4** at 60 °C for 60 h, we observed the gradual consumption of **5** with the concomitant formation of a new compound that exhibits a signal at δ = 56.3 ppm in ^{31}P NMR (this reaction does not occur in the absence of **4**) (Scheme 3). In fact, the process is base-catalyzed, but with 10 mol % of **4**, the reaction time is slower and needs 90 h [Note: catalytic amounts (15 mol %) of alternative Lewis bases such as DMAP or Et$_3$N can be used but the reactions are less selective, see Supplementary Materials for more details]. The structure of the new product **7**, determined by X-ray diffraction analysis (Figure 3), involves the 1,3-migration of a phenyl group from the sulfur to the germanium atom. Considering the ligand moiety, this isomerization transforms a bis-ylide (carbone) to an original yldiide [44]. Unfortunately, because of the presence of **4** in the media, product **7** could not be isolated in pure form for complete characterization despite several attempts.

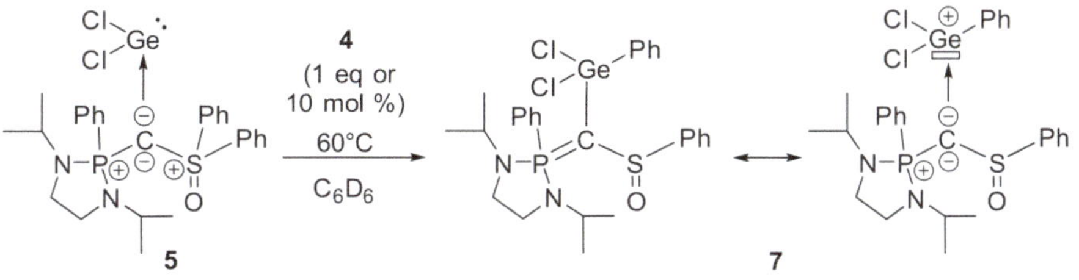

Scheme 3. Evolution of **5** in presence of **4** upon heating at 60 °C.

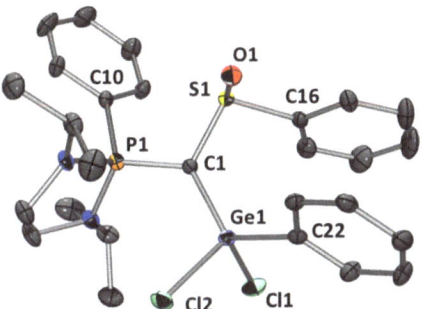

Figure 3. Molecular structure of **7**. Ellipsoids are drawn at the 30% probability level; hydrogen atoms are omitted for clarity. Selected bond lengths (Å) and angles (°): P1-C1 1.707(3), C1-S1 1.744(3), C1-Ge1 1.891(3), Ge1-C22 1.927(3), Ge1-Cl2 2.172(1), Ge1-Cl1 2.173(1), P1-C10 1.805(3), S1-O1 1.499(2), S1-C16 1.800(4), P1-C1-S1 114.48(18), S1-C1-Ge1 120.89(17), Ge1-C1-P1 122.37(19), C1-Ge1-C22 119.52(14), C1-Ge1-Cl2 111.27(10), C22-Ge1-Cl2 104.77(10), C1-Ge1-Cl1 111.72(10), C22-Ge1-Cl1 106.65(11), Cl2-Ge1-Cl1 101.15(4), O1-S1-C1 112.64(15), O1-S1-C16 105.28(16), C1-S1-C16 100.04(16).

2.3. Conclusions

In summary, the excellent coordination ability of the phosphine/sulfoxide-supported carbone ligand **4** allows the preparation of Ge(II)-complex **5**. The strong donation of **4** results in an enriched germylene **5**, which becomes sufficiently nucleophilic to coordinate a second GeCl$_2$ unit. The two original and stable coordination complexes **5** and **6** were fully characterized by NMR spectroscopy and X-ray diffraction analysis. Interestingly, the Ge(II)-complex **5** shows an original isomerization in the presence of **4** that transforms the bis-ylide ligand into an yldiide, thanks to a phenyl migration. Efforts are currently underway to extend the diversity of organometallic complexes that can be obtained with **4** to consider its application in catalysis.

3. Materials and Methods

3.1. General Comments

All manipulations were performed under an inert atmosphere of argon by using standard Schlenk techniques or high-pressure NMR tube techniques. Dry and oxygen-free solvents were used. ^{1}H, ^{13}C, ^{19}F and ^{31}P NMR spectra were recorded on Brucker Avance II 300 MHz, Avance III HD 400 MHz and Avance I and II 500 MHz spectrometers (Brucker, Karlsruhe, Germany). Chemical shifts are expressed in parts per million with residual solvent signals as internal reference (^{1}H and ^{13}C{^{1}H}). ^{19}F and ^{31}P NMR chemical shifts were reported in ppm relative to CFCl$_3$ and 85% H$_3$PO$_4$, respectively. The following abbreviations and their combinations are used: br, broad; s, singlet; d, doublet; t, triplet; q, quartet; hept, heptuplet; m, multiplet. ^{1}H and ^{13}C resonance signals were attributed by means of 2D COSY, HSQC and HMBC experiments. Mass spectra were recorded on a Hewlett Packard 5989A spectrometer (Hewlett-Packard, Palo Alto, CA, USA). All commercially available reagents were used without further purification otherwise noted. Preparation of diphenylsulfonium, **2** and **4** were prepared following previously reported procedures [39].

3.2. Synthesis

Diphenylmethylsulfoxonium triflate **1**: A suspension of diphenylmethylsulfonium triflate (14.96 g, 42.7 mmol, 1 eq.), Na_2CO_3 (13.58 g, 128.1 mmol, 3 eq.) and meta-chloroperbenzoic acid (MCPBA) (22.13 g, 128.1 mmol, 3 eq.) in water (400 mL) was stirred at RT for three days. Na_2CO_3 (4.53 g, 42.7 mmol, 1 eq.) and MCPBA (7.28 g, 42.7 mmol, 1 eq.) were added and the mixture was stirred at RT for one additional day. A 37% aqueous solution of HCl was added to the solution until pH = 1. White solid was filtrated off and washed with an aqueous solution of HCl at pH = 1 (3 × 20 mL). The product was then extracted with CH_2Cl_2 (3 × 20 mL). The solution was dried then the solvent was removed under reduced pressure. The residue was purified by successive crystallizations in acetone/pentane, yielding **1** as colorless crystals (8.30 g, 22.6 mmol, 53%). ^1H NMR (300 MHz, 298 K, Acetone-d_6): δ = 4.86 (s, 3H, CH_3), 7.91–7.98 (m, 4H, CH_{ar}), 8.04–8.11 (m, 2H, CH_{para}), 8.31–8.37 (m, 4H, CH_{ar}). $^{13}C\{^1H\}$ NMR (75 MHz, 298 K, Acetone-d_6): δ = 39.7 (s, CH_3), 128.4 (s, CH_{ar}), 132.0 (s, CH_{ar}), 132.9 (s, C_{ipso}), 138.1 (s, CH_{para}). The signal of the triflate could not be detected. ^{19}F NMR (282 MHz, 298 K, DMSO-d_6) δ = −77.7 (s). Mp = 157 °C. HRMS (ES +): m/z $[M]^+$ calculated for $C_{13}H_{13}OS$ = 217.0687, found = 217.0690.

Protonated phosphine/sulfoxide precursor **3**: In situ prepared LDA (18.2 mmol, 2 eq.) in THF (20 mL) was added dropwise to a suspension of **1** (4 g, 10.9 mmol, 1.2 eq.) in THF (100 mL) at −80 °C and the reaction was stirred at this temperature for 2 h. A suspension of **2** (2.92 g, 9.1 mmol, 1 eq.) in THF (50 mL) was then added dropwise to the solution at −80 °C. The solution was allowed to warm up to RT then heated at 60 °C for two days. The solution was concentrated (2/3 of the solvent removed) and a white precipitate was observed. The solvent was filtered off and the white solid was washed with small volumes of THF (4 × 2 mL). The remaining solid was extracted in CH_2Cl_2 then dried under a high vacuum. Ylide **3** was obtained as a white powder (3.9 g, 6.37 mmol, 70%). $^{31}P\{^1H\}$ NMR (202 MHz, 298 K, $CDCl_3$): δ = 45.0 ppm (s). ^1H NMR (300 MHz, 298 K, $CDCl_3$): δ = 0.76 (d, J_{HH} = 6.5 Hz, 12H, CH_{3iPr}), 3.08–3.24 (m, 4H, CH_2), 3.40 (hept, J_{HH} = 6.5 Hz, 1H, CH_{iPr}), 3.43 (hept, J_{HH} = 6.5 Hz, 1H, CH_{iPr}), 3.80 (d, J_{PH} = 13.7 Hz, 1H, PCHS), 7.57 (m, 9H, CH_{ar}), 8.05–8.16 (m, 2H, CH_{ar}), 8.18–8.25 (m, 4H, CH_{ar}). $^{13}C\{^1H\}$ NMR (75 MHz, 298 K, $CDCl_3$): δ = 19.9–20.1 (m, CH_{3iPr}), 31.6 (d, J_{CP} = 137.2 Hz, PCHS), 39.1 (d, J_{PC} = 8.6 Hz, CH_2), 45.1 (d, J_{PC} = 5.7 Hz, CH_{iPr}), 121.2 (q, J_{CF} = 318.9 Hz, CF_3), 126.7 (d, J_{PC} = 121.1 Hz, $C_{ipso\,P\,side}$), 127.1 (s, CH_{ar}), 130.0 (d, J_{PC} = 13.7 Hz, CH_{ar}), 130.4 (s, CH_{ar}), 132.8 (d, J_{PC} = 11.7 Hz, CH_{ar}), 134.4 (s, CH_{ar}), 134.5 (d, J_{PC} = 3.1 Hz, CH_{ar}), 140.4 ppm (d, J_{PC} = 2.4 Hz, $C_{ipso\,S\,side}$). ^{19}F NMR (282 MHz, 298 K $CDCl_3$): δ = −78.1 (s). HRMS (ES +): m/z $[M]^+$ calculated for $C_{27}H_{34}ON_2PS$ = 465.2130, found = 465.2133. The elemental analysis calculated (%) for $C_{28}H_{34}F_3N_2O_4PS_2$: C 54.71, H 5.58, N 4.56; found: C 54.63, H 5.47, N 4.51.

Phosphine/sulfoxide-carbone-$GeCl_2$ complex **5**: To a solution of **4** (37.1 mg, 0.08 mmol, 1 eq.) in C_6D_6 (0.6 mL), $GeCl_2$•dioxane (9 mg, 0.08 mmol, 1 eq.) was added. The reaction is complete after a few minutes. C_6D_6 was removed under reduced pressure and the residue afforded crystals (38.9 mg, 0.064 mmol, 80% yield) from a saturated solution of CH_2Cl_2/pentane. $^{31}P\{^1H\}$ NMR (202 MHz, 298 K, C_6D_6): δ = 49.5 ppm (s). $^{31}P\{^1H\}$ NMR (162 MHz, 298 K, CD_2Cl_2): δ = 50.9 ppm (s). ^1H NMR (500 MHz, 298 K, CD_2Cl_2): δ = 0.70 (d, J_{HH} = 6.5 Hz, 6H, CH_{3iPr}), 0.81 (d, J_{HH} = 6.5 Hz, 6H, CH_{3iPr}), 3.08–3.18 (m, 2H, CH_2), 3.19–3.28 (m, 2H, CH_2), 3.58–3.69 (m, 2H, CH_{iPr}), 7.59–7.71 (m, 9H, CH_{ar}), 8.07–8.14 (m, 6H, CH_{ar}). $^{13}C\{^1H\}$ NMR (126 MHz, 298 K, CD_2Cl_2): δ = 19.9 (m, CH_{3iPr}), 39.3 (d, J_{PC} = 8.9 Hz, CH_2), 46.0 (d, J_{PC} = 4.6 Hz, CH_{iPr}), 47.0 (d, J_{PC} = 77.3 Hz, PCS), 129.1 (s, CH_{ar}) 129.9 (d, J_{PC} = 125.5 Hz, $C_{ipso\,P\,side}$), 130.1 (d, J_{PC} = 13.9 Hz CH_{ar}), 130.3 (s, CH_{ar}) 132.9 (d, J_{PC} = 11.8 Hz, CH_{ar}), 134.2 (d, J_{PC} = 3.1 Hz, CH_{ar}), 134.7(s, CH_{ar}), 140.7 (d, J_{PC} = 3.1 Hz, $C_{ipso\,S\,side}$). HRMS (DCI-CH_4): m/z $[M + H]^+$ calcd for $C_{27}H_{34}Cl_2GeN_2OPS$: 609.0713; found: 609.0715.

Phosphine/sulfoxide-carbone-GeCl$_2$-GeCl$_2$ complex **6**: To a solution of **4** (37.1 mg, 0.08 mmol, 1 eq.) in C$_6$D$_6$ (0.6 mL), GeCl$_2$•dioxane (18 mg, 0.16 mmol, 2 eq.) was added. Product **6** directly crystallized in C$_6$D$_6$ (45.0 mg, 0.06 mmol, 75% yield). ^{31}P {^{1}H} NMR (202 MHz, 298 K, C$_6$D$_6$): δ = 51.2 ppm (s). ^{31}P {^{1}H} NMR (202 MHz, 298 K, CD$_2$Cl$_2$): δ = 51.2 ppm (s). ^{1}H NMR (300 MHz, 298 K, CD$_2$Cl$_2$): δ = 0.70 (d, J_{HH} = 6.4 Hz, 6H, CH$_{3iPr}$), 0.82 (d, J_{HH} = 6.5 Hz, 6H, CH$_{3iPr}$), 3.09–3.18 (m, 2H, CH$_2$), 3.18–3.28 (m, 2H, CH$_2$), 3.60–3.70 (m, 2H, CH$_{iPr}$), 7.60–7.71 (m, 9H, CH$_{ar}$), 8.06–8.13 (m, 3H, 6CH$_{ar}$). ^{13}C{^{1}H} NMR (126 MHz, 298 K, CD$_2$Cl$_2$): δ = 19.7–20.3 (m, CH$_{3iPr}$), 39.3 (d, J_{PC} = 9.2 Hz, CH$_2$), 46.1 (d, J_{PC} = 5.3 Hz, CH$_{iPr}$), 46.6 (d, J_{PC} = 79.1 Hz, PCS), 129.1 (s, CH$_{ar}$), 129.7 (d, J_{PC} = 125.0 Hz, C$_{ipso}$ deduced from J-Mod), 130.2 (d, J_{PC} = 13.9 Hz, CH$_{ar}$), 130.4 (s, CH$_{ar}$), 132.8 (d, J_{PC} = 11.8 Hz, CH$_{ar}$), 134.4 (d, J_{PC} = 3.1 Hz, CH$_{ar}$), 134.8 (s, CH$_{ar}$), 140.5 (d, J_{PC} = 2.95 Hz, C$_{ipso\,S\,side}$). HRMS for **6** did not afford satisfactory results.

Isomer **7**: To a solution of **5** (48.6 mg, 0.08 mmol, 1 eq.) in C$_6$D$_6$ (0.6 mL), one equivalent of **4**, 37.1 mg, 0.08 mmol, 1 eq.) was added. The reaction was heated at 60 °C until complete consumption of **5** (after 60 h). Crystals of **7** could be obtained from the crude mixture. Unfortunately, despite several attempts, **7** was only analyzed by spectroscopy as a mixture. The spectroscopic data were extracted from a mixture containing **7** and **4** in a 51% to 45% ratio (4% of protonated phosphine/sulfoxide precursor **3**). The reaction can also be performed with 10 mol% of **4** (3.7 mg, 0.008 mmol). ^{31}P {^{1}H} NMR (121 MHz, 298 K, C$_6$D$_6$): δ = 56.3 ppm (s). ^{1}H NMR (300 MHz, 298 K, C$_6$D$_6$): δ = 0.45 (d, J_{HH} = 6.5 Hz, 3H, CH$_{3iPr}$), 0.83 (d, J_{HH} = 6.6 Hz, 3H, CH$_{3iPr}$), 1.34–1.50 (m, 6H, CH$_{3iPr}$), 2.40–2.70 (m, 2H, CH$_2$), 3.05–3.15 (m, 2H, CH$_2$), 4.10–4.40 (m, 2H, CH$_{iPr}$), 6.75–7.25 (m, 9H, CH$_{ar}$), 7.75–7.85 (m, 2H, CH$_{ar}$), 7.85–8.15 (m, 4H, CH$_{ar}$). ^{13}C{^{1}H} NMR (126 MHz, 298 K, C$_6$D$_6$): δ = 20.6 (d, J_{PC} = 2.4 Hz, CH$_{3iPr}$), 20.7 (d, J_{PC} = 5.7 Hz, CH$_{3iPr}$), 21.7 (d, J_{PC} = 6.1 Hz, CH$_{3iPr}$), 38.0 (d, J_{PC} = 12.3 Hz, CH$_2$), 38.1 (d, J_{PC} = 12.7 Hz, CH$_2$), 44.5 (d, J_{PC} = 7.4 Hz, CH$_{iPr}$), 44.9 (d, J_{PC} = 5.0 Hz, CH$_{iPr}$), 59.1 (d, J_{PC} = 121.5 Hz, PCS), 127.2 (s, CH$_{ar}$), 128.0 (s, CH$_{ar}$), 128.3 (s, CH$_{ar}$), 128.7 (d, J_{PC} = 12.1 Hz), 128.9 (s, CH$_{ar}$), 130.2 (d, J_{PC} = 109.6 Hz C$_{ipso\,P\,side}$), 130.3 (s, CH$_{ar}$), 132.6 (d, J_{PC} = 2.9 Hz, CH$_{ar}$), 133.4 (s, CH$_{ar}$), 133.8 (d, J_{PC} = 10.3 Hz, CH$_{ar}$), 140.4 (d, J_{PC} = 6.2 Hz, C$_{ipso\,S\,side}$), 147.8 (d, J_{PC} = 21.9 Hz, C$_{ipso\,Ge\,side}$). HRMS (DCI-CH$_4$): m/z [M + H]$^+$ calcd for C$_{27}$H$_{34}$Cl$_2$GeN$_2$OPS: 609.0713; found: 609.0721.

3.3. X-ray Data

The data of the structures for **5**, **6** and **7** were collected at 193 K on a Bruker-AXS APEX II CCD Quazar diffractometer (**7**) equipped with a 30 W air-cooled microfocus source or on a Brucker-AXS D8-Venture diffractometer (**5** and **6**) equipped with a CMOS area detector with MoKα radiation (wavelength = 0.71073 Å) by using phi- and omega-scans. The data were integrated with SAINT, and an empirical absorption correction with SADABS was applied [45]. The structures were solved using an intrinsic phasing method (ShelXT) [46] and refined using the least–squares method on F^2 (ShelXL-2014) [47]. All non-H atoms were treated anisotropically. All H atoms attached to C atoms were fixed geometrically and treated as riding on their parent atoms with C-H = 0.95 Å (aromatic), 0.98 Å (CH$_3$), 0.99 Å (CH$_2$) or 1.0 Å (CH) with U$_{iso}$(H) = 1.2U$_{eq}$(CH, CH$_2$) or U$_{iso}$(H) = 1.5U$_{eq}$(CH$_3$).

Supplementary crystallographic data for CCDC-2068304 (**5**), CCDC-2068305 (**6**), CCDC-2068306 (**7**) can be obtained free of charge from The Cambridge Crystallographic Data Centre via https://www.ccdc.cam.ac.uk/structures/ accessed on 25 March 2021.

Supplementary Materials: The following are available online. NMR spectra and crystallographic data.

Author Contributions: Conceptualization, S.H., E.M. and D.M.; Investigation, U.A., S.H. and A.D.; X-ray structural studies: N.S.-M.; writing—original draft preparation, U.A. and E.M.; writing—review and editing, all authors; supervision, A.B., D.M. and E.M. All authors have read and agreed to the published version of the manuscript.

Funding: This research was funded by The Agence Nationale de la Recherche, ANR-19-CE07-0013.

Institutional Review Board Statement: Not applicable.

Informed Consent Statement: Not applicable.

Data Availability Statement: Not applicable.

Acknowledgments: The Agence Nationale de la Recherche (ANR-16-CE07-0018-01) and the Ministère de l'Enseignement Supérieur et de la Recherche are gratefully acknowledged for Ph.D. grant to U.A. The authors would like to thank the CNRS and the Université de Toulouse, UPS for financial support. The authors would like to thank the reviewers for all their useful and helpful comments.

Conflicts of Interest: The authors declare no conflict of interest. The funders had no role in the design of the study; in the collection, analyses, or interpretation of data; in the writing of the manuscript, or in the decision to publish the results.

Sample Availability: Samples of the compounds are not available from the authors.

References

1. Mortreux, A.; Petit, F. *Industrial Applications of Homogeneous Catalysis*; Springer: Dordrecht/Holland, The Netherlands, 1988.
2. Igau, A.; Grützmacher, H.; Baceiredo, A.; Bertrand, G. Analogous α,α'-Bis-Carbenoid Triply Bonded Species: Synthesis of a Stable λ^3-Phosphinocarbene-λ^5-Phosphaacetylene. *J. Am. Chem. Soc.* **1988**, *110*, 6463–6466. [CrossRef]
3. Arduengo, A.J.; Harlow, R.L.; Kline, M. A Stable Crystalline Carbene. *J. Am. Chem. Soc.* **1991**, *113*, 361–363. [CrossRef]
4. Glorius, F. *N-Heterocyclic Carbenes in Transition Metal Catalysis*; Springer: Berlin/Heidelberg, Germany, 2007; Volume 21.
5. Nolan, S.P. *N-Heterocyclic Carbenes in Synthesis*; Wiley-VCH: Weinheim, Germany, 2006.
6. Herrmann, W.A. N-Heterocyclic Carbenes: A New Concept in Organometallic Catalysis. *Angew. Chem. Int. Ed.* **2002**, *41*, 1290–1309. [CrossRef]
7. César, V.; Bellemin-Laponnaz, S.; Gade, L.H. Chiral N-heterocyclic carbenes as stereodirecting ligands in asymmetric catalysis. *Chem. Soc. Rev.* **2004**, *33*, 619–636. [CrossRef]
8. Ramirez, F.; Desai, N.B.; Hansen, B.; McKelvie, N. Hexaphenylcarbodiphosphorane, $(C_6H_5)_3PCP(C_6H_5)_3$. *J. Am. Chem. Soc.* **1961**, *83*, 3539–3540. [CrossRef]
9. Tonner, R.; Öxler, F.; Neumüller, B.; Petz, W.; Frenking, G. Carbodiphosphoranes: The Chemistry of Divalent Carbon(0). *Angew. Chem. Int. Ed.* **2006**, *45*, 8038–8042. [CrossRef] [PubMed]
10. Tonner, R.; Frenking, G. C(NHC)$_2$: Divalent Carbon(0) Compounds with N-Heterocyclic Carbene Ligands—Theoretical Evidence for a Class of Molecules with Promising Chemical Properties. *Angew. Chem. Int. Ed.* **2007**, *46*, 8695–8698. [CrossRef]
11. Tonner, R.; Frenking, G. Divalent Carbon(0) Chemistry, Part 1: Parent Compounds. *Chem. Eur. J.* **2008**, *14*, 3260–3272. [CrossRef]
12. Tonner, R.; Frenking, G. Divalent Carbon(0) Chemistry, Part 2: Protonation and Complexes with Main Group and Transition Metal Lewis Acids. *Chem. Eur. J.* **2008**, *14*, 3273–3289. [CrossRef]
13. Kaska, W.C.; Mitchell, D.K.; Reichelderfer, R.F. Transition metal complexes of hexaphenylcarbodiphosphorane. *J. Organomet. Chem.* **1973**, *47*, 391–402. [CrossRef]
14. Fujii, T.; Ikeda, T.; Mikami, T.; Suzuki, T.; Yoshimura, T. Synthesis and structure of (MeN)Ph2S=C=SPh2(NMe). *Angew. Chem. Int. Ed.* **2002**, *41*, 2576–2578. [CrossRef]
15. Alcarazo, M.; Lehmann, C.W.; Anoop, A.; Thiel, W.; Fürstner, A. Coordination chemistry at carbon. *Nat. Chem.* **2009**, *1*, 295–301. [CrossRef]
16. Dellus, N.; Kato, T.; Bagan, X.; Saffon, N.; Branchadell, V.; Baceiredo, A. An isolable mixed P,S-bis(ylide) as an asymmetric carbon atom source. *Angew. Chem. Int. Ed.* **2010**, *49*, 6798–6801. [CrossRef]
17. Alcarazo, M.; Radkowski, K.; Mehler, G.; Goddard, R.; Fürstner, A. Chiral heterobimetallic complexes of carbodiphosphoranes and phosphinidene–carbene adducts. *Chem. Commun.* **2013**, *49*, 3140–3142. [CrossRef] [PubMed]
18. Schmidbaur, H.; Schier, A. Coordination Chemistry at Carbon: The Patchwork Family Comprising $(Ph_3P)_2C$, $(Ph_3P)C(C_2H_4)$, and $(C_2H_4)_2C$. *Angew. Chem. Int. Ed.* **2013**, *52*, 176–186. [CrossRef] [PubMed]
19. Morosaki, T.; Suzuki, T.; Wang, W.W.; Nagase, S.; Fujii, T. Syntheses, Structures, and Reactivities of Two Chalcogen-Stabilized Carbones. *Angew. Chem. Int. Ed.* **2014**, *53*, 9569–9571. [CrossRef]
20. Morosaki, T.; Wang, W.-W.; Nagase, S.; Fujii, T. Synthesis, Structure, and Reactivities of Iminosulfane- and Phosphane-Stabilized Carbones Exhibiting Four-Electron Donor Ability. *Chem. Eur. J.* **2015**, *21*, 15405–15411. [CrossRef]
21. Chen, W.-C.; Shen, J.-S.; Jurca, T.; Peng, C.-J.; Lin, Y.-H.; Wang, Y.-P.; Shih, W.-C.; Yap, G.P.A.; Ong, T.-G. Expanding the Ligand Framework Diversity of Carbodicarbenes and Direct Detection of Boron Activation in the Methylation of Amines with CO_2. *Angew. Chem. Int. Ed.* **2015**, *54*, 15207–15212. [CrossRef] [PubMed]
22. Troadec, T.; Wasano, T.; Lenk, R.; Baceiredo, A.; Saffon-Merceron, N.; Hashizume, D.; Saito, Y.; Nakata, N.; Branchadell, V.; Kato, T. Donor-Stabilized Silylene/Phosphine-Supported Carbon(0) Center with High Electron Density. *Angew. Chem. Int. Ed.* **2017**, *56*, 6891–6895. [CrossRef]
23. Corberan, R.; Marrot, S.; Dellus, N.; Merceron-Saffon, N.; Kato, T.; Peris, E.; Baceiredo, A. First Cyclic Carbodiphosphoranes of Copper(I) and Gold(I) and Their Application in The Catalytic Cleavage of X-H bonds (X = N and O). *Organometallics* **2009**, *28*, 326–330. [CrossRef]

24. Goldfogel, M.J.; Roberts, C.C.; Meek, S.J. Intermolecular hydroamination of 1,3-dienes catalyzed by bis(phosphine)carbodicarbene-rhodium complexes. *J. Am. Chem. Soc.* **2014**, *136*, 6227–6230. [CrossRef] [PubMed]
25. Hsu, Y.-C.; Shen, J.-S.; Lin, B.-C.; Chen, W.-C.; Chan, Y.-T.; Ching, W.-M.; Yap, G.P.A.; Hsu, C.-P.; Ong, T.-G. Synthesis and isolation of an acyclic tridentate bis(pyridine)carbodicarbene and studies on its structural implications and reactivities. *Angew. Chem. Int. Ed.* **2015**, *54*, 2420–2424. [CrossRef] [PubMed]
26. Roberts, C.C.; Matias, D.M.; Goldfogel, M.J.; Meek, S.J. Lewis Acid Activation of Carbodicarbene Catalysts for Rh-Catalyzed Hydroarylation of Dienes. *J. Am. Chem. Soc.* **2015**, *137*, 6488–6491. [CrossRef]
27. Pranckevicius, C.; Fan, L.; Stephan, D.W. Cyclic Bent Allene Hydrido-Carbonyl Complexes of Ruthenium: Highly Active Catalysts for Hydrogenation of Olefins. *J. Am. Chem. Soc.* **2015**, *137*, 5582–5589. [CrossRef]
28. Marcum, J.S.; Roberts, C.C.; Manan, R.S.; Cervarich, T.N.; Meek, S.J. Chiral Pincer Carbodicarbene Ligands for Enantioselective Rhodium-Catalyzed Hydroarylation of Terminal and Internal 1,3-Dienes with Indoles. *J. Am. Chem. Soc.* **2017**, *139*, 15580–15583. [CrossRef] [PubMed]
29. Liberman-Martin, A.L.; Grubbs, R.H. Ruthenium Olefin Metathesis Catalysts Featuring a Labile Carbodicarbene Ligand. *Organometallics* **2017**, *36*, 4091–4094. [CrossRef]
30. Inés, B.; Patil, M.; Carreras, J.; Goddard, R.; Thiel, W.; Alcarazo, M. Synthesis, Structure, and Reactivity of a Dihydrido Borenium Cation. *Angew. Chem. Int. Ed.* **2011**, *50*, 8400–8403. [CrossRef]
31. Xiong, Y.; Yao, S.; Tan, G.; Inoue, S.; Driess, M. A cyclic Germadicarbene ("Germylone") from Germyliumylidene. *J. Am. Chem. Soc.* **2013**, *135*, 5004–5007. [CrossRef]
32. Li, Y.; Mondal, C.; Roesky, H.W.; Zhu, H.; Stollberg, P.; Herbst-Irmer, R.; Stalke, D.; Andrada, D. Acyclic Germylones: Congeners of Allenes with a CentralGermanium. *J. Am. Chem. Soc.* **2013**, *135*, 12422–12428. [CrossRef]
33. Khan, S.; Gopakumar, G.; Thiel, W.; Alcarazo, M. Stabilization of a two-Coordinate [GeCl]+ Cation by Simultaneous s and p Donation from a Monodentate Carbodiphosphorane. *Angew. Chem. Int. Ed.* **2013**, *52*, 5644–5647. [CrossRef]
34. Roy, M.M.D.; Lummis, P.A.; Ferguson, M.J.; McDonald, R.; Rivard, E. Accessing Low-Valent Inorganic Cations by Using an Extremely Bulky N-Heterocyclic Carbene. *Chem. Eur. J.* **2017**, *23*, 11249–11252. [CrossRef] [PubMed]
35. Chu, T.; Belding, L.; Van der Est, A.; Dudding, T.; Korobkov, I.; Nikonov, G.I. A coordination Compound of Ge0 Stabilized by a Diiminopyridine Ligand. *Angew. Chem. Int. Ed.* **2014**, *53*, 2711–2715. [CrossRef] [PubMed]
36. Shan, Y.-L.; Yim, W.-L.; So, C.-W. An N-Heterocyclic Silylene-Stabilized Digermanium(0) Complex. *Angew. Chem. Int. Ed.* **2014**, *53*, 13155–13158. [CrossRef]
37. Zhou, Y.-P.; Karni, M.; Yao, S.; Apeloig, Y.; Driess, M. A Bis(silylenyl)pyridine Zero-Valent Germanium Complex and Its Remarkable Reactivity. *Angew. Chem. Int. Ed.* **2016**, *55*, 15096–15099. [CrossRef] [PubMed]
38. Nguyen, M.T.; Gusev, D.; Dmitrienko, A.; Gabidullin, B.M.; Spasyuk, D.; Pilkington, M.; Nikonov, G.I. Ge(0) Compound Stabilized by a Diimino-Carbene Ligand: Synthesis and Ambiphilic Reactivity. *J. Am. Chem. Soc.* **2020**, *142*, 5852–5861. [CrossRef]
39. Gonzalez, M.L.; Bousquet, L.; Hameury, S.; Alvarez Toledano, C.; Saffon-Merceron, N.; Branchadell, V.; Maerten, E.; Baceiredo, A. Phosphine/Sulfoxide-Supported Carbon(0) Complex. *Chem. Eur. J.* **2018**, *24*, 2570–2574. [CrossRef]
40. Meiners, F.; Saak, W.; Weidenbruch, M. Reaction of a diarylgermylene with a phosphaalkyne: Formation of a germadiphosphacyclobutene with an exocyclic C=Ge double bond. *Chem. Commun.* **2001**, 215–216. [CrossRef]
41. Alabugin, I.V.; Bresch, S.; Manoharan, M. Hybridization Trends for Main Group Elements and Expanding the Bent's Rule beyond Carbon: More than Electronegativity. *J. Phys. Chem. A* **2014**, *118*, 3663–3677. [CrossRef]
42. Amadoruge, M.L.; Weinert, C.S. Singly Bonded Catenated Germanes: Eighty Years of Progress. *Chem. Rev.* **2008**, *108*, 4253–4294. [CrossRef]
43. Ibrahim Al-Rafia, S.M.; Momeni, M.R.; McDonald, R.; Ferguson, M.J.; Brown, A.; Rivard, E. Controlled Growth of Dichlorogermanium Oligomers from Lewis Basic Hosts. *Angew. Chem. Int. Ed.* **2013**, *52*, 6390–6395. [CrossRef]
44. Fustier-Boutignon, M.; Nebra, N.; Mézailles, N. Geminal Dianions Stabilized by Main Group Elements. *Chem. Rev.* **2019**, *119*, 8555–8700. [CrossRef] [PubMed]
45. SADABS. *Program for Data Correction, Version 2016/2*; Bruker–AXS: Madison, WI, USA, 2016.
46. Sheldrick, G.M. *SHELXT*—Integrated space-group and crystal-structure determination. *Acta Crystallogr. Sect. A* **2015**, *71*, 3–8. [CrossRef] [PubMed]
47. Sheldrick, G.M. Crystal structure refinement with *SHELXL*. *Acta Crystallogr. Sect. C* **2015**, *71*, 3–8. [CrossRef] [PubMed]

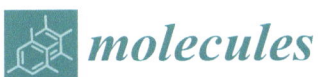

Article

Cu(I) Complexes of Multidentate *N,C,N*- and *P,C,P*-Carbodiphosphorane Ligands and Their Photoluminescence

Marius Klein [1], Nemrud Demirel [1], Alexander Schinabeck [2], Hartmut Yersin [2] 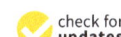 and Jörg Sundermeyer [1,*]

1. Department of Chemistry and Science, Materials Sciences Center, Philipps University of Marburg, 35043 Marburg, Germany; kleinma8@staff.uni-marburg.de (M.K.); Demireln@students.uni-marburg.de (N.D.)
2. Institute for Physical Chemistry, University of Regensburg, 93040 Regensburg, Germany; alexander.schinabeck@chemie.uni-regensburg.de (A.S.); Hartmut.Yersin@chemie.uni-regensburg.de (H.Y.)
* Correspondence: jsu@staff.uni-marburg.de; Tel.: +49-6421-2825693

Academic Editor: Yves Canac
Received: 20 July 2020; Accepted: 29 August 2020; Published: 1 September 2020

Abstract: A series of dinuclear copper(I) *N,C,N*- and *P,C,P*-carbodiphosphorane (CDP) complexes using multidentate ligands CDP(Py)$_2$ (**1**) and (CDP(CH$_2$PPh$_2$)$_2$ (**13**) have been isolated and characterized. Detailed structural information was gained by single-crystal XRD analyses of nine representative examples. The common structural motive is the central double ylidic carbon atom with its characteristic two lone pairs involved in the binding of two geminal L-Cu(I) fragments at Cu–Cu distances in the range 2.55–2.67 Å. In order to enhance conformational rigidity within the characteristic Cu–C–Cu triangle, two types of chelating side arms were symmetrically attached to each phosphorus atom: two 2-pyridyl functions in ligand CDP(Py)$_2$ (**1**) and its dinuclear copper complexes **2–9** and **11**, as well as two diphenylphosphinomethylene functions in ligand CDP(CH$_2$PPh$_2$)$_2$ (**13**) and its di- and mononuclear complexes **14–18**. Neutral complexes were typically obtained via the reaction of **1** with Cu(I) species CuCl, CuI, and CuSPh or via the salt elimination reaction of [(CuCl)$_2$(CDP(Py)$_2$] (**2**) with sodium carbazolate. Cationic Cu(I) complexes were prepared upon treating **1** with two equivalents of [Cu(NCMe)$_4$]PF$_6$, followed by the addition of either two equivalents of an aryl phosphine (PPh$_3$, P(C$_6$H$_4$OMe)$_3$) or one equivalent of bisphosphine ligands bis[(2-diphenylphosphino)phenyl] ether (DPEPhos), 4,5-bis(diphenylphosphino)-9,9-dimethylxanthene (XantPhos), or 1,1'-bis(diphenyl-phosphino) ferrocene (dppf). For the first time, carbodiphosphorane CDP(CH$_2$PPh$_2$)$_2$ (**13**) could be isolated upon treating its precursor [CH(dppm)$_2$]Cl (**12**) with NaNH$_2$ in liquid NH$_3$. A protonated and a deprotonated derivative of ligand **13** were prepared, and their coordination was compared to neutral CDP ligand **13**. NMR analysis and DFT calculations reveal that the most stable tautomer of **13** does not show a CDP (or carbone) structure in its uncoordinated base form. For most of the prepared complexes, photoluminescence upon irradiation with UV light at room temperature was observed. Quantum yields (Φ_{PL}) were determined to be 36% for dicationic [(CuPPh$_3$)$_2$(CDP(Py)$_2$)](PF$_6$)$_2$ (**4**) and 60% for neutral [(CuSPh)$_2$(CDP(CH$_2$PPh$_2$)$_2$] (**16**).

Keywords: carbodiphosphorane; phosphorus ylides; pincer ligands; coordination chemistry; Cu(I) complex; photoluminescence

1. Introduction

In 1961, hexaphenyl-carbodiphosphorane, the first carbodiphosphorane (CDP), was synthesized by Ramirez et al. [1]. Despite this early discovery, the interest in such double ylide carbon (or carbone) compounds is still evolving. One reason for attracting interest is the bonding description of carbodiphosphoranes. Next to a classical ylide valence bond description, the bonding in carbodiphosphoranes can be decribed as a formal carbon(0) atom stabilized by two dative phosphine ligands with C–P retro dative bonding components, which is a model discussed earlier but quantified by a theoretical approach of Frenking and co-workers [2–6]. The central carbon atom is best described in its excited singlet (^{1}D) state [7]. It acts as an acceptor and is stabilized by the σ donating phosphine ligands. The two characteristic occupied lone pairs (HOMO and HOMO+1) centered at this carbon atom (therefore named "carbone") are either capable of binding two metals via two σ bonds in a close to tetrahedral configuration P_2CM_2 or one metal in a trigonal–planar P_2CM configuration via a σ- and a π dative bond of very strong π,σ-donor character [8]. For this reason, the coordination chemistry of carbodiphosphoranes has experienced a renaissance [9–11]. A topic of current interest is introducing secondary ligand functions into the CDP frame: Cyclometalation with noble metals rhodium and platinum gave rise to the characterization of C,C,C-pincer ligand complexes with two cyclometalated phenyl rings [12–17], and an ortho-directed double lithiation of hexaphenyl-carbodiphosphorane leads to lithium complexes that are capable of transfering the C,C,C-pincer ligand synthon $[CDP]^{2-}$ to any other element of the periodic table [17]. P,C,P-chelate complexes of a phosphine functionalized CDP ligand $CDP(CH_2PPh_2)_2$ (13), formally a carbone $C(dppm)_2$ (dppm = bis-diphenylphosphinomethane), were characterized, but the free ligand 13 was not isolated so far [18–24]. Only recently, complexes of 2-pyridyl functionalized N,C,N-carbodiphosphorane $CDP(Py)_2$ (1) have been reported [25,26]. The isolation of the free ligand base 1 [25] enabled the synthesis of Cu(I) CPD complexes, which are discussed in this work. Cu(I) complexes [27–43] can be used as cost-efficient luminescent materials, which potentially can replace highly phosphorescent Ir [44–50] or Pt [47,51–58] complexes in OLED technology. For example, OLED devices with internal quantum efficiencies of up to 100% could be realized based on the thermally activated delayed fluorescence *(TADF) singlet-harvesting* mechanism [28–31,41]. According to this mechanism, both the singlet and triplet excitons formed in an OLED emission layer can be harvested, and emission occurs via the S_1 state.

Very frequently, Cu(I) complexes exhibit low-lying metal-to-ligand charge transfer (MLCT) transitions that are related to small energy separations $\Delta E(S_1–T_1)$ between the lowest singlet S_1 and the lowest triplet T_1 state due to small HOMO–LUMO overlap. As a consequence, efficient up-intersystem crossing ($T_1 \rightarrow S_1$), also designated as reverse intersystem crossing RISC, can occur at near ambient temperature [28,41,45,59,60], thus resulting in thermally activated delayed fluorescence (TADF). This is also related to a small transition dipole moment, and thus, a small radiative rate $k^r(S_1 \rightarrow S_0)$ [31,32]. The described MLCT formally corresponds to the oxidation of Cu(I) to Cu(II) and leads to photo-induced structural rearrangements in the excited state(s) being connected to large Franck–Condon factors [61], and as a consequence, to competing non-radiative relaxations. Therefore, the design of rigid structures with small reorganization energy between the ground state and excited states is essential.

While the first luminescent behavior of an Au(I) N-heterocyclic carbene (NHC) complex was already described in 1999 [62], it took another 10 years until the first photoluminescent Cu(I) NHC complexes were characterized [63] followed by further studies more recently [64–70]. In contrast to the π-acidic NHCs ligands, the π-donating CDP ligands have not yet been considered in luminescent materials. Herein, we report such luminescent Cu(I) CDP complexes, their synthesis, X-ray structure data, and photoluminescence properties. We demonstrate, that high emission quantum yields can be obtained with selected materials of this class.

2. Results

2.1. Synthesis and Characterization of N,C,N-CDP Complexes

The N,C,N-carbodiphosphorane pincer ligand $CDP(Py)_2$ (1) was synthesized as reported previously [25] and used as a ligand in order to synthesize neutral and cationic dinuclear copper (I) complexes. Complexes 2, 3, and 9 were conveniently prepared by stirring ligand

1 with two equivalents of the respective copper(I) salts CuX in THF at room temperature for 18 h. Moderate yields of 86% and 63% for **2** and **3**, as well as 27% for **9** were achieved in form of orange powders. Dicationic complexes **4–8** were prepared in an in situ two-step protocol by the reaction of CDP(Py)$_2$ (**1**) with tetrakis(acetonitrile)copper(I) hexafluorophosphate (2 eq.) in THF, followed by the addition of either two equivalents of monodentate triaryl phosphine or one equivalent of a bisphosphine ligand: triphenylphosphine, tris(o-methoxyphenyl)phosphine, bis[(2-diphenylphosphino)phenyl] ether (DPEPhos), 4,5-bis(diphenylphosphino)-9,9-dimethylxanthene (XantPhos), and 1,1′-bis(diphenyl-phosphino)ferrocene (dppf) were chosen as ligands. The dicationic Cu(I) complexes were isolated and crystallized in yields of 47–90% (Scheme 1). Additionally, a neutral Cu(I) CDP complex was obtained via the deprotonation of carbazole (**10**) in THF using sodium *tert*-butoxide and the addition of [(CuCl)$_2$(CDP(Py)$_2$)] (**2**) to this solution. [(CuCarb)$_2$(CDP(Py)$_2$)] (**11**) was obtained as light orange powder in a yield of 56%. Complexes **2–9** and **11** have been characterized via ^{31}P{^{1}H} NMR, ^{1}H-NMR, ^{13}C{^{1}H} NMR, and by elemental analyses. Due to the typically poor volatility of ionic and zwitterionic Cu(I) complexes **2–9** and **11**, no mass spectra with molecular ions were obtained under EI, FD, and ESI ionization techniques.

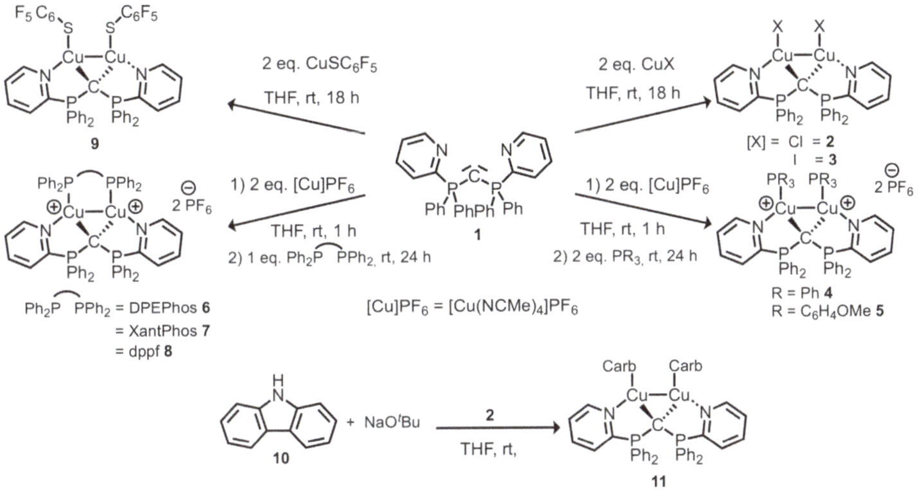

Scheme 1. Synthesis of a wide variety of novel dinuclear N,C,N-carbodiphosphorane complexes **2–9** and **11**.

Single crystals suitable for X-ray diffraction analysis were obtained upon layering THF or DCM solutions of the complexes with *n*-pentane. Crystal structures for **2**, **4**, **6**, **7**, **9**, and **11** are shown in Figure 1, selected bond distances and angles are shown in Table 1. Further details of the XRD analyses of **3**, **5**, and **8** are described in the Supplementary Materials. The molecular structures of **2–9** reveal that the central carbon atom within the CDP ligand is capable of coordinating two copper atoms in a geminal fashion. Each copper atom is additionally coordinated by one 2-pyridyl unit of ligand **1**. If the Cu–Cu interaction is disregarded, the two copper atoms per molecule are coordinated in a planar fashion, which is more T-shaped than trigonal planar. Each copper atom is interacting with one of the two carbone lone pairs of the central carbon atom C1, each by one nitrogen atom of a 2-pyridyl chelate ring and by the variable neutral ligand L or anionic ligand X. The strongest ligand interactions (C and X/phosphine) define a Cu(I) archetypical close to the linear axis. The geminal nature of both copper(I) centers leads Cu–Cu distances in the range of 2.55–2.67 Å (Table 1). These distances are smaller than twice the size of the covalent radius of Cu (1.32 Å) [71] or twice the size of the van der Waals radius of Cu (1.4 Å) [72]. Twice the size of the Cu(I) covalent radius (1.27 Å) [73] is close to the observed Cu–Cu distance. Similar trends are observed in dinuclear Cu(I) CDP complexes without any constraints of additional chelating CDP functions [74]. The Cu–Cu interaction leads to a formally coordinatively saturated pseudo tetrahedral coordination around each copper atom. This dinuclear entity is intramolecularly stabilized by a neutral 4-electron donor carbone ligand bridging the two Cu atoms. This rather rigid ligand template is characterized by characteristic torsion angles X–Cu–Cu–X in the range 41.9° (**2**)–76.0° (**3**) for anionic ligands X (X = Cl, I, S(C_6F_6)) or L–Cu–Cu–L in the range 62.4° (**8**)–82.9° (**4**) for phosphine and the bridging bisphosphine ligands. The rather rigid frame of this N,C,N-ligand backbone seems to be privileged to stabilize this 8-electron-5-center inner Cu_2CN_2 core.

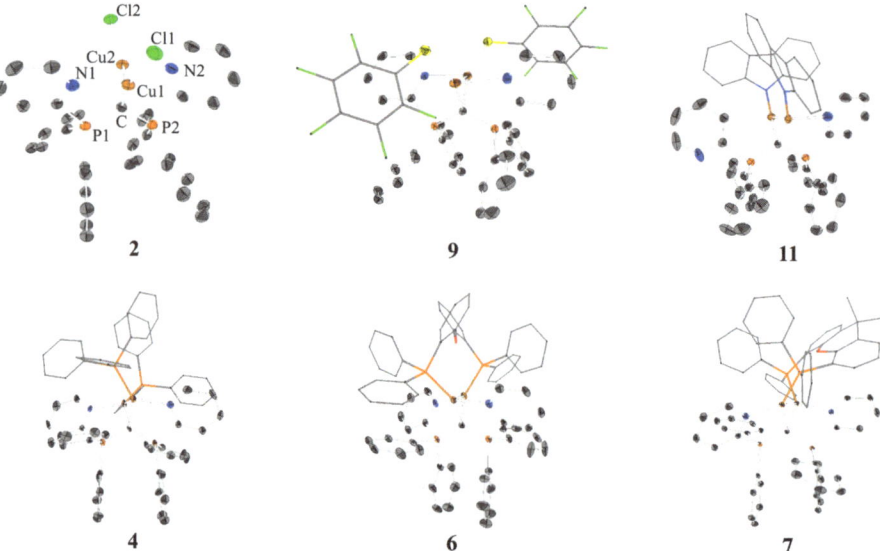

Figure 1. XRD molecular structures of [(CuCl)$_2$(CDP(Py)$_2$)] (**2**), [Cu$_2$(PPh$_3$)(CDP(Py)$_2$)](PF$_6$)$_2$ (**4**), [Cu$_2$(DPEPhos)(CDP(Py)$_2$)](PF$_6$)$_2$ (**6**), [Cu$_2$(XantPhos)(CDP(Py)$_2$)](PF$_6$)$_2$ (**7**), [(CuS(C$_6$F$_5$))$_2$(CDP(Py)$_2$)] (**9**), and [(CuCarb)$_2$(CDP(Py)$_2$)] (**11**). Hydrogen atoms and solvent molecules have been omitted for clarity; thermal ellipsoids are given at 50% probability. For **4**, **6**, and **7**, the counter anions [PF$_6$]$^-$ are omitted for clarity. The labeling of **2** is identical for all species. For details and further XRD molecular structures of **3**, **5**, and **8**, see the Supplementary Materials.

Table 1. Selected bond distances [Å] and angles [°] for **2**–**9** and **11**.

	Cu–Cu	C–P1	C–P2	Cu–X [1]	Cu–C–Cu	P1–C–P2
2	2.5525(5)	1.714(3)	1.718(2)	2.1504	80.26(9)	121.51(14)
3	2.5727(10)	1.679(5)	1.702(5)	2.4501	78.64(19)	128.5(3)
4	2.6039(16)	1.709(10)	1.693(9)	2.186	79.3(3)	126.8(6)
5	2.5768(5)	1.707(3)	1.710(3)	2.2024	78.29(10)	123.64(18)
6	2.5798(6)	1.710(4)	1.712(4)	2.1903	78.77(13)	124.0(2)
7	2.5580(3)	1.7064(19)	1.7211(18)	2.1920	77.73(6)	122.10(11)
8	2.5882(16)	1.730(6)	1.717(6)	2.1915	80.0(2)	121.8(4)
9	2.6667(7)	1.710(3)	1.710(3)	2.1881	83.01(11)	123.70(17)
11	2.671(2)	1.726(2)	1.728(2)	1.886	86.14(12)	120.45(15)

[1] Average value of the distances of Cu1–X1 and Cu2–X2. X = Cl, I, S, P or N.

Representative parent complex **2** crystallizes in a triclinic crystal system with a crystallographic point group of P-1 and with four units and two unique molecules in the unit cell. One of the two independent molecules is slightly disordered, and both have very similar geometric parameters. The angles (°) around copper are almost identical for the two Cu atoms, but crystallographically, they are not strictly identical: C–Cu–Cl 162.11(8)°, C–Cu–N 89.45(9)°, and N–Cu–Cl 106.95(6)°. Each copper atom deviates only marginally from the plane defined by C, N, and X = Cl to which copper(I) is bound. Cu–Cu distances, which indicate weak Cu–Cu interactions, e.g., 2.5525(5) Å for **2**. The C–Cu–Cu angles of **2** and related species are typically sharp, e.g., 49.98(7)° in case of **2**. A comparable coordination scenario can be found for the other complexes **3–9**. Only small differences for the C–P distances as well for the Cu–C–Cu and the P–C–C angles are observed within the series **2–9**.

Complex **11** crystallizes in a monoclinic crystal system with a space group of $P2_1/n$ and four units in its unit cell. In contrast to the described XRD molecular structures of **2–9**, the neutral complex **11** shows only one pyridine copper interaction, while the remaining pyridyl unit stays in a dangling nonbonding situation. The carbazolyl anions display a perpendicular orientation with respect to each other. Both steric and electronic factors are probably responsible for the dangling pyridyl unit in **11**. As expected, the Cu–N$_{carb}$ distance 1.911(3) Å for copper with the higher coordination number due to additional pyridine interaction is longer than Cu–N$_{carb}$ 1.861(2) Å for the other one. According to NMR spectroscopy, there is a dynamic exchange process of bonded and dangling pyridine ligands in solution.

2.2. Synthesis and Characterization of P,C,P–CDP Complexes

Peringer et al. developed *P,C,P*–CDP pincer complexes of a formal carbone ligand C(dppm)$_2$, which was not isolated and characterized, but trapped in the form of its complexes [18–24]. The synthetic strategy involved complex redox reactions. It is limited to the characterization of Ni(II), Pd(II), Pt(II), or Au(III) complexes so far. Our synthetic approach was to isolate the free CDP base. Thus, [CH(dppm)$_2$]Cl (**12**) [18,19] was treated with an excess of sodium amide (6.5 eq.) in liquid ammonia at −78 °C. Since the basicity of sodium amide leads to the deprotonation of only one proton, CDP(CH$_2$PPh$_2$)$_2$ (**13**) could be isolated in 98% yield as an intense yellow powder. No further deprotonation products and no adduct formation with lithium salts were observed as in the case of using organolithium bases. The isolation of **13** was the precondition to access the coordination chemistry of Cu(I) with this *P,C,P*–CDP ligand base. Dinuclear copper complexes **14–16** were synthesized and characterized via NMR spectroscopy and mass spectrometry (Scheme 2).

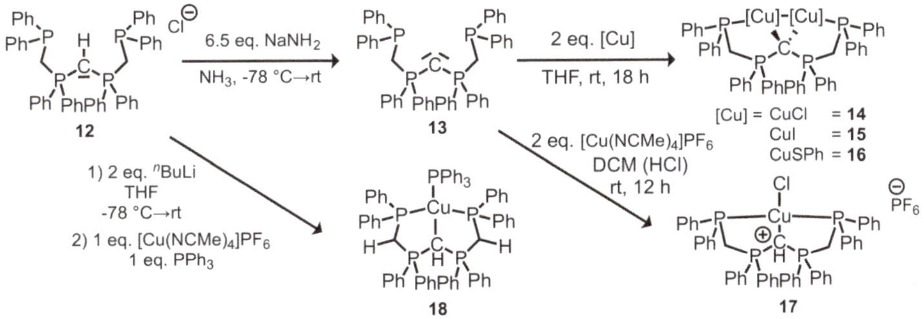

Scheme 2. Synthesis of dinuclear *P,C,P*–CDP complexes **14–16** via the isolation of previously non-characterized CDP(CH$_2$PPh$_2$)$_2$ (**13**). A monoprotonated form of **13** was trapped and characterized in **17** and a monodeprotonated form of **13** was trapped and characterized in **18**.

Upon treating **13** with tetrakis(acetonitrile)copper(I) hexafluorophosphate in DCM, a cationic complex [CuCl(H-CDP(CH$_2$PPh$_2$)$_2$]PF$_6$ (**17**) was obtained. The enhanced basicity of alkyl-substituted CDP **13** compared to pyridyl-substituted CDP **1** leads to a protonation of a Lewis acid-activated acetonitrile ligand. Therefore, monoprotonated **13** is acting as a ligand in mononuclear copper complex **17** with hexafluorophosphate as a counter ion. While searching for adequate bases for the deprotonation of **12**, we observed the ability of *n*-BuLi (2 eq.) to further deprotonate CDP **13**, generating an anionic CDP ligand **20** (Scheme 3) as lithium salt. Trapping this anion with one equivalent of tetrakis(acetonitrile)copper(I) hexafluorophosphate and one equivalent of triphenylphosphine leads to neutral copper(I) complex **18** as a light yellow powder in 73% yield. **18** was characterized via ^{31}P{^{1}H} NMR, ^{1}H-NMR, and elemental and XRD analysis.

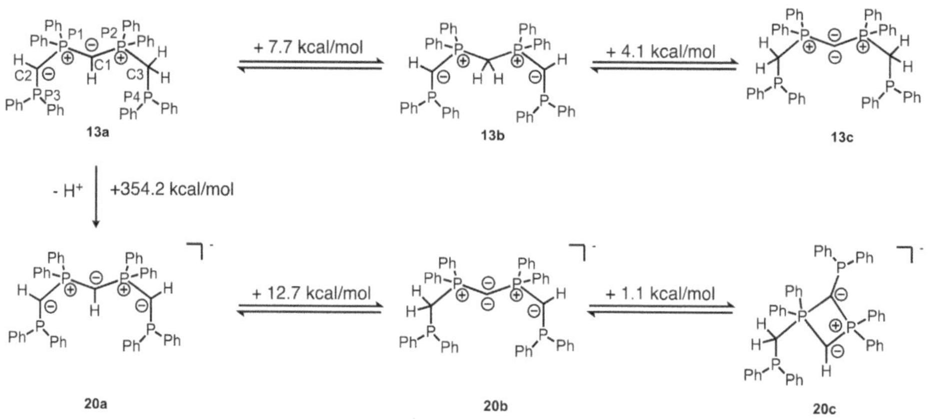

Scheme 3. Results of quantum chemical calculations on the deprotonation of [H-CDP(CH$_2$PPh$_2$)$_2$]Cl (**12**) and formation of different more or less stable tautomers of CDP(CH$_2$PPh$_2$)$_2$ (**13**). The positive value of the energy corresponds to the energy that has to be applied in order to convert one molecule into the other. The most stable tautomer **13a** and its deprotonation product **20a** are shown on the left side of the scheme.

After the deprotonation of symmetric protonated CDP form **12**, ^{31}P{^{1}H} NMR spectra of the product (or products) become temperature and solvent-dependent. We presumed that this observation could be an indication of the presence of more than one tautomer, at least two with definitely chemically non-equivalent ^{31}P nuclei of monodeprotonated base **13** (see Figure S-28). As there were no literature data available on this particular carbodiphosphorane **13**, even though it was used as a ligand in several publications, we decided to investigate the tautomeric forms of **13** via computational methods (Scheme 3). Geometry optimizations were performed at the PBE-D3(BJ)/def2-TZVPP level of theory, which were followed by single-point calculations and a natural bond orbital (NBO) analysis at the PBE0-D3(BJ)/def2-TZVPP level of theory. Interestingly, the results reveal that the free ligand base **13** cannot be acknowledged as a carbodiphosphorane, but rather as tautomer **13a**. Due to the high first proton affinity (PA) and drastically lower second PA of the alkyl-substituted central CDP carbon atom and due to the enhanced CH acidity of the methylene group placed in between a phosphanyl and a phosphionio functionality, the ground state of **13** is not represented by tautomer **13c** or **13b** but by asymmetric tautomer **13a**. This equilibrium explains the highly complex ^{31}P{^{1}H} NMR spectra obtained from solutions of pure **13**. Symmetric tautomer **13b** is 4.1 kcal/mol more stable than **13c**, but asymmetric **13a** is 7.7 kcal/mol more stable than **13b**. Therefore, **13b** seems to be observable at very low concentration in a dynamic equilibrium ratio next to **13a** but not symmetric carbodiphosphorane form **13c**.

Our results from solution and gas phase investigation and very clear results from XRD solid-state investigations of ligand **13** complexes indicate that the equilibrium of tautomers displayed in Scheme 3 is shifted toward **13c**, if the free base **13** is trapped by coordination with two Cu(I) ions. The further deprotonation of **13a** leads to symmetric carbanion **20** as the most stable tautomer: **20a** with equally CH-functionalized C1, C2, and C3 is 12.7 kcal/mole more stable than asymmetric tautomer **20b** retaining a carbodiphosphorane structure. A hypothetical 1λ^5,3λ^3 diphosphete derivate **20c** is just 1.1 kcal/mole less stable than **20b** in the gas phase. The charge distribution of the tautomers can be monitored via NBO analysis. While the atomic partial charge q(C) of C1 of **13a** is −1.38 e, which corresponds to q(C) of the protonated hexaphenyl-carbodiphosphorane (−1.33 e) [6], the one of **13c** reveals as −1.45 e and therefore is in the same order of magnitude as for the hexaphenyl-carbodiphosphorane (−1.43 e) [6]. For **20a**, the $q(C)$ values of C1, C2, and C3 are −1.39 e, 1.37 e, and 1.37 e, while the $q(C)$ values of P1, P2, P3 and P4 are 1.68 e, 1.68 e, 0.83 e and 0.83 e. For more information regarding the atomic partial charges and for a detailed deprotonation of **12**, see Tables S-1–S-8, as well as Scheme S-1 in the Supplementary Materials.

Single crystals suitable for X-ray diffraction analysis were obtained upon layering a THF or a DCM solution of the complexes **14**–**18** with *n*-pentane. The XRD molecular structures are depicted in Figure 2, while selected bond distances and angles are shown in Tables 2 and 3. For dinuclear complexes **14**–**16**, a very similar trend is observed, as discussed in Chapter 2.1. The central CDP carbon atom acts as 4-electron donor involving two geminal copper atoms into a Cu–C–Cu triangle. Each copper atom is further coordinated to one chelating phosphine group. While **14** and **16** crystalize in a triclinic crystal system with space group *P*-1 and two units in the unit cell, **15** crystalizes in a monoclinic crystal system with space group *C*2/*c* and four units in the unit cell. In contrast to dinuclear Cu(I) complexes of pyridyl-CDP **1**, complexes **14**–**16** of phosphanyl-CDP **13** reveal significantly longer Cu–Cu distances (Å). 2.8681(5) (**14**), 2.8816(12) (**15**), and 2.989(2) (**16**) compared to 2.5525(5) (**2**) and 2.671(2) (**11**). This is in accord with the higher steric demand of the phosphine and an increased freedom of motion in CDP ligand **13** compared to the more rigid and compact CDP **1** (also compare the XYZ.file of the SI). In contrast to **2**–**9**, disregarding the Cu–Cu interaction, a less pronounced T-shape but more trigonal planar coordination sphere of the copper(I) ions is observed for **14**–**16**. This is probably due to the fact that phosphines, carbones, and the anions X are more similar in their donor strength and Cu(I) affinity compared to weaker pyridine ligands in the first series of compounds. For **14**, the angles (°) around copper are 128.57(7) (C–Cu–Cl), 99.71(7) (C–Cu–P) and 129.61(3) (P–Cu–Cl) and therefore closer to the ideal 120° of a trigonal coordination sphere compared to **2**. This rather rigid ligand template is characterized by characteristic torsion angles X–Cu–Cu–X in the range 119.9° (**15**)–140.2 (**16**) and are therefore larger compared to the complexes of **2**. The less rigid frame of this *P,C,P* ligand backbone stabilizes an 8-electron-5-center inner Cu_2CP_2 core.

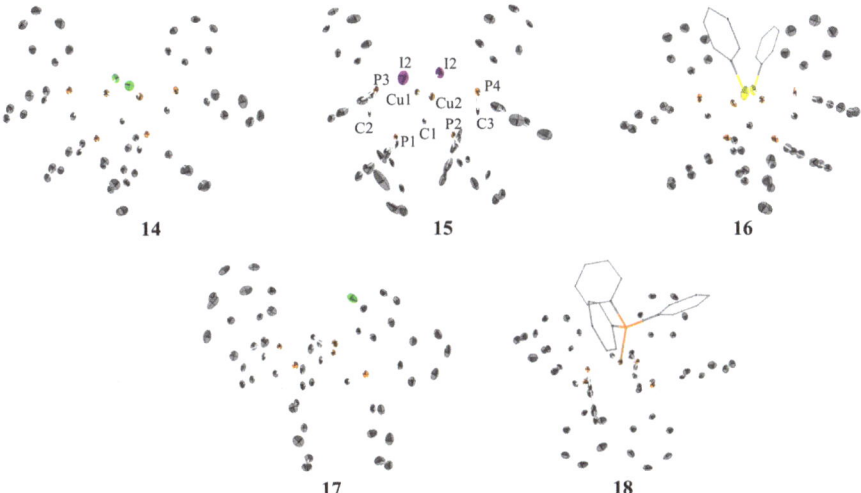

Figure 2. XRD molecular structures of $[(CuCl)_2(CDP(CH_2PPh_2)_2]$ (**14**), $[(CuI)_2(CDP(CH_2PPh_2)_2]$ (**15**), $[(CuSPh)_2(CDP(CH_2PPh_2)_2]$ (**16**), $[CuCl(H\text{-}CDP(CH_2PPh_2)_2]PF_6$ (**17**), and $[CuPPh_3(CH(PPh_2CHPPh_2)_2]$ (**18**). Hydrogen atoms and solvent molecules have been omitted for clarity; thermal ellipsoids are given at 50% probability. For **17**, the counter anion $[PF_6]^-$ is omitted for clarity. The labeling of **15** is identical for all species. For more details, see the Supplementary Materials.

Table 2. Selected bond distances [Å] and angles [°] for 14–16.

	14	15	16
Cu–Cu	2.8681(5)	2.8816(12)	2.989(2)
C–P1	1.718(2)	1.716(3)	1.707(12)
C–P2	1.717(2)	1.717(2)	1.718(12)
Cu–X [1]	2.2041	2.4396(7)	2.195
Cu–C–Cu	90.02(9)	90.02(9)	92.0(4)
P1–C–P2	122.86(14)	126.3(4)	126.9(7)

[1] Average value of the distances of Cu1–X1 and Cu2–X2. X=Cl, I or S.

Table 3. Selected bond distances [Å] and angles [°] for 14, 17 and 18.

	17	18	14
C1–Cu	2.304(2)	2.196(3)	2.0275 [a]
C1–P1	1.745(2)	1.761(3)	1.718(2)
C1–P2	1.745(2)	1.777(3)	1.717(2)
C2–P1	1.745(2)	1.700(3)	1.824(2)
C2–P3	1.846(2)	1.699(3)	1.846(2)
C3–P2	1.800(2)	1.742(3)	1.823(2)
C3–P4	1.847(2)	1.737(3)	1.847(2)
P3–Cu(1)	2.2588(6)	2.2774(9)	2.2649(7)
P4–Cu(2)	2.2629(6)	2.2767(9)	2.2701(7)
Cu–X	2.2753(6)	2.2509(9)	2.204 [a]
P1–C1–P2	125.26(14)	124.26(17)	122.86(14)
P1–C2–P3	107.70(12)	115.90(19)	108.03(12)
P2–C3–P4	109.53(12)	120.13(18)	108.17(12)
P3–Cu–P4	113.07(2)	116.76(3)	-
C1–Cu–P3	94.80(6)	95.17(8)	99.71(7)
C1–Cu–P4	94.87(6)	94.41(8)	98.92(7)
C1–Cu–X	108.08(6)	118.49(3)	129.95 [a]
P3–Cu–X	118.72(2)	113.48(8)	129.61(3)
P4–Cu–X	120.21(2)	113.87(3)	127.98(3)

X=Cl or P. [a] Average value of the distances.

Selected bond distances and angles of **14–16** can be found in Table 2, which demonstrates an increase of the Cu–C–Cu angle of about 10° in addition to the increased Cu–Cu distances relating to the increasing freedom of motion of **13** compared to **1**. The P–C–P angles of the CDP complexes **14–16** are comparable to the ones of ligand **1**.

Selected bond distances and angles of **17** and **18** are displayed in Table 3 and are compared to the ones of complex **14**. While [CuCl(H-CDP(CH$_2$PPh$_2$)$_2$]PF$_6$ (**17**) can be considered as a complex of a cationic ligand, [CuPPh$_3$(CH(PPh$_2$CHPPh$_2$)$_2$] (**18**) has to be considered as an example of a complex with the deprotonated, anionic form of ligand **13**. The charge distribution of the corresponding ligand is also reflected in the C–P distances within the complexes **14**, **17**, and **18**. While C1–P1 and C1–P2 are distinctly shorter for **14**, an increase in C–P bond distance is observed for **17** and **18** due to the protonation of C1. Furthermore, the deprotonation of C2 and C3 of complex **18** leads to a shortening of the distances C2–P1, C2–P3 and C3–P2, C3–P4 compared to **14** and **17**, where C2 and C3 are considered as methylene groups. This also corresponds to the P1–C2–P3 and P2–C3–P4 angles, which are significantly larger for the anionic ligand complex **18** compared to **14** and **17**.

2.3. Photophysical Characterization of Selected CDP Complexes

Since the photophysical properties of carbodiphosphorane Cu(I) complexes have not yet been considered, the first investigations were performed in this report. The Cu(I) complexes **2–7**, **9** and **14–16** show photoluminescence upon irradiation with UV light at room temperature. As proof of concept, we investigated emission spectra and quantum yields of [(CuPPh$_3$)$_2$(CDP(Py)$_2$)](PF$_6$)$_2$ (**4**) and [(CuSPh)$_2$(CDP(CH$_2$PPh$_2$)$_2$] (**16**). Figure 3 illustrates the normalized room-temperature emission spectra of these materials. Compound **4** shows an emission maximum at 541 nm, corresponding to green/yellow color, along with a quantum yield (Φ_{PL}) of 36% for the powder sample. The emission maximum of [(CuSPh)$_2$(CDP(CH$_2$PPh$_2$)$_2$] (**16**) (powder) is found at 510 nm (green color) showing Φ_{PL} = 60%. The high quantum yields indicate the relatively high rigidity of the complexes in powder form. Moreover, these materials are chemically robust: After exposing the complexes to air for two months, the compounds still show their characteristic photoluminescence upon irradiation with UV light at room temperature.

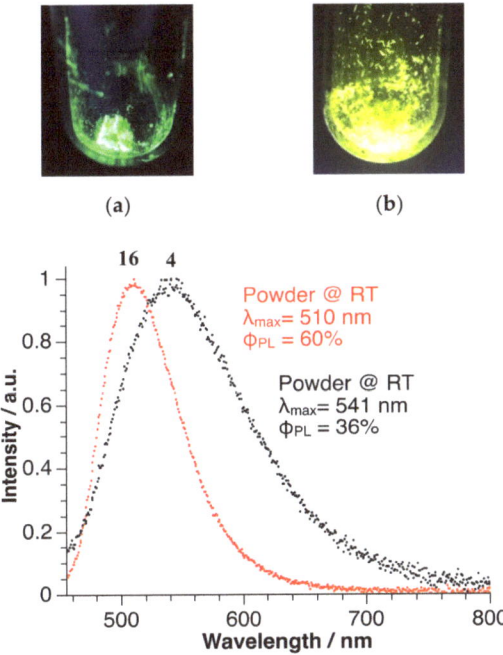

Figure 3. Normalized room-temperature emission spectra for [(CuPPh$_3$)$_2$(CDP(Py)$_2$)](PF$_6$)$_2$ (**4**) and [(CuSPh)$_2$(CDP(CH$_2$PPh$_2$)$_2$] (**16**). (**a**) illustrates the photoluminescence upon irradiation with UV light at room temperature of **16**, (**b**) of complex **4**.

First insight in the electronic structure of the emitting compounds **4** and **16** is obtained from consideration of the HOMO and LUMO distributions. Figure 4 displays that the HOMO shows for both compounds significant participation of metal d character as well as a marginal contribution of the central carbon. The LUMO, on the other hand, is primarily localized at the pyridyl units of the ligand backbone as well as on the phenyl groups attached to P1 and P2 for **16**. Considering HOMO→LUMO transitions, the excitations can be ascribed to metal-to-ligand charge transfer (MLCT) transitions. According to the relatively small HOMO-LUMO overlap, it is indicated that the energy separations $\Delta E(S_1-T_1)$ between the lowest singlet S_1 and triplet T_1 states are small enough to allow for up-inter-system crossing at ambient temperature [28,31,32]. Therefore, we tentatively assign the emission observed as TADF emission. Details will be reported in a subsequent study.

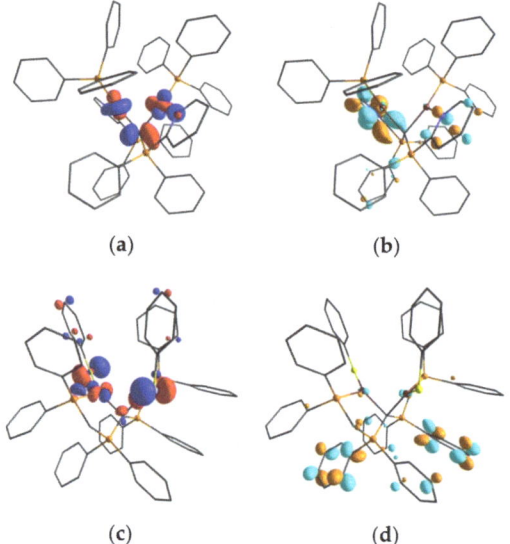

Figure 4. Kohn–Sham orbitals of HOMO (a), LUMO (b) of [(CuPPh$_3$)$_2$(CDP(Py)$_2$)](PF$_6$)$_2$ (**4**) and HOMO (c), LUMO (d) of [(CuSPh)$_2$(CDP(CH$_2$PPh$_2$)$_2$] (**16**) calculated for the optimized S$_0$ state geometry (isovalue = 0.05). Calculations were performed at the PBE-D3(BJ)/def2-TZVPP level of theory. For more details of the MOs, compare Figure S-43 and Figure S-44 in the Supplementary Materials.

For completeness, it is mentioned that also complexes **17** and **18** exhibit photoluminescence upon irradiation with UV light at room temperature. This was not the case for [Cu$_2$(dppf)(CDP(Py)$_2$)](PF$_6$)$_2$ (**8**) and [(CuCarb)$_2$(CDP(Py)$_2$)] (**11**). For **8**, quenching of the ferrocenyl ligand could be responsible for the lack of photoluminescence. In case of **11**, a reason could be the asymmetric coordination found in the crystal structure. The reduced rigidity could lead to larger geometry rearrangement after excitation and thus to quenching.

3. Conclusions

We successfully isolated and characterized a series of dinuclear copper(I) complexes of two so far poorly investigated, multidentate pyridyl and phosphanyl functionalized *N,C,N*- and *P,C,P*-carbodiphosphorane ligands. A series of neutral complexes of CDP(Py)$_2$ (**1**) with anionic coligands X and a series of dicationic complexes with monodentate and bridging bidentate bisphosphine ligands DPEPhos, XantPhos, and dppf were fully characterized, including their XRD molecular structures. In order to prepare unprecedented dinuclear copper complexes with a previously discovered *P,C,P*-carbodiphosphorane ligand backbone, it was necessary to isolate the free ligand base CDP(CH$_2$PPh$_2$)$_2$ (**13**), which has not been demonstrated before. **13** can be obtained from [CH(dppm)$_2$]Cl (**12**) and an excess of sodium amide in liquid ammonia. DFT calculations reveal that the ground state of **13** has no CDP structure in the gas phase, but rather an unsymmetric tautomer form **13a**. However, upon reaction with CuX, the CDP tautomer is trapped from the tautomeric equilibrium and neutral dinuclear Cu(I) CDP complexes are isolated and fully characterized. In addition, a protonated and a deprotonated ligand form of **13** was characterized in mononuclear complexes [CuCl(H-CDP(CH$_2$PPh$_2$)$_2$]PF$_6$ (**17**) and [CuPPh$_3$(CH(PPh$_2$CHPPh$_2$)$_2$] (**18**). With the exception of [Cu$_2$(dppf)(CDP(Py)$_2$)](PF$_6$)$_2$ (**8**) and [(CuCarb)$_2$(CDP(Py)$_2$)] (**11**), the complexes studied show photoluminescence upon irradiation with UV light at room temperature. Photophysical measurements reveal quantum yields Φ_{PL} of 36% and 60% for [(CuPPh$_3$)$_2$(CDP(Py)$_2$)](PF$_6$)$_2$ (**4**) and [(CuSPh)$_2$(CDP(CH$_2$PPh$_2$)$_2$] (**16**). As found in the crystal structure, the formal central carbon(0) atom is capable of coordinating two copper atoms relatively close to each other. They are further coordinated in a chelating manner to the chelating side arms of the CDPs. This rigid ligand design leads to high-emission quantum yields and makes the CDP complexes relatively stable under air. Therefore, it is proposed to test the compound's OLED suitability.

Supplementary Materials: The following are available online. Experimental section, NMR spectra, IR spectra, crystal data tables of **2** (2017394), **3** (2017392), **4** (2017399), **5** (2017397), **6** (2017398), **7** (2017400), **8** (2017406), **9** (2017395), **11** (2017393), **14** (2017408), **15** (2017410), **16** (2017409), **17** (2017407) and **18** (2017411) and DFT calculations (PDF). Cartesian coordinates of calculated structures (XYZ).

Author Contributions: Conceptualization, M.K. and J.S.; Formal analysis, H.Y. and J.S.; Structural Analysis and DFT Calculations, M.K.; Synthesis, M.K. and N.D.; Luminescence Investigation and Metology, A.S. and H.Y.; Project administration, J.S.; Writing—original draft, M.K. and H.Y.; Writing—review & editing, J.S. All authors have read and agreed to the published version of the manuscript.

Funding: Financial support by TransMIT GmbH, Gesellschaft für Technologietransfer (Gießen, Germany) is acknowledged.

Conflicts of Interest: The authors declare no conflict of interest.

References

1. Ramirez, F.; Desai, N.B.; Hansen, B.; McKelvie, N. HEXAPHENYLCARBODIPHOSPHORANE, $(C_6H_5)_3PCP(C_6H_5)_3$. *J. Am. Chem. Soc.* **1961**, *83*, 3539–3540. [CrossRef]
2. Tonner, R.; Frenking, G. Divalent Carbon(0) Chemistry, Part 1: Parent Compounds. *Chem. Eur. J.* **2008**, *14*, 3260–3272. [CrossRef]
3. Tonner, R.; Frenking, G. Divalent Carbon(0) Chemistry, Part 2: Protonation and Complexes with Main Group and Transition Metal Lewis Acids. *Chem. Eur. J.* **2008**, *14*, 3273–3289. [CrossRef] [PubMed]
4. Tonner, R.; Frenking, G. C(NHC)2: Divalent Carbon(0) Compounds with N-Heterocyclic Carbene Ligands-Theoretical Evidence for a Class of Molecules with Promising Chemical Properties. *Angew. Chem. Int. Ed.* **2007**, *46*, 8695–8698. [CrossRef] [PubMed]
5. Frenking, G.; Tonner, R. Divalent carbon(0) compounds. *Pure Appl. Chem.* **2009**, *81*, 597–614. [CrossRef]
6. Tonner, R.; Öxler, F.; Neumüller, B.; Petz, W.; Frenking, G. Carbodiphosphoranes: The Chemistry of Divalent Carbon(0). *Angew. Chem. Int. Ed.* **2006**, *45*, 8038–8042. [CrossRef]
7. Appel, R.; Knoll, F.; Schöler, H.; Wihler, H.-D. Vereinfachte Synthese von Bis(triphenylphosphoranyliden)methan. *Angew. Chem.* **1976**, *88*, 769–770. [CrossRef]
8. Sundermeyer, J.; Weber, K.; Peters, K.; Von Schnering, H.G. Modeling Surface Reactivity of Metal Oxides: Synthesis and Structure of an Ionic Organorhenyl Perrhenate Formed by Ligand-Induced Dissociation of Covalent Re_2O_7. *Organometallics* **1994**, *13*, 2560–2562. [CrossRef]
9. Petz, W.; Frenking, G. ChemInform Abstract: Carbodiphosphoranes and Related Ligands. *J. Nat. Prod.* **2010**, *42*, 49–92. [CrossRef]
10. Petz, W. Addition compounds between carbones, CL_2, and main group Lewis acids: A new glance at old and new compounds. *Coord. Chem. Rev.* **2015**, *291*, 1–27. [CrossRef]
11. Gessner, V.H. *Modern Ylide Chemistry*, 1st ed.; Springer International Publishing AG: Oxford, UK, 2018.
12. Kubo, K.; Jones, N.D.; Ferguson, M.J.; McDonald, R.; Cavell, R.G. Chelate and Pincer Carbene Complexes of Rhodium and Platinum Derived from Hexaphenylcarbodiphosphorane, Ph_3PCPPh_3. *J. Am. Chem. Soc.* **2005**, *127*, 5314–5315. [CrossRef] [PubMed]
13. Cavell, R.G. Pincer and Chelate Carbodiphosphorane Complexes of Noble Metals. In *The Chemistry of Pincer Compounds*, 1st ed.; Morales-Morales, D., Jensen, C.M., Eds.; Elsevier Science: Amsterdam, The Netherlands, 2007; pp. 347–355.
14. Kubo, K.; Okitsu, H.; Miwa, H.; Kume, S.; Cavell, R.G.; Mizuta, T. Carbon(0)-Bridged Pt/Ag Dinuclear and Tetranuclear Complexes Based on a Cyclometalated Pincer Carbodiphosphorane Platform. *Organometallics* **2017**, *36*, 266–274. [CrossRef]

15. Petz, W.; Neumuüller, B.; Klein, S.; Frenking, G. Syntheses and Crystal Structures of [Hg{C(PPh$_3$)$_2$}$_2$][Hg$_2$I$_6$] and [Cu{C(PPh$_3$)$_2$}$_2$]I and Comparative Theoretical Study of Carbene Complexes [M(NHC)$_2$] with Carbone Complexes [M{C(PH$_3$)$_2$}$_2$] (M = Cu$^+$, Ag$^+$, Au$^+$, Zn^{2+}, Cd^{2+}, Hg^{2+}). *Organometallics* **2011**, *30*, 3330–3339. [CrossRef]
16. Petz, W.; Neumüller, B. New platinum complexes with carbodiphosphorane as pincer ligand via ortho phenyl metallation. *Polyhedron* **2011**, *30*, 1779–1784. [CrossRef]
17. Böttger, S.C.; Poggel, C.; Sundermeyer, J. Ortho-directed Dilithiation of Hexaphenyl- carbodiphosphorane. *Preprints* **2020**. [CrossRef]
18. Stallinger, S.; Reitsamer, C.; Schuh, W.; Kopacka, H.; Wurst, K.; Peringer, P. Novel route to carbodiphosphoranes producing a new P,C,P pincer carbene ligand. *Chem. Commun.* **2007**, *5*, 510–512. [CrossRef]
19. Reitsamer, C.; Schuh, W.; Kopacka, H.; Wurst, K.; Peringer, P. Synthesis and Structure of the First Heterodinuclear PCP–Pincer–CDP Complex with a Pd–Au d8–d10Pseudo-Closed-Shell Interaction. *Organometallics* **2009**, *28*, 6617–6620. [CrossRef]
20. Reitsamer, C.; Schuh, W.; Kopacka, H.; Wurst, K.; Ellmerer, E.P.; Peringer, P. The First Carbodiphosphorane Complex with Two Palladium Centers Attached to the CDP Carbon: Assembly of a Single-Stranded di-Pd Helicate by the PCP Pincer ligand C(dppm)2. *Organometallics* **2011**, *30*, 4220–4223. [CrossRef]
21. Reitsamer, C.; Stallinger, S.; Schuh, W.; Kopacka, H.; Wurst, K.; Obendorf, D.; Peringer, P. Novel access to carbodiphosphoranes in the coordination sphere of group 10 metals: Template synthesis and protonation of PCP pincer carbodiphosphorane complexes of C(dppm)2. *Dalton Trans.* **2012**, *41*, 3503. [CrossRef]
22. Reitsamer, C.; Hackl, I.; Schuh, W.; Kopacka, H.; Wurst, K.; Peringer, P. Gold(I) and Gold(III) complexes of the [CH(dppm)$_2$]$^+$ and C(dppm)$_2$ PCP pincer ligand systems. *J. Organomet. Chem.* **2017**, *830*, 150–154. [CrossRef]
23. Maser, L.; Herritsch, J.; Langer, R. Carbodiphosphorane-based nickel pincer complexes and their (de)protonated analogues: Dimerisation, ligand tautomers and proton affinities. *Dalton Trans.* **2018**, *47*, 10544–10552. [CrossRef]
24. Maser, L.; Vondung, L.; Langer, R. The ABC in pincer chemistry—From amine- to borylene- and carbon-based pincer-ligands. *Polyhedron* **2018**, *143*, 28–42. [CrossRef]
25. Klein, M.; Xie, X.; Burghaus, O.; Sundermeyer, J. Synthesis and Characterization of a N,C,N-Carbodiphosphorane Pincer Ligand and Its Complexes. *Organometallics* **2019**, *38*, 3768–3777. [CrossRef]
26. Su, W.; Pan, S.; Sun, X.; Zhao, L.; Frenking, G.; Zhu, C. Cerium–carbon dative interactions supported by carbodiphosphorane. *Dalton Trans.* **2019**, *48*, 16108–16114. [CrossRef]
27. Kwon, J.H.; Yoo, S.; Lampande, R.; Kim, S. Vacuum Deposition. In *Handbook of Organic Light-Emitting Diodes*; Adachi, C., Hattori, R., Kaji, H., Tsujimura, T., Eds.; Springer: Tokyo, Japan, 2019. [CrossRef]
28. Yersin, H. *Highly Efficient OLEDs: Materials Based on Thermally Activated Delayed Fluorescence*; WILEY-VCH: Weinheim, Germany, 2019.
29. Deaton, J.C.; Switalski, S.C.; Kondakov, D.Y.; Young, R.H.; Pawlik, T.D.; Giesen, D.J.; Harkins, S.B.; Miller, A.J.M.; Mickenberg, S.F.; Peters, J.C. E-Type Delayed Fluorescence of a Phosphine-Supported Cu$_2$(μ-NAr$_2$)$_2$ Diamond Core: Harvesting Singlet and Triplet Excitons in OLEDs‖. *J. Am. Chem. Soc.* **2010**, *132*, 9499–9508. [CrossRef]
30. Leitl, M.J.; Zink, D.M.; Schinabeck, A.; Baumann, T.; Volz, D.; Yersin, H. Copper(I) Complexes for Thermally Activated Delayed Fluorescence: From Photophysical to Device Properties. *Top. Curr. Chem.* **2016**, *374*, 25. [CrossRef] [PubMed]
31. Czerwieniec, R.; Leitl, M.J.; Homeier, H.H.H.; Yersin, H. Cu(I) complexes. Thermally activated delayed fluorescence. Photophysical approach and material design. *Coord. Chem. Rev.* **2016**, *325*, 2–28. [CrossRef]
32. Yersin, H.; Czerwieniec, R.; Shafikov, M.Z.; Suleymanova, A.F. TADF Material Design: Photophysical Background and Case Studies Focusing on CuI and AgI Complexes. *Chem. Phys. Chem.* **2017**, *18*, 3508–3535. [CrossRef]

33. Chen, J.; Yu, R.; Zhang, Q.-K.; Zhou, L.-J.; Wu, X.-Y.; Zhang, Q.; Lu, C.-Z. Rational Design of Strongly Blue-Emitting Cuprous Complexes with Thermally Activated Delayed Fluorescence and Application in Solution-Processed OLEDs. *Chem. Mater.* **2013**, *25*, 3910–3920. [CrossRef]
34. Gneuß, T.; Leitl, M.J.; Finger, L.H.; Yersin, H.; Sundermeyer, J. A new class of deep-blue emitting Cu(I) compounds—Effects of counter ions on the emission behavior. *Dalton Trans.* **2015**, *44*, 20045–20055. [CrossRef]
35. Gneuß, T.; Leitl, M.J.; Finger, L.H.; Rau, N.; Yersin, H.; Sundermeyer, J. A new class of luminescent Cu(I) complexes with tripodal ligands—TADF emitters for the yellow to red color range. *Dalton Trans.* **2015**, *44*, 8506–8520. [CrossRef] [PubMed]
36. Volz, D.; Chen, Y.; Wallesch, M.; Liu, R.; Fléchon, C.; Zink, D.M.; Friedrichs, J.; Flügge, H.; Steininger, R.; Göttlicher, J.; et al. Bridging the Efficiency Gap: Fully Bridged Dinuclear Cu(I)-Complexes for Singlet Harvesting in High-Efficiency OLEDs. *Adv. Mater.* **2015**, *27*, 2538–2543. [CrossRef]
37. Salehi, A.; Ho, S.; Chen, Y.; Peng, C.; Yersin, H.; So, F. Highly Efficient Organic Light-Emitting Diode Using A Low Refractive Index Electron Transport Layer. *Adv. Opt. Mater.* **2017**, *5*, 1700197. [CrossRef]
38. Igawa, S.; Hashimoto, M.; Kawata, I.; Yashima, M.; Hoshino, M.; Osawa, M. Highly efficient green organic light-emitting diodes containing luminescent tetrahedral copper(i) complexes. *J. Mater. Chem. C* **2013**, *1*, 542–551. [CrossRef]
39. Hashimoto, M.; Igawa, S.; Yashima, M.; Kawata, I.; Hoshino, M.; Osawa, M. Highly Efficient Green Organic Light-Emitting Diodes Containing Luminescent Three-Coordinate Copper(I) Complexes. *J. Am. Chem. Soc.* **2011**, *133*, 10348–10351. [CrossRef]
40. Zhang, Q.; Komino, T.; Huang, S.; Matsunami, S.; Goushi, K.; Adachi, C. Triplet Exciton Confinement in Green Organic Light-Emitting Diodes Containing Luminescent Charge-Transfer Cu(I) Complexes. *Adv. Funct. Mater.* **2012**, *22*, 2327–2336. [CrossRef]
41. Czerwieniec, R.; Yu, J.; Yersin, H. Blue-Light Emission of Cu(I) Complexes and Singlet Harvesting. *Inorg. Chem.* **2011**, *50*, 8293–8301. [CrossRef]
42. Chen, J.; Yu, R.; Wu, X.-Y.; Liang, D.; Jia, J.-H.; Lu, C.-Z. A strongly greenish-blue-emitting Cu_4Cl_4 cluster with an efficient spin–orbit coupling (SOC): Fast phosphorescence versus thermally activated delayed fluorescence. *Chem. Commun.* **2016**, *52*, 6288–6291. [CrossRef]
43. Schinabeck, A.; Rau, N.; Klein, M.; Sundermeyer, J.; Yersin, H. Deep blue emitting Cu(I) tripod complexes. Design of high quantum yield materials showing TADF-assisted phosphorescence. *Dalton Trans.* **2018**, *47*, 17067–17076. [CrossRef]
44. Lamansky, S.; Djurovich, P.; Murphy, D.; Abdel-Razzaq, F.; Lee, H.-E.; Adachi, C.; Burrows, P.E.; Forrest, S.R.; Thompson, M. Highly phosphorescent bis-cyclometalated iridium complexes: Synthesis, photophysical characterization, and use in organic light emitting diodes. *J. Am. Chem. Soc.* **2001**, *123*, 4304–4312. [CrossRef]
45. Yersin, H.; Rausch, A.F.; Czerwieniec, R.; Hofbeck, T.; Fischer, T. The triplet state of organo-transition metal compounds. Triplet harvesting and singlet harvesting for efficient OLEDs. *Coord. Chem. Rev.* **2011**, *255*, 2622–2652. [CrossRef]
46. Yersin, H. Triplet Emitters for OLED Applications. Mechanisms of Exciton Trapping and Control of Emission Properties. *Top. Curr. Chem.* **2012**, *241*, 1–26. [CrossRef]
47. Yersin, H.; Finkenzeller, W.J. Triplet Emitters for Organic Light-Emitting Diodes: Basic Properties. In *Highly Efficient OLEDs*; Wiley: Weinheim, Germany, 2008; pp. 1–97.
48. Adachi, C.; Baldo, M.A.; Thompson, M.; Forrest, S.R. Nearly 100% internal phosphorescence efficiency in an organic light-emitting device. *J. Appl. Phys.* **2001**, *90*, 5048–5051. [CrossRef]
49. Deaton, J.C.; Castellano, F.N. Archetypal Iridium(III) Compounds for Optoelectronic and Photonic Applications. In *Iridium(III) in Optoelectronic and Photonics Applications*; Wiley: Hoboken, NJ, USA, 2017; Volume 83, pp. 1–69.
50. Liang, X.; Zhang, F.; Yan, Z.-P.; Wu, Z.-G.; Zheng, Y.-X.; Cheng, G.; Wang, Y.; Zuo, J.-L.; Pan, Y.; Che, C.-M. Fast Synthesis of Iridium(III) Complexes Incorporating a Bis(diphenylphorothioyl)amide Ligand for Efficient Pure Green OLEDs. *ACS Appl. Mater. Interfaces* **2019**, *11*, 7184–7191. [CrossRef]
51. Cheng, G.; Chow, P.-K.; Kui, S.C.F.; Kwok, C.-C.; Che, C.-M. High-Efficiency Polymer Light-Emitting Devices with Robust Phosphorescent Platinum(II) Emitters Containing Tetradentate Dianionic O∧N∧C∧N Ligands. *Adv. Mater.* **2013**, *25*, 6765–6770. [CrossRef]
52. Li, G.; Fleetham, T.; Li, J. Efficient and Stable White Organic Light-Emitting Diodes Employing a Single Emitter. *Adv. Mater.* **2014**, *26*, 2931–2936. [CrossRef] [PubMed]

53. Yersin, H.; Rausch, A.F.; Czerwieniec, R. Organometallic Emitters for OLEDs: Triplet Harvesting, Singlet Harvesting, Case Structures, and Trends. In *Physics of Organic Semiconductors*; Wiley: Hoboken, NJ, USA, 2013; pp. 371–424.
54. Baldo, M.A.; O'Brien, D.F.; You, Y.; Shoustikov, A.; Sibley, S.; Thompson, M.; Forrest, S.R. Highly efficient phosphorescent emission from organic electroluminescent devices. *Nature* **1998**, *395*, 151–154. [CrossRef]
55. Che, C.-M.; Kwok, C.-C.; Lai, S.-W.; Rausch, A.; Finkenzeller, W.; Zhu, N.; Yersin, H. Photophysical Properties and OLED Applications of Phosphorescent Platinum(II) Schiff Base Complexes. *Chem. Eur. J.* **2010**, *16*, 233–247. [CrossRef]
56. Williams, J.A.G. Photochemistry and Photophysics of Coordination Compounds: Platinum. In *Photochemistry and Photophysics of Coordination Compounds II*; Balzani, V., Campagna, S., Eds.; Springer: Berlin, Germany, 2007; pp. 205–268.
57. Murphy, L.; Williams, J.A.G. Luminescent Platinum Compounds: From Molecules to OLEDs. In *Molecular Organometallic Materials for Optics*; Bozec, H., Guerchais, V., Eds.; Springer: Berlin, Germany, 2010; pp. 75–111.
58. Cheng, G.; Kui, S.C.F.; Ang, W.-H.; Ko, M.-Y.; Chow, P.-K.; Kwong, C.-L.; Kwok, C.-C.; Ma, C.; Guan, X.; Low, K.-H.; et al. Structurally robust phosphorescent [Pt(O^N^C^N)] emitters for high performance organic light-emitting devices with power efficiency up to 126 lm W−1 and external quantum efficiency over 20%. *Chem. Sci.* **2014**, *5*, 4819–4830. [CrossRef]
59. Cui, L.; Nomura, H.; Geng, Y.; Kim, J.U.; Nakanotani, H.; Adachi, C. Controlling Singlet–Triplet Energy Splitting for Deep-Blue Thermally Activated Delayed Fluorescence Emitters. *Angew. Chem. Int. Ed.* **2017**, *56*, 1571–1575. [CrossRef]
60. Samanta, P.K.; Kim, D.; Coropceanu, V.; Brédas, J.-L. Up-Conversion Intersystem Crossing Rates in Organic Emitters for Thermally Activated Delayed Fluorescence: Impact of the Nature of Singlet vs Triplet Excited States. *J. Am. Chem. Soc.* **2017**, *139*, 4042–4051. [CrossRef] [PubMed]
61. Turro, N.J. *Modern Molecular Photochemistry of Organic Molecules*; Benjamin/Cummings Pub. Co.: Melon Park, CA, USA, 1978.
62. Wang, H.M.J.; Chen, C.Y.L.; Lin, I.J.B. Synthesis, Structure, and Spectroscopic Properties of Gold(I)-Carbene Complexes. *Organometallics* **1999**, *18*, 1216–1223. [CrossRef]
63. Matsumoto, K.; Matsumoto, N.; Ishii, A.; Tsukuda, T.; Hasegawa, M.; Tsubomura, T. Structural and spectroscopic properties of a copper(I)–bis(N-heterocyclic)carbene complex. *Dalton Trans.* **2009**, 6795. [CrossRef] [PubMed]
64. Krylova, V.A.; Djurovich, P.I.; Whited, M.T.; Thompson, M. Synthesis and characterization of phosphorescent three-coordinate Cu(i)–NHC complexes. *Chem. Commun.* **2010**, *46*, 6696. [CrossRef]
65. Catalano, V.J.; Munro, L.B.; Strasser, C.E.; Samin, A.F. Modulation of Metal–Metal Separations in a Series of Ag(I) and Intensely Blue Photoluminescent Cu(I) NHC-Bridged Triangular Clusters. *Inorg. Chem.* **2011**, *50*, 8465–8476. [CrossRef]
66. Krylova, V.A.; Djurovich, P.I.; Aronson, J.W.; Haiges, R.; Whited, M.T.; Thompson, M. Structural and Photophysical Studies of Phosphorescent Three-Coordinate Copper(I) Complexes Supported by an N-Heterocyclic Carbene Ligand. *Organometallics* **2012**, *31*, 7983–7993. [CrossRef]
67. Hamze, R.; Shi, S.; Kapper, S.C.; Sylvinson, D.; Estergreen, L.; Jung, M.; Tadle, A.; Haiges, R.; Djurovich, P.I.; Peltier, J.L.; et al. "Quick-Silver" from a Systematic Study of Highly Luminescent, Two-Coordinate, d10 Coinage Metal Complexes. *J. Am. Chem. Soc.* **2019**, *141*, 8616–8626. [CrossRef]
68. Shi, S.; Jung, M.C.; Coburn, C.; Tadle, A.; Sylvinson, M.R.D.; Djurovich, P.I.; Forrest, S.R.; Thompson, M. Highly Efficient Photo- and Electroluminescence from Two-Coordinate Cu(I) Complexes Featuring Nonconventional N-Heterocyclic Carbenes. *J. Am. Chem. Soc.* **2019**, *141*, 3576–3588. [CrossRef]
69. Hamze, R.; Peltier, J.L.; Sylvinson, D.; Jung, M.; Cardenas, J.; Haiges, R.; Soleilhavoup, M.; Jazzar, R.; Djurovich, P.I.; Bertrand, G.; et al. Eliminating nonradiative decay in Cu(I) emitters: >99% quantum efficiency and microsecond lifetime. *Sciences* **2019**, *363*, 601–606. [CrossRef]
70. Leitl, M.J.; Krylova, V.A.; Djurovich, P.I.; Thompson, M.; Yersin, H. Phosphorescence versus Thermally Activated Delayed Fluorescence. Controlling Singlet–Triplet Splitting in Brightly Emitting and Sublimable Cu(I) Compounds. *J. Am. Chem. Soc.* **2014**, *136*, 16032–16038. [CrossRef]
71. Cordero, B.; Gómez, V.; Platero-Prats, A.E.; Revés, M.; Echeverría, J.; Cremades, E.; Barragán, F.; Alvarez, S. Covalent radii revisited. *Dalton Trans.* **2008**, 2832. [CrossRef] [PubMed]
72. Bondi, A. van der Waals Volumes and Radii. *J. Phys. Chem.* **1964**, *68*, 441–451. [CrossRef]

73. Soloveichik, G.L.; Eisenstein, O.; Poulton, J.T.; Streib, W.E.; Huffman, J.C.; Caulton, K.G. Multiple structural variants of LnCuI(.mu.-X)2CuILn (n = 1, 2). Influence of halide on a "soft" potential energy surface. *Inorg. Chem.* **1992**, *31*, 3306–3312. [CrossRef]
74. Ma, G.; Ferguson, M.J.; McDonald, R.; Cavell, R.G. Rare, Hexatomic, Boat-Shaped, Cross-Linked Bis(iminodiphenylphosphorano)methanediide Pincer Carbon Bridged Photoluminescent Copper Clusters Capped with Methyl or Halide Bridges. *Organometallics* **2010**, *29*, 4251–4264. [CrossRef]

Sample Availability: Samples of the selected compounds might be available from the authors.

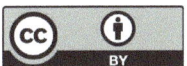
© 2020 by the authors. Licensee MDPI, Basel, Switzerland. This article is an open access article distributed under the terms and conditions of the Creative Commons Attribution (CC BY) license (http://creativecommons.org/licenses/by/4.0/).

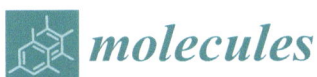

Review

Carbones and Carbon Atom as Ligands in Transition Metal Complexes

Lili Zhao [1], Chaoqun Chai [1], Wolfgang Petz [2],* and Gernot Frenking [1,2],*

[1] Institute of Advanced Synthesis, School of Chemistry and Molecular Engineering, Jiangsu National Synergetic Innovation Center for Advanced Materials, Nanjing Tech University, Nanjing 211816, China; ias_llzhao@njtech.edu.cn (L.Z.); 201861205094@njtech.edu.cn (C.C.)

[2] Fachbereich Chemie, Philipps-Universität Marburg, Hans-Meerwein-Strasse 4, D-35043 Marburg, Germany

* Correspondence: petz@chemie.uni-marburg.de (W.P.); frenking@chemie.uni-marburg.de (G.F.)

Academic Editors: Yves Canac and Carlo Santini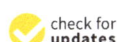
Received: 23 August 2020; Accepted: 15 October 2020; Published: 26 October 2020

Abstract: This review summarizes experimental and theoretical studies of transition metal complexes with two types of novel metal-carbon bonds. One type features complexes with carbones CL_2 as ligands, where the carbon(0) atom has two electron lone pairs which engage in double (σ and π) donation to the metal atom $[M]\Leftarrow CL_2$. The second part of this review reports complexes which have a neutral carbon atom C as ligand. Carbido complexes with naked carbon atoms may be considered as endpoint of the series $[M]\text{-}CR_3 \to [M]\text{-}CR_2 \to [M]\text{-}CR \to [M]\text{-}C$. This review includes some work on uranium and cerium complexes, but it does not present a complete coverage of actinide and lanthanide complexes with carbone or carbide ligands.

Keywords: carbone complexes; carbido complexes; transition metal complexes; chemical bonding

1. Introduction

Transition metal compounds with metal-carbon bonds are the backbone of organometallic chemistry. Molecules with M-C single bonds are already known since 1849 when Frankland reported the accidental synthesis of diethyl zinc while attempting to prepare free ethyl radicals [1,2]. Molecules with a $[M]=CR_2$ double bond (carbene complexes) or a $[M]\equiv CR$ triple bond (carbyne complexes) were synthesized much later [3–6]. Two types of compounds with metal-carbon double or triple bonds having different types of bonds are generally distinguished, which are named after the people who isolated them first. Fischer-type carbene and carbyne complexes are best described in terms of dative bonds following the Dewar–Chatt–Duncan (DCD) model [7,8] $[M]\rightleftarrows CR_2$ and $[M^{(-)}]\rightleftarrows CR^{(+)}$, whereas Schrock-type alkylidenes and alkylidynes are assumed to have electron-sharing double and triple bonds $[M]=CR_2$ and $[M]\equiv CR$ [9–11].

This review deals with transition metal complexes with metal-carbon bonds to two types of ligands, which have only recently been isolated and theoretically studied. One type of ligand are carbones CL_2 [12], which are carbon(0) compounds with two dative bonds to a carbon atom in the excited ^1D state $L\to \underaccent{\smile}{C} \leftarrow L$ where the carbon atom retains its four valence electrons as two lone pairs that can serve as four-electron donors [13,14]. Thus, carbones CL_2 are four-electron donor ligands whereas carbenes CR_2 are two-electron donors. Carbenes have a formally [15] vacant $p(\pi)$ orbital that can accept electrons in donor-acceptor complexes $M\rightleftarrows CR_2$ whereas carbones are double (σ and π) donors in complexes $[M]\rightleftarrows CL_2$. A good Lewis acid acceptor fragment A for a carbene complex has a vacant σ orbital and an occupied π orbital whereas a suitable acceptor for a carbone is a double Lewis acid with vacant σ and π orbitals as shown in Figure 1a,b. If the Lewis acid A has an occupied π orbital, it would lead to π repulsion with the π lone pair of the carbone CL_2, whereby the repulsive interaction is reduced if L is a good π acceptor (Figure 1c). The two electron lone pairs of a carbone may bind to one or two monodentate Lewis acids A or protons or to a single bidentate Lewis acid as shown in Figure 1. The large second proton affinity is a characteristic feature of carbones, which distinguishes them from carbenes [16]. Examples of all cases are known and are described below.

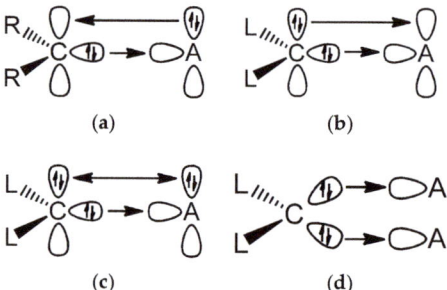

Figure 1. Schematic representation of the most important orbital interactions between carbene ligands CR_2 and carbones CL_2 with Lewis acids A. (a) Carbene complex with a monodentate Lewis acid; (b) Carbone with a bidentate Lewis acid; (c) Carbone with a monodentate Lewis acid; (d) Carbone with two monodentate Lewis acids.

It is important to realize that the two electron lone-pairs of a carbone CL_2 may additionally engage in π-backdonation to the ligands L whose strength depends on the availability of vacant π orbitals of the ligands L. Stronger π acceptor ligands L enhance the π-backdonation L← $\bar{C}$ →L which leads to wider bending angles at the carbon atom (Figure 2). The significant bending of free $C(CO)_2$ [17,18] can straightforwardly be explained in terms of dative bonding in carbon suboxide C_3O_2 [19,20]. The π-acceptor strength of ligands L thus modulates the donor interaction of the carbone CL_2.

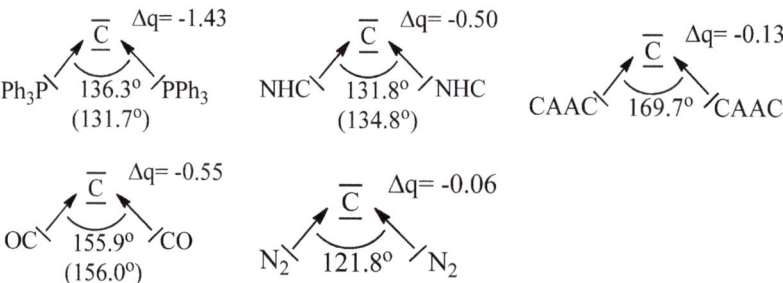

Figure 2. Calculated and (in parentheses) experimental bond angles of carbones CL_2 with different ligands L and partial charges Δq of the divalent carbon atom. The data are taken from [19].

The following list gives some essential features of carbones and their differences to carbenes. At the same time we want to stress that the distinction between carbenes and carbones are just a useful classification of compounds, which are a helpful model to explain the structures and reactivity of molecules. Nature does not exhibit a strict distinction line and there are complexes with electronic structures that have intermediate features between both classes of compounds. Carbenes and carbones are two ordering principles like ionic and covalent bonding. Intermediate cases are common and yet, the two concepts are essential ingredients of chemistry. The first part of this review summarizes experimental and theoretical work about transition metal complexes with carbone ligands [M]-CL_2.

1. Carbones are neutral carbon(0) compounds of the general formula CL_2, which possess two electron lone pairs of electrons of σ and π symmetry, respectively.
2. Carbones CL_2 have dative σ bonds L→ $\bar{C}$ ←L and weaker π backdonation L← $\bar{C}$ →L which resemble donor-acceptor bonds in transition metal complexes.

3. The carbon atom of carbones has very large electron densities and thus, unusually large negative partial charges.
4. In contrast to carbenes, carbones exhibit high first and second proton affinities (PAs) in the region of about 290 and 150–190 kcal/mol, respectively. The second PA is a sensitive probe for the divalent C(0) character of a CL_2 molecule. Carbones can take up one and two protons with formation of $[HCL_2]^+$ cations or $[H_2CL_2]^{2+}$ dications, respectively.
5. Carbones have a bent equilibrium geometry where the bending angle becomes wider when the ligand L is a better π acceptor.
6. Carbones can take up one or two monodentate Lewis acids A building the complexes A←C(L$_2$) and A←C(L$_2$)→A or one bidentate Lewis acid A⇇C(L$_2$).

To the thematic of carbones several review articles were reported previously; A general overview on species that bear two lone pairs of electrons at the same C-center are summarized in [21], transition metal adducts of carbones are described in [22], and those of main group fragments in [23]. Two contributions, [24] and [25], in the series Structure and Bonding (Springer Edition) also deal with carbone transition metal addition compounds.

The second type of transition metal complexes with a carbon ligand features species with a naked neutral carbon atom as a ligand [M]-C, which can be considered as endpoint of the series [M]-CR$_3$ → [M]-CR$_2$ → [M]-CR → [M]-C. Complexes with negatively charged carbon ligands [M]-C^{--}, which are isoelectronic to nitride complexes [M]-N and are termed as carbides, were synthesized in 1997 by Cummins [26]. The first neutral carbon complex [M]-C, which was prepared and structurally characterized was reported in 2002 by by Heppert and co-workers [27]. They isolated the diamagnetic 16 valence electron ruthenium complexes [(PCy$_3$)LCl$_2$Ru(C)] (L = PCy$_3$ and 1,3-dimesityl-4,5-dihydroimidazol-2-ylidene; Cy = Cyclohexyl) by a metathesis facilitated reaction. Quantum chemical calculations of model compounds suggested that the Ru-C bond in the complexes is best described by an electron-sharing double bond like in Schrock carbenes, which is reinforced by a donor bond [Ru]⇌C| [28]. The field of neutral carbon complexes was systematically explored in recent years by Bendix [29]. This review summarizes in its second part the research in transition metal complexes with a naked carbon atom as ligand [M]-C that has been accomplished since 2002. The review includes some work on uranium and cerium complexes, but it does not present a complete coverage of actinide and lanthanide complexes with carbone or carbide ligands.

2. Transition Metal Complexes with Carbone Ligands [M]-CL$_2$

2.1. Transition Metal Addition Compounds of Symmetrical Carbones C(PR$_3$)$_2$

Among the existing carbones with a symmetric P-C-P skeleton, five species (**1a**–**1e**) are known today as donor ligands to various transition metal fragments as outlined in Figure 3. From other linear or bent carbones with this skeleton, no transition metal complexes are described so far.

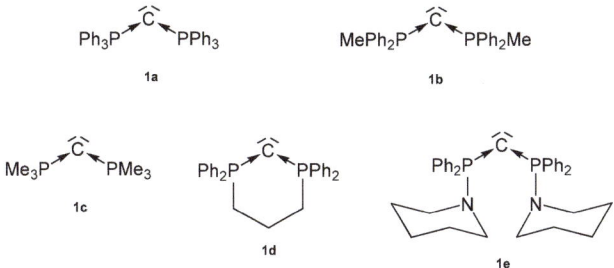

Figure 3. Symmetric carbones **1a**–**1e** as ligands for transition metal complexes.

In 1961, **1a** was detected by Ramirez [30], and 1b–1d stem from the laboratory of Schmidbaurs group [31]. Later on, a series of related carbones were synthesized, but for which transition metal complexes are unknown so far. Quite recently the new amino substituted carbone **1e** was published together with Zn and Rh addition compounds (See Scheme 1) [32]. In the 31P NMR spectra singlets at about −4.50 (**1a**), −6.70 (**1b**), −29.6 (**1c**), −22.45 (**1d**), and 12.5 ppm (**1e**) confirm the symmetric array of the compounds. All carbones have a bent structure but a linear form of **1a** is realized if crystallized from benzene [33,34]. **1a** has a short P-C distance of 1.633(4) Å and the P-C-P angle amounts to 130.1(6)° [35]. The carbone **1b** exhibits a slightly longer P-C distance of 1.648(4) Å and the introduction of two less bulky methyl groups allows a more acute P-C-P angle of 121.8(3)° [36]. **1d** has similar P-C bond distances of 1.645(12) Å 1.653(14) Å and the acutest P-C-P angle in this series of 116.7(7)° [37,38]. For **1c**, gas phase electron diffraction studies result in a P-C distance of 1.594(3) Å and a P-C-P angle of 147.6(5)° assuming an apparent non-linearity but linearity in the average structure [37]. All structural parameters of **1e** are close to those of **1a** (P-C = 1.632(2) Å, P-C-P angle = 136.5(3)° [32]).

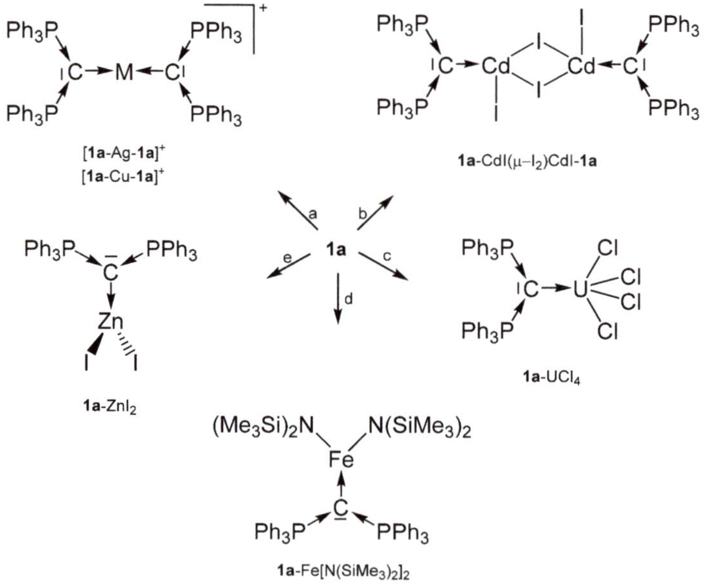

Scheme 1. Selected transition metal compounds with the carbone **1a** as two electron donor ligand; (a) MI, (b) CdI$_2$, (c) UCl$_4$, (d) Fe(N{SiMe$_3$}$_2$)$_2$, (e) ZnI$_2$.

In Table 1, transition metal addition compounds between carbones with the P-C-P core are collected. All compounds show longer P-C bonds than the basic carbones as consequence of the competition of the occupied p orbital at C(0) between the two P-σ* orbitals and those of A.

Table 1. Transition metal complexes with the carbones **1a** to **1e** including C-M and P-C bond lengths and P-C-P angles and ^{31}PNMR shifts in ppm.

1-M	^{31}P NMR	C-M	P-C	P-C-P	Ref
Transition metal complexes with the carbone **1a**					
1a-Ni(CO)$_2$	19.20	1.990(3)	1.677(3) 1.676(3)	132.13(16)	[39]
1a-Ni(CO)$_3$	9.92	2.110(3)	1.681(3) 1.674(3)	124.58(19)	[39]
1a-ZnI$_2$	17.8	2.000(9)	1.691(9) 1.703(8)	128.3(6)	[40]
1a-CdI(μ I$_2$)CdI-1a	18.5	2.25(1)	1.700(9) 1.68(1)	124.8(7)	[40]
[1a-Hg-1a][Hg$_2$Cl$_6$]	21.2	2.057(6) 2.082(7)	1.731(6) 1.706(6) 1.737(6) 1.702(7)	124.2(4) 125.7(3)	[41]
[1a-Ag-1a]I	13.6	2.115(8) 2.134(7)	1.656(7) 1.690(7) 1.667(5) 1.663(7)	128.5(5) 129.1(5)	[42]
[1a-Cu-1a]I	15.8	1.944(5) 1.951(5)	1.683(6) 1.688(6) 1.673(6) 1.694(5)	125.6(3) 128.3(3)	[41]
[1a-ReO$_3$][ReO$_4$]	29.5	1.997(7)	1.771(8)	123.1(4)	[43]

Table 1. Cont.

1-M	^{31}P NMR	C-M	P-C	P-C-P	Ref
1a-CuCl	16.5	1.906(2)	nr	123.8(1)	[44]
1a-Cu-C$_5$H$_5$	8.5	nr	nr	nr	[45]
1a-Cu-C$_5$Me$_5$	7.5	1.922(6)	1.668(5) 1.660(6)	136.0(4)	[45]
1a-CuPPh$_3$	3.7	nr	nr	nr	[45]
1a-AgCl	16.5	nr	nr	nr	[44]
1a-AgCp*	6.5	nr	nr	nr	[45]
1a-Au-C≡C-R R = C$_6$H$_4$NO$_2$-p	nr	2.082(2)	1.688(2) 1.682(2)	133.64(13)	[46]
1a-Au-CH(COMe)$_2$	nr	nr	nr	nr	[46]
1a-AuCl	13.7 14.4	nr	nr	nr	[44]
[1a-Ir(COD)]PF$_6$	nr	nr	nr	nr	[47]
1a-VCl$_3$	21.13	2.050(3)	1.712(2) 1.722(2)	123.6(2)	[48]
1a-FeCl (µCl$_2$)FeCl-1a	par	2.043(7)	1.689(7) 1.712(7)	121.3(4)	[49]
1a-Fe[N(SiMe$_3$)$_2$]$_2$	par	2.147(2)	1.702(2) 1.720(2)	120.0(1)	[50]
1a-FeCl$_2$	par	2.055(8)	1.709(7) 1.702(7)	122.7(5)	[49]
1a-Fe(CH$_2$Ph)$_2$	par	2.097(5)	1.694(5) 1.671(5)	124.5(3)	[49]
1a-FeCl[N(TMS)$_2$]	par	nr	nr	nr	[49]
1a-FeOTf[N(TMS)$_2$]	par	2.040(3)	1.701(3) 1.704(3)	122.1(2)	[49]
1a-UCl$_4$	nr	2.411(3)	1.705(3) 1.719(3)	125.05(16)	[51]
1a-(AuCl)$_2$	21.2	2.078(3) 2.074(3)	1.776(3) 1.776(3)	117.30(15)	[46]
[1aH-Ag-1aH](BF$_4$)$_3$	23.6	2.221(5)	1.770(7) 1.779(7)	119.9(4)	[52]
[1aH-Au-1aH](OTf)$_3$	26.1	nr	nr	nr	[46]
[1aH-AuCl](OTf)	22.1	nr	nr	nr	[46]
Transition metal complexes with the carbone 1b					
1b-Fe[N(SiMe$_3$)$_2$]$_2$	par	2.100(2)	1.694(2) 1.696(1)	120.8(9)	[50]
1b-Ni(CO)$_3$	2.6	2.091(2)	1.683(2) 1.673(2)	122.3(1)	[53]
1b-Ni$_2$(CO)$_5$	12.1	2.080(5) 2.070(5)	1.742(5) 1.743(5)	117.1(3)	[53]
[1bH-AuC$_6$F$_5$](CF$_3$SO$_3$)	22.7	2.029(6)	1.781(2) 1.792(2)	119.1	[54]
[1bH-AuCl](CF$_3$SO$_3$)	22.1	nr	nr	nr	[54]
Transition metal complexes with the carbone 1c					
[1c-W(CO)$_2$(Tp*)]PF$_6$	36	2.11(1)	1.75(2) 1.77(1)	114.5(8)	[55]
1c-(AuMe)$_2$	nr	nr	nr	nr	[56]
Transition metal complexes with the carbone 1d					
1d-Ni(CO)$_3$	3.5	2.0661(9)	1.712(2) 1.722(2)	117.19(9)	[48]
Transition metal complexes with the carbone 1e					
1e-ZnCl$_2$	28.9	1.994(2)	1.686(2)	125.3(1)	[32]
1e-Rh(CO)(acac)	32.9	2.092(3)	1.685(3)	128.56(17)	[32]

Occupied d orbitals of Ni in the 1a-Ni(CO)$_3$ complex elongate the C-Ni bond to a carbone (2.110 Å) [39] but this leads to a relative short bond length to a NHC (1.971 Å) moiety [57]. In contrast, UCl$_4$ leads to a short bond to a carbone (2.411 Å) [51] indicating an appreciable U-C double bond character and a long one to a NHC base (2.612 Å) [58,59].

The cation [1a-ReO$_3$]$^+$ holds the longest one with 1.771(8) Å indicating an appreciable C=Re double bond character. This feature applies also in part to **1a**-UCl$_4$ and **1c**-W(CO)$_2$N$_3$ with elongated P-C bonds(See Scheme 2); a partial C-U double bond is confirmed by theoretical calculations. Similar long P-C bonds are found in the trication [**1aH**-Ag-**1aH**]$^{3+}$, in **1a**-(AuCl)$_2$(See Scheme 3), and in **1b**-Ni$_2$(CO)$_5$(See Scheme 4), where the carbone provides each two electrons to two accepting Lewis acids as depicted in Figure 1d.

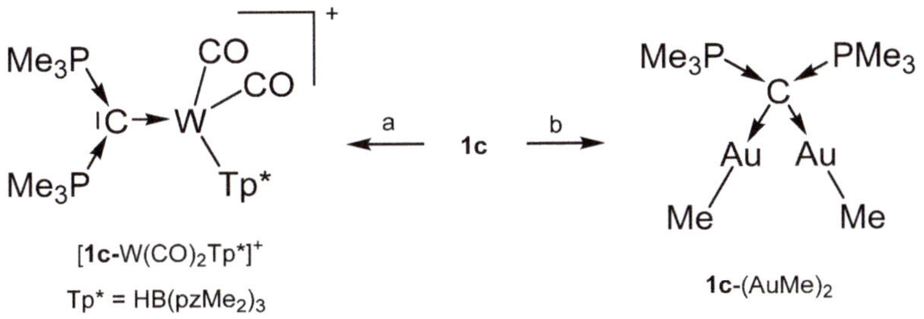

Scheme 2. Transition metal complex with the carbone **1c** as two and four electron donor ligand. (**a**) [Tp*(CO)$_2$W≡CPMe$_3$]$^+$/PMe$_3$, (**b**) 1c/2 MeAuPMe$_3$.

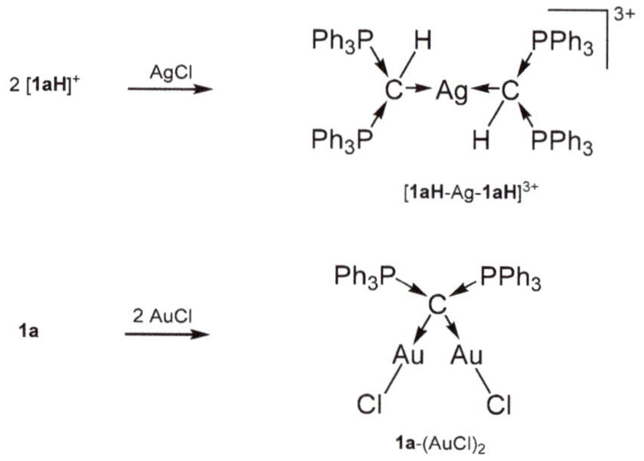

Scheme 3. Selected transition metal compounds with the carbone **1a** as four electron donor ligand.

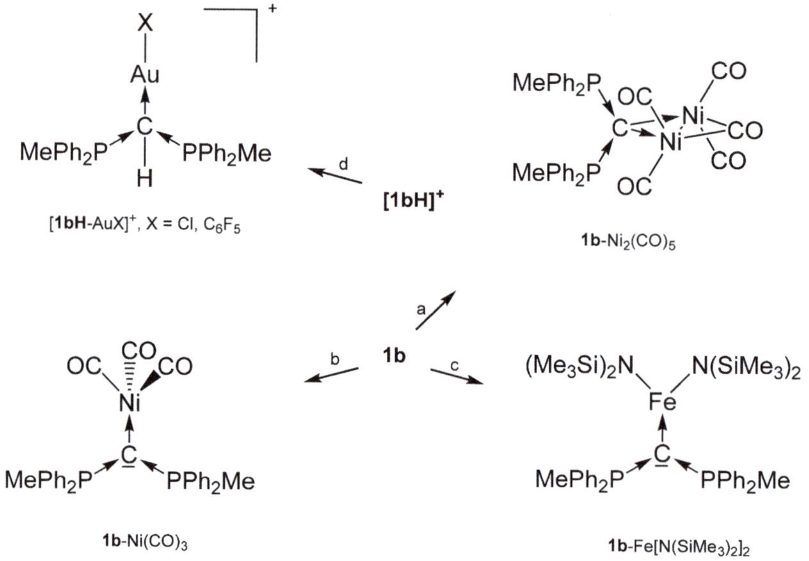

Scheme 4. Selected transition metal complexes with the carbone **1b** as two and four electron donor ligand. (**a**) Ni(CO)$_4$, (**b**) Ni(CO)$_4$ under CO atm, (**c**) Fe(N{SiMe$_3$}$_2$)$_2$, (**d**) AuX(tht).

The P-C-P angles are in the range between 115° and 132° reflecting the required space of the appropriate Lewis acid. The ^{31}P NMR shift of the carbone **1a** amounts to about −5 ppm and those of the related addition compounds are shifted to lower fields and range between 4 ppm and 30 ppm. All iron(II) complexes of **1a** and **1b** are paramagnetic and ^{31}P NMR spectra could not be obtained.

For the ^{31}P NMR spectrum of the carbone **1b**, a shift of −6.70 ppm was recorded [31]. With exception of **1b**-Ni(CO)$_3$ which resonate at 2.6 ppm, low field shifts between 12 and 22 ppm were found when **1b** act as a four electron donor [40].

Further, **1e**-ZnCl$_2$ (See Scheme 5) [32] and **1a**-ZnI$_2$ [53] have closely related structural parameters but exhibit shorter C-Zn bond lengths than to related NHC-addition compounds (Δ = 0.051 Å) [60]. In both compounds a nearly perpendicular array of the ZnX$_2$ and the PCP plane are found. No tendency for an additional N-coordination to the amino ligand of **1e** is recorded for the ZnCl$_2$ addition compound. In contrast the Rh-C distances in **1e**-Rh(CO)$_2$(acac) are longer (Δ = 0.117 Å) than in the corresponding

NHC compound [61] and a partial π interaction was found by DFT calculation. Rh also shows no tendency for coordination of the adjacent amino groups [32].

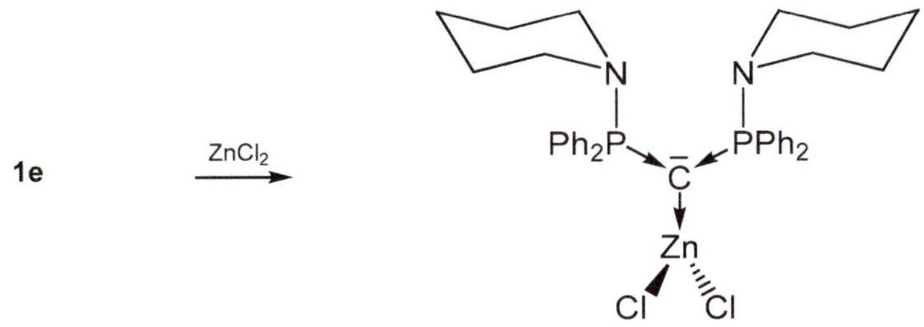

Scheme 5. Selected transition metal complex with the carbone **1e** as two electron donor ligand.

2.2. Transition Metal Addition Compounds of Carbones C(PR$_3$)$_2$ with an Additional Pincer Function

Starting material for **2a** is not the free carbone Ph$_2$P-CH$_2$-PPh$_2$-C-PPh$_2$-CH$_2$-PPh$_2$, which could not be prepared so far, but the dication [Ph$_2$P-CH$_2$-PPh$_2$-CH$_2$-PPh$_2$-CH$_2$-PPh$_2$]$^{2+}$ as reported by Peringer [62]. Later on, Sundermeyer studied the deprotonation of the cation [Ph$_2$P-CH$_2$-PPh$_2$-CH-PPh$_2$-CH$_2$-PPh$_2$]$^+$ by quantum chemical methods giving more or less stable tautomers of **2a**, see Figure 4. Deprotonation of the tautomer C of **2a** generates the anionic pincer ligand [Ph$_2$P-CH-PPh$_2$-CH-PPh$_2$-CH-PPh$_2$]$^-$ [**2c**]$^-$ [63]. The same working group also published the X-ray structure of the pincer ligand **2b** with the P-C-P angle of 133.76(13)° and P-C distances of 1.633(2) and 1.642(2) Å; the ^{31}P NMR shift δ = −5.6 ppm [64].

Various cationic complexes where reported with the pincer ligand **2a** (See Figure 4) and group 10 metal halides and one dication with the group 11 metal Au. The ^{31}P NMR shifts range between 32 and 41 ppm(See Table 2). As with **1a** the carbone carbon atom of **2a** is basic enough to accept a proton to generate complexes of the type **2aH**-MCl dications with all group 10 elements (See Scheme 6).

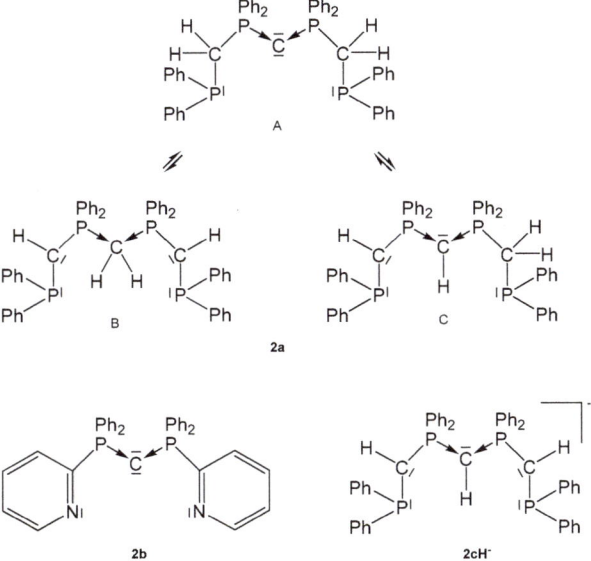

Figure 4. Tripodal basic pincer ligand **2a** with its tautomers, the anionic pincer ligand **2cH**$^-$ and the pyridyl pincer ligand **2b**.

Table 2. Transition metal complexes with the phosphine based pincer ligands **2a** and the pyridyl based pincer ligand **2b**; C-M and P-C distances are included and ^{31}P NMR shifts in ppm.

	^{31}P NMR	C-M	P-C	P-C-P	Ref
	Transition metal complexes with the tripodal carbone **2a**				
[**2a**-(PdCl)]Cl	34.5	2.062(2)	1.694(3)	124.9(2)	[62,65]
[**2a**-(NiCl)]Cl	36.4	1.942(4)	1.6925(18)	125.1(2)	[65]
[**2a**-(NiCl)]$_2$NiCl$_4$	nr	1.930(7)	1.696(7) 1.701(7)	126.3(4)	[65]
[**2a**-(PtCl)]Cl	35.7	2.060(4)	1.692(5)	124.86(15)	[65]
[**2a**-(NiMe)][AlCl$_2$Me$_2$]	31.8	1.959	1.697	120.9	[66]
[**2a**-(AuCl)]TfO$_2$	nr	2.080(8)	1.723(8)	124.5(5)	[67]
[**2a**-(AuCl)](NO$_3$)$_2$	40.8	2.060(3)	1.721(3)	125.1(2)	[67]
[**2a**-(AuI)](TfO)$_2$	41.1	2.082(8)	1.723(8)	124.9(5)	[67]
[**2aH**-PdCl]Cl$_2$	42.4	2.102(3)	1.803(3)	121.9(2)	[62]
[**2aH**-PtCl]Cl$_2$	44.4	2.106(4)	1.811(4) 1.823(4)	120.4(2)	[62]
[**2aH**-NiCl]Cl$_2$	32.7	1.990	1.801–1.834	121.1	[65,66]
[**2aH**-(CuCl)]PF$_6$	nr	2.304(2)	1.745(2)	125.26(14)	[63]
2a-(CuCl)$_2$	20.4	2.2041	1.718	122.86(14)	[63]
2a-(CuI)$_2$	22.5	2.4936	1.717	126.3(4)	[63]
2a-(CuSPh)$_2$	19.8–19.0	2.195	1.712	126.9(7)	[63]
	Transition metal complexes with the tripodal carbone **2b**				
2b-(CeBr$_3$THF)	−10.2	2.597(6)	1.672(6)	122.5(4)	[68]
2b-(CeBr)-**2b**	nr	2.573(6) 2.597(6)	1.684(7)	120.5(4)	[68]
2b-(UCl$_4$)	nr	2.471(7)	1.696(7)	121.3(4)	[41]
2b-(TiCl$_3$) [57]	18.24	2.144(6)	1.670(3) 1.670(3)	129.9(4)	[64]
2b-(Cr(CO)$_3$)	6.97	2.212(2)	1.651(3) 1.650(3)	133.6(2)	[64]
2b-(MnCl$_2$)	par	2.1843(14)	1.6671(17) 1.6636(17)	127.70(9)	[64]
2b-(CoCl$_2$)	par	2.015(6)	1.680(7) 1.661(7)	127.5(3)	[64]
2b-[Mo$_2$(CO)$_7$]	9.49	2.355(4)	1.722(4) 1.724(4)	120.4(2)	[64]
[**2b**-(PdCl)]Cl	31.6	2.004(4)	1.689(4) 1.676(4)	132.4	[64]
2b-[Ni$_2$(CO)$_4$]	34.20	2.0635(18) 2.0912(18)	1.7142(18) 1.7146(18)	nr	[64]
2b-(Cu$_2$Cl$_2$)	21.4	nr	1.714(3) 1.718(2)	121.51(14)	[63]
2b-(Cu$_2$I$_2$)	21.5	nr	1.679(5) 1.702(5)	128.5(3)	[63]
[**2b**-Cu$_2$(PPh$_3$)$_2$](PF$_6$)$_2$	32.9	nr	1.709(10) 1.693(9)	126.8(6)	[63]
2b-Cu$_2$(PC$_6$H$_4$OMe)$_2$](PF$_6$)$_2$	32.8	nr	1.707(3) 1.710(3)	123.64(18)	[63]
[**2b**-Cu$_2$(DPEPhos)](PF$_6$)$_2$	29.7	nr	1.710(4)	124.0(2)	[63]
[**2b**-Cu$_2$(XantPhos)](PF$_6$)$_2$	34.9	nr	1.712(4)		[63]
[**2b**-Cu$_2$(dppf)](PF$_6$)$_2$	36.5	nr	1.7064(19) 1.7211(18)	122.10(11)	[63]
2b-Cu$_2$(SC$_6$F$_5$)$_2$	23.1	nr	1.730(6) 1.717(6) 1.710(3)	121.8(4) 123.70(17)	[63]
2b-Cu$_2$(Carb)$_2$	22.8	nr	1.710(3) 1.726(2) 1.728(2)	120.45(15)	[63]
	Transition metal complex with **2cH**				
2cH-(CuPPh$_3$)	23.6	2.196(3)	1.761(3) 1.777(3)	124.26(17)	[63]

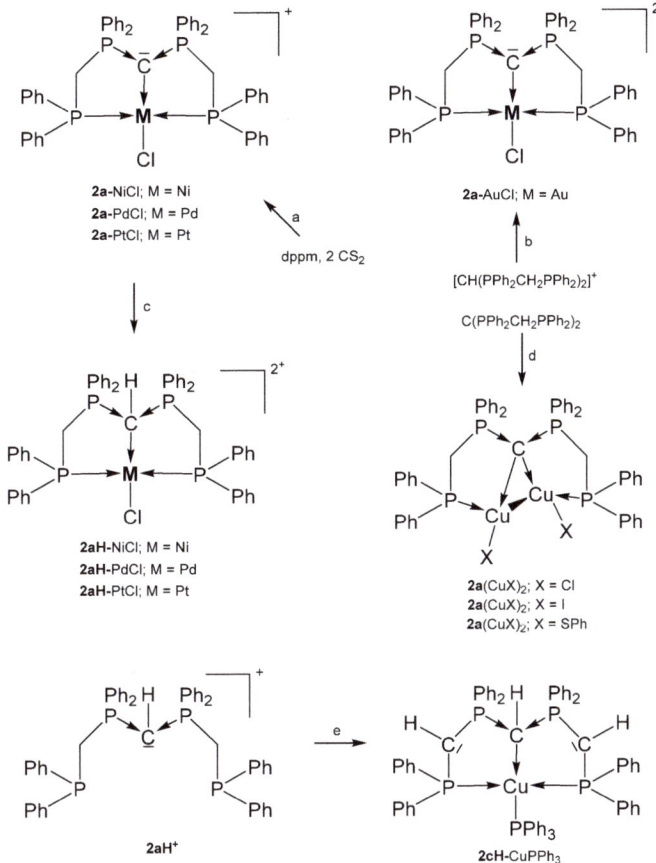

Scheme 6. Selected compounds with the pincer ligands **2a** and **2aH**. (**a**) MCl$_2$ with a mixture of dppm and 2 eq. of CS$_2$, (**b**) AuCl(tht)/HNO$_3$, (**c**) HCl. (**d**) two eq. of CuX. (**e**) 2 ^{n}BuLi, [Cu(NCMe)$_4$]PF$_6$/PPh$_3$.

A series of complexes with the N,C,N pincer ligand *sym*-bis(2-pyridyl) tetraphenylcarbodiphosphorane (**2b**) were reported recently by the group of Sundermeyer. Remarkable is the molybdenum complex **2b**-[Mo$_2$(CO)$_7$] in which **2b** provides four pairs of electrons for donation to a Mo$_2$ unit with an Mo-Mo separation of 3.0456(5) Å [64]. This coordination mode is continued in a series of dicopper complexes presented by the same working group and prepared as depicted in Scheme 7. The addition of [Cu]PF$_6$ to **2b** followed by treatment with two eq. of PR$_3$ generated the cationic complexes [**2b**-(CuPPh$_3$)](PF$_6$)$_2$ and [**2b**-(CuP{C$_6$H$_4$OMe}$_3$)](PF$_6$)$_2$, respectively; **2b**-(CuCarb)$_2$ was obtained from **2b**-(CuCl)$_2$ and two eq. of CarbH/NaO^{t}Bu (CarbH = carbazol) [63].

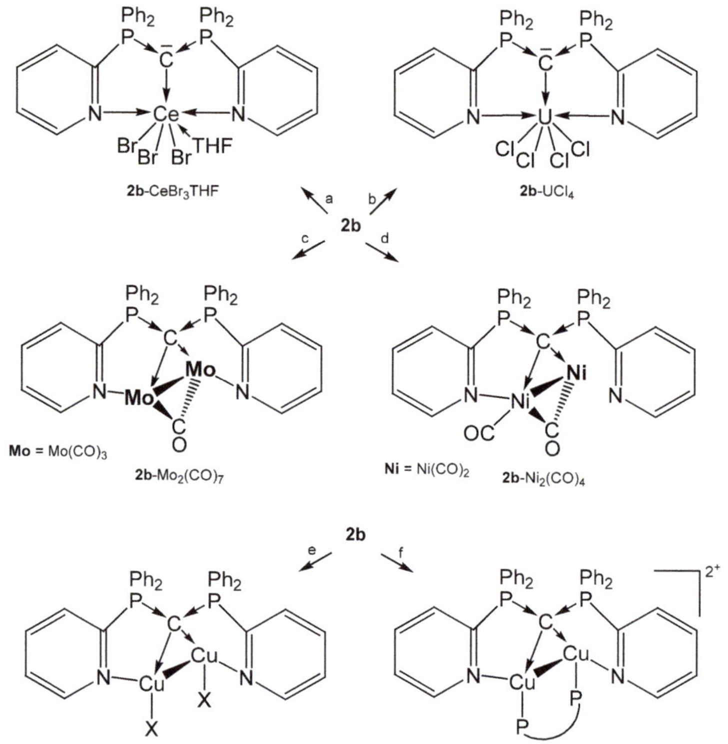

Scheme 7. Selected compounds with the pincer ligand **2b** as two and four electron donor. (**a**) CeBr$_3$ in THF, (**b**) UCl$_4$, (**c**) 2 eq. of Mo(CO)$_3$(NCMe)$_3$, (**d**) 2 eq. of Ni(CO)$_4$, (**e**) 2 eq. of CuX, (**f**) 2 eq. of [Cu]PF$_6$/1 eq. of P-P.

For the cationic complexes [**2b**-Cu$_2$(P-P)]$^{2+}$ the chelating ligands are: DPEPhos = bis[(2-diphenylphosphino)phenyl] ether, XantPhos = 4,5-bis(diphenylphosphino)-9,9-dimethylxanthene, dppf = 1,10-bis(diphenyl-phosphino)ferrocene. The germinal nature of both Cu(I) centers leads to Cu-Cu distances in the range of 2.55–2.67 Å. Most of the Cu(I) complexes show photoluminescence upon irradiation with UV light at room temperature [63].

Further, **2cH**-CuPPh$_3$ is an example of a complex with a deprotonated form of **2a** and longer P-C distances are observed due to the protonation of the central carbon atom [63].

2.3. Transition Metal Addition Compounds of Carbones C(PR$_3$)$_2$ with an Additional Ortho Metallated Pincer Function

The source for the Rh complex **3a**-Rh(PMe$_3$)$_2$H was the half pincer compound **5a**-Rh(C$_6$H$_8$) (vide infra) upon reacting with PMe$_3$ under loss of cod (see Scheme 8). **3a**-Pt(SMe$_2$) forms upon reacting **1a** with [Me$_2$Pt(SMe$_2$)]$_2$ and loss of 4 molecules of CH$_4$ [69]. PEt$_3$ replaces the labile bonded SMe$_2$ group of **3a**-Pt(SMe$_2$) to produce **3a**-PtEt$_3$, which is transformed with P(OPh)$_3$ into **3a**-Pt(OPh)$_3$. The dication [**3a**-PtEt$_3$(µ-Ag$_2$)Et$_3$PPt-**3a**]$^{2+}$ was obtained upon addition of AgOTf to **3a**-PtEt$_3$. According to the carbone C atom as four electron donor the Pt complexes with µ-Ag functions show long Pt-C distances between 1.737 and 1.749 Å (mean values) and the ^{31}PNMR shifts are in the narrow range of 33 and 36 ppm (See Table 3) [70]. More complicated is the formation of **3a**-Pt(CO), which stems from the hydrolysis of the related **3a**-Pt(CCl$_2$) complex (not isolated) [71].

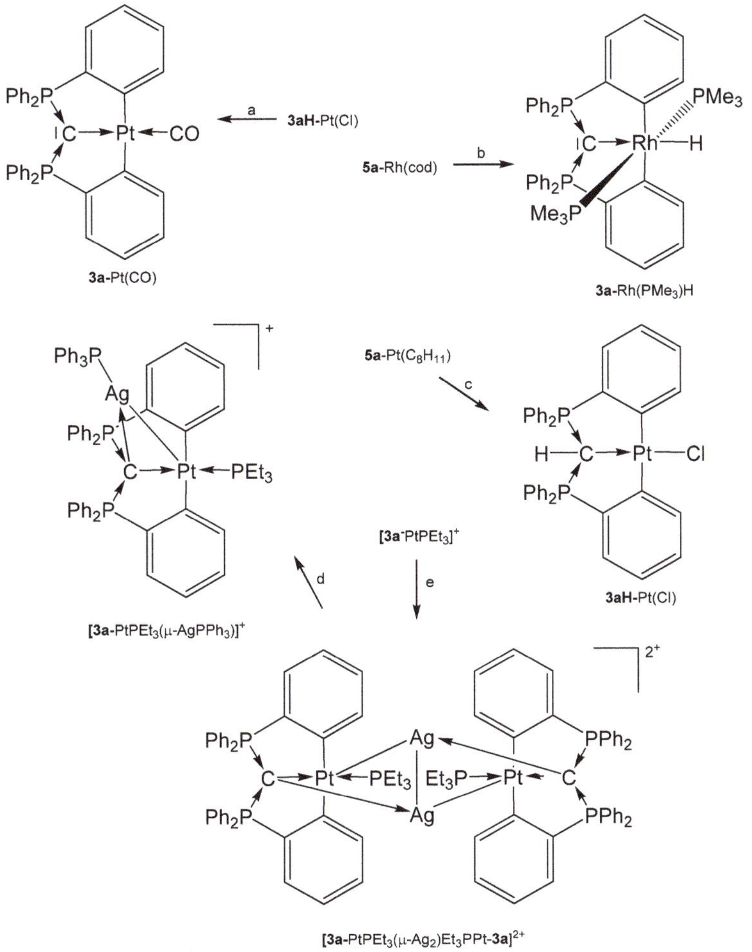

Scheme 8. Selected addition compounds with the pincer ligand 3a and 3aH and those with the Ag-bridged cations or dication, respectively. (a) from 3aH-PtCl via 3a-Pt(CCl$_2$) and H$_2$O, (b) PMe$_3$, (c) from 5a-Pt(C$_8$H$_{11}$) (see Scheme 11) and CHCl$_3$, (d) PPh$_3$, (e) 2 AgOTf.

Table 3. Transition metal complexes with ortho metallated tripodal pincer ligand **3a** derived from **1a** and the related pincer ligand **3b** and ^{31}P NMR shifts.

3-M	^{31}P NMR	C-M	P-C	P-C-P	Ref
Transition metal complexes with the tripodal ligand **3a**					
3a-Rh(PMe$_3$)$_2$H	8.56	2.203(3)	1.674(3)	138.32(18)	[69]
3a-PtSMe$_2$	30.42	nr	nr	nr	[69]
3a-PtCO	41.5	2.037(5)	1.706(3)	128.4(3)	[71]
3a-PtPEt$_3$	28.5	2.067(2)	1.697(2)	124.88(14)	[70]
3a-PtP(OPh)$_3$	nr	nr	nr	nr	[70]
[3a-PtPEt$_3$(µ-AgPPh$_3$)$_3$](OTf)	32.5	2.130(4)	1.737	126.0(2)	[70]
[3a-PtP(OPh)$_3$(µ-AgPEt$_3$)](OTf)	36.0	2.105(3)	1.743	122.9(2)	[70]
[3a-PtPEt$_3$(µ-Ag$_2$)Et$_3$PPt-3a](OTf)$_2$	33.4	2.128(3)	1.749	125.29(18)	[70]
3aH-PtCl	27.9	2.077(6)	1.796(6)	123.4(4)	[71]
Transition metal complexes with the tripodal ligand **3b**					
3b-Pt(CO)	46.9	2.002(5)	nr	133.3(3)	[72]

The carbone complex **3b**-Pt(CO) was obtained from reacting the yldiide platinum complex (see Scheme 9) with 1 atm CO that inserts into the N-Si bond of the yldiide.

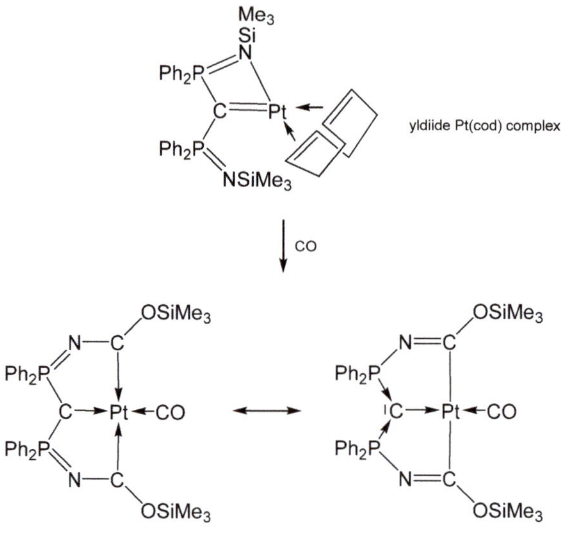

Scheme 9. Two mesomeric forms of **3b**-Pt(CO); **3ba** favors a tricarbene coordination at Pt(0) whereas **3bb** is consistent Pt(II) forming two C-Pt s-bonds similar to **3a**-Pt(CO). The short central C-Pt bond length of 2.002 Å indicates a partial doubly donation of the carbone C atom as shown in Figure 5. The planar environment at Pt is typical for Pt(II) and supports this view [72].

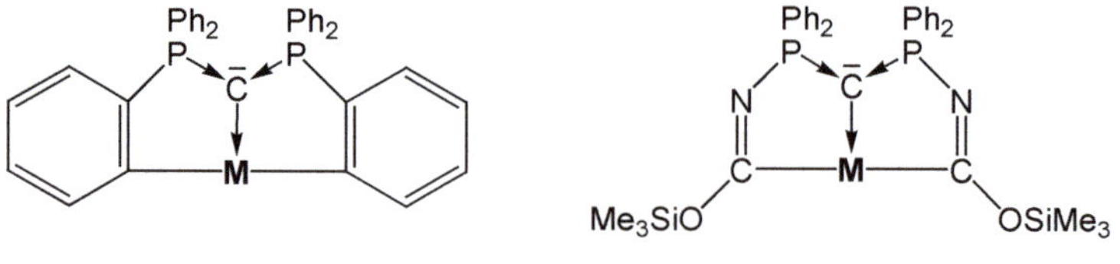

Figure 5. Bis-ortho metallated pincer complexes **3a** and **3b**.

2.4. Transition Metal Complexes with P-C-P Five Membered Ring

The carbone **4** (see Figure 6) was obtained by deprotonation of the cation [**4H**]$^+$. According to two P atoms in different chemical environments two doublets in the ^{31}P NMR spectrum were recorded at δ = 60.0 and 71.5 ppm; $^2J_{PP}$ = 153 Hz. From X-ray determination stem the P-C(1) and P-C(2) distances of 1.644(19) and 1.657(17) Å, respectively, and the P-C-P angle amounts to 104.82(10)° [73]. The bond lengths (see Table 4) are close to that reported for the carbone **1a**.

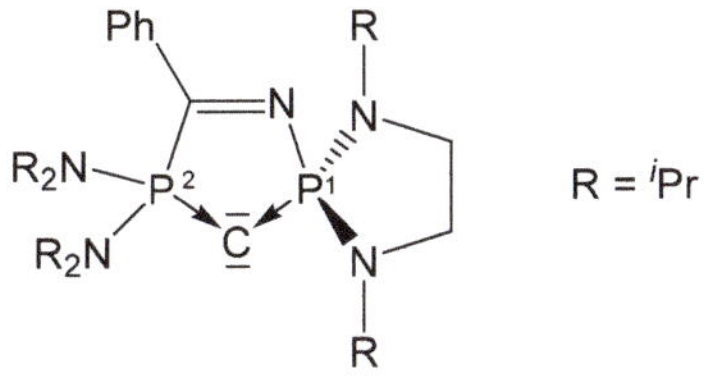

Figure 6. Structure of compound **4**.

Table 4. Transition metal complexes with the cyclic carbone **4**, containing ^{31}P NMR shifts and relevant structural parameters.

4-M	^{31}P NMR	M-C	P^1-C P^2-C	P-C-P	Ref
4-PdCl(π-C3H5)	61.2 71.9 (225)	2.120(2)	1.673(2) 1.694(2)	106.66(13)	[73]
4-RhCl(nbd)	64.6 75.7 (230)	2.115(18)	1.676(18) 1.702(18)	106.86(10)	[73]
4-Rh(CO)2Cl	68.2 75.6 (224)	nr	nr	nr	[73]
4-AuOBut	64.1 60.4 (225)	2.018(6)	1.674(7) 1.687(7)	108.5(4)	[74]
4-CuOBut	69.8 62.6 (195)	1.8923(15)	1.6763(15) 1.6887(15)	106.90(8)	[74]
4-CuCl	63.2 70.6 (186)	1.8914(19)	1.6700(19) 1.6869(19)	107.20(11)	[74]

From the cyclic and asymmetric carbone **4** six transition metal complexes (see Scheme 10) are known in which the ligand acts as two electron donor via the C atom. As in the starting compound **4** the P^2-C bond distances are slightly longer than P^1-C bond. Addition of CuCl and AuCl(SMe$_2$) to **4H$^+$**/*t*BuOK generates the compounds **4-CuO*t*Bu** and **4-AuO*t*Bu**, respectively. In CH$_3$Cl$_2$ or CHCl$_3$ **4-CuO*t*Bu** is converted into **4-CuCl** [74]. **4-Rh(CO)$_2$Cl** stems from the reaction of **4** with [{RhCl(CO)$_2$}$_2$] [73]. **4-CuO*t*Bu** and **4-AuO*t*Bu** catalyze the hydroamination or hydroalkoxylation of acrylonitrile [74].

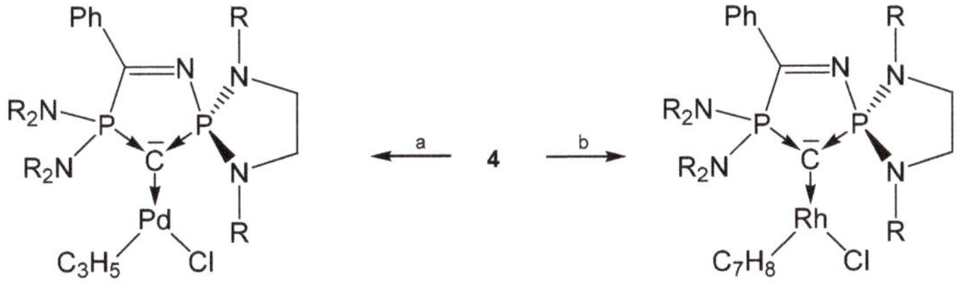

Scheme 10. Selected complexes with the cyclic carbone **4**. R = ^{i}Pr. a) [{PdCl(allyl)}$_2$], b) [{RhCl(nbd)}$_2$].

2.5. Transition Metal Complexes with Asymmetric P-C-P Ligands

Several asymmetric carbones with orthometallation (**5a-M**, **5d-M**), with an additional donor function (**5c**), or with a functionalized phenyl ring (**5b**) were reported that form TM complexes (see Figure 7).

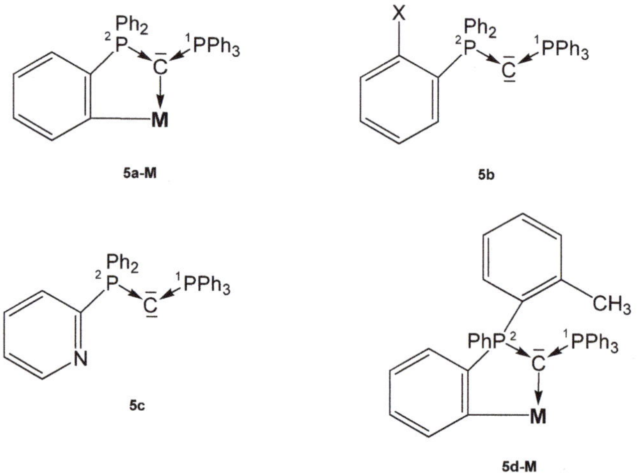

Figure 7. Structures of compounds **5a-M**, **5b**, **5c** and **5d-M**.

The neutral asymmetric carbone **5b** (X = PPh$_2$) has the structural parameters P^1-C = 1.642(2), P^2-C = 1.636(1) Å, and a P-C-P angle of 140.74(8)° (see Table 5); the P atoms resonate at δ = −6.9 and −3.4 ppm (^{2}J$_{PP}$ = 93 Hz) [75]. Those of **5c** are P^1-C = 1.6416(16) Å, P^2-C = 1.6398(17) Å, and P-C-P = 133.25(10)° [76]. Three complexes in which the carbone **1a** is half-side orthometallated forming **5a-M** complexes are described [69,73,77].

Table 5. Transition metal complexes with the unsymmetrical carbones **5a–5d**; ^{31}P NMR shifts in ppm.

5-M	^{31}P NMR (^{2}J$_{PP}$)	M-C	P^1-C P^2-C	P-C-P	Ref.
	Transition metal complexes of **5a-M**				
5a-Ptcod(C$_8$H$_{11}$)	14.9 5.7 (59.8)	2.072(3)	1.694(4) 1.716(4)	114.8(2)	[77]
5a-Rhcod(p)	10.15 12.40 (50.9)	2.165(2)	1.693(2) 1.692(2)	124.50(13)	[69]
5a-PdC$_3$H$_5$	39.8 9.9 (54)	nr	nr	nr	[73]
	Transition metal complexes with the carbone **5b**				
5b-AuCl (X = PPh$_2$)	8.6 18.7 (52)	2.043	1.701(4) 1.696(2)	126.0(2)	[75]
5b-AuCl (X = PPh$_2$-AuCl)	25.6 20.2 (47)	2.037(3)	1.690(3) 1.689(3)	131.4(2)	[75]
5b-(AuCl)$_2$ (X = PPh$_2$-AuCl)	25.4 26.9	2.089 2.064	1.774(5) 1.763(5)	123.6(3)	[75]
5b-PtMe$_2$ (X = Me)	19.3	nr	nr	nr	[78]
	Transition metal complexes with the carbone **5c**				
5c-UCl$_4$	par	2.461(5)	1.699(5) 1.711(5)	120.6(3)	[41]
[**5c**AuPPh$_3$)]$^+$	19.70 15.03 (30.7)	2.067(9)	1.688(9) 1.707(9)	124.3(5)	[76]
[**5c**(CuCl)(AuPPh$_3$)]$^+$	39.7 26.2 (m)	2.111(4) Au 1.981(5) Cu	1.732(5) 1.750(5)	120.2(3)	[76]
[**5c**(AuCl)(AuPPh$_3$)]$^+$	35.4 27.5 (m)	2.080(9) Au^2 2.127(8) Au^1	1.756(9)	119.3(5)	[76]
	Transition metal complexes with the carbone **5d-M**				
5d-Pt-**5d**	19.3	nr	nr	nr	[78]

As depicted in Scheme 11, three neutral complexes of **1a** are known in which one of its phenyl group is orthometallated to produce the **5a-M** core. The ^{31}P NMR shift of the unchanged PPh$_3$ group range between about 6 and 13 ppm whereas for the orthometallated side shifts between 15 and 40 ppm where recorded. Both P-C distances do not differ markedly and amount to about 1.700 Å.

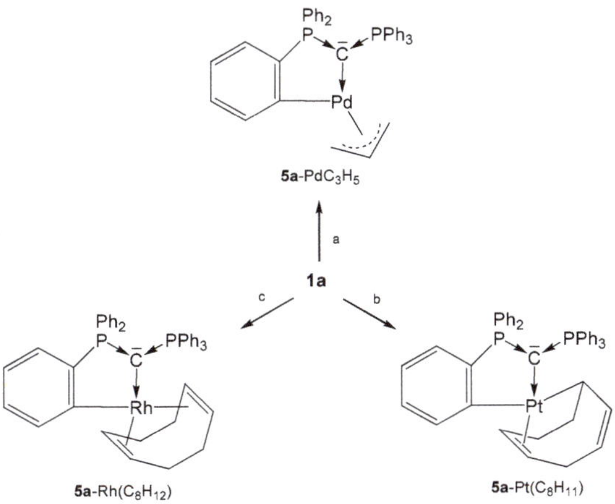

Scheme 11. Selected structures of transition metal complexes with the carbone **5a**; (a) $\frac{1}{2}$ [PdCl(allyl)]; (b) 1/3 [PtI$_2$(cod)]; (c) $\frac{1}{4}$ [RhCl(cod)]. All complexes are formed upon release of the cation [**1aH**]$^+$.

All complexes shown in Scheme 12 have a further PPh$_2$ function at the ortho position of one phenyl group of **1a**. In the complex **5b**-(AuCl)$_2$ the carbone provides four electrons for donation with typical long P-C distances of about 1.770 Å [75].

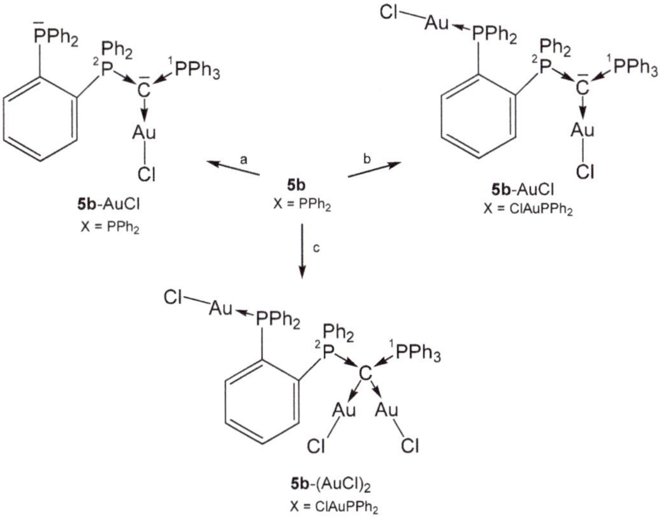

Scheme 12. Selected structures of transition metal complexes with the carbone **5b**. (a) [AuCl(tht)], (b) 2 [AuCl(tht), 3 [AuCl(tht)].

The paramagnetic **5c**-UCl$_4$ exhibits a short C-U distance indicative for a double dative bond of the carbone C atom as in **2b**-UCl$_4$ and was obtained by reacting UCl$_4$ with the dication **5c**-H$_2$/NaHMDS. Upon further coordination of the pyridyl group (U-N = 2.537(4) Å) the U atom attains the coordination number 6 [41].

[**5c**-AuPPh$_3$]$^+$ was obtained from reacting the carbone **5c** with [PPh$_3$AuCl]/Na[SbCl$_6$] (see Scheme 13). In the cationic complex [**5c**-(CuCl)((AuPPh$_3$)]SbF$_6$, the carbone **5c** acts as a six-electron donor with a Cu-N distance of 2.267(6) Å and Cu-Au separation of 2.8483(10) Å. The Cu and Cl atoms are each disordered over two positions with occupancy of about 0.8 to 0.2. If CuCl is replaced by AuCl as in [**5c**-(AuCl)(AuPPh$_3$)]SbF$_6$ the C-AuPPh$_3$ distance is slightly elongated and no coordination of the pyridyl N atom is observed. The Au-Au separation is with 3.1274(6) Å too long for a metallophilic interaction. In both compounds, the carbone C atom constitutes a chiral center according to four chemical different substituents and acts as a four-electron donor. The PPh$_3$ group resonates between 15 and 27 ppm [76]. In the related symmetric pyridyl-free complex **1a**-(AuCl)$_2$, slightly shorter C-Au (2.076(3) Å) were recorded accompanied by longer P-C (1.776(3) Å) bond lengths [51].

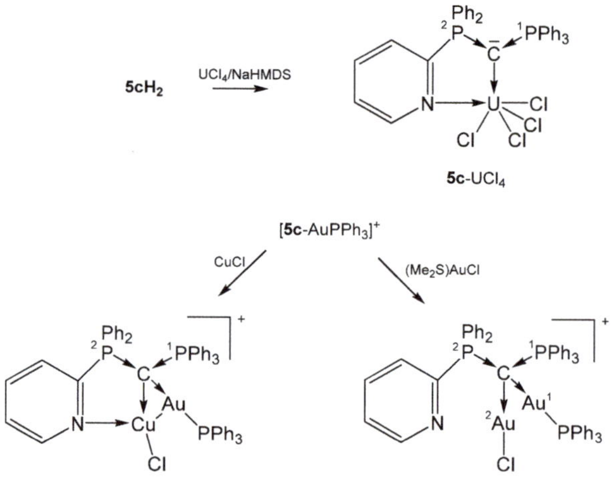

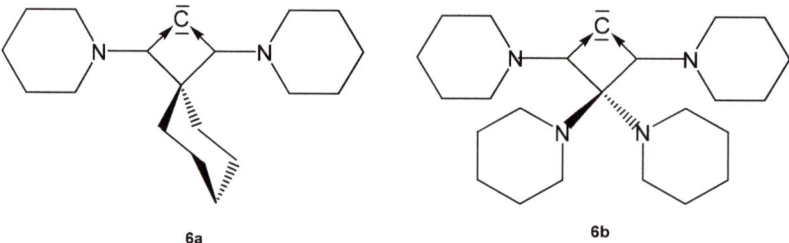

Scheme 13. Selected structures of transition metal complexes with the mono pyridyl substituted carbone **5c**.

2.6. Transition Metal Complexes of Carbones with Cyclobutadiene

The carbones **6a** and **6b** (see Figure 8) can also be seen as an all-carbon four-membered ring bent allene (CBA); **6a** is stable for several hours at −20° but decomposes when warmed up to −5°. The optimized geometry reveals a very acute allene bond angle of 85.0° and coplanarity of the ring carbon atoms including the two nitrogen atoms. The C=C bonds of the allene fragment amount to 1.423 Å and are significantly longer than in typical linear allenes (1.31 Å). Short CN bonds of 1.36 Å indicate some double bond character. The CCC carbon atom resonates in the ^{13}C NMR spectrum at 151 ppm. The first and second proton affinities (PAs) are very high amounting to 307 and 152 kcal/mol [79].

Figure 8. Structures of compounds **6a** and **6b**.

The molecular orbitals show that the HOMO and HOMO-1 have clearly the largest coefficients at the central carbon atom and exhibit the typical shape of lone-pair molecular orbitals with σ (HOMO) and π (HOMO-1) symmetry; however, with reversed order with respect to CDPs and CDCs. To emphasize the proximity of **6** to CDP carbones, we use the same symbolism mimicking a metal.

The free CBA **6b** could not be obtained, but only the cationic **6bH$^+$** and **6bH$_2^{2+}$** are known and used as starting compounds for the syntheses of the related transition metal complexes [80].

The ^{13}C NMR shifts of the central carbon atom are shifted to higher fields relative to the starting free carbone ranging between 124 and 139 ppm (see Table 6).

Table 6. Transition metal complexes with the all carbon ligand **6**; ^{13}C NMR shifts (in ppm) of the donating carbon atom. Distances in Å, angles in deg.

	^{13}C NMR	C-M	C-C	C-C-C	Ref.
Transition metal complexes with the carbone **6a**					
6a-RhCl(cod)	136.6	2.038(5)	1.405(6)	88.4(3)	[79]
6a-IrCl(cod)	138.6	nr	nr	nr	[79]
6a-RhCl(CO)$_2$	124.7	nr	nr	nr	[79]
6a-IrCl(CO)$_2$	129.2	nr	nr	nr	[79]
Transition metal complexes with the carbone **6b**					
6b-W(CO)$_5$	130.1	2.319(3)	1.419(4)	88.0(2)	[80]
6b-AuCl	123.6	2.001(4)	1.409(5)	90.5(3)	[80]
6b-RhCl(CO)$_2$	131.2	2.0602(14)	1.4102(19)	89.73(11)	[80]

All complexes of the CBA **6a** where obtained by reacting the freshly prepared free carbone **6a** at −20° with [{MCl(cod)}$_2$] complexes (M = Rh, Ir). The cod ligand can be replaced by bubbling CO through solutions of **6a**-MCl(cod) to produce the related **6a**-MCl(CO)$_2$ compounds (see Scheme 14) [79].

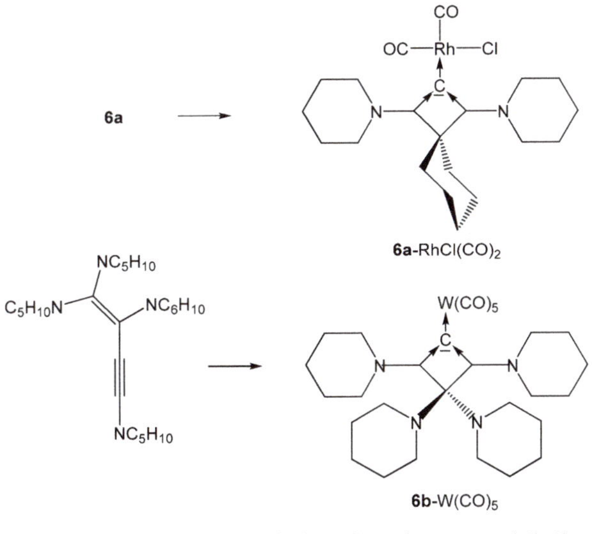

Scheme 14. Selected structures of complexes with the cyclic carbones **6a** and **6b**. Preparation see text.

Transition metal complexes with **6b** as ligand were obtained by reacting 1,1,2,4-tetrapiperidino-1-buten-3-yne with (a) [(tht)AuCl], (b) [RhCl(CO)$_2$]$_2$, and (c) [(NMe$_3$)W(CO)$_5$] during the reaction rearrangement of the starting buten-3-yne to **6b** has occurred [80].

2.7. Carbodicyclopropenylidene

Stephan described the first carbodicarbene stabilized by flanking cyclopropylidenes, named carbodicyclopropylidene **7** (see Figure 9) [81].

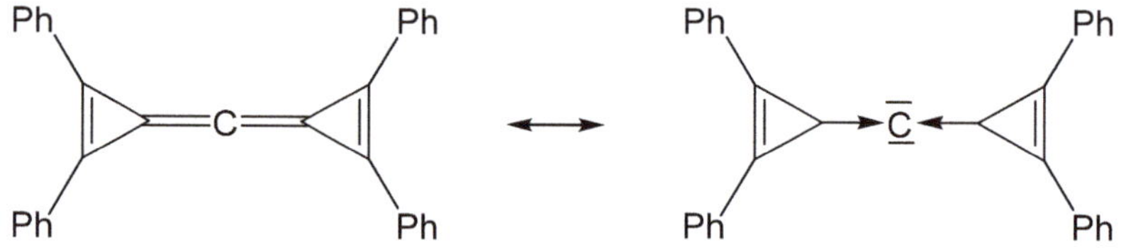

Figure 9. Possible description of the bonding in the carbone **7**.

Neither the neutral singlet 1,2-diphenylcyclopropenylidene as carbene ligand L in **7** nor the carbone tetraphenylcarbodicyclopropenyliden (CDC) **7** itself are stable compounds at room temperature. The free carbene L has only been observed in an argon matrix isolated at 10 K and **7** could be characterized in solution by low temperature NMR spectroscopy; for the central carbon atom a ^{13}C NMR shift at δ = 133 ppm was recorded at −60 °C.

The first and second proton affinities of **7** were determined to be 283 and 153 kcal/mol, respectively. The molecular structure of **7** was determined by computational methods. Calculations reveal that the central carbon atom is in a linear environment the C-C distances were calculated at 1.308 Å and the C-C-C angle to 180°. The energy difference between the linear allenic structure and the bent arrangement is shallow amounting to 6.6 kcal/mol for a bending angle of 140° and 10 kcal/mol for 130°. The highest occupied molecular orbital (HOMO) and HOMO-1 of **7** are degenerate and incorporate the p(π) orbitals of the C2-C1-C2a fragment.

The central C atom is more negatively charged (−0.19 a.u.) than the adjacent C atoms, suggesting nucleophilic character [81].

The addition compounds [**7**-AuNHC-Ad](OTf) and [**7**-AuNHC-Dipp](OTf) (see Table 7) were prepared from reacting [**7H**]$^+$ with KHMDS and the related (NHC)AuOTf at −45°(see Scheme 15) [81].

Table 7. Complexes with the carbone **7**. ^{13}C NMR shifts (in ppm) of the donating carbon atom.

7-M	^{13}C NMR	M-C	C-C	C-C-C	Ref.
[7-AuNHC-Ad](OTf)	92.7	2.071(6) 2.047(6)	nr	nr	[81]
[7-AuNHC-Dipp](OTf)	98.0	nr	nr	nr	[81]

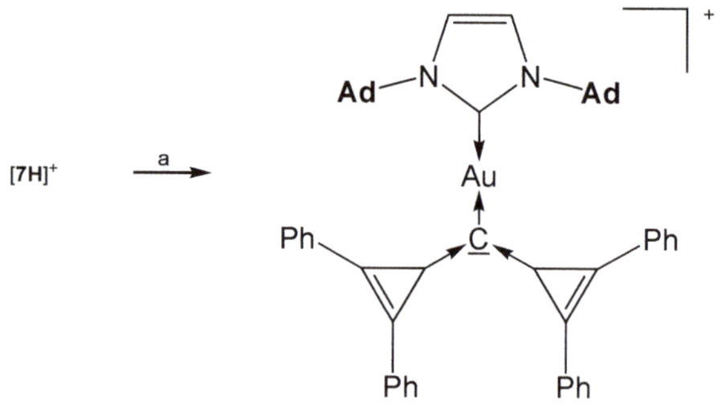

Scheme 15. Selected structures of complexes with the cyclo propylidene stabilized carbone **7**. (a) KHMDS/(NHC)AuOTf.

2.8. Carbodicarbenes

Carbodicarbenes, CDCs, are neutral compounds where a bare carbon atom with its four electrons is stabilized by two NHC ligands which plays the role of a phosphine group as in carbodiphosphoranes, CDPs. Theoretical studies have demonstrated that this class of compounds could be stable and their existence was predicted by Frenking [82] and short times later realized by the group of Bertrand [83].

Structural and spectroscopic parameters of the following symmetric CDCs (see Figure 10) are available: **8a**, C-C = 1.343(2) Å, C-C-C = 134.8(2)°, ^{13}C NMR 110.2 ppm [83]; **8b**, C-C = 1.333(2) Å and 1.324(2) Å, C-C-C = 143.61(15)° [84]; **8c**, C-C = 1.335(5) Å, C-C-C = 136.6(5)° (see Table 8) [85].

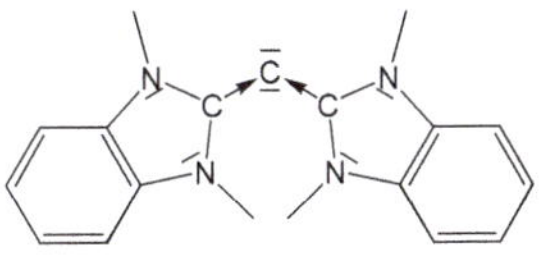

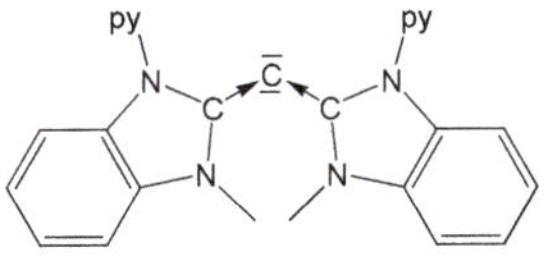

Figure 10. Symmetrical CDCs from which transition metal complexes are known.

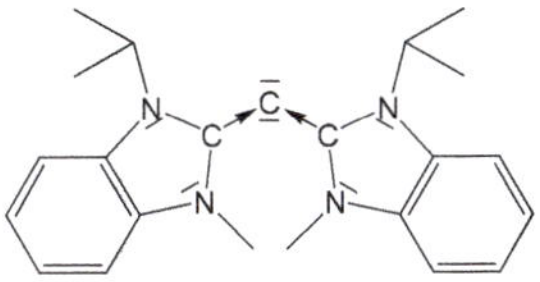

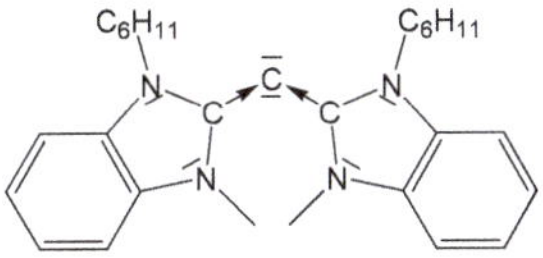

Table 8. Collection of transition metal complexes with the CDCs **8a–8h**. ^{13}C NMR shifts of the central carbon atom (in ppm).

	^{13}C NMR	M-C	C-C	C-C-C	Ref.
	Transition metal complexes with the CDC **8a**				
8a-RhCl(CO)$_2$	64.1	2.089(7)	1.398(10)	121.2(7)	[83]
8a-RuCl$_2$(=CHPh)NHC	73.01 mes	2.2069(18)	1.352(3) 1.429(3)	119.84(17)	[86]
8a-RuCl$_2$(=CHPh)NHC	73.4 ^{i}Pr	2.210(7)	1.345(11) 1.439(9)	116.9(6)	[86]
	Transition metal complexes with the CDC **8b**				
[**8b**-PdCl]$^+$	nr	1.973(3)	1.369(5) 1.398(5)	126.5(3)	[84]
[**8b**-Fe$_{0.5}$]$^{2+}$		2.018(3)	1.374(3)	128.4(3)	[87]
[**8b**-Fe$_{0.5}$]$^{3+}$		1.968(4)	1.387(6)	125.2(4)	[87]
[**8b**-Fe$_{0.5}$]$^{4+}$		1.928(3)	1.407(4)	125.4(2)	[87]
	Transition metal complexes with the CDC **8c**				
8c-PdClC$_3$H$_5$	nr	2.207(4)	1.404(5) 1.377(5)	119.7(4)	[85]
8c-RhCl(CO)$_2$	63.7	2.109(2)	1.411(3) 1.385(3)	117.4(2)	[85]
	Transition metal complexes with the CDC **8d**				
8d--RhCl(CO)$_2$		2.123(2)	1.416(3) 1.368(3)	116.8(2)	[85]
	Transition metal complexes with the asymmetric CDC **8e**				
8e-PdCl$_2$(POR)$_3$	nr	2.0398(18)	1.395(3) 1.328(3)	119.20(16)	[88]
8e-PdCl$_2$PPh$_3$	nr	2.063(2)	1.383(3) 1.409(3) tP	115.63(19)	[89]
8e-PdCl$_2$PTol$_3$	nr	2.049(4)	1.374(7) 1.412(8) tP	117.7(4)	[89]
8e-PdCl$_2$PCy$_3$	nr	2.111(2)	1.343(3) 1.415(4) tP	123.6(2)	[89]
	Transition metal complexes with the asymmetric CDC **8f**				
8f-RhCl(CO)$_2$	67.1	2.117(2)	1.369(3) 1.424(3)	117.8(2)	[90]
	Transition metal complexes with the asymmetric CDC **8g**				
8g-RhCl(CO)$_2$	63.2	2.1164(17)	1.374(2)$_{NHC}$ 1.420(3)	118.77(16)	[90]
	Transition metal complexes with the asymmetric CDC **8h**				
8h-IrCl(CO)$_2$	nr	nr	nr	nr	[91]
8h-IrCl(cod)	166.4	nr	nr	nr	[91]

Structural parameters of the unsymmetrical CDCs (see Figure 11) are: **8e**, C-C = 1.3401(16) Å and 1.3455(16), C-C-C 137.55(12)°. For **8f**, no data are available [90]. **8g**: C-C = 1.344(3) Å and, 1.318(3) Å, C-C-C = 146.11(19)° [90]. **8h** was obtained at −60° by reacting **8hH⁺** with KMDS, and characterized spectroscopically. On warming to room temperature, it dimerizes. ^{13}C NMR: δ = 105.5 ppm (see Table 8) [91].

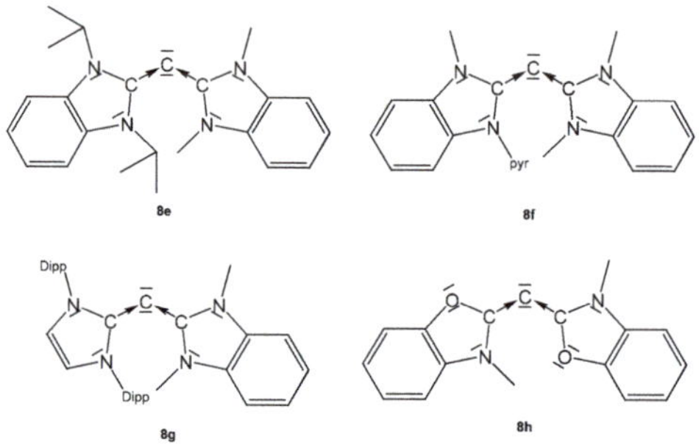

Figure 11. Unsymmetrical CDCs from which transition metal complexes are reported.

Further, **8a**-RhCl(CO)$_2$ was prepared by addition of a suspension of **8a** (see Scheme 16) in benzene to a solution of [RhCl(CO)$_2$]$_2$ [83]. [**8b**-Fe$_{0.5}$]$^{2+}$ contains Fe^{2+} in octahedral environment coordinated by two molecules of **8b**. Fe(II) can be successively oxidized to the corresponding tri-, tetra-, and pentacationic species [87].

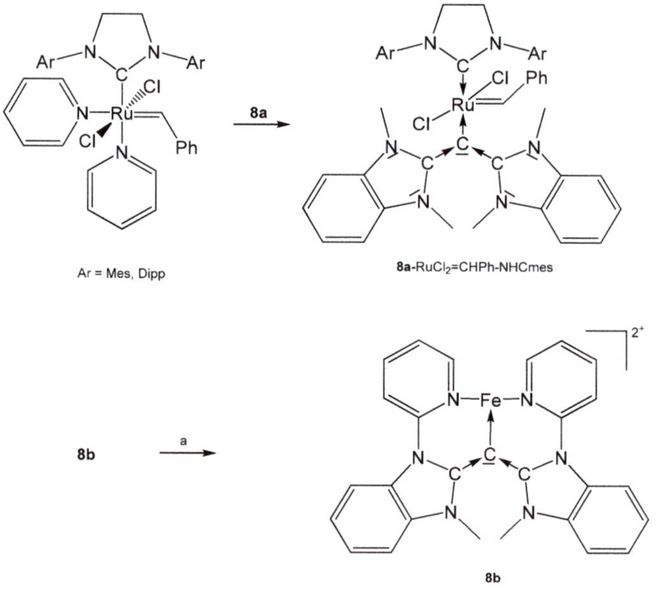

Scheme 16. Selected structures of transition metal complexes with symmetric CDCs **8a** and **8b**; (a) Fe(OTf)$_2$(MeCN)$_2$.

The addition compounds **8c**-RhCl(CO)$_2$ and **8d**-RhCl(CO)$_2$ where obtained upon reacting the appropriate carbone **8c** or **8d** with [RhCl(CO)$_2$]$_2$. Similarly, the addition of [Pd(allyl)Cl]$_2$ to **8c** leads to the allyl complex **8c**-PdCl(C$_3$H$_5$) [85].

As depicted in Scheme 17, introduction of PdCl$_2$P(OiPr)$_3$ to **8e** afforded the complex **8e**-PdCl$_2$P(OiPr)$_3$; it features a square planar Pd center with a short interatomic distance of one phosphite oxygen atom and the carbon atom of the NHC molecule of 2.890 Å that is smaller than the sum of van der Waals radii. This indicates strong attractive interaction between the atoms [88]. The three Pd complexes **8e**-PdCl$_2$PPh$_3$, **8e**-PdCl$_2$PTol$_3$, and **8e**-PdCl$_2$PCy$_3$ were obtained by reacting the carbone **8e** with the appropriate PdCl$_2$PR$_3$; between the NHC and the aromatic phosphine substituents (Ph or Tol) an unexpected π-π interaction was detected. One Ph and one Tol group are nearly parallel to the imidazole rings with centroid-centroid distances of 3.25 Å (Ph) and 3.30 Å (Tol), respectively [89].

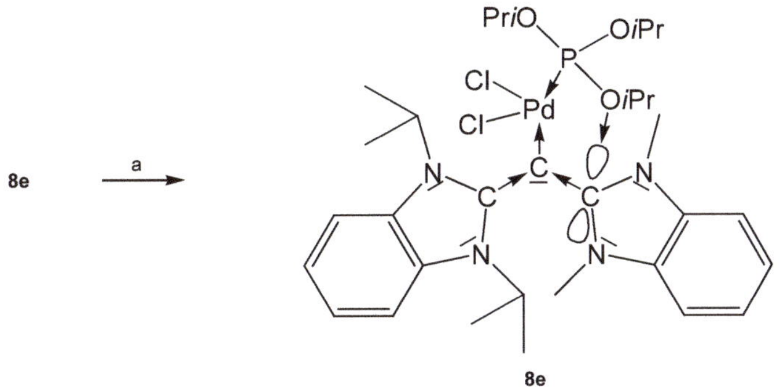

Scheme 17. Selected structural representation of **8e**-PdCl$_2$P(OiPr)$_3$ (a) PdCl$_2$P(OiPr)$_3$.

8f-RhCl(CO)$_2$ and **8g**-RhCl(CO)$_2$ stem from reacting the appropriate carbone with [RhCl(CO)$_2$]$_2$ [90]. The cod ligand of [Ir(cod)Cl]$_2$ was replaced by bubbling CO through a mixture with **8h** to generate the complex **8h**-IrCl(CO)$_2$ [91].

Some experimental findings indicate that carbodicarbenes also have catalytic properties for a wide range of transformations, which are currently being actively studied by several groups. Examples have been reported such as hydrogenation of inert olefins [92], C-C cross-coupling reactions [84], intermolecular hydroamination [93] and hydroheteroarylation [94]. It seems that this area is still in an infant stadium and it can be expected that CDCs may be found useful as catalyst for other reactions.

2.9. Tridentate Cyclic Diphosphino CDCs

The carbones **9a** and **9b** in Figure 12 are functionalized carbodicarbene in which the donating carbon atom is part of a seven membered ring.

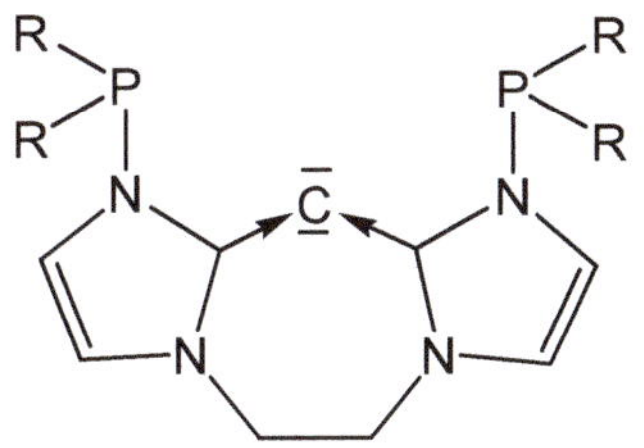

9a, R = Ph
9b, R = ^{i}Pr

Figure 12. Hypothetical free carbones **9a** and **9b**.

The neutral **9a** and **9b** could not be isolated, source for transition metal complexes are the related cations **9aH$^+$** and **9bH$^+$** (see Table 9) [93].

Table 9. Transition metal complexes with the carbones **9a** and **9b**; ^{13}C NMR signal of the central donating carbon atom.

9-M	^{13}C NMR	M-C	C-C	C-C-C	Ref.
Transition metal complexes with the carbone **9a**					
9a-RhCl	73.0	nr	nr	nr	[93]
[**9a**-RhNCMe]$^+$	nr	2.043	1.398 1.387	nr	[93]
[**9a**-Rh(CO)]BF$_4$	nr	nr	nr	nr	[93]
[**9a**-Rh(styrene)]BF$_4$	nr	2.075(2)	1.404(3) 1.391(3)	121.7(2)	[94]
[**9aH**-Rh(CO)](BF$_4$)$_2$	nr	nr	nr	nr	[94]
Transition metal complexes with the carbone **9b**					
9b-RhCl	73.4	nr	nr	nr	[93]
[**9b**-RhNCMe]BF$_4$	nr	nr	nr	nr	[93]
[**9b**-Rh(CO)]BF$_4$	nr	nr	nr	nr	[93]

The neutral complexes **9a**-RhCl and **9b**-RhCl (see Scheme 18) where prepared upon reacting the cations **9aH**$^+$ or **9bH**$^+$, respectively with [Rh(cod)Cl]$_2$/NaOMe; if treated with AgBF$_4$/MeCN the cationic spezies [**9a**-Rh(MeCN)]BF$_4$ and [**9b**-Rh(MeCN)]BF$_4$, respectively, were isolated. The related carbonyl complexes [**9a**-Rh(CO)]BF$_4$ and [**9b**-Rh(CO)]BF$_4$ formed similarly upon reaction with [Rh(CO)$_2$Cl]$_2$/NaOMe [93]. The styrene complex [**9a**-Rh(styrene)]$^+$ was obtained upon treating the related chloro complex with styrene/NaBAr$_4$; the styrene complex catalyzes the hydroarylation of dienes. Protonation of [**9a**-Rh(CO)]$^+$ with HBF$_4$·OEt$_2$ generates [**9aH**-Rh(CO)]$^{2+}$ in which the carbone acts as four-electron donor [94].

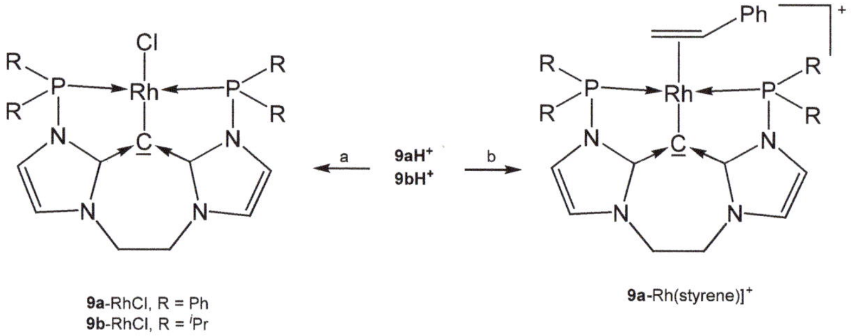

Scheme 18. Selected structures of transition metal complexes with the carbones **9a** and **9b**. (**a**) [Rh(cod)Cl]$_2$/NaOMe, (**b**) **9a**-RhCl/styrene/NaBF$_4$.

2.10. Tetraaminoallene (TAA) Transition Metal Complexes

The ^{13}C NMR shift of the central carbon atom amounts to 142.8 ppm. The first and second PAs of **10** are 282.5 and 151.6 kcal/mol, respectively [16,82].

The salt [**10**-AuPPh$_3$]SbF$_6$ in Scheme 19 is the only transition metal complex of TAA (see Figure 13), which has been reported so far. Both carbene moieties are planar, but are tilted relative to each other, to relieve allylic strain. The Au-C bond lengths amounts to 2.072(3) Å and the slightly different C-C dative bonds has interatomic distances of 1.406(5) and 1.424(5) Å. The central C-C-C bond angle is reported with 118.5(3)° [95].

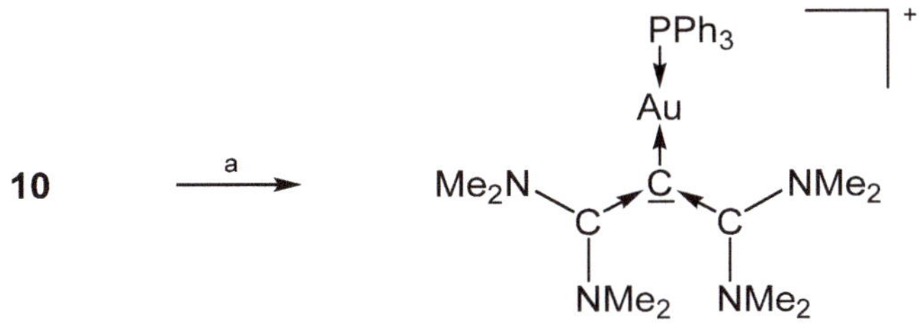

Scheme 19. Preparation of [**10**-AuPPh$_3$]SbF$_6$; a) AuClPPh$_3$/NaSbF$_6$.

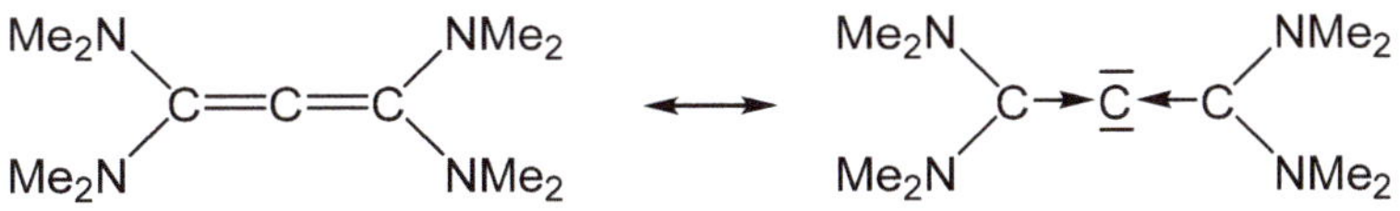

Figure 13. Bonding description of tetraaminoallene (TAA) (**10**). TAA's may have a bent geometry with hidden or masked pairs of electrons, which are delocalized but serve as double donor orbitals in complexes with CO$_2$ and CS$_2$ [96].

2.11. Transition Metal Complexes of Carbones with the P-C-C Skeleton

Mixed carbene-phosphine stabilized carbones from the working group of Bestmann (1974) and Alkarazo (2009).

The crystal structure of **11a** in Figure 14 reveals a planar configuration of the carbene ligand C(OEt)$_2$. Short P-C and C-C distances indicate some p back donation; P-C = 1.682(4)Å, C-C = 1.316(10) Å, C-C-C 125.6° (see Table 10) [97].

Figure 14. In compounds **11** the C(0) atoms are stabilized by a phophine or a carbene ligand.

Table 10. Transition metal complexes with the mixed carbones **11a** and **11b**. ^{31}P NMR shifts in ppm.

11-M	^{31}P NMR	M-C	P-C C-C	P-C-C	Ref.
	Transition metal complexes with the carbone **11a**				
11a-RhCl(CO)$_2$	25.1	nr	nr	nr	[98]
11a-AuCl	26.7	2.014(16)	1.7449(16) 1.362(2)	114.30(12)	[98]
11a-(AuCl)$_2$	28.1	2.081(4) 2.103(4)	1.785(4) 1.425(6)	114.2(3)	[98]
	Transition metal complexes with the carbone **11b**				
11b-AuCl	22.2	nr	nr	nr	[98]

The neutral Rh complex **11a**-RhCl(CO)$_2$ was obtained from reacting the carbone **11a** with [Rh(CO)$_2$Cl]$_2$. Similarly, the complex **11b**-AuCl results from reaction of **11b** with AuCl(SMe$_2$) (Scheme 20) [98].

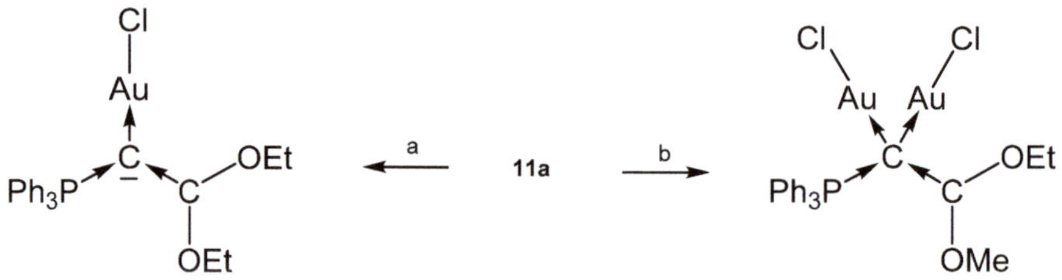

Scheme 20. Selected structural representation of transition metal complexes of **11a**. (**a**) one equiv. of AuCl(SMe$_2$), (**b**) two equiv. of AuCl(SMe$_2$).

2.12. Transition Metal Complexes of Carbones with the P-C-Si Skeleton

The neutral compound **12** in Figure 15 is a carbone in which the C(0) atom is stabilized by a donor stabilized silylene and a phosphine ligand.

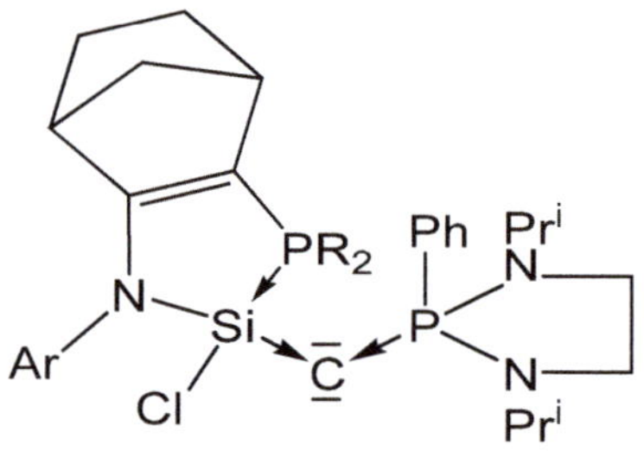

Figure 15. Carbone complex reported by Kato et al. [99].

The crystal structure of a related compound to **12** (a cyclopentene instead of a cyclohexene ring) shows a P-C distance of 1.6226(4) Å and Si-C distance of 1.6844(4) Å; the Si-C-P angle amounts to 140.03(3)°.

Addition of CuCl generates the complex **12**-CuCl. No spectroscopic or structural details are available [99].

2.13. Transition Metal Complexes of Carbones with the P-C-S Skeleton

A series of carbones (**13a**, **13b**) in Figure 16 based on a P-C-S core containing the neutral S(IV) ligands SPh$_2$=NMe (Figure 16) were reported by Fujii [100].

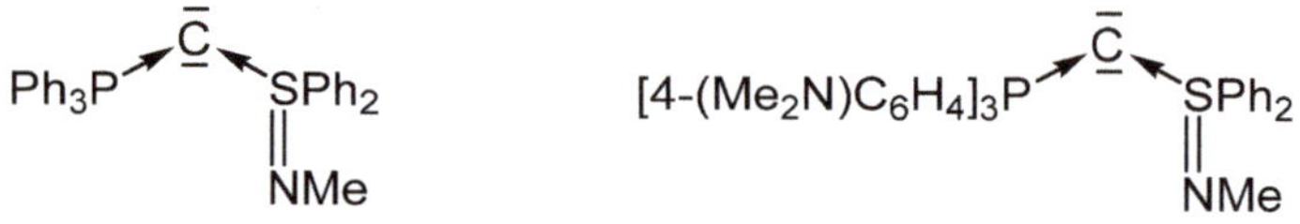

Figure 16. Carbone complexes reported by Fujii et al. [100].

Crystal structures and ^{31}P NMR shifts of the following basic carbones are available (see Table 11): **13a**, δ = −2.64 ppm; **13b**, δ = −1.39 ppm, P-C = 1.663(2) Å, S-C = 1.602(2) Å, P-C-S = 125.59(15)°. The authors revealed a high electron density at the central carbon atom.

Table 11. Collection of transition metal complexes with the carbones **13a** and **13b**. ^{31}P NMR signals (in ppm) are given.

13-M	^{31}P NMR	M-C	P-C S-C	P-C-S	Ref
Transition metal complexes with the carbone **13a** based on a P-C-S core					
13a-AgCl	10.8	2.131	1.711 1.648	121.9	[100]
[**13a**-AuPPh₃](OTf)	15.2	nr	nr	nr	[100]
[**13a**-(AuPPh₃)₂](OTf)₂	29.7	nr	nr	nr	[100]
Transition metal complexes with the carbone **13b** based on a P-C-S core					
13b-AgCl	9.13	2.098	1.728 1.636	119.1	[100]
[**13b**-AuPPh₃](SbF₆)	12.88	nr	nr	nr	[100]
[**13b**-(AuPPh₃)₂](SbF₆)₂	27.45	2.127 2.118	1.788 1.737	115.6	[100]
[**13b**-Ag-**13b**][OTf]	8.43	2.160	1.707 1.635	121.8 127.0	[100]
[**13bH**-AuPPh₃](OTf)₂	17.1	2.106	1.817 1.782	116.3	[100]

The addition products **13a**-AgCl and **13b**-AgCl were obtained from reacting [**13aH**]⁺ or [**13bH**]⁺, respectively with ion exchange resin (Cl⁻ form) and Ag₂O/CH₂Cl₂. For the other products see Scheme 21 [100].

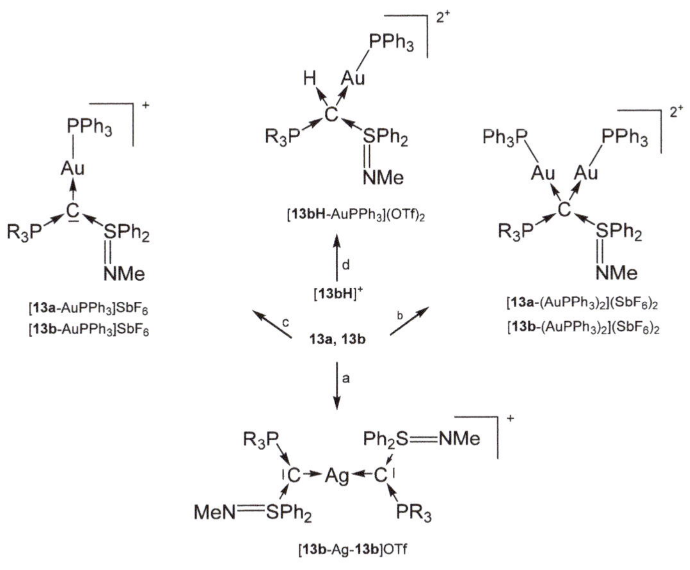

Scheme 21. Selected structures with the carbones **13a** und **13b**: (**a**) 0.5 eq. of AgOTf, (**b**) 2 eq. of AuCl(PPh₃)/2 eq. of AgSbF₆, (**c**) 1 eq. of AuCl(PPh₃)/1 eq. of AgSbF₆, (**d**) ion exchange (OH⁻ form), 1 eq. of AuClPPh₃/1 eq. of AgOTf [100].

Addition of TM fragments to **13a** or **13b** in Scheme 21 elongates P-C and S-C bond length as reported for **1a**. That of [**13bH**-AuPPh₃](OTf)₂ in which **13b** acts as four-electron donor are elongated to normal single bonds [100].

2.14. Transition Metal Complex with a P-C-S Core Possessing a Neutral S(II) Ligand

The carbone **14** in Figure 17 contains a phosphine and a S(II) ligand with a free pair of electrons to stabilize the C(0) atom. However, the bare **14** could not be isolated, but only the protonated cation [**14H**]⁺ and used as starting material [101].

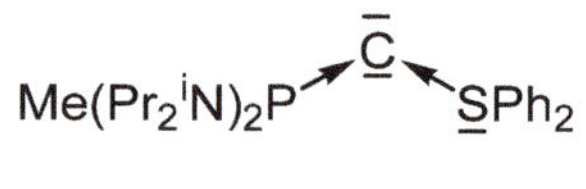

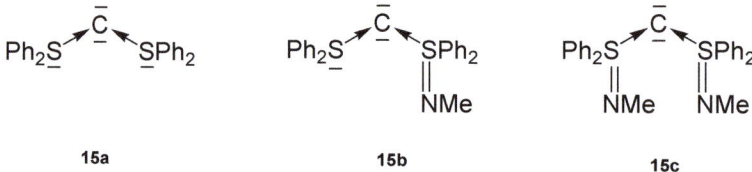

14

Figure 17. Mixed P and S stabilized carbone **14**.

The transition metal complex [**14**-CuN(SiMe$_3$)$_2$](OTf) was prepared upon reacting [**14**H]+ with KHMDS/CuCl. X-ray analysis reveals a Cu-C distance of 1.903(4) Å and the P-C and S-C distances amount to 1.709(5) and 1.677(5) Å, respectively. As found in carbone addition compounds of **13a** and **13b** the P-C distance is longer than the S-C distance. An acute P-C-S angle of 115.3(2)° was recorded. The ^{31}P NMR signal is shifted to lower fields at 66.5 ppm [101].

2.15. Transition Metal Complexes of Carbones with the S-C-S Skeleton

In the carbones **15** (carbodisulfanes, CDS) the central carbon atom is stabilized by two neutral S(II) ligands (**15a**), or S(II), S(IV) groups (**15b**), or two S(IV) (**15c**) ligands (see Figure 18).

Figure 18. Sulfur based carbones **15** as ligands for transition metal complexes.

The molecular structure of **15a** was investigated computationally (see Table 12) [102]. For the carbones the following parameters were recorded: **15b**, C-S^{II} 1.707(2), C-S^{IV} 1.648(2), S-C-S 106.67(14). ^{13}C NMR, δ = 35.4 ppm [103]. **15c**, S-C 1.635(4), 1.636(2); S-C-S 116.8(2) [104]. Similar to CDCs the first and second PAs of **15b** amount to 288.0 and 184.4 kcal/mol, respectively.

Table 12. Transition metal complexes with selected bond length (Å) and angles (deg) of the carbone ligands **15a** to **15c**. ^{13}C NMR signal (in ppm) of the central carbon atom.

15-M	^{13}C NMR	C-M	S^{II}-C	S^{II}-M-S^{II}	Ref.
15a-AgCl	not obs	2.058(8)	1.707(8) 1.698(8)	107.3(5)	[102]
[**15a**-AuPPh$_3$]OTf	65.4	nr	nr	nr	[102]
[**15a**-(AuPPh$_3$)$_2$]$^{2+}$	not obs	2.116(6) 2.084(5)	1.782(6) 1.767(6)	115.4(3)	[102]
[**15a**H-AuPPh$_3$]$^{2+}$	66.0	2.090(7)	1.837(7) 1.805(7)	104.4	[102]
Transition metal complexes with the CDS **15b**					
		C-M	S^{II}-C S^{IV}-C	S^{II}-M-S^{IV}	
[**15b**-AuPPh$_3$]OTf	67.4	nr	nr	nr	[102]
[**15b**-Ag-**15b**]OTf	not obs	2.111(7) 2.097(7)	1.718(6) 1.664(7)	106.3(6)	[102,105]
[**15b**-(AuPPh$_3$)$_2$](OTf)$_2$	not obs	2.130(3) 2.103(3)	1.792(3) 1.746(3)	106.27(18)	[102]
[**15b**-Ag$_2$-**15b**](OTf)$_2$	not obs	nr	nr	nr	[105]
[**15b**-Ag$_4$-**15b**](OTf)$_4$	not obs	2.192 2.187	nr	nr	[105]
[**15b**H-AuPPh$_3$](OTf)$_2$	72.1	2.098(3)	1.796(3) 1.789(3)	106.83(17)	[102]
Transition metal complexes with the CDS **15c**					
		C-M	S^{IV}-C	S^{IV}-M-S^{IV}	
[**15c**-AuPPh$_3$]OTf	65.1	nr	nr	nr	[102]
15c-AgCl	not obs	2.134(3)	1.690(3) 1.678(3)	112.16(14)	[102]
[**15c**-(AuPPh$_3$)$_2$](OTf)$_2$	not obs	2.126(4) 2.125(4)	1.789(4) 1.735(5)	112.5(2)	[102]
[**15c**-Ag-**15c**]OTf	40.0	2.116 2.127	1.671–1.696	114.6 115.6	[105]
[**15c**-Ag$_2$-**15c**](OTf)$_2$	43.1	2.147	1.666 1.696	114.7	[105]
[**15c**-Ag$_4$-**15c**](OTf)$_4$	nr	2.228 2.193	nr	nr	[105]
{[**15c**-(AuPPh$_3$)$_2$AgOTf](OTf)$_4$}$_2$	nr	2.139 2.108	1.757 1.747	116.8	[102]

15a-AgCl was obtained from [**15aH**]⁺ upon treating with Ag₂O/CH₂Cl₂. The salt [**15a**-AuPPh₃]OTf formed reacting the bare **15a** with AuCl(PPh₃) followed by addition of NaTfO in THF. [**15a**-(AuPPh₃)₂](OTf)₂ and [**15aH**-AuPPh₃](SbF₆) are sketched in Scheme 22 [102].

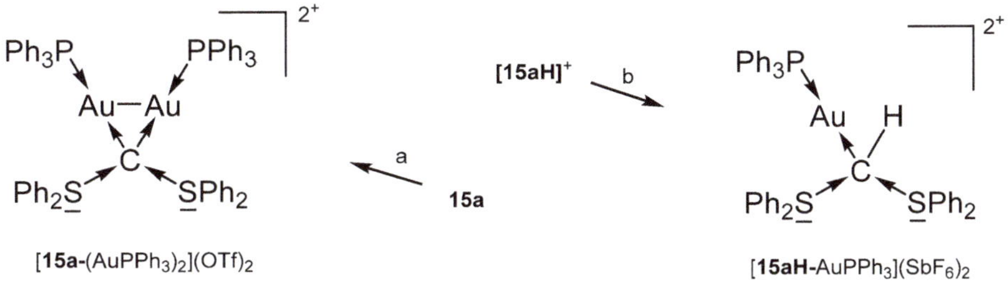

Scheme 22. Selected of complexes with the carbone **15a**. (**a**) 2 eq AuCl(PPh₃), (**b**) AuCl(PPh₃)₂.

[**15b**-AuPPh₃]OTf was obtained analogously formed from reacting **15b** with AuCl(PPh₃) followed by addition of NaTfO in THF. For the other compounds, see Scheme 23 [102].

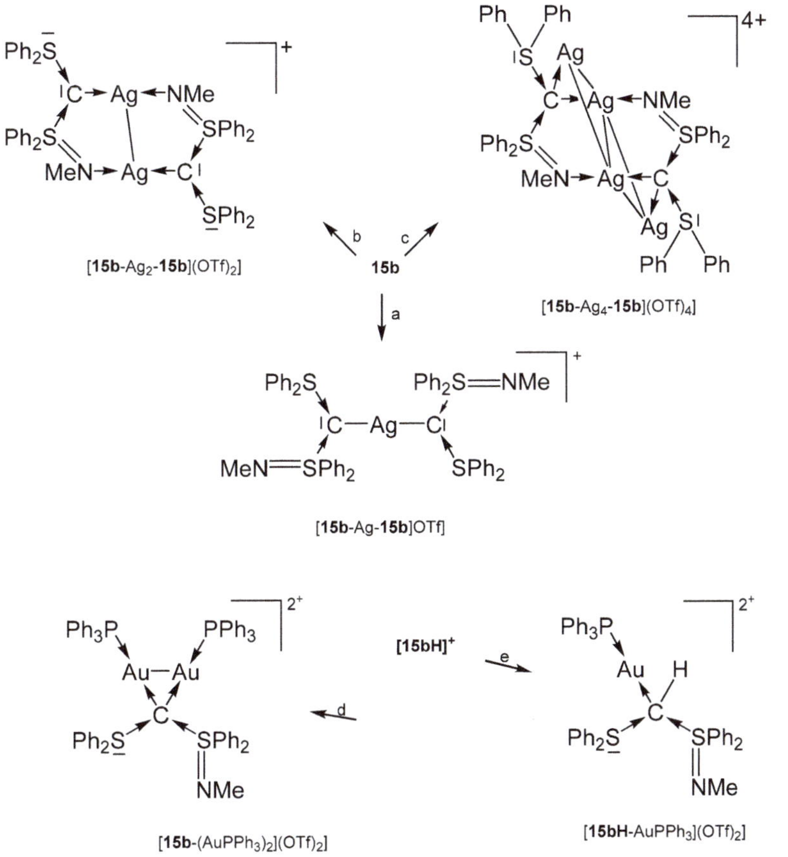

Scheme 23. Selected of complexes with the carbone **15b**. (**a**) 0.5 eq AgOTf, (**b**) 1.0 eq AgOTf, (**c**) 2.0 eq AgOTf, (**d**) 2 eq AuCl(PPh₃), (**e**) AuCl(PPh₃).

The preparation of [**15c**-AuPPh$_3$]OTf and **15c**-AgCl follows the procedure outlined for the related **15b** compounds [102]. For the other compounds, see Scheme 24 [102,105]. The hetero hexametallic cluster {[**15c**-(AuPPh$_3$)$_2$AgOTf](OTf)$_4$}$_2$ is supported by two carbone ligands that adopt a $\kappa^4 C,C',N,N'$ coordination mode. The Au-Ag separation amounts to 3.003 Å [102].

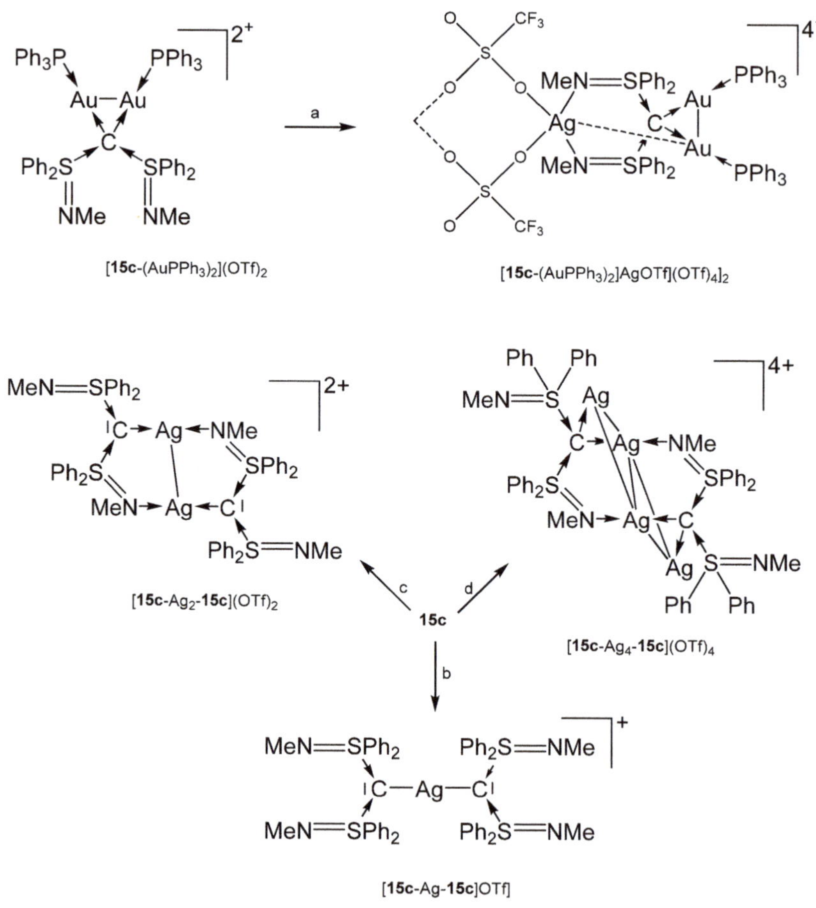

Scheme 24. Selected complexes with the carbone ligand **15c**; (a) AgOTf, (b) 0.5 eq AgOTf, (c) 1.0 eq AgOTf, (d) 2.0 eq AgOTf. {[**15c**-(AuPPh$_3$)$_2$AgOTf](OTf)$_4$}$_2$ is dimeric linked by two OTf anions.

^{13}C NMR signals of the donating C(0) atoms (if available) of all addition compounds of **15a** to **15c** are less shielded than that of the basic carbones [102].

2.16. *Transition Metal Complexes of Carbones with the S-C-Se Skeleton (16)*

Compound **16** in Figure 19 is the first carbone containing a Se(II) compound together with a S(IV) one as ligand for stabilization of a C(0) atom.

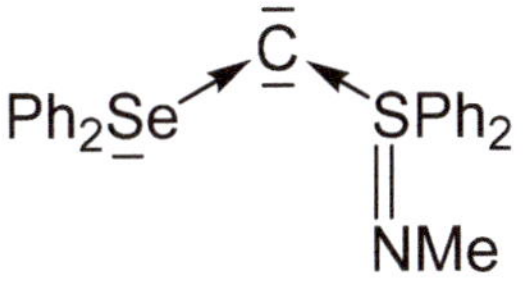

Ph$_2$Se—C—SPh$_2$
        ‖
        NMe

16

Figure 19. Carbone with Se and S based ligands L.

The tetranuclear complex [16-Ag$_4$-16]$^{4+}$ contains a rhomboidal [Ag$_4$]$^{4+}$ core surrounded by two carbones **16** (see Table 13). In this and in [16H-Ag-16H]$^{3+}$ the donating C(0) acts as a four-electron donor (see Scheme 25) [105].

Table 13. Transition metal complexes with selected bond length (Å) and angles (deg) of the carbone **16**. ^{13}C NMR signal (in ppm) of the central carbon atom.

16-M	^{13}C NMR	C-M	C-S C-Se	S-C-Se	Ref.
[16-Ag-16](OTf)	not obs.	nr	nr	nr	[105]
[16-Ag$_2$-16](OTf)$_2$	52.7	nr	nr	nr	[105]
[16-Ag$_4$-16](OTf)$_4$	not obs	2.174(5)	1.714(5) 1.923(6)	106.4(3)	[105]
[16H-Ag-16H](BF$_4$)$_3$	not obs	2.164(4) 2.177(4)	1.772(5) 1.771(5) 1.936(4) 1.948(5)	103.8(2)	[103]

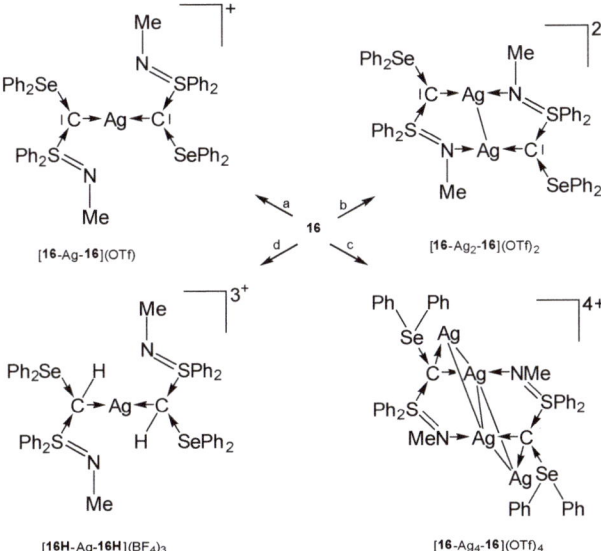

Scheme 25. Transition metal complexes with the carbone **16** as two and four electron donor. (a) 0.5 eq AgOTf, (b) 1 eq AgOTf, (c) 2.0 eq AgOTf, (d) AgBF$_4$/CH$_2$Cl$_2$.

3. Transition Metal Carbido Complexes [M]-C

The second part of this review summarizes the research of transition metal complexes with a naked carbon atom as ligand [M]-C. They are often termed as carbides, but the bonding situation is clearly different from well-known carbides of the alkaline and alkaline earth elements E, which are salt compounds of acetylene E$_n$C$_2$. The electron configuration of carbon atom in the ^{1}D state

($2s^2 2p_x^2 2p_y^0 2p_z^0$) is perfectly suited for dative bonding with a transition metal following the DCD model [7] in terms of σ donation and π backdonation [M]⇌C]. Carbon complexes [M]-C may thus be considered as carbone complexes [M]-CL$_2$ without the ligands L at the carbon atoms. A theoretical study showed in 2000 that the 18 valence electron (VE) complex [(CO)$_4$Fe(C)] is an energy minimum structure with a rather strong Fe-C bond [106]. However, such 18 VE systems could not be synthesized as isolated species but were only found as ligands where the lone-pair electron at the carbon atom serves as donor (see below). It seems that the electron lone-pair at carbon in the 18 VE complexes [M]-C makes the adducts too reactive to become isolated.

It came as a surprise when Heppert and co-workers reported in 2002 the first neutral adducts with a naked carbon atom as a ligand, which are the formally 16 VE diamagnetic ruthenium complexes [(PCy$_3$)LCl$_2$Ru(C)] (L= PCy and 1,3-dimesityl-4,5-dihydroimidazol-2-ylidene; Cy = Cyclohexyl) [27]. A subsequent bonding analysis of the model compound [(Me$_3$P)$_2$Cl$_2$Ru-C] considered five different models A–E for the Ru-C bonds that are shown in Figure 20 [28]. It turned out that the best description for the bonding interactions is a combination of electron-sharing and dative bonds. An energy decomposition analysis [107] suggested that the model B provides the most faithful account of the bond, where the σ bond and the π bond in the Cl$_2$M plane come from electron-sharing interactions Cl$_2$M=C whereas the π bond in the P$_2$M plane is due to backdonation (Me$_3$P)$_2$Ru→C. The compounds [(PCy$_3$)LCl$_2$Ru(C)] should therefore be considered as 18 VE Ru(IV) adducts. The following section summarizes the research of transition metal complexes with a naked carbon atom as ligand [M]-C that has been accomplished since 2002.

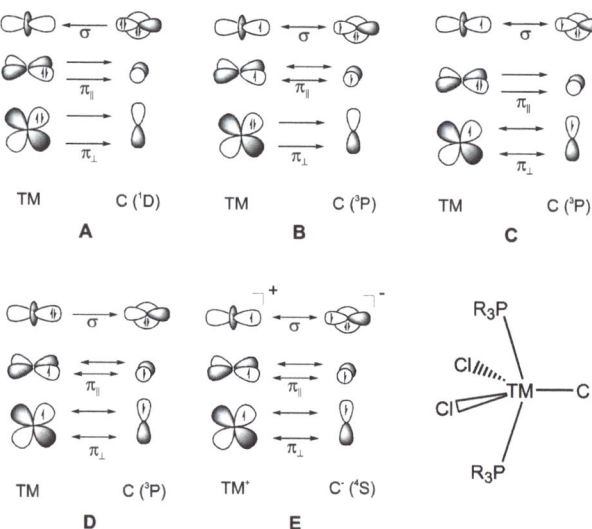

Figure 20. Bonding models (**A–E**) for the bonding between a transition metal (TM) and a naked carbon atom in the compound [(R$_3$P)$_2$Cl$_2$Ru-C].

3.1. The System RuCl$_2$(PCy$_3$)$_2$C ([Ru]C)

By far the most known complexes with carbido ligands that have been synthesized and structurally characterized are ruthenium adducts. The progress in the chemistry of ruthenium carbido complexes was reviewed in 2012 by Takemoto and Matsuzaka [108]. In the following, we summarize the present knowledge on ruthenium carbido complexes which has been reported in the literature.

The X-ray analysis of [Ru]C in Figure 21 exhibits a Ru-C distance of 1.632(6) Å. A signal at 471.8 ppm was attributed to the ligand carbon atom [109]. A general route to carbon complexes is described in [110].

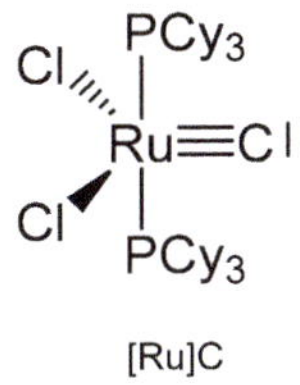

Figure 21. The [Ru]C core.

Addition of PdCl$_2$(SMe$_2$)$_2$ gives the complex [Ru]C→PdCl$_2$(SMe$_2$), while with Mo(CO)$_5$(NMe$_3$) the carbonyl complex [Ru]C→Mo(CO)$_5$ is generated (see Table 14) [29,109]. A series of [Ru]C→PtCl$_2$L complexes were obtained by Bendix from reacting the dimeric complex {[Ru]C→PtCl$_2$}$_2$ with various ligands L (L = PPh$_3$, PCy$_3$, P(OPh)$_3$, AsPh$_3$, CN^{t}Bu, CNCy). Complexes with bridging ligands L such as {[Ru]C→PtCl$_2$}$_2$bipy, {[Ru]C→PtCl$_2$}$_2$pyz, and {[Ru]C→PtCl$_2$}$_2$pym formed upon displacing ethylene from the related (C$_2$H$_4$)PtCl$_2$-L-PtCl$_2$(C$_2$H$_4$) by [Ru]C. {[Ru]C→PtCl]$_2$(μ-Cl)pz results from an ethylene complex and [Ru]C as depicted in Scheme 26 [111]. A series of Pt, Pd, Rh, Ir, Ag, Ru complexes were presented by Bendix with X-ray data and ^{13}C NMR shifts of the ligand carbon atom ranging between 340 and 412 ppm [112]. Sulfur containing TM complexes with the metals Pd, Pt, Au, and Cu stem from the same laboratory. The sulfur ligands are ttcn = 1,4,7-trithiacyclononane and S$_4$(MCp*)$_3$ (see Figure 22) [113].

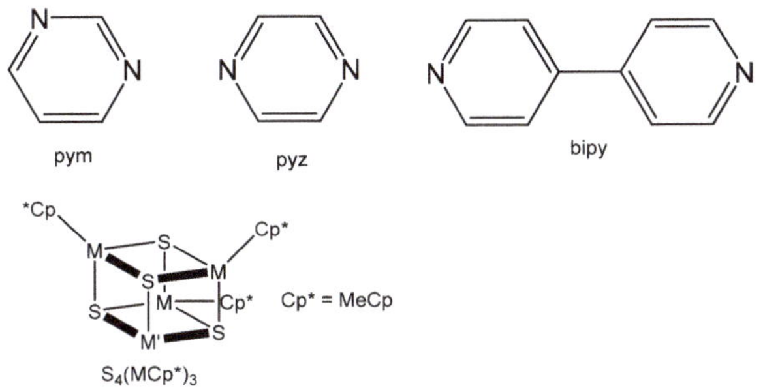

Figure 22. Spezification of ligands of Table 14.

Table 14. Selected structural (in Å and deg) and spectroscopic (^{13}C NMR in ppm) details of [Ru]C addition compounds.

	^{13}C NMR	Ru-C	M-C	Ru-C-M	Ref
[Ru]C→PdCl$_2$(SMe$_2$)	381.23	1.662(2)	1.946(2)	175.1(1)	[109]
{[Ru]C→PdCl$_3$}$^-$	380.9	nr	nr	nr	[112]
[Ru]C→Mo(CO)$_5$	446.31	nr	nr	nr	[109]
[Ru]C→PtCl$_2$Py	350.34	nr	nr	nr	[29,111]
[Ru]C→PtCl$_2$NCr(dbm)$_2$	nr	1.676(2)	1.899(2)	174.5(1)	[29]
{[Ru]C→PtCl$_3$}$^-$	344.7	nr	nr	nr	[29,112]
{[Ru]C→PtCl$_2$}$_2$	326.23	1.676(8)	1.871(8)	1796(4)	[29,111]
[Ru]C→PtCl$_2$PPh$_3$	388.81	1672(2)	1.983(2)	173.7(1)	[111]
[Ru]C→PtCl$_2$P(OPh)$_3$	387.54	1.659(2)	2.001(2)	179.3(2)	[111]
[Ru]C→PtCl$_2$AsPh$_3$	374.68	1.670(2)	1.949(2)	171.9(2)	[111]
[Ru]C→PtCl$_2$CN^{t}Bu	376.26	1.661(2)	1.967(6)	176.5(3)	[111]
[Ru]C→PtCl$_2$CNCy	376.04	nr	nr	nr	[111]
[Ru]C→PtCl$_2$PCy$_3$	396.77	1.666(3)	1.971(2)	174.5(2)	[111]
[Ru]C→PtCl$_2$(dmso)	349.0				[112]
{[Ru]C→PtCl$_2$}$_2$bipy	348.27	1.679(3)	1.891(4)	171.4(2)	[111]
{[Ru]C→PtCl$_2$}$_2$pyz	342.48	1.668(6)	1.895(6)	176.3(3)	[111]

Table 14. Cont.

	^{13}C NMR	Ru-C	M-C	Ru-C-M	Ref
{[Ru]C→PtCl$_2$}$_2$pym	341.36	1.678(3)	1.893(3)	176.0(2)	[111]
{[Ru]C→PtCl}$_2$(μ-Cl)pz	355.09	1.678(4)	1.909(4)	169.9(2)	[111]
[Ru]C→AuCl	395.3	nr	nr	nr	[112]
{[Ru]C→Au←C[Ru]}$^+$	395.3	nr	nr	nr	[112]
{[Ru]C→IrCl(CO)←C[Ru]}	397.4	nr	nr	nr	[112]
{[Ru]C→Rh(CO)}$_2$(μ-Cl)$_2$	396.4	nr	nr	nr	[112]
[Ru]C→RhCl(cod)	411.7	nr	nr	nr	[112]
[Ru]C→IrCl(cod)	387.6	nr	nr	nr	[112]
{[Ru]C→Ag(4′-H-terpy)}	433.5	nr	nr	nr	[112]
{[Ru]C→Ag(4′-Ph-terpy)}	433.1	nr	nr	nr	[112]
[Ru]C→Ag(ttcn)	nr	1.653(4)	1.876(4)	177.3(2)	[112]
[Ru]C→Cu(ttcn)	nr	1.622(7)	2.098(7)	176.9(5)	[112]
[Ru]C→Pd-S$_4$(MoCp*)$_3$	nr	1.672(3)	1.971(3	178.3(2)	[112]
[Ru]C→Pt-S$_4$(MoCp*)$_3$	nr	1.689(7)	1.896(7)	178.2(5)	[112]
[Ru]C→Pd-S$_4$(WCp*)$_3$	nr	1.668(5)	1.959(5)	178.1(3)	[112]
[Ru]C→Pt-S$_4$(WCp*)$_3$	nr	1.699(9)	1.874(9)	178.8(6)	[112]

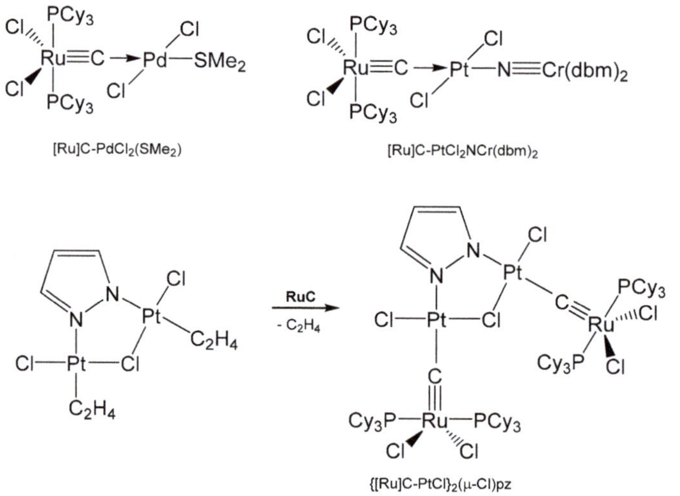

Scheme 26. Selected [Ru]C→M carbido complexes and synthesis of {[Ru]C→PtCl}$_2$(μ-Cl)pz.

3.2. The System RuCl$_2$(PCy$_3$)(NHC)C (^{NHC}[Ru]C)

The X-ray analysis of ^{NHC}[Ru]C in Figure 23 exhibits a Ru-C distance of 1.605(2) Å. A signal at 471.5 ppm was attributed to the ligand carbon atom. No addition compounds were described so far [27].

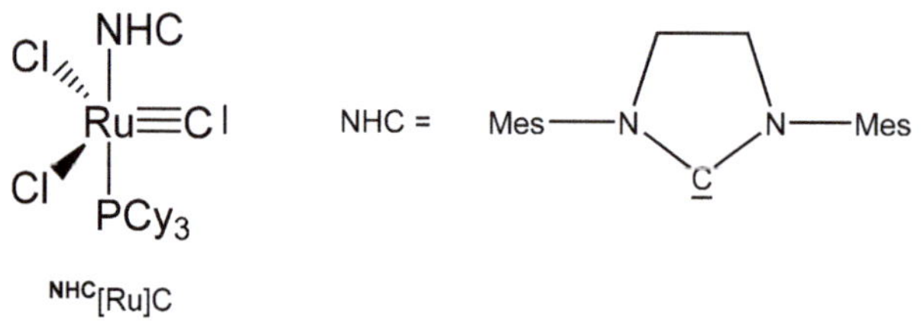

Figure 23. The ^{NHC}[Ru]C core.

3.3. The System (NHC)Cl₃RuC⁻ (^NHC[Ru]⁻C)

Treating the carbene complex (NHC)Cl₂(PCy₃)Ru=CH₂ in Figure 24 at 55° in benzene generated the neutral complex depicted in Figure 25. X-ray analysis revealed a Ru¹-C distance of 1.698(4) Å and the Ru²-C distance of 1.875(4) Å with a Ru-C-Ru angle of 160.3(2)°. In the ^{13}C NMR the bridging C atom resonates at the typical value of 414.0 ppm [114].

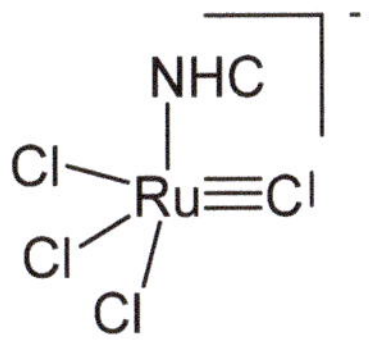

Figure 24. The ^{NHC}[RuCl₃]⁻C core.

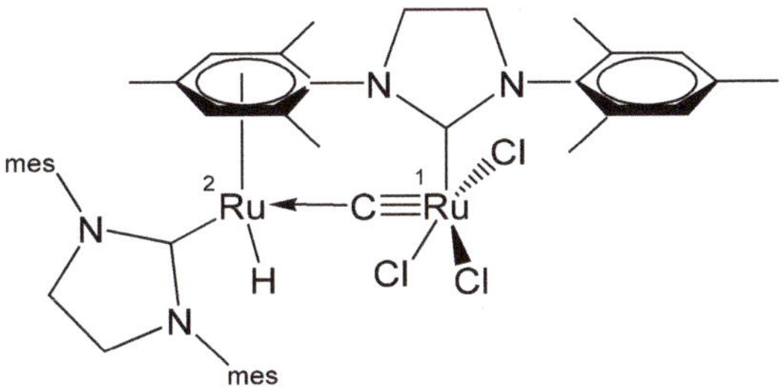

Figure 25. Structural representation of the Ru carbido complex Ru₂(NHC)₂(≡C)Cl₃H.

3.4. The system RuClX(PCy₃)₂C ([Ru]XC)

Various carbido complexes were reported in which one or both chloride ions in [Ru]C are replaced by X (X = Br, I, CN, NCO, NCS) (see Figure 26). {[Ru](MeCN)C}OTf is the first cationic carbido complex which is also starting point for most of the substituted carbido complexes. X-ray data for {[Ru](MeCN)C}OTf, [Ru](CN)₂C, [Ru](Br)C, and [Ru](NCO)C are available (see Table 15) [115].

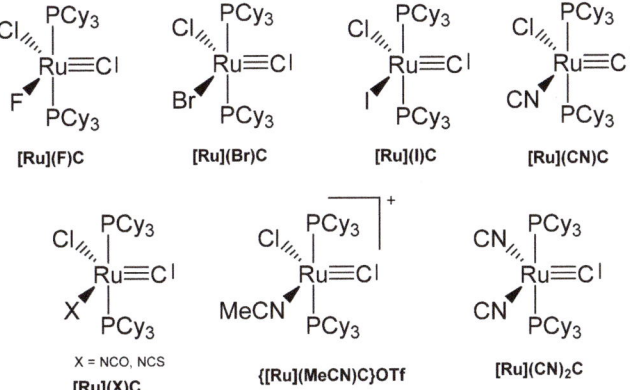

Figure 26. Carbido compounds of [Ru]XC with various X.

Table 15. Carbido complexes with the [Ru]XC core.

	^{13}C NMR	Ru-C	M-C	Ru-C-M	Ref
{[Ru](MeCN)C}OTf	464.75	nr	nr	nr	[115]
[Ru](CN)$_2$C	464.70	nr	nr	nr	[115]
[Ru](F)C	474.58	nr	nr	nr	[115]
[Ru](Br)C	471.38	nr	nr	nr	[115]
[Ru](I)C	469.74	nr	nr	nr	[115]
[Ru](CN)C	474.91	nr	nr	nr	[115]
[Ru](NCO)C	473.51	nr	nr	nr	[115]
[Ru](NCS)C	477.50	nr	nr	nr	[115]

3.5. The Systems OsCl$_2$(PCy$_3$)$_2$C and OsI$_2$(PCy$_3$)$_2$C ([OsX]C)

The carbido complexes [OsX]C in Figure 27 were studied by X-ray analysis. The most important structural parameter is the Os-C separation, which for X = Cl amounts to 1.689(5) Å [116]. Single-crystal X-ray diffraction reveals that molecular [OsX]C adopts an approximately square-pyramidal core geometry, with the carbido ligand occupying the apical position and a short Os-C bond. In the ^{13}C NMR spectrum the signal at 471.8 ppm for X = Cl was attributed to the ligand carbon atom. It was synthesized via S-atom abstraction from the thiocarbonyl complex Os(CS)(PCy$_3$)$_2$Cl$_2$ by Ta(OSi-*t*-Bu$_3$)$_3$. The diiodo derivative was synthesized from [OsCl]C upon reacting with 10 eq of Me$_3$SiI and exhibits a ^{13}C NMR signal at 446.14 ppm.

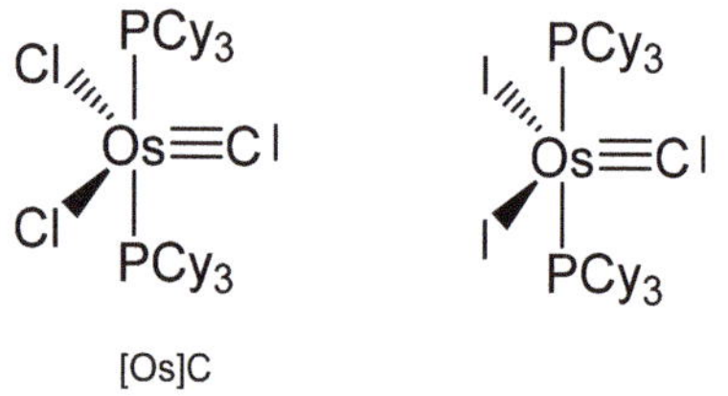

Figure 27. The [Os]C core.

3.6. The System [Tp*Mo(CO)$_3$≡C]$^-$ ([Mo]$^-$C)

The reaction between Tp*Mo(CO)$_2$CCl (see Figure 28) and KFeCp(CO)$_2$ generates the carbido complex [Mo]C→FeCp(CO)$_2$ (see Table 16) [117]; see alternative synthesis from Tp*Mo(CO)$_2$C-Li and ClFeCp(CO)$_2$ [118]. When Tp*Mo(CO)$_2$CSe was allowed to react with [Ir(NCMe)(CO)(PPh$_3$)$_2$]BF$_4$ the tetranuclear carbido complex (μ-Se$_2$)[Ir$_2$-{[Mo]C}$_2$(CO)$_2$(PPh$_3$)$_2$] was obtained (see Figure 29) [119]. A solution of Tp*Mo(CO)$_2$CBr in THF was treated with BuLi followed by addition of HgCl$_2$ resulted in the formation of the carbido complex [Mo]C→Hg←C[Mo] [120]. The platinum complex [Mo]C→Pt(PPh$_3$)$_2$Br was prepared from reacting [(HB(pz)$_3$)Mo(CO)$_2$CBr with [(PPh$_3$)$_2$Pt(C$_2$H$_4$)] [121].

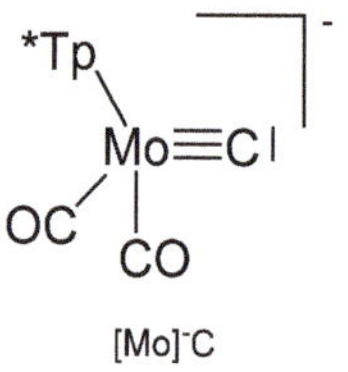

Figure 28. The [Mo]$^-$C core. Tp* = tris(3,5-dimethylpyrazolyl)borate, [HB(pzMe$_2$)$_3$]$^-$ or [HB(pz)$_3$]$^-$.

Table 16. Compounds with [Mo]⁻C core with Tp* = [HB(pzMe$_2$)$_3$]⁻ or [HB(pz)$_3$]⁻.

	Mo-C	M-C	Mo-C-M	^{13}C NMR	Ref
	Tp* is [HB(pzMe$_2$)$_3$]⁻				
[Mo]C→FeCp(CO)$_2$	1.819(6)	1.911(8)	172.2(5)	381	[117]
(µ-Se$_2$)[Ir$_2$-{[Mo]C}$_2$(CO)$_2$(PPh$_3$)$_2$]	1.843(5)	1.974(5)	171.3(3) 168.2(3)	286.1	[119]
[Mo]C→Hg←C[Mo]	nr	nr	nr	373	[120]
[Mo]C→AuPPh$_3$	nr	nr	nr	nr	[122]
	Tp* is [HB(pz)$_3$]⁻				
[Mo]C→Pt(PPh$_3$)$_2$Br	nr	nr	nr	339.0	[121]

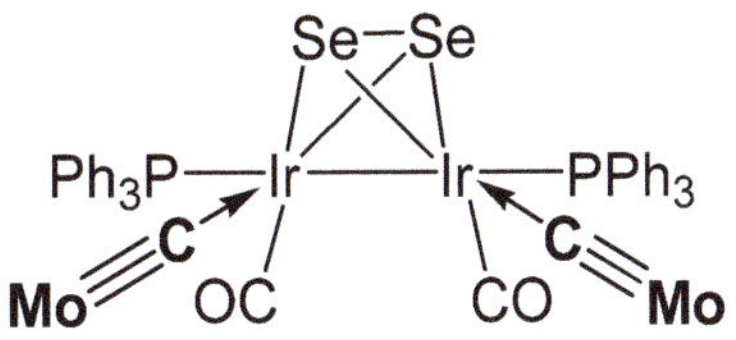

Figure 29. Selected structure of compounds with the [Mo]⁻C moiety.

3.7. Unique Mo Carbido Complex

A further unique carbido complex was described recently as shown in Figure 30. A signal at 360.8 ppm in the ^{13}C NMR spectrum was assigned to the ligand carbon atom [123].

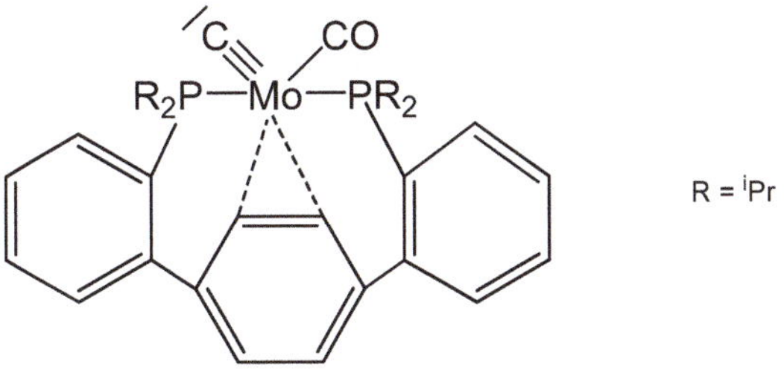

Figure 30. The carbido complex with the P$_2$(CO)Mo≡C core.

3.8. The System [Tp*W(CO)$_3$≡C]⁻ ([W]⁻C)

Reaction of [W]C-Li(THF) with NiCl$_2$(PEt$_3$)$_2$ produced the complex [W]C→NiCl(PEt$_3$)$_2$ in Figure 31 [124]. Similarly, with [W]C-Li(THF) and FeCl(CO)$_2$Cp or HgCl$_2$ the compounds [W]C→Fe(CO)$_2$Cp and [W]C→Hg←C[W], respectively, were obtained. [W]C→AuPEt$_3$ was prepared from reacting [W]C→SnMe$_3$ with AuCl(SMe$_2$) followed by addition of PEt$_3$. A similar reaction with AuCl(PPh$_3$) yielded [W]C→AuPPh$_3$. [W]C→AuAsPh$_3$ and [W]C→AuPPh$_3$ form a tetrameric assembly as depicted in Figure 32. The X-ray analysis of the tetrameric unit revealed Au-C distances of 1.995 and 2.078 Å and the W-C distance is 1.877 Å [122].

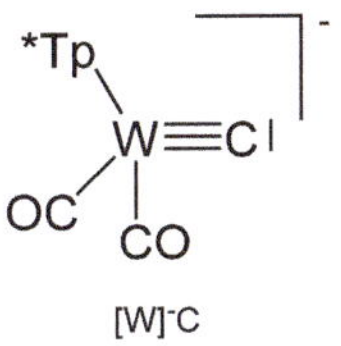

Figure 31. The [W]⁻C core. T* = tris(3,5-dimethylpyrazolyl)borate, [HB(pzMe$_2$)$_3$]⁻.

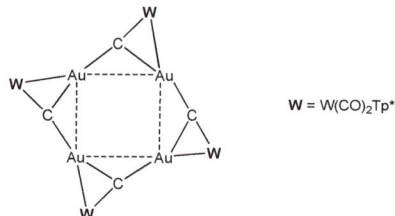

Figure 32. Tetrameric unit from [W]C→AuAsPh$_3$ and [W]C→AuPPh$_3$ [122].

The terpyridine complex salt {[W]C→Pt(terpy)}PF$_6$ was obtained from [W]C-Li and [PtCl(terpy)]PF$_6$; the neutral complex [W]C→PtCl(terpyC[W]) (see Figure 33) was prepared from the same starting material and [PtCl$_2$(phen)] (see Table 17) [125].

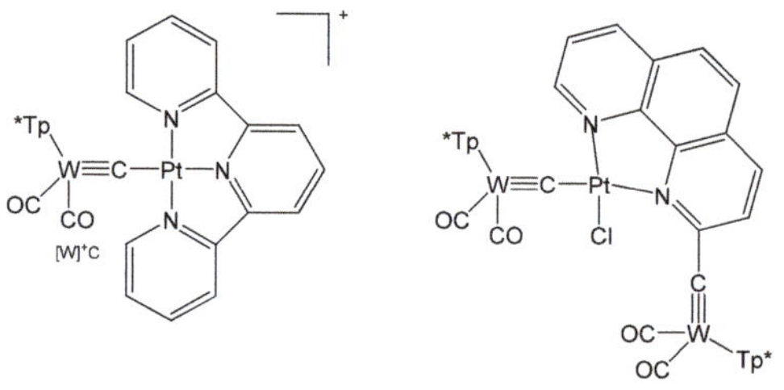

Figure 33. Structural representation of [W]C→Pt complexes [125].

Table 17. Compounds with [W]$^-$C core. Tp* = [HB(pzMe$_2$)$_3$]$^-$.

	W-C	M-C	W-C-M	^{13}C NMR	Ref
[W]C→NiCl(PEt$_3$)$_2$	nr	nr	nr	nr	[124]
[W]C→Fe(CO)$_2$Cp	nr	nr	nr	nr	[122]
[W]C→Hg←C[W]	nr	nr	nr	nr	[122]
[W]C→AuAsPh$_3$	nr	nr	nr	nr	[122]
[W]C→AuPPh$_3$	nr	nr	nr	nr	[122]
[W]C→AuPEt$_3$	nr	nr	nr	397.7	[122]
{[W]C→Pt(terpy)}PF$_6$	1.835(5)	1.938(5)	176.3(3)	368	[125]
[W]C→PtCl(terpyC[W])	1.853(14)	1.890(14)	173.4(9)	331.3	[125]

3.9. The Systems N$_3$MoC and O$_3$MoC

The potassium salt of ^{N}MOC$^-$ in Figure 34 is dimeric with two K$^+$ ions bridging two anions and can be transformed with the crown ethers 2.0-benzo-15-crown-5 and 1.0 2,2,2-crypt into the related ion pairs. X-ray analysis of the crown ether salt revealed a Mo-C distance of 1.713(9) Å [26,126].

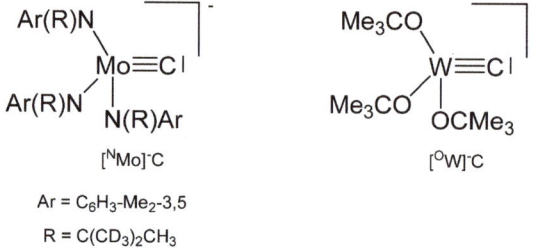

Ar = C$_6$H$_3$-Me$_2$-3,5
R = C(CD$_3$)$_2$CH$_3$

Figure 34. The [^{N}Mo]$^-$C and [^{O}W]$^-$C core.

The complex [^{O}W]C→Ru(CO)$_2$Cp was prepared from reacting [^{O}W]C-Et with Ru(C≡CMe)(CO)$_2$Cp under loss of MeCCEt. The ligand C atom resonates at 237.3 ppm ($^1J_{WC}$ = 290.1 Hz). Distances are W-C = 1.75(2) Å, Ru-C = 2.09(2) Å and the W-C-Ru angle amounts to 177(2) ° [127].

3.10. Symmetrically Bridged Carbido Complexes M=C=M

3.10.1. The Fe=C=Fe Core

[Fe(TPP)]$_2$C was obtained from Fe^{III}(TPP)Cl in the presence of iron powder by reacting with CI$_4$ (TPP = 5, 10, 15, 20-tetraphenylporphyrin; according to Fe^{II} the complex is diamagnetic [128]. The complex was also obtained upon reacting Fe(TPP) with Me$_3$SiCCl$_3$ [129]; see also [130]. An X-ray analysis was performed in [131] and later in [130]. The Mössbauer spectrum is published in [132]. [Fe(TTP)]$_2$C (TTP = tetratolylporphyrine) was similarly obtained from Fe(TTP) with Me$_3$SiCCl$_3$ [129]. [Fe(oep)]$_2$C (oep = octaethylporphyrine) was prepared from [ClFe(oep)] and HCCl$_3$ and studied by X-ray analysis ans Mössbauer spectroscopy (see Table 18) [132].

Table 18. Fe-C distances (in Å) and Fe-C-Fe angles (in deg). ^{13}C NMR of the bridging carbon atom in ppm.

	^{13}C NMR	Fe-C	Fe-C	Fe-C-Fe	Ref
[Fe(TPP)]$_2$C	nr	1.683(1)	1.675	180	[130,131]
[Fe(TTP)]$_2$C	nr	nr	nr	nr	[129]
[Fe(oep)]$_2$C	nr	1.6638(9)	1.6638(9)	179.5(3)	[132]
(TPP)Fe–C–Fe(CO)$_4$	nr	nr	nr	nr	[121]
(TCNP)Fe=C=Fe(CO)$_4$	nr	nr	nr	nr	[121]
[Fe(pc)]$_2$C	nr	nr	nr	nr	[95]
{[Fe(pc)]$_2$C}(I$_3$)$_{0.66}$	nr	nr	nr	nr	[95]
[(py)Fe(pc)]$_2$C	nr	1.69(2)	1.69(2)	177.5(8)	[133]
[(1-meim)Fe(pc)]$_2$C	nr	1.70(1)	1.70(1)	178(1)	[134]
[(4-Mepy)Fe(pc)]$_2$C	nr	nr	nr	nr	[133]
[(pip)Fe(pc)]$_2$C	nr	nr	nr	nr	[133]
[(thf)Fe(pc)]$_2$C	nr	1.71(2)	1.64(2)	180(1)	[130]
[(thf)(TPP)Fe=C=Fe(pc)(thf)]	nr	1.71(1)	1.65(1)	179(1)	[130]
(Bu$_4$N)$_2${[(F)Fe(pc)]$_2$C}	nr	1.687(4)	1.687(4)	179.5(3)	[135]
(Bu$_4$N)$_2${[(Cl)Fe(pc)]$_2$C}	nr	nr	nr	nr	[135]
(Bu$_4$N)$_2${[(Br)Fe(pc)]$_2$C}	nr	nr	nr	nr	[135]

The mixed carbido compounds (TPP)Fe=C=Fe(CO)$_4$, and (TCNP)Fe=C=Fe(CO)$_4$ (TCNP = Tetrakis-p-cyanophenylporphyrinate) were synthesized from [(TPP)FeCCl$_2$] or (TCNP)FeCCl$_2$ and [Na$_2$Fe(CO)$_4$]; characterization proceeded via IR spectroscopy [121].

[Fe(pc)]$_2$C was prepared from [ClFe(pc)]$^-$ and KOH/HCCl$_3$ [132], or from Fe(pc) and CI$_4$ in the presence of sodium dithionite [95,136], see also [134]. It also forms upon hydrolysis of (Bu$_4$N)$_2$ {[(F)Fe(pc)]$_2$C}in acetone [135]. Oxidation with I$_2$ generates {[Fe(pc)]$_2$C}(I$_3$)$_{0.66}$ which was characterized by IR, Mössbauer spectroscopy and powder X-ray diffraction [95].

A series of six-coordinate N-Base adducts of μ-carbido phthalocyanine complexes were reported. The pyridine adduct [(py)Fe(pc)]$_2$C was obtained y dissolution of [Fe(pc)]$_2$C in warm pyridine [133] and characterized by Mössbauer spectroscopy [136] and X-ray analysis [133]. [Fe(pc)(1-meim)]$_2$C was similarly obtained as the TPP derivate; starting with pcFe and CI$_4$ followed by addition of sodium dithionite gave the μ-carbido bridged dimer; an X-ray diffraction analysis was reportedd (1-meim = 1-methylimidazole, pc = phthalocyanine) [134]. [(4-Mepy)Fe(pc)]$_2$C and [(pip)Fe(pc)]$_2$C were similarly obtained and studied by IR and Mössbauer spectroscopy [136].

[(thf)Fe(pc)]$_2$C forms on dissolving [Fe(pc)] in THF. The asymmetric μ-carbido complex [(thf)(TPP)Fe=C=Fe(pc)(thf)] stems from the reaction of [FeCCl$_2$(TPP)] with [Fe(pc)]-; both compounds were characterized by X-ray analyses [130].

Anionic six-coordinate μ-carbido complexes (Bu$_4$N)$_2${[(hal)Fe(pc)]$_2$C} were reported (hal = F. Cl. Br) and obtained from reacting [Fe(pc)]$_2$C with (Bu$_4$N)(hal) (F: RT, Cl: 115°, Br: 140°) in solution (F) and in a melt [135].

3.10.2. The Rh=C=Rh Core

[Rh(PEt$_3$)$_2$(SGePh$_3$)]$_2$C was obtained upon reacting Rh(PEt$_3$)$_2$(SGePh$_3$)CS with Rh(PEt$_3$)$_3$(Bpin) via the intermediate mixed carbido complex (SGePh$_3$)(PEt$_3$)$_2$Rh=C=Rh(PEt$_3$)$_2$(SBpin) which rearranges to this complex and [Rh(PEt$_3$)$_2$(SBpin)]$_2$. The X-ray analysis was performed (see Table 19) [137] [Rh(PEt$_3$)$_2$(SBpin)]$_2$C was prepared earlier by the same working group from Rh(PEt$_3$)$_3$(Bpin) and 0,5 eq of CS$_2$ (X-ray data (see Table 19). Addition of MeOH generated the carbido complex [Rh(PEt$_3$)$_2$(SH)]$_2$C [138]. [Rh(Cl)(PPh$_3$)$_2$]$_2$C resulted from reacting the thiocarbonyl complex Rh(Cl)(PPh$_3$)$_2$CS with HBCat. The central C atom resonates at 424 ppm (t, $^1J_{RhC}$ = 47 Hz). In the chloro complex the chloride ion can be replaced with K[(H$_2$B(pz)$_2$], K[(H$_2$B(pzMe$_2$)$_2$], or K[(HB(pz)$_3$] to produce the carbido complexes [Rh(H$_2$B(pz)$_2$)(PPh$_3$)]$_2$C, [Rh(H$_2$B(pzMe$_2$)$_2$)(PPh$_3$)]$_2$C, and [Rh(HB(pz)$_3$)(PPh$_3$)]$_2$C, respectively (see Figure 35). The unusual asymmetric carbido complex [Rh$_2$H(μ-C)(μ-C$_6$H$_4$PPh$_2$-2){HB(pzMe$_2$)$_3$}$_2$] contains a Rh^I atom with a shorter Rh-C distance, while the Rh^{III} –C distance is longer [139].

Table 19. Rh-C distances (in Å) and Rh-C-Rh angles (in deg). ^{13}C NMR of the bridging carbon atom in ppm.

	^{13}C NMR	Rh-C	Rh-C	Rh-C-Rh	Ref
[Rh(PEt$_3$)$_2$(SGePh$_3$)]$_2$C	425.8, $^1J_{RhC}$ = 47	1.788(4)	1.798(4)	175.6(2)	[137]
[Rh(PEt$_3$)$_2$(SBpin)]$_2$C	nr	1.790(7)	1.766(7)	176.1(4)	[137,138]
[Rh(PEt$_3$)$_2$(SH)]$_2$C	nr	nr	nr	nr	[137]
[Rh(Cl)(PPh$_3$)$_2$]$_2$C	424.4, $^1J_{RhC}$ = 47	1.7828(19)	1.7828(19)	nr	[139]
[Rh(H$_2$B(pz)$_2$)(PPh$_3$)]$_2$C	nr	1.7644(11)	1.7644(11)	169.1(7)	[139]
[Rh(H$_2$B(pzMe$_2$)$_2$)(PPh$_3$)]$_2$C	nr	1.7794(9)	1.7794(9)	168.8(6)	[139]
[Rh(HB(pz)$_3$)(PPh$_3$)]$_2$C	nr	1.7761(7)	1.7761(7)	163.7(4)	[139]
[Rh$_2$H(μ-C)(μ-C$_6$H$_4$PPh$_2$-2){HB(pzMe$_2$)$_3$}$_2$]	447.2 $^1J_{RhC}$ = 40, 50	1.740(6)	1.818(6)	165.9(3)	[139]

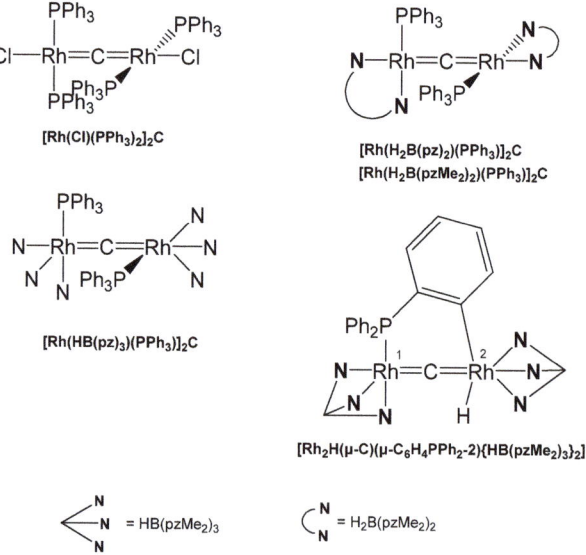

Figure 35. Selected structures of Rh=C=Rh complexes.

3.10.3. The Ru=C=Ru Core

The tetranuclear carbido complex [Ru(PEt$_3$)Cl(µ-Cl$_3$)RuAr]$_2$C was prepared from the reaction of [(p-cymene)Ru(µ-Cl)$_3$RuCl(C$_2$H$_4$)-(PCy$_3$)] with HCCH in THF. X-ray analysis adopts Ru-C distances of 1.877(9) Å and a Ru-C-Ru angle of 178.8(9)°(see Figure 36) [140].

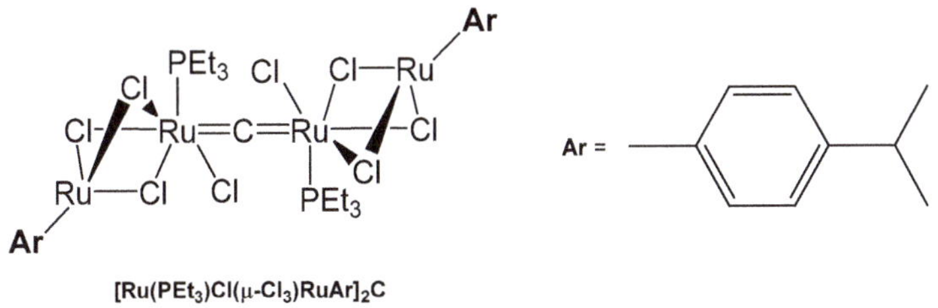

Figure 36. Structural representation of the Ru carbido complex [Ru(PEt$_3$)Cl(µ-Cl$_3$)RuAr]$_2$C.

Five coordinate [Ru(pc)]$_2$C with pc = phthalocyaninate was obtained from H[RuCl$_2$(pc)] and CCl$_2$ (in situ from KOH/HCCl$_3$) [132]. The related pyridine adduct with six-coordinate Ru(IV) [(py)Ru(pc)]$_2$C was obtained upon dissolution of [Ru(pc)]$_2$C in warm pyridine. X-ray analysis revealed a Ru-C distance of 1.77(1) Å and a Ru-C-Ru angle of 174.5(8)° [136].

3.10.4. The Re=C=Re Core

The unique carbido complex [Re(CO)$_2$Cp]$_2$C in Figure 37 results from reaction of [Re(thf)(CO)$_2$(η-C$_5$H$_5$)], CS$_2$, and PPh$_3$ (with the aim of the thiocarbonyl complex [Re(CS)(CO)(η-C$_5$H$_5$)]) as by-product in small amounts. X-ray analysis revealed Re-C distances of 1.882(14) and 1.881(14) Å and a Re-C-Re angle of 173.3(7)°. A ^{13}C NMR shift for the bridging carbon atom at δ = 436.4 ppm was measured [141].

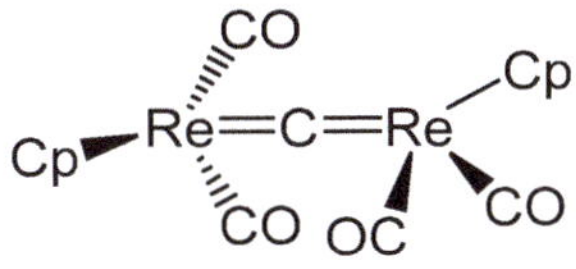

Figure 37. Structural representation of the Re carbido complex [Re(CO)$_2$Cp]$_2$C.

3.10.5. The W=C=W Core

The oxo complex (^{t}Bu$_3$SiO)$_2$(O)W=C=WCl$_2$(OSi^{t}Bu$_3$)$_2$ in Figure 38 formed in high yield from thermolysis of [(siloxo)$_2$Cl(CO)W]$_2$ in toluene with loss of CO; in the ^{13}C NMR spectrum the carbide C atom resonates at δ = 379.14 ppm (J$_{WC}$ = 200, 180 Hz). Degradation of the (silox)$_4$Cl$_2$W$_2$(CNAr) complex afforded the imido µ-carbido compound (^{t}Bu$_3$SiO)$_2$(NR)W=C=WCl$_2$(OSi^{t}Bu$_3$)$_2$; the ^{13}C NMR shift of the µ-C atom appears at δ = 406.25 ppm. X-ray analysis revealed a tetrahedral tungsten core with a W-C distance of 1.994(17) Å (W$_1$) and a distorted square-pyramidal tungsten core with a shorter distance of 1.796(17) Å (W$_2$). The W-C-W bond angle amounts to 176.0(12)° [142].

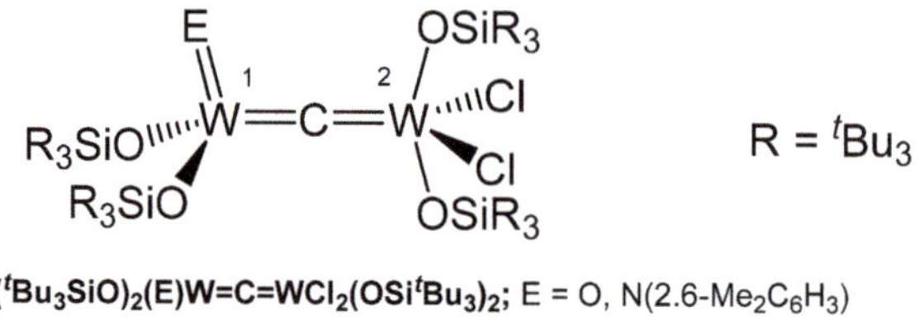

$$(^tBu_3SiO)_2(E)W=C=WCl_2(OSi^tBu_3)_2;\ E = O,\ N(2.6\text{-}Me_2C_6H_3)$$

Figure 38. Structural representation of the W carbido complexes $(^tBu_3SiO)_2(NR)W=C=WCl_2(OSi^tBu_3)_2$ and $(^tBu_3SiO)_2(O)W=C=WCl_2(OSi^tBu_3)_2$.

3.11. Asymmetrically Bridged Carbido Complex Fe=C=M

3.11.1. The Fe=C=Re Core

The asymmetrical carbido complex $(TPP)Fe=C=Re(CO)_4Re(CO)_5$ in Figure 39 was prepared upon reacting the dichlorocarbene complex $(TPP)Fe=CCl_2$ with 2 eq of pentacarbonylrhenate, $[Re(CO)_5]^-$, under release of CO and 2 Cl$^-$; TPP is tetraphenylporphyrin. Crystals were analyzed by X-ray diffraction and revealed a Fe=C distance of 1.605(13) Å and a C=Re distance of 1.957(12) Å. The Fe-C-Re angle amounts to 173.3(9)°; the Fe-C distance is somewhat smaller than in $[(TPP)Fe]_2C$ and the Re-C distance is appreciable longer than in $[Re(CO)_2Cp]_2C$. In the ^{13}C NMR spectrum the central carbido C atom resonates at 211.7 ppm [143].

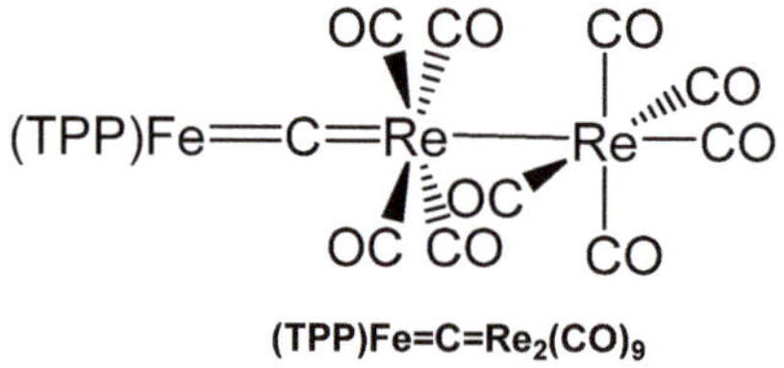

$$(TPP)Fe=C=Re_2(CO)_9$$

Figure 39. Structural representation of the Fe=C=Re carbido complex $(TPP)Fe=C=Re_2(CO)_9$.

3.11.2. The Fe=C=Mn Core

The carbido bridged di-manganese complex $(TCNP)Fe=C=Mn_2(CO)_9$ (TCNP = tetrakis (p-cyanophenyl)porphyrinate) (see Figure 40) was synthesized from $[(TCNP)Fe=CCl_2]$ and two eq. of $Na(Mn(CO)_5)$ in THF and characterized with elemental analysis, IR, and UV spectroscopy [121].

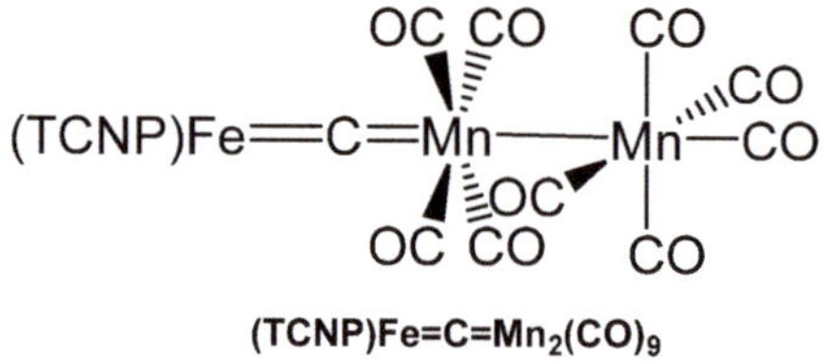

$$(TCNP)Fe=C=Mn_2(CO)_9$$

Figure 40. Structural representation of the Fe=C=Mn carbido complex $(TCNP)Fe=C=Mn_2(CO)_9$.

3.11.3. The Fe=C=Cr Core

Two compounds with the Fe=C=Cr core have been reported by the group of Beck and characterized by elemental analysis, IR, and UV spectroscopy. Thus, $(TPP)Fe=C=Cr(CO)_5$ and $(TAP)Fe=C=Cr(CO)_5$ (see Figure 41) were prepared upon reacting the related dichlorocarbene iron complexes $[(L)Fe=CCl_2]$ with $Na_2[Cr(CO)_5]$ in THF (TAP = tetrakis(p-methoxyphenyl)porphyrinate) [121].

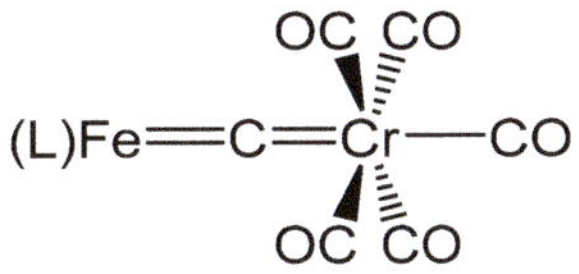

$$(L)Fe=C=Cr(CO)_5;\ L = TPP,\ TAP$$

Figure 41. Structural representation of the Fe=C=Cr carbido complexes (TPP)Fe=C=Cr(CO)$_5$ and (TAP)Fe=C=Cr(CO)$_5$.

4. Conclusions

The experimental and theoretical research with regard transition metal complexes with carbone ligands [M]-CL$_2$ and carbido complexes [M]-C has blossomed in the recent past and it can be foreseen that it will remain a very active area of organometallic chemistry in the future. The well-known family of transition metal complexes with C1-bonded carbon ligands that comprise alkyl (CR$_3$), carbene (CR$_2$), and carbyne (CR) groups has been extended by carbones (CL$_2$) and carbido (C) ligands. The summary of recent work, which is described in this review, indicates that carbone and carbido complexes are still largely terra incognita and that many new discoveries can be expected.

Author Contributions: Conceptualization and writing of the first draft, W.P. and G.F. Checking and partial visualization L.Z. and C.C. All authors have read and agreed to the published version of the manuscript.

Funding: The work at Marburg was financially supported by the Deutsche Forschungsgemeinschaft. L.Z. and G.F acknowledge the financial support from Nanjing Tech University (grant number 39837132 and 39837123), National Natural Science Foundation of China (Grant No. 21703099 and 21993044), Natural Science Foundation of Jiangsu Province for Youth (Grant No: BK20170964), and SICAM Fellowship from Jiangsu National Synergetic Innovation Center for Advanced Materials.

Conflicts of Interest: The authors declare no conflict of interest.

References

1. Frankland, E. Über die Isolierung der Organischen Radicale. *Justus Liebigs Ann. Chem.* **1849**, *71*, 171–213. [CrossRef]
2. Seyferth, D. Zinc Alkyls, Edward Frankland, and the Beginnings of Main-Group Organometallic Chemistry. *Organomet. Chem.* **2001**, *20*, 2940–2955. [CrossRef]
3. Fischer, E.O.M. A Zur Frage eines Wolfram-Carbonyl-Carben Komplexes. *Angew. Chem.* **1964**, *76*, 645. [CrossRef]
4. Fischer, E.O.; Kreis, G.; Kreiter, C.G.; Müller, J.; Huttner, G.; Lorenz, H. Trans-Halogeno[alkyl(aryl)carbyne] tetracarbonyl Complexes of Chromium, Molybdenum, and Tungsten—A New Class of Compounds Having a Transition Metal-Carbon Triple Bond. *Angew. Chem. Int. Ed.* **1973**, *12*, 564–565. [CrossRef]
5. Schrock, R.R. Alkylcarbene Complex of Tantalum by Intramolecular Alpha-Hydrogen Abstraction. *J. Am. Chem. Soc.* **1974**, *96*, 6796–6797. [CrossRef]
6. McLain, S.J.; Wood, C.D.; Messerle, L.W.; Schrock, R.R.; Hollander, F.J.; Youngs, W.J.; Churchill, M.R. Multiple Metal-Carbon Bonds. Thermally Stable Tantalum Alkylidyne Complexes and the Crystal Structure of Ta(.eta.5-C$_5$Me$_5$)(CPh)(PMe$_3$)$_2$Cl. *J. Am. Chem. Soc.* **1978**, *100*, 5962–5964. [CrossRef]
7. Dewar, M.J.S. A Review of Π Complex Theory. *Bull. Soc. Chim. Fr.* **1951**, *18*, C79.
8. Chatt, J.; Duncanson, L.A. 586. Olefin Co-Ordination Compounds. Part III. Infra-Red Spectra and Structure: Attempted Preparation of Acetylene Complexes. *J. Chem. Soc.* **1953**, *1*, 2939–2947. [CrossRef]
9. Vyboishchikov, S.F.; Frenking, G. Theoretical Studies of Organometallic Compounds, Part 29-Structure and Bonding of Low-Valent (Fischer-Type) and High-Valent (Schrock-Type) Transition Metal Carbene Complexes. *Chem. Eur. J.* **1998**, *4*, 1428–1438. [CrossRef]
10. Vyboishchikov, S.F.; Frenking, G. Structure and Bonding of Low-Valent (Fischer-Type) and High-Valent (Schrock-Type) Transition Metal Carbyne Complexes. *Chem. Eur. J.* **1998**, *4*, 1439–1448. [CrossRef]
11. Jerabek, P.; Schwerdtfeger, P.; Frenking, G. Dative and Electron-Sharing Bonding in Transition Metal Compounds. *J. Comput. Chem.* **2019**, *40*, 247–264. [CrossRef] [PubMed]

12. Frenking, G.; Tonner, R. Divalent Carbon(0) Compounds. *Pure Appl. Chem.* **2009**, *81*, 597–614. [CrossRef]
13. Frenking, G.; Tonner, R.; Klein, S.; Takagi, N.; Shimizu, T.; Krapp, A.; Pandey, K.K.; Parameswaran, P. New Bonding Modes of Carbon and Heavier Group 14 Atoms Si–Pb. *Chem. Soc. Rev.* **2014**, *43*, 5106–5139. [CrossRef] [PubMed]
14. Frenking, G.; Hermann, M.; Andrada, D.M.; Holzmann, N. Donor–Acceptor Bonding in Novel Low-Coordinated Compounds of Boron and Group 14 Atoms C–Sn. *Chem. Soc. Rev.* **2016**, *45*, 1129–1144. [CrossRef]
15. Frenking, G.; Solà, M.; Vyboishchikov, S.F. Chemical bonding in transition metal carbene complexes. *J. Organomet. Chem.* **2005**, *690*, 6178–6204. [CrossRef]
16. Tonner, R.; Heydenrych, G.; Frenking, G. First and Second Proton Affinities of Carbon Bases. *Chem. Phys. Chem.* **2008**, *9*, 1474–1481. [CrossRef] [PubMed]
17. Jensen, P.; Johns, J.W.C. The Infrared Spectrum of Carbon Suboxide in the ν6 Fundamental Region: Experimental Observation and Semirigid Bender Analysis. *J. Mol. Spectrosc.* **1986**, *118*, 248–266. [CrossRef]
18. Koput, J. An ab Initio Study on the Equilibrium Structure and CCC Bending Energy Levels of Carbon Suboxide. *Chem. Phys. Lett.* **2000**, *320*, 237–244. [CrossRef]
19. Tonner, R.; Frenking, G. Divalent Carbon(0) Chemistry, Part 1: Parent Compounds. *Chem. Eur. J.* **2008**, *14*, 3260–3272. [CrossRef]
20. Frenking, G. Dative Bonds in Main-Group Compounds: A Case for More Arrows! *Angew. Chem. Int. Ed.* **2014**, *53*, 6040–6046. [CrossRef]
21. Fustier-Boutignon, M.; Nebra, N.; Mézailles, N. Geminal Dianions Stabilized by Main Group Elements. *Chem. Rev.* **2019**, *119*, 855–8700. [CrossRef] [PubMed]
22. Petz, W.; Frenking, G. Carbodiphosphoranes and Related Ligands. *Top. Organomet. Chem.* **2010**, *30*, 49–92.
23. Petz, W. Addition Compounds between Carbones, CL_2, and Main Group Lewis Acids: A New Glance at Old and New Compounds. *Coord. Chem. Rev.* **2015**, *291*, 1–27. [CrossRef]
24. Alcarazo, M. Synthesis, Structure, and Reactivity of Carbidiphosphoranes, Carbodicarbenes and Related Species. *Struct. Bond.* **2018**, *177*, 25–50.
25. Liu, S.; Chen, W.C.; Ong, T.G. Synthesis and Structure of Carbodicarbenes and Their Application in Catalysis. *Struct. Bond.* **2018**, *177*, 51–72.
26. Peters, J.C.; Odom, A.L.; Cummins, C.C. A Terminal Molybdenum Carbide Prepared by Methylidyne Deprotonation. *Chem. Commun.* **1997**, *20*, 1995–1996. [CrossRef]
27. Carlson, R.G.; Gile, M.A.; Heppert, J.A.; Mason, M.H.; Powell, D.R.; Velde, D.V.; Vilain, J.M. The Metathesis-Facilitated Synthesis of Terminal Ruthenium Carbide Complexes: A Unique Carbon Atom Transfer Reaction. *J. Am. Chem. Soc.* **2002**, *124*, 1580–1581. [CrossRef]
28. Krapp, A.; Pandey, K.K.; Frenking, G. Transition Metal–Carbon Complexes. A Theoretical Study. *J. Am. Chem. Soc.* **2007**, *129*, 7596–7610. [CrossRef]
29. Reinholdt, A.; Bendix, J. Platinum(ii) as an Assembly Point for Carbide and Nitride Ligands. *Chem. Commun.* **2019**, *55*, 8270–8273. [CrossRef]
30. Ramirez, F.; Desai, N.B.; Hansen, B.; McKelvie, N. Hexaphenylcarbodiphosphorane, $(C_6H_5)_3PCP(C_6H_5)_3$. *J. Am. Chem. Soc.* **1961**, *83*, 3539–3540. [CrossRef]
31. Hussain, M.S.; Schmidbaur, H. Ein Gemischt Methyl/Phenyl-Substituiertes Carbodiphosphoran. Darstellung, Reaktionen und verwandte Verbindungen. *Z. Nat. B* **1976**, *31*, 721–726.
32. Kroll, A.; Steinert, H.; Scharf, L.T.; Scherpf, T.; Mallick, B.; Gessner, V.H. A Diamino-Substituted Carbodiphosphorane as Strong C-Donor and Weak N-Donor: Isolation of Monomeric Trigonal-Planar $L·ZnCl_2$. *Chem. Commun.* **2020**, *56*, 8051–8054. [CrossRef] [PubMed]
33. Quinlivan, P.J.; Parkin, G. Flexibility of the Carbodiphosphorane, $(Ph_3P)_2C$: Structural Characterization of a Linear Form. *Inorg. Chem.* **2017**, *56*, 5493–5497. [CrossRef]
34. Böttger, S.; Gruber, M.; Münzer, J.E.; Bernard, G.M.; Kneusels, N.-J.H.; Poggel, C.; Klein, M.; Hampel, F.; Neumülöler, B.; Sundermeyer, J.; et al. Solvent-Induced Bond-Bending Isomerism in Hexaphenyl Carbodiphosphorane: Decisive Dispersion Interactions in the Solid State. *Inorg. Chem.* **2020**, *59*, 12054–12064.
35. Vincent, A.T.; Wheatley, P.J. Crystal Structure of Bis(triphenylphosphoranylidene)methane [hexaphenylcarbodiphosphorane, $Ph_3P:C:PPh_3$]. *J. Chem. Soc. Dalton Trans.* **1972**, *5*, 617–622. [CrossRef]
36. Schmidbaur, H.; Hasslberger, G.; Deschler, U.; Schubert, U.; Kappenstein, C.; Frank, A. Problem of the Structure of Carbodiphosphoranes, R_3PCPR_3—New Aspects. *Angew. Chem. Int. Ed.* **1979**, *18*, 408–409. [CrossRef]

37. Schubert, U.; Kappenstein, C.; Milewskimahrla, B.; Schmidbaur, H. Molecular and Crystal-Structures of 2 Carbodiphosphoranes with P-C-P Bond Angles near 120-Degrees. *Chem. Ber. Recl.* **1981**, *114*, 3070–3078. [CrossRef]

38. Schmidbaur, H.; Costa, T.; Milewskimahrla, B.; Schubert, U. Ring-Strained Carbodiphosphoranes. *Angew. Chem. Int. Ed.* **1980**, *19*, 555–556. [CrossRef]

39. Petz, W.; Weller, F.; Uddin, J.; Frenking, G. Reaction of Carbodiphosphorane Ph$_3$P=C=PPh$_3$ with Ni(CO)$_4$. Experimental and Theoretical Study of the Structures and Properties of (CO)$_3$NiC(PPh$_3$)$_2$ and (CO)$_2$NiC(PPh$_3$)$_2$. *Organometallics* **1999**, *18*, 619–626. [CrossRef]

40. Flosdorf, K.; Jiang, D.D.; Zhao, L.L.; Neumüller, B.; Frenking, G.; Kuzu, I. An Experimental and Theoretical Study of the Structures and Properties of CDPMe-Ni(CO)$_3$ and Ni-2(CO)$_4$(μ^2-CO)(μ^2-CDPMe). *Eur. J. Inorg. Chem.* **2019**, *2019*, 4546–4554. [CrossRef]

41. Petz, W.; Neumüller, B.; Klein, S.; Frenking, G. Syntheses and Crystal Structures of [Hg{C(PPh$_3$)$_2$}$_2$][Hg$_2$I$_6$] and [Cu{C(PPh$_3$)$_2$}$_2$]I and Comparative Theoretical Study of Carbene Complexes [M(NHC)$_2$] with Carbone Complexes [M{C(PH$_3$)$_2$}$_2$] (M = Cu$^+$, Ag$^+$, Au$^+$, Zn^{2+}, Cd^{2+}, Hg^{2+}). *Organometallics* **2011**, *30*, 3330–3339. [CrossRef]

42. Petz, W.; Öxler, F.; Neumüller, B. Syntheses and Crystal Structures of Linear Coordinated Complexes of Ag$^+$ with the Ligands C(PPh$_3$)$_2$ and (HC{PPh$_3$}$_2$)$^+$. *J. Organomet. Chem.* **2009**, *694*, 4094–4099. [CrossRef]

43. Sundermeyer, J.; Weber, K.; Peters, K.; von Schnering, H.G. Modeling Surface Reactivity of Metal Oxides: Synthesis and Structure of an Ionic Organorhenyl Perrhenate Formed by Ligand-Induced Dissociation of Covalent Re$_2$O$_7$. *Organometallics* **1994**, *13*, 2560–2562. [CrossRef]

44. Schmidbaur, H.; Zybill, C.E.; Müller, G.; Krüger, C. Coinage Metal Complexes of Hexaphenylcarbodiphosphorane–Organometallic Compounds with Coordination Number 2. *Angew. Chem. Int. Ed.* **1983**, *22*, 729–730. [CrossRef]

45. Zybill, C.; Mueller, G. Mononuclear Complexes of Copper(I) and Silver(I) Featuring the Metals Exclusively Bound to Carbon. Synthesis and Structure of (.eta.5-Pentamethylcyclopentadienyl)[(triphenylphosphonio) (triphenylphosphoranylidene)methyl]Copper(I). *Organometallics* **1987**, *6*, 2489–2494. [CrossRef]

46. Vicente, J.; Singhal, A.R.; Jones, P.G. New Ylide–, Alkynyl–, and Mixed Alkynyl/Ylide–Gold(I) Complexes. *Organometallics* **2002**, *21*, 5887–5900. [CrossRef]

47. Kaska, W.C.; Reichelderfer, R.F. The Interaction of Hexaphenylcarbodiphosphorane with Iridium Olefin Cations. Metalation of Coordinated Ligands. *J. Organomet. Chem.* **1974**, *78*, C47–C50. [CrossRef]

48. Münzer, J.E.; Kuzu, I.; Philipps-Universität Marburgdisabled, Marburg, Germany. Unpublished results. Private communication to WP.

49. Pranckevicius, C.; Iovan, D.A.; Stephan, D.W. Three and Four Coordinate Fe Carbodiphosphorane Complexes. *Dalton Trans.* **2016**, *45*, 16820–16825. [CrossRef]

50. Kneusels, N.J.H.; Münzer, J.E.; Flosdorf, K.; Jiang, D.; Neumüller, B.; Zhao, L.; Eichhöfer, A.; Frenking, G.; Kuzu, I. Double Donation in Trigonal Planar Iron–Carbodiphosphorane Complexes—A Aoncise Study on Their Spectroscopic and Electronic Properties. *Dalton Trans.* **2020**, *49*, 2537–2546. [CrossRef]

51. Su, W.; Pan, S.; Sun, X.; Wang, S.; Zhao, L.; Frenking, G.; Zhu, C. Double Dative Bond between Divalent Carbon(0) and Uranium. *Nat. Commun.* **2018**, *9*, 4997. [CrossRef]

52. Tonner, R.; Oexler, F.; Neumuller, B.; Petz, W.; Frenking, G. Carbodiphosphoranes: The Chemistry of Divalent Carbon(0). *Angew. Chem. Int. Ed.* **2006**, *45*, 8038–8042. [CrossRef] [PubMed]

53. Petz, W.; Neumüller, B. Reaction of C(PPh$_3$)$_2$ with MI$_2$ Compounds (M = Zn, Cd) - Formation and Crystal Structures of [I$_2$Zn{C(PPh$_3$)$_2$}], [(I$_2$Cd{C(PPh$_3$)$_2$})$_2$] and the Salt-Like Compounds (HC{PPh$_3$}$_2$)[MI$_3$(THF)] and (HC{PPh$_3$}$_2$)$_2$[ZnI$_4$]. *Eur. J. Inorg. Chem.* **2011**, *31*, 4889–4895. [CrossRef]

54. Romeo, I.; Bardají, M.; Concepción Gimeno, M.; Laguna, M. Gold(I) Complexes Containing the Cationic Ylide Ligand Bis(methyldiphenylphosphonio)methylide. *Polyhedron* **2000**, *19*, 1837–1841. [CrossRef]

55. Bruce, A.E.; Gamble, A.S.; Tonker, T.L.; Templeton, J.L. Cationic Phosphonium Carbyne and Bis(phosphonium) Carbene Tungsten Complexes: [Tp'(OC)$_2$WC(PMe$_3$)n][PF$_6$] (n = 1, 2). *Organometallics* **1987**, *6*, 1350–1352. [CrossRef]

56. Schmidbaur, H.; Gasser, O. The Ambident Ligand Properties of Bis(trimethylphosphoranylidene)methan. *Angew. Chem. Int. Ed.* **1976**, *15*, 502–503. [CrossRef]

57. Dorta, R.; Stevens, E.D.; Scott, N.M.; Costabile, C.; Cavallo, L.; Hoff, C.D.; Nolan, S.P. Steric and Electronic Properties of N-Heterocyclic Carbenes (NHC): A Detailed Study on Their Interaction with Ni(CO)$_4$. *J. Am. Chem. Soc.* **2005**, *127*, 2485–2495. [CrossRef]
58. Pugh, D.; Wright, J.A.; Freeman, S.; Danopoulos, A.A. 'Pincer' Dicarbene Complexes of Some Early Transition Metals and Uranium. *Dalton Trans.* **2006**, *6*, 775–782. [CrossRef]
59. Gardner, B.M.; McMaster, J.; Liddle, S.T. Synthesis and Structure of a Dis-N-Heterocyclic Carbene Complex of Uranium Tetrachloride Exhibiting Short Cl···C Carbene Contacts. *Dalton Trans.* **2009**, *35*, 6924–6926. [CrossRef]
60. Doddi, A.; Gemel, C.; Seidel, R.W.; Winter, M.; Fischer, R.A. Coordination Complexes of TiX$_4$ (X = F, Cl) with a Bulky N-Heterocyclic Carbene: Syntheses, Characterization and Molecular Structures. *Polyhedron* **2013**, *52*, 1103–1108. [CrossRef]
61. Datt, M.S.; Nair, J.J.; Otto, S. Synthesis and Characterisation of Two Novel Rh(I) Carbene Complexes: Crystal Structure of [Rh(acac)(CO)(L$_1$)]. *J. Organomet. Chem.* **2005**, *690*, 3422–3426. [CrossRef]
62. Stallinger, S.; Reitsamer, C.; Schuh, W.; Kopacka, H.; Wurst, K.; Peringer, P. Novel Route to Carbodiphosphoranes Producing a New P,C,P Pincer Carbene Ligand. *Chem. Commun.* **2007**, 510–512. [CrossRef]
63. Klein, M.; Demirel, N.; Schinabeck, A.; Yersin, H.; Sundermeyer, J. Cu(I) Complexes of Multidentate N,C,N- and P,C,P-Carbodiphosphorane Ligands and Their Photoluminescence. *Molecules* **2020**, *25*, 3990. [CrossRef]
64. Klein, M.; Xie, X.; Burghaus, O.; Sundermeyer, J. Synthesis and Characterization of a N,C,N-Carbodiphosphorane Pincer Ligand and Its Complexes. *Organometallics* **2019**, *38*, 3768–3777. [CrossRef]
65. Reitsamer, C.; Stallinger, S.; Schuh, W.; Kopacka, H.; Wurst, K.; Obendorf, D.; Peringer, P. Novel Access to Carbodiphosphoranes in the Coordination Sphere of Group 10 Metals: Template Synthesis and Protonation of PCP Pincer Carbodiphosphorane Complexes of C(dppm)$_2$. *Dalton Trans.* **2012**, *41*, 3503–3514. [CrossRef]
66. Maser, L.; Herritsch, J.; Langer, R. Carbodiphosphorane-Based Nickel Pincer Complexes and Their (de)Protonated Analogues: Dimerisation, Ligand Tautomers and Proton Affinities. *Dalton Trans.* **2018**, *47*, 10544–10552. [CrossRef] [PubMed]
67. Reitsamer, C.; Hackl, I.; Schuh, W.; Kopacka, H.; Wurst, K.; Peringer, P. Gold(I) and Gold(III) Complexes of the [CH(dppm)$_2$]$^+$ and C(dppm)$_2$ PCP Pincer Ligand Systems. *J. Organomet. Chem.* **2017**, *830*, 150–154. [CrossRef]
68. Su, W.; Pan, S.; Sun, X.; Zhao, L.; Frenking, G.; Zhu, C. Cerium–Carbon Dative Interactions Supported by Carbodiphosphorane. *Dalton Trans.* **2019**, *48*, 16108–16114. [CrossRef]
69. Kubo, K.; Jones, N.D.; Ferguson, M.J.; McDonald, R.; Cavell, R.G. Chelate and Pincer Carbene Complexes of Rhodium and Platinum Derived from Hexaphenylcarbodiphosphorane, Ph$_3$PCPPh$_3$. *J. Am. Chem. Soc.* **2005**, *127*, 5314–5315. [CrossRef] [PubMed]
70. Kubo, K.; Okitsu, H.; Miwa, H.; Kume, S.; Cavell, R.G.; Mizuta, T. Carbon(0)-Bridged Pt/Ag Dinuclear and Tetranuclear Complexes Based on a Cyclometalated Pincer Carbodiphosphorane Platform. *Organometallics* **2017**, *36*, 266–274. [CrossRef]
71. Petz, W.; Neumüller, B. New Platinum Complexes with Carbodiphosphorane as Pincer Ligand via Ortho Phenyl Metallation. *Polyhedron* **2011**, *30*, 1779–1784. [CrossRef]
72. Lin, G.; Jones, N.D.; Gossage, R.A.; McDonald, R.; Cavell, R.G. A Tris(carbene) Pincer Complex: Monomeric Platinum Carbonyl with Three Bound Carbene Centers. *Angew. Chem. Int. Ed.* **2003**, *42*, 4054–4057. [CrossRef]
73. Marrot, S.; Kato, T.; Gornitzka, H.; Baceiredo, A. Cyclic Carbodiphosphoranes: Strongly Nucleophilic σ-Donor Ligands. *Angew. Chem. Int. Ed.* **2006**, *45*, 2598–2601. [CrossRef] [PubMed]
74. Corberán, R.; Marrot, S.; Dellus, N.; Merceron-Saffon, N.; Kato, T.; Peris, E.; Baceiredo, A. First Cyclic Carbodiphosphoranes of Copper(I) and Gold(I) and Their Application in the Catalytic Cleavage of X–H Bonds (X = N and O). *Organometallics* **2009**, *28*, 326–330. [CrossRef]
75. Yogendra, S.; Schulz, S.; Hennersdorf, F.; Kumar, S.; Fischer, R.; Weigand, J.J. Reductive Ring Opening of a Cyclo-Tri(phosphonio)methanide Dication to a Phosphanylcarbodiphosphorane: In Situ UV-Vis Spectroelectrochemistry and Gold Coordination. *Organometallics* **2018**, *37*, 748–754. [CrossRef]
76. Alcarazo, M.; Radkowski, K.; Mehler, G.; Goddard, R.; Fürstner, A. Chiral Heterobimetallic Complexes of Carbodiphosphoranes and Phosphinidene–Carbene Adducts. *Chem. Commun.* **2013**, *49*, 3140–3142. [CrossRef] [PubMed]

77. Petz, W.; Kutschera, C.; Neumüller, B. Reaction of the Carbodiphosphorane Ph$_3$PCPPh$_3$ with Platinum(II) and -(0) Compounds: Platinum Induced Activation of C−H Bonds. *Organometallics* **2005**, *24*, 5038–5043. [CrossRef]

78. Baldwin, J.C.; Kaska, W.C. The Interaction of Hexaphenylcarbodiphosphorane with the Trimethylplatinum(IV) Cation. *Inorg. Chem.* **1979**, *18*, 686–691. [CrossRef]

79. Melaimi, M.; Parameswaran, P.; Donnadieu, B.; Frenking, G.; Bertrand, G. Synthesis and Ligand Properties of a Persistent, All-Carbon Four-Membered-Ring Allene. *Angew. Chem. Int. Ed.* **2009**, *48*, 4792–4795. [CrossRef]

80. Hackl, L.; Petrov, A.R.; Bannenberg, T.; Freytag, M.; Jones, P.G.; Tamm, M. Dimerisation of Dipiperidinoacetylene: Convenient Access to Tetraamino-1,3-Cyclobutadiene and Tetraamino-1,2-Cyclobutadiene Metal Complexes. *Chem. Eur. J.* **2019**, *25*, 16148–16155. [CrossRef]

81. Pranckevicius, C.; Liu, L.; Bertrand, G.; Stephan, D.W. Synthesis of a Carbodicyclopropenylidene: A Carbodicarbene Based Solely on Carbon. *Angew. Chem. Int. Ed.* **2016**, *55*, 5536–5540. [CrossRef]

82. Tonner, R.; Frenking, G. C(NHC)$_2$: Divalent Carbon(0) Compounds with N-Heterocyclic Carbene Ligands—Theoretical Evidence for a Class of Molecules with Promising Chemical Properties. *Angew. Chem. Int. Ed.* **2007**, *46*, 8695–8698. [CrossRef] [PubMed]

83. Dyker, C.A.; Lavallo, V.; Donnadieu, B.; Bertrand, G. Synthesis of an Extremely Bent Acyclic Allene (A "Carbodicarbene"): A Strong Donor Ligand. *Angew. Chem. Int. Ed.* **2008**, *47*, 3206–3209. [CrossRef]

84. Hsu, Y.C.; Shen, J.S.; Lin, B.C.; Chen, W.C.; Chan, Y.T.; Ching, W.M.; Yap, G.P.A.; Hsu, C.P.; Ong, T.G. Synthesis and Isolation of an Acyclic Tridentate Bis(pyridine)carbodicarbene and Studies on Its Structural Implications and Reactivities. *Angew. Chem. Int. Ed.* **2015**, *54*, 2420–2424. [CrossRef]

85. Chen, W.C.; Hsu, Y.C.; Lee, C.Y.; Yap, G.P.A.; Ong, T.G. Synthetic Modification of Acyclic Bent Allenes (Carbodicarbenes) and Further Studies on Their Structural Implications and Reactivities. *Organometallics* **2013**, *32*, 2435–2442. [CrossRef]

86. Liberman-Martin, A.L.; Grubbs, R.H. Ruthenium Olefin Metathesis Catalysts Featuring a Labile Carbodicarbene Ligand. *Organometallics* **2017**, *36*, 4091–4094. [CrossRef]

87. Chan, S.C.; Gupta, P.; Engelmann, X.; Ang, Z.Z.; Ganguly, R.; Bill, E.; Ray, K.; Ye, S.F.; England, J. Observation of Carbodicarbene Ligand Redox Noninnocence in Highly Oxidized Iron Complexes. *Angew. Chem. Int. Ed.* **2018**, *57*, 15717–15722. [CrossRef]

88. Chen, W.C.; Shih, W.C.; Jurca, T.; Zhao, L.L.; Andrada, D.M.; Peng, C.J.; Chang, C.C.; Liu, S.K.; Wang, Y.P.; Wen, Y.S.; et al. Carbodicarbenes: Unexpected π-Accepting Ability during Reactivity with Small Molecules. *J. Am. Chem. Soc.* **2017**, *139*, 12830–12836. [CrossRef] [PubMed]

89. Shih, W.C.; Chiang, Y.T.; Wang, Q.; Wu, M.C.; Yap, G.P.A.; Zhao, L.; Ong, T.G. Invisible Chelating Effect Exhibited between Carbodicarbene and Phosphine through π–π Interaction and Implication in the Cross-Coupling Reaction. *Organometallics* **2017**, *36*, 4287–4297. [CrossRef]

90. Chen, W.C.; Shen, J.S.; Jurca, T.; Peng, C.J.; Lin, Y.H.; Wang, Y.P.; Shih, W.C.; Yap, G.P.A.; Ong, T.G. Expanding the Ligand Framework Diversity of Carbodicarbenes and Direct Detection of Boron Activation in the Methylation of Amines with CO$_2$. *Angew. Chem. Int. Ed.* **2015**, *54*, 15207–15212. [CrossRef] [PubMed]

91. Ruiz, D.A.; Melaimi, M.; Bertrand, G. Carbodicarbenes, Carbon(0) Derivatives, Can Dimerize. *Chem. Asian J.* **2013**, *8*, 2940–2942. [CrossRef]

92. Pranckevicius, C.; Fan, L.; Stephan, D.W. Cyclic Bent Allene Hydrido-Carbonyl Complexes of Ruthenium: Highly Active Catalysts for Hydrogenation of Olefins. *J. Am. Chem. Soc.* **2015**, *137*, 5582–5589. [CrossRef]

93. Goldfogel, M.J.; Roberts, C.C.; Meek, S.J. Intermolecular Hydroamination of 1,3-Dienes Catalyzed by Bis(phosphine)carbodicarbene–Rhodium Complexes. *J. Am. Chem. Soc.* **2014**, *136*, 6227–6230. [CrossRef]

94. Roberts, C.C.; Matías, D.M.; Goldfogel, M.J.; Meek, S.J. Lewis Acid Activation of Carbodicarbene Catalysts for Rh-Catalyzed Hydroarylation of Dienes. *J. Am. Chem. Soc.* **2015**, *137*, 6488–6491. [CrossRef]

95. Fürstner, A.; Alcarazo, M.; Goddard, R.; Lehmann, C.W. Coordination Chemistry of Ene-1,1-diamines and a Prototype "Carbodicarbene". *Angew. Chem. Int. Ed.* **2008**, *47*, 3210–3214. [CrossRef] [PubMed]

96. Paoletti, A.M.; Pennesi, G.; Rossi, G.; Ercolani, C. A New Approach to Cofacially Assembled Partially Oxidized Metal Phthalocyanine Low Dimensional Solids: Synthesis, Structure, and Electrical Conductivity Properties of the Fe(IV) Containing Species [(PcFe)$_2$C](I$_3$)$_{0.66}$ Obtained by I$_2$ Doping of (m-Carbido)bis[phthalocyaninatoiron(IV)]. *Inorg. Chem.* **1995**, *34*, 4780–4784.

97. Burzlaff, H.; Voll, U.; Bestmann, H.J. Die Kristall- und Molekülstruktur des (2,2-Diäthoxyvinyliden) -triphenylphosphorans. *Chem. Ber.* **1974**, *107*, 1949–1956. [CrossRef]

98. Alcarazo, M.; Lehmann, C.W.; Anoop, A.; Thiel, W.; Furstner, A. Coordination Chemistry at Carbon. *Nat. Chem.* **2009**, *1*, 295–301. [CrossRef]
99. Troadec, T.; Wasano, T.; Lenk, R.; Baceiredo, A.; Saffon-Merceron, N.; Hashizume, D.; Saito, Y.; Nakata, N.; Branchadell, V.; Kato, T. Donor-Stabilized Silylene/Phosphine-Supported Carbon(0) Center with High Electron Density. *Angew. Chem. Int. Ed.* **2017**, *56*, 6891–6895. [CrossRef] [PubMed]
100. Morosaki, T.; Wang, W.W.; Nagase, S.; Fujii, T. Synthesis, Structure, and Reactivities of Iminosulfane- and Phosphane-Stabilized Carbones Exhibiting Four-Electron Donor Ability. *Chem. Eur. J.* **2015**, *21*, 15405–15411. [CrossRef] [PubMed]
101. Pascual, S.; Asay, M.; Illa, O.; Kato, T.; Bertrand, G.; Saffon-Merceron, N.; Branchadell, V.; Baceiredo, A. Synthesis of a Mixed Phosphonium-Sulfonium Bisylide $R_3P=C=SR_2$. *Angew. Chem. Int. Ed.* **2007**, *46*, 9078–9080. [CrossRef]
102. Morosaki, T.; Iijima, R.; Suzuki, T.; Wang, W.W.; Nagase, S.; Fujii, T. Synthesis, Electronic Structure, and Reactivities of Two-Sulfur-Stabilized Carbones Exhibiting Four-Electron Donor Ability. *Chem. Eur. J.* **2017**, *23*, 8694–8702. [CrossRef]
103. Morosaki, T.; Suzuki, T.; Wang, W.W.; Nagase, S.; Fujii, T. Syntheses, Structures, and Reactivities of Two Chalcogen-Stabilized Carbones. *Angew. Chem. Int. Ed.* **2014**, *53*, 9569–9571. [CrossRef]
104. Fujii, T.; Ikeda, T.; Mikami, T.; Suzuki, T.; Yoshimura, T. Synthesis and Structure of $(MeN)Ph_2S=C=SPh_2(NMe)$. *Angew. Chem. Int. Ed.* **2002**, *41*, 2576–2578. [CrossRef]
105. Morosaki, T.; Suzuki, T.; Fujii, T. Syntheses and Structural Characterization of Mono-, Di-, and Tetranuclear Silver Carbone Complexes. *Organometallics* **2016**, *35*, 2715–2721. [CrossRef]
106. Chen, Y.; Petz, W.; Frenking, G. Is It Possible to Synthesize a Low-Valent Transition Metal Complex with a Neutral Carbon Atom as Terminal Ligand? A Theoretical Study of $(CO)_4FeC$. *Organometallics* **2000**, *19*, 2698–2706. [CrossRef]
107. Zhao, L.; von Hopffgarten, M.; Andrada, D.M.; Frenking, G. Energy Decomposition Analysis. *Wires Comput. Mol. Sci.* **2018**, *8*, e1345. [CrossRef]
108. Takemoto, S.; Matsuzaka, H. Recent Advances in the Chemistry of Ruthenium Carbido Complexes. *Coord. Chem. Rev.* **2012**, *256*, 574–588. [CrossRef]
109. Hejl, A.; Trnka, T.M.; Day, M.W.; Grubbs, R.H. Terminal Ruthenium Carbido Complexes as σ-Donor Ligands. *Chem. Commun.* **2002**, *21*, 2524–2525. [CrossRef]
110. Caskey, S.R.; Stewart, M.H.; Kivela, J.E.; Sootsman, J.R.; Johnson, M.J.A.; Kampf, J.W. Two Generalizable Routes to Terminal Carbido Complexes. *J. Am. Chem. Soc.* **2005**, *127*, 16750–16751. [CrossRef]
111. Reinholdt, A.; Bendix, J. Weakening of Carbide–Platinum Bonds as a Probe for Ligand Donor Strengths. *Inorg. Chem.* **2017**, *56*, 12492–12497. [CrossRef]
112. Reinholdt, A.; Vibenholt, J.E.; Morsing, T.J.; Schau-Magnussen, M.; Reeler, N.E.A.; Bendix, J. Carbide Complexes as π-Acceptor Ligands. *Chem. Sci.* **2015**, *6*, 5815–5823. [CrossRef]
113. Reinholdt, A.; Herbst, K.; Bendix, J. Delivering Carbide Ligands to Sulfide-Rich Clusters. *Chem. Commun.* **2016**, *52*, 2015–2018. [CrossRef] [PubMed]
114. Hong, S.H.; Day, M.W.; Grupps, R.H. Decomposition of a Key Intermediate in Ruthenium-Catalyzed Olefin Metatesis Reactions. *J. Am. Chem. Soc.* **2004**, *126*, 7414–7415. [CrossRef] [PubMed]
115. Morsing, T.J.; Reinholdt, A.; Sauer, S.P.A.; Bendix, J. Ligand Sphere Conversions in Terminal Carbide Complexes. *Organometallics* **2016**, *35*, 100–105. [CrossRef]
116. Stewart, M.H.; Johnson, M.J.A.; Kampf, J.W. Terminal Carbido Complexes of Osmium: Synthesis, Structure, and Reactivity Comparison to the Ruthenium Analogues. *Organometallics* **2007**, *26*, 5102–5110. [CrossRef]
117. Etienne, M.; White, P.S.; Templeton, J.L. An Agostic.mu.-Methyne Molybdenum-Iron Complex from Protonation of a.mu.-Carbide Precursor, $Tp'(CO)_2Mo.tplbond.CFe(CO)_2Cp$. *J. Am. Chem. Soc.* **1991**, *113*, 2324–2325. [CrossRef]
118. Cordiner, L.R.; Hill, A.F.; Wagler, J. Facil Generation of Lithiocarbyne Complexes; $[M(\equiv CLi)(CO)_2\{HB(pzMe_2)_3\}]$ (M = Mo, W; pz = Pyrazol-1-yl). *Organometallics* **2008**, *27*, 5177–5179. [CrossRef]
119. Cade, I.A.; Hill, A.F.; McQueen, C.M.A. Iridium–Molybdenum Carbido Complex via C–Se Activation of a Selenocarbonyl Ligand: $(\mu\text{-}Se_2)[Ir_2\{C\equiv Mo(CO)_2(Tp^*)\}_2(CO)_2(PPh_3)_2]$ (Tp* = Hydrotris (dimethylpyrazolyl)borate). *Organometallics* **2009**, *28*, 6639–6641. [CrossRef]

120. Colebatch, A.L.; Cordiner, R.L.; Hill, A.F.; Nguyen, K.T.H.D.; Shang, R.; Willis, A.C. A Bis-Carbyne (Ethanediylidyne) Complex via the Catalytic Demercuration of a Mercury Bis(carbido) Complex. *Organometallics* **2009**, *28*, 4394–4399. [CrossRef]

121. Knauer, W.; Beck, W. Carbide Bridged Complexes [HB(pz)$_3$(OC)$_2$Mo=C-Pt(PPh$_3$)$_2$Br], [(TPP)Fe=C-M (CO)$_4$-M(CO)$_5$] (M = Mn, Re), [(TPP)Fe=C=Cr(CO)$_5$], TPP)Fe=C=Fe(CO)$_4$] (pz- 3,5-dimethylpyrazol-1-yl; TPP Tetraphenylporphyrinate) from Halogeno-Carbyne and -Carbene Complexes. *Z. Anorg. Allg. Chem.* **2008**, *634*, 2241–2245. [CrossRef]

122. Borren, E.S.; Hill, A.F.; Shang, R.; Sharma, M.; Willis, A.C. A Golden Ring: Molecular Gold Carbido Complexes. *J. Am. Chem. Soc.* **2013**, *135*, 4942–4945. [CrossRef]

123. Buss, J.A.; Agapie, T. Mechanism of Molybdenum-Mediated Carbon Monoxide Deoxygenation and Coupling: Mono- and Dicarbyne Complexes Precede C–O Bond Cleavage and C–C Bond Formation. *J. Am. Chem. Soc.* **2016**, *138*, 16466–16477. [CrossRef] [PubMed]

124. Hill, A.F.; Sharma, M.; Willis, A.C. Heterodinuclear Bridging Carbido and Phosphoniocarbyne Complexes. *Organometallics* **2012**, *31*, 2538–2542. [CrossRef]

125. Frogley, B.J.; Hill, A.F. Tungsten–Platinum μ-Carbido and μ-Methylidyne Complexes. *Chem. Commun.* **2019**, *55*, 12400–12403. [CrossRef] [PubMed]

126. Agapie, T.; Diaconescu, P.L.; Cummins, C.C. Methine (CH) Transfer via a Chlorine Atom Abstraction/Benzene-Elimination Strategy: Molybdenum Methylidyne Synthesis and Elaboration to a Phosphaisocyanide Complex. *J. Am. Chem. Soc.* **2002**, *124*, 2412–2413. [CrossRef] [PubMed]

127. Latesky, S.L.; Selegue, J.P. Preparation and Structure of [(Me$_3$CO)$_3$W.tplbond.C-Ru(CO)$_2$(Cp)], a Heteronuclear,.mu.$_2$-Carbide Complex. *J. Am. Chem. Soc.* **1987**, *109*, 4731–4733. [CrossRef]

128. Mansuy, D.; Lecomte, J.P.; Chottard, J.C.; Bartoli, J.F. Formation of a Complex with a Carbide Bridge between Two Iron Atoms from the Reaction of (Tetraphenylporphyrin)iron(II) with Carbon Tetraiodide. *Inorg. Chem.* **1981**, *20*, 3119–3121. [CrossRef]

129. Battioni, J.-P.; Dupre, D.; Mansuy, D. Reactions du Trichloromethyl-Trimethyl-Silane avec des Ferrotetra-Aryl-Porphyrines. *J. Organometal. Chem.* **1981**, *414*, 303–309. [CrossRef]

130. Galich, L.; Kienast, A.; Hückstädt, H.; Homborg, H. Syntheses, Spectroscopical Properties, and Crystal Structures of Binuclear Homo- and Heteroleptic μ-Carbido Complexes of Iron(IV) with Phthalocyaninate and Tetraphenylporphyrinate Ligands. *Z. Anorg. Allg. Chem.* **1998**, *624*, 1235–1242. [CrossRef]

131. Goedken, V.L.; Deakin, M.R.; Bottomley, L.A. Molecular Stereochemistry of a Carbon-Bridged Metalloporphyrin: μ-Carbido-Bid(5,10,15,20-tetraphenylporphinatoiron). *J. Chem. Soc. Chem. Commun.* **1982**, *11*, 607–608. [CrossRef]

132. Kienast, A.; Galich, L.; Murray, K.S.; Moubaraki, B.; Lazarev, G.; Cashion, J.D.; Homborg, H. M-Carbido Dipophyrinates and Diphthalocyaninates of Iron and Ruthenium. *J. Porphyr. Phthalocyanines* **1997**, *1*, 141–157. [CrossRef]

133. Kienast, A.; Bruhn, C.; Homborg, H. Synthesis, Properties, and Crystal Structure of μ-Carbidodi (pyridinephthalocyaninato(2-)Iron(IV)) and -Ruthenium(IV). *Z. Anorg. Allg. Chem.* **1997**, *623*, 967–972. [CrossRef]

134. Rossi, G.; Goedken, V.L.; Ercolani, C. μ-Carbido-Bridged Iron Phthalocyanine Dimers: Synthesis and Characterization. *J. Chem. Soc. Chem. Commun.* **1988**, *1*, 46–47. [CrossRef]

135. Kienast, A.; Homborg, H. Synthese und Eigenschaften von Bis(tetra(n-butyl)ammonium)-l-carbidodi(halogenophthalocyaninato(2-)ferraten(IV)); Kristallstruktur von Bis(tetra(n-butyl)ammonium)-μ-carbidodi(fluorophthalocyaninato(2-)ferrat(IV))-Trihydrat. *Z. Anorg. Allg. Chem.* **1998**, *624*, 107–112. [CrossRef]

136. Ercolani, C.; Gardini, M.; Goedken, V.L.; Pennesi, G.; Rossi, G.; Russo, U.; Zanonato, P. High-Valent Iron Phthalocyanine Five- and Six-Coordinated μ-Carbido Dimers. *Inorg. Chem.* **1989**, *28*, 3097–3099. [CrossRef]

137. Ahrens, T.; Schmiedecke, B.; Braun, T.; Herrmann, R.; Laubenstein, R. Activation of CS$_2$ and COS at a Rhodium(I) Germyl Complex: Generation of CS and Carbido Complexes. *Eur. J. Inorg. Chem.* **2017**, *3*, 713–722. [CrossRef]

138. Kalläne, S.I.; Braun, T.; Teltewskoi, M.; Braun, B.; Herrmann, R.; Laubenstein, R. Remarkable Reactivity of a Rhodium(i) Boryl Complex Towards CO$_2$ and CS$_2$: Isolation of a Carbido Complex. *Chem. Commun.* **2015**, *51*, 14613–14616. [CrossRef]

139. Barnett, H.J.; Burt, L.K.; Hill, A.F. Simple Generation of a Dirhodium μ-Carbido Complex via Thiocarbonyl Reduction. *Dalton Trans.* **2018**, *47*, 9570–9574. [CrossRef]

140. Solari, E.; Antonijevic, S.; Gauthier, S.; Scopelliti, R.; Severin, K. Formation of a Ruthenium mu-Carbide Complex with Acetylene as the Crbon Source. *Eur. J. Inorg. Chem.* **2007**, *3*, 367–371. [CrossRef]
141. Young, R.D.; Hill, A.F.; Cavigliasso, G.E.; Stranger, R. [(μ-C){Re(CO)$_2$(η-C$_5$H$_5$)}$_2$]: A Surprisingly Simple Bimetallic Carbido Complex. *Angew. Chem. Int. Ed.* **2013**, *52*, 3699–3702. [CrossRef]
142. Miller, R.L.; Wolczanski, P.T.; Rheingold, A.L. Carbide Formation via Carbon Monoxide Dissociation Across a W≡W Bond. *J. Am. Chem. Soc.* **1993**, *115*, 10422–10423. [CrossRef]
143. Beck, W.; Knauer, W.; Robl, C. Synthesis and Structure of the Novel μ-Carbido Complex [(TPP)Fe=C=Re(CO)$_4$Re(CO)$_5$]. *Angew. Chem. Int. Ed.* **1990**, *29*, 318–320. [CrossRef]

Publisher's Note: MDPI stays neutral with regard to jurisdictional claims in published maps and institutional affiliations.

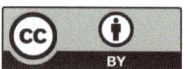

© 2020 by the authors. Licensee MDPI, Basel, Switzerland. This article is an open access article distributed under the terms and conditions of the Creative Commons Attribution (CC BY) license (http://creativecommons.org/licenses/by/4.0/).

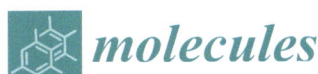

Review

Selenonium Ylides: Syntheses, Structural Aspects, and Synthetic Applications

Józef Drabowicz [1,2,*], **Aneta Rzewnicka [1,*]** and **Remigiusz Żurawiński [1,*]**

1   Division of Organic Chemistry, Centre of Molecular and Macromolecular Studies, Polish Academy of Sciences, Sienkiewicza 112, 90-363 Łódź, Poland
2   Institute of Chemistry, Jan Dlugosz University in Czestochowa, Armii Krajowej 13/15, 42–200 Czestochowa, Poland
*   Correspondence: draj@cbmm.lodz.pl (J.D.); anetrzew@cbmm.lodz.pl (A.R.); remzur@cbmm.lodz.pl (R.Ż.); Tel.: +48-510812551 (J.D.)

Academic Editor: Yves Canac
Received: 30 April 2020; Accepted: 19 May 2020; Published: 22 May 2020

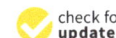

Abstract: The goals of this mini review constitute (a) a presentation of the synthetic protocols applied to the preparation of achiral and non-racemic selenonium ylides; (b) discussion of their basic structural features, including their optical activity; and (c) a description of their synthetic applications in general synthetic methodology and in asymmetric synthesis.

Keywords: selenonium ylides; selenonium salts; chirality; stereogenic selenium atom; asymmetric synthesis; optical resolution; reactivity

1. Introduction

A large family of organic selenium derivatives showing various reactivities and structural properties can be classified by different criteria. A general systematic scheme proposed by Martin and coworkers [1,2], based on simultaneous consideration of the formal oxidation state and number (*N*) of ligands bonded to selenium, allows a description of selenonium ylides, for which two resonance structures **1** and **2** can be considered, as 8-Se-3 or 10-Se-3 species, respectively (Figure 1).

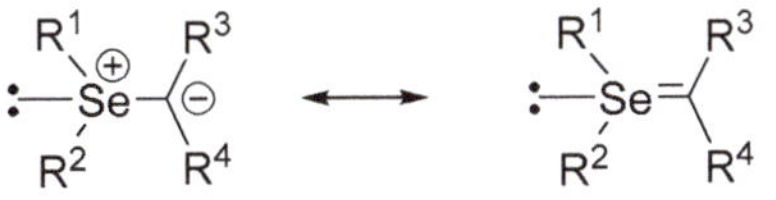

Figure 1. Resonance structures of selenonium ylides **1** and **2**.

It is worth noting that for this family of selenoorganic derivatives, adopting resonance structure **1** allows formal consideration of these compounds as the group of trivalent tri-coordinated onium salts. On the other hand, considering structure **2**, in which the central selenium atom has expanded its valence shell from 8 to 10 electrons, allows them to be treated formally as hypervalent compounds (concept first proposed by Musher in 1969 [3]). Due to the importance of the charged structure **1**, polarized from selenium to carbon, selenonium ylides are not considered as hypervalent compounds and they represent 8-Se-3 species. In our review, both resonance structures of selenonium ylides are used.

After looking at the structure of sulfonium ylides (Figure 2), which constitute the basic group of sulfur ylides [4–8], it is obvious to consider them as a reference point for selenonium ylides (Figure 1). This is due to the fact that their reactivity is dominated mainly by the presence of a highly polarized heteroatom–carbon bond, and their chirality is associated with their tetrahedral geometry, which induces the optical activity of compounds in which three different carbon chains or/and rings are bonded to a stereogenic heteroatom.

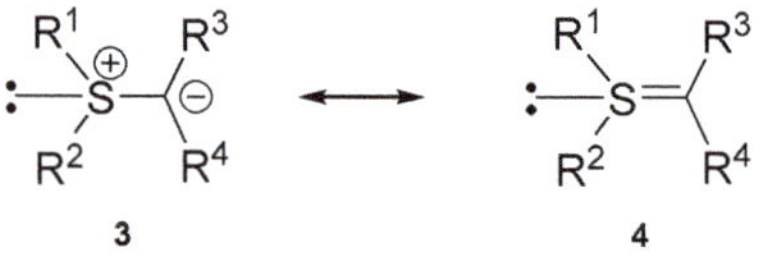

Figure 2. Resonance structures of sulfur ylides **3** and **4**.

The tetrahedral geometry of chiral sulfur and selenium ylides can also be represented alternatively as an irregular trigonal pyramid in which the selenium atom occupies the top of the pyramid (Figure 3).

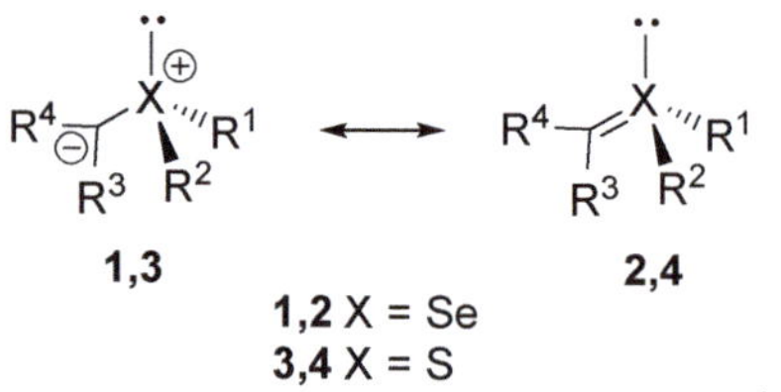

1,2 X = Se
3,4 X = S

Figure 3. Stereo presentation of resonance structures of selenium(sulfur) ylides **1–4**.

In fact, studies devoted to sulfur ylides, especially optically active derivatives, are much richer compared to selenium analogues [4–8]. The best illustration of this phenomenon may be the comparison of the number of documents, which can be obtained by entering the terms "sulfur ylides" and "selenium ylides" or their general drawings to SciFinder or Reaxys databases (close 1 to 6, i.e., around 500 for sulfur ylides and 85 for selenium ylides).

The purpose of this mini review is to provide, as much as possible, available information on the preparation of selenium ylides, including the isolation of optically active species, their chemical and optical stabilities, basic reactivity, and their use in organic and asymmetric synthesis. It is our hope that this paper will stimulate additional research on this topic. It should be noted here that this topic has not yet been presented in a dedicated review. It has usually been discussed as a part of review articles or book chapters devoted to the chemistry of organic chalcogen derivatives, the co-authors of which were researchers conducting research in this field. A list of such, usually short, literature compilations opens a mini review based on the lecture given by Lloyd and published in a special issue of Chemica Scripta devoted to selenium chemistry in 1975 [9]. For the next few years in a row, a brief discussion devoted to selenonium ylides was included into the chapters from Specialist Periodical Reports, Organic Compounds of Sulfur, Selenium, and Tellurium [10–14]. A few years later, similar discussion was included into Chapter 17 of The Chemistry of Organic Selenium and Tellurium Compounds from Patai's Chemistry of Functional Groups [15]. An update of this information can be found in an analogous chapter entitled "Synthesis of selenium and tellurium ylides and carbanions: application to organic synthesis" again included in "The Chemistry of Organic Selenium and Tellurium Compounds" from Patai's "Chemistry of Functional Groups" series published in 2014 [16]. There are also brief accounts that describe experiments on the synthesis, stereochemical aspects, and the application in asymmetric synthesis of optically active tricoordinated selenium and tellurium compounds in which optically active selenonium ylides are also mentioned [17,18]. A piece of information related to the chemistry of selenonium ylides can be found in a review article entitled "Twice stabilized chalcogen ylides" written in the Russian language and published in Uspekhi Khimii in 1981 [19]. Below, we are going to discuss the synthesis of selenonium ylides (achiral, racemic, and optically active), their structural parameters and selected reactivities, and their application in general and asymmetric syntheses.

2. Structural Features

The basic geometrical parameters of selenonium ylides (tetrahedral arrangement of three substituents and a lone electron pair) were not mentioned in two pioneering papers devoted to this group of selenoorganic derivatives. In fact, the first attempt to isolate selenonium ylide as a stable chemical entity was unsuccessful. It was found that the action of aqueous alkali or ammonia on fluorenyl-9-dimethylselenonium bromide **5** gave the expected selenonium ylide **6** as a black solid product, which after dissolving in organic solvents, decomposed rapidly with the evolution of dimethyl selenide even at room temperature (Scheme 1) [20].

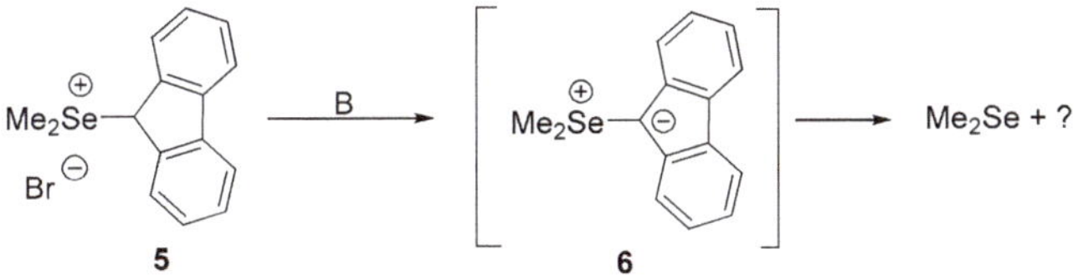

Scheme 1. Unsuccessful attempt to isolate fluorenyl-9-dimethyl selenonium ylide **6**.

It was not until more than 30 years ago that the first stable selenonium ylide **7** (Figure 4) was isolated and fully characterized (for details, see Section 3—Synthesis) [21]. However, also in this article, the geometrical features of a chemically stable compound are not mentioned.

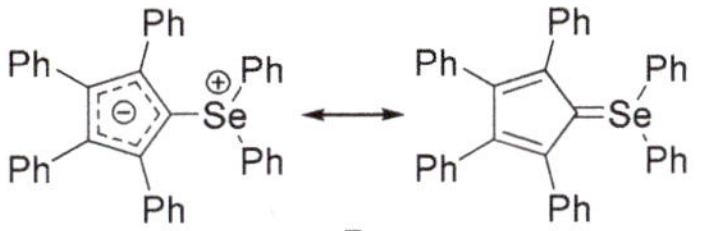

Figure 4. The first isolated selenonium ylide **7**.

Only the first crystallographic data obtained in 1972 for the selenonium ylide **8** fully supported the aforementioned geometrical framework of this family of ylides (Figure 5) [22].

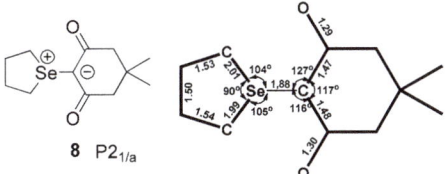

Figure 5. Selected cystallographic data of selenonium ylide **8** (taken from [22]).

Namely, it was found [22] that in the structure of this solid ylide, which crystallizes in the P2$_1$/a space group, the selenium atom occupies the top of the irregular trigonal pyramid with angles C-Se-C 90, 104, 105°. The value of the first angle (90°) results from the rigidity of the cycle, as in the free ion (CH$_3$)$_3$Se$^+$ the corresponding angles are 98, 98, and 99° [23]. The distance Se-C (endocyclic) 1.88 Å practically does not differ from the length of the corresponding bonds in dibenzoselenophene 1.90 Å [24]. It is shorter than the weighted average distances Se-C$_{arom}$ 1.92(2) Å and Se-C$_{alif}$ 1.98(2) Å [24], as well as distances Se-C 1.95 Å in trimethylselenonium iodide [23] but longer than a double Se=C bond of 1.80 Å in the structure of [1,2,5]oxaselenazolo[2,3-b][1,2,5]oxaselenazole-7-Se^{IV} [25]. Over the next few years, the determination of the molecular geometry was achieved by an X-ray structure analysis for two other cyclic selenonium ylides **9** and **10** [26] and acyclic diacetylmethylenediphenylselenurane **11** [27] and acetylnitromethylenediphenylselenurane **12** [28] (Figure 6). Similar parameters were observed in all cases.

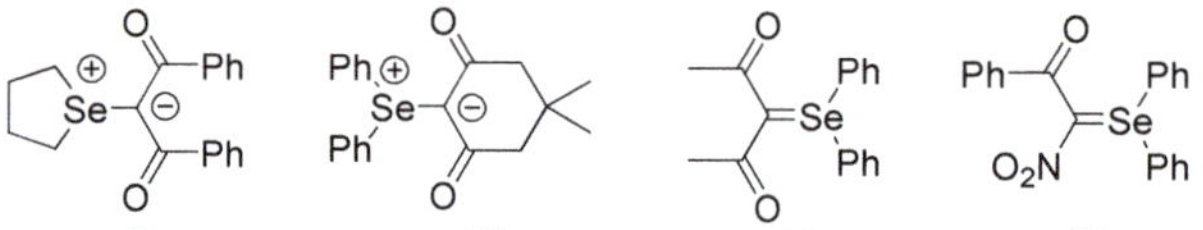

Figure 6. Selenonium ylides **9–12**.

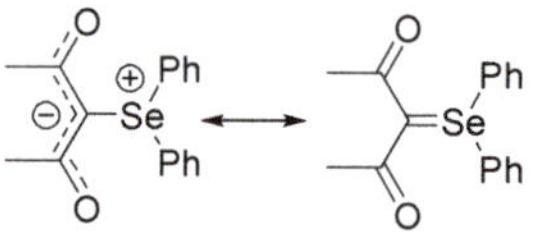

Thus, the detailed analysis [27] of the data collected for the orange crystals of **11** showed that they are monocyclic with four molecules in the unit cell. The space group is P2$_1$/c and the configuration at selenium in **11** is pyramidal with Se lying 0.78 Å out of the plane of the three substituents. The Se-C[C(CO)Me)]$_2$ bond length is 1.906(8) Å, and the Se-C(phenyl) bond lengths are 1.898(9) and 1.926(9) Å. The long Se-C[C(CO)Me)]$_2$ bond and the configuration at selenium was suggested to indicate a large contribution of the ylide resonance structure **11a**. The importance of resonance structure **11a**, in which the delocalization afforded the carbanion by the carbonyl groups, is evident from the IR spectrum of the selenonium ylide **11**, in which the carbonyl group gave a broad absorption at 1520 cm^{-1}.

The X-ray structural analysis of a remarkably stable crystals of the selenonium ylide **13** (monoclinic, space group P2$_1$) (Figure 7) [29] shows the strong transannular contact between oxygen and selenium atoms [O(1)-Se contact is 2.70 Å]. The approximately collinear C(3)-Se-O(1) angle of 170.3° indicates that the cationic species generated on the selenium atom strongly interacts with the oxygen atom of the ether linkage. In addition, the bond length of Se-C(3), 1.887 Å, supports a strongly polarized resonance structure (since the calculated double Se-C bond is close to 1.84 Å [30,31] and the C(1)-Se-C(2) angle, 107.7°, supports the pyramidal geometry.

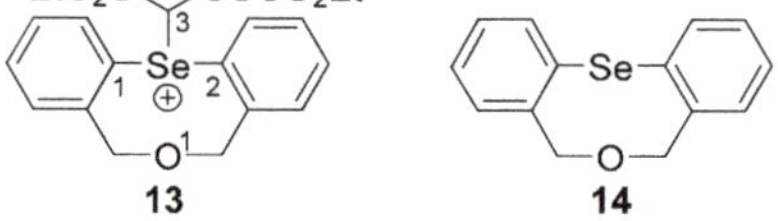

Figure 7. Selenonium ylide **13** and its precursor **14**.

From a set of four diastereomeric selenonium ylides, [(menthyloxycarbonyl)phenyl] (methyl)selenonium 4,4-dimethyl-2,6-dioxocyclohexylides **15a,b** and **16a,b** prepared with the use of (−)-(1R,2S,5R)-menthol or (+)-(1S,2R,5S)-menthol as a chiral auxiliary (Figure 8) diastereoisomerically pure, dextrorotatory selenonium ylide, (+)-{4′-[(−)-menthyloxycarbonyl]}phenyl](methyl)selenonium 4,4-dimethyl-2,6-dioxocyclohexylide **15a**, was isolated by multiple fractional recrystallizations [27,28]. The X-ray crystallographic analysis allowed determination of its *R* absolute configuration at the stereogenic selenium atom. [32,33]. This analysis also showed that the bond length Se-C(2) (1.873 Å) in this diastereoisomer is much shorter than the standard Se-C bond length (1.95–2.04 Å) [25,26] and slightly shorter than that observed in diphenylselenonium diacetylmethylide **11a** (1.906 Å) [27]. This suggests the important resonance contribution from an ylene structure in ylide **15a**. This is additionally supported by the shortening of the bond lengths C(2)-C(3) and C(2)-C(7) (1.41 Å) in isomer **15a**. They are shorter than the usual C-C single-bond [25,26]. The bond angles around the stereogenic selenium in **15a** equal to C(1)-Se-C(2) 103.8(4)°, C(1)-Se-C(l0) 98.6(4)°, and C(2)-Se-C(10) 102.1(4)° are smaller than the values of 100.8, 105.0, and 107.5° observed in diphenylselenonium diacetylmethylide **11** [27]. These changes suggest that selenonium ylide **15a** has a 'sharper' pyramidal structure than diacetylmethylide **11** [27].

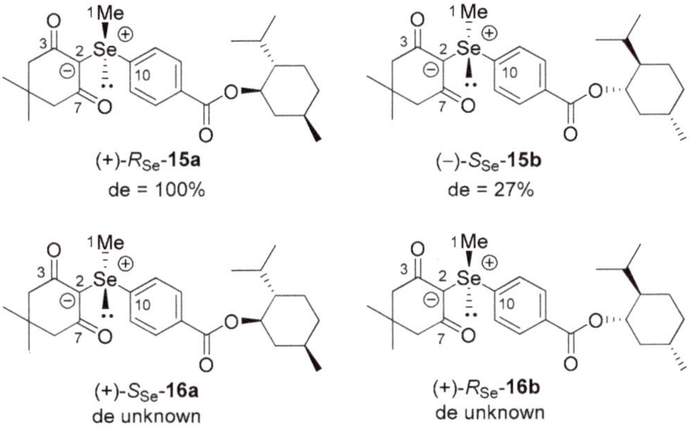

Figure 8. Diasteroisomerically pure selenonium ylide **15a** and diastereoisomerically enriched ylides **15b** and **16a,b**.

The X-ray crystallographic analysis also allowed determination of its *R* absolute configuration at the stereogenic selenium atom in the selenonium ylide **17a** designed using the 2-*exo*-hydroxy 10-bornyl moiety as a chiral frame (Figure 9) [34]. This analysis also showed that the bond length and bond angels of **17a** are similar to those presented above for **15a**.

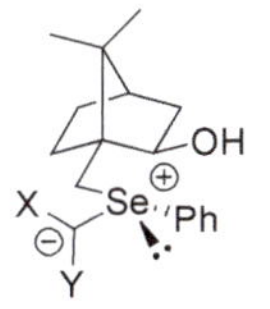

17a: X = COMe, Y = CO$_2$Me

Figure 9. Selenonium ylide **17a** containing the 2-*exo*-hydroxy 10-bornyl moiety.

In addition to the use of X-ray analysis to confirm the solid state structures of selected selenonium ylides, including the assignment of the absolute configuration of a stereogenic selenium atom of two optically active diastereoisomerically pure ylides, other spectroscopic techniques were used and are still applied in the determination of other structural features of achiral and chiral selenonium ylides. Of the various spectroscopies used for these purposes, ^{77}Se-NMR spectroscopy can be formally considered as natural. Its utility, however, is limited because it only allows the incorporation of the tested compound into a given family of selenoorganic derivatives, taking into account its chemical shift. This is most probably the reason why there is only one publication, in the available chemical literature, devoted specifically to ^{77}Se-NMR spectroscopy. The basic topic of this paper, published in Russian as early as 1982, is a brief discussion on the relationship between the structure of selected selenonium ylides and their ^{77}Se chemical shift [35]. The table prepared based on the original data is placed below (Figure 10). We also prepared a plot showing the relationship between the chemical shift and the structure of various selenoorganic groups (Figure 11).

Ylide	R¹	R²	R³	R⁴	δ (^{77}Se): ppm	Solvent
a	CH_3	CH_3	b)	b)	259.9	DMSO-d_6
a	CH_3	CH_3	b)	b)	249.4	$CHCl_3$
b	CH_3	CH_3	$COCH_3$	$COCH_3$	301.5	$CHCl_3$
c	CH_3	Ph	c)	c)	338.9	DMSO-d_6
c	CH_3	Ph	c)	c)	329.5	$CHCl_3$
d	CH_3	CH_3	$COCH_3$	CONHPh	328.3	DMSO-d_6
d	CH_3	CH_3	$COCH_3$	CONHPh	318.6	$CHCl_3$
e	CH_3	CH_3	c)	c)	233.5	$CHCl_3$
f	Ph	Ph	c)	c)	431.2	$CHCl_3$
g	Ph	Ph	b)	b)	448.7	DMSO-d_6
h	CH_3	CH_3	COPh	$COCH_3$	303.0	$CHCl_3$
i	CH_3	CH_3	COPh	COPh	310.0	$CHCl_3$
j	d)	d)	$COCH_3$	CONHPh	452.1	$CHCl_3$
k	Ph	Ph	CN	CN	538.3	$CHCl_3$

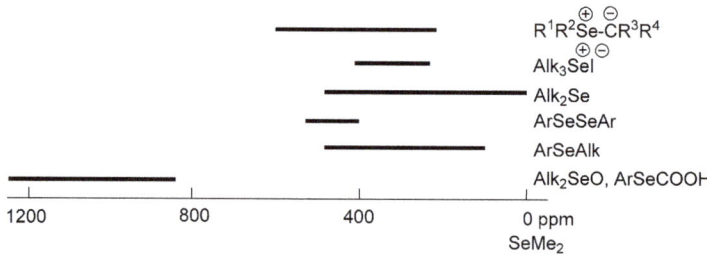

a) 20% mol solution, 25 °C; b) CR^3R^4 = (cyclohexane-1,3-dione); c) CR^3R^4 = (indane-1,3-dione); d) R^1R^2Se = (tetrahydroselenophene)

Figure 10. ^{77}Se chemical shifts of selenonium ylides **1** a) ($R^1R^2Se^+$-$^-CR^3R^4$) (Me_2Se as a reference).

```
                                           ⊕ ⊖
                                    R¹R²Se-CR³R⁴
                                        ⊕ ⊖
                                    Alk₃SeI
                                    Alk₂Se
                                    ArSeSeAr
                                    ArSeAlk
                                    Alk₂SeO, ArSeCOOH
   1200        800        400        0 ppm
                                    SeMe₂
```

Figure 11. Figure presenting the relationship between the structure and chemical shift for the different groups of selenoorganic derivatives.

The analysis of the relationship between the structure and chemical shift for the various groups of selenoorganic derivatives shown in both figures indicates that the range of ^{77}Se chemical shifts observed for selenonium ylides is not very characteristic for this group of selenoorganic derivatives, because it is imposed with the range that is characteristic for trialkylselenonium iodides, dialkyl selenides, alkyl aryl selenides, diaryl diselenides, and aryl alkyl selenides. In this context, it is interesting to note that the ^{77}Se chemical shift for the selenonium ylide **13** in $CDCl_3$ shows a downfield shift to σ = 504.1 from σ = 367.1 observed for its precursor **14** (relative to Me_2Se) [24].

As a rule, ^{1}H-NMR spectroscopy is used as a standard tool for the structural determination of selenonium ylides, which provides information on the numbers of chemically nonequivalent protons, which appear in the spectra of given compounds as typical multiplets. However, sometimes, in addition to standard applications, it is also used to solve more specific structural problems associated with, for example, dynamic processes occurring in the test molecule or to determine the enantiomeric or diastereomeric excesses of chiral derivatives. Thus, based on the ^{1}H-NMR spectrum of the selenonium ylide **13**, in which the methylene protons peaks absorb at σ = 4.79 and 5.03 (ABq J = 14.0 Hz), the existence of the boat conformation of an eight-membered selenium-containing ring was suggested [29].

The lack of broadening of the methyl peak in the ^{1}H-NMR spectrum of the selenonium ylide **11** upon cooling to −60 °C indicates that the equilibration of the two methyl groups proceeds via an energy barrier of <10 kcal/mol [27]. This value is lower than that of the sulfonium ylide $Me_2SC(COCMe)_2$ for which a barrier of 12 kcal/mol (based on C-methyl signals broadening at −25 °C) was reported [36]. The ^{1}H-NMR spectra were used for the determination of the diastereoisomeric excesses of selenonium ylides **15a** and **15b**. Unexpectedly, only one singlet signal of MeSe group was observed, at δ = 3.22, not only in diastereoisomerically pure ylide (+)-**15a** but also in diastereoisomeric mixture of selenonium ylides **15a,b**. However, two singlets for the MeSe group were observed, at δ = 4.01 and 4.16, for the diastereoisomeric mixture of selenonium ylides **15a,b** when the ^{1}H-NMR spectrum was recorded in the presence of europium trisheptafluorobutyrylcamphorate [Eu(hfc)$_3$] as a chiral shift reagent. Moreover, the *ortho*-aromatic hydrogen (from Ar-selenium ring) in diastereoisomers **15a,b** appeared as two AB quartets at δ = 7.724 and 7.732. Thus, the diastereoisomeric purity of the diastereoisomeric mixture of ylide **15** was determined from the integration of their ^{1}H-NMR signals at the ortho-position of the aromatic ring or at the MeSe signal using the shift reagent [32]. The analysis of the ^{1}H-NMR spectra of the cyclic *exo*-ylides, (3,4-dihydro-1*H*-2-benzoselenin-2-io)methanides **18a–e** (Figure 12), which showed AB quartets assigned to 1-H of the methanide entities occupying the sterically relaxed pseudo-equatorial positions, allowed the suggestion of the preference for the given conformation of the 6-membered saturated selenocyclohexane, as the protons *cis* to the 1- and 4-positions of the methanide groups appear at lower magnetic fields as a result of the anisotropic effects of the methanide entities [37].

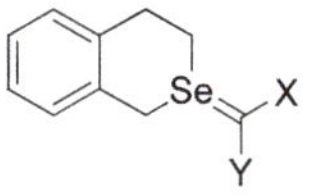

a, X = COMe, Y = COMe
b, X = COMe, Y = CO$_2$Me
c, X = CO$_2$Me, Y = CO$_2$Me
d, X = CO$_2$Me, Y = CN
e, X = CN, Y = CN

Figure 12. Cyclic *exo*-selenonium ylides **18a–e** based on the dihydro-2-benzoselenin cycle.

There are only very few reports on the application of ^{13}C- and ^{19}F-NMR spectroscopies as a standard tool for the structural determination of selenonium ylides, which provides information on the numbers of chemically nonequivalent carbon or fluorine atoms, which appear in the spectra of given compounds as typical multiplets. The data for a series of selenonium ylides **19a–f**, which were extracted from the supporting information of a very recent publication [38], are given in Figure 13. Similar values were observed for the ethyl analogue of the selenonium ylide **19a** [39].

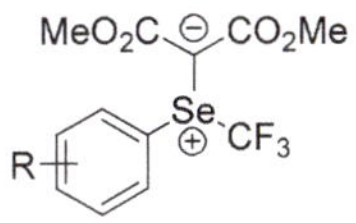

No	R	^{19}F-NMR CF$_3$	^{13}C-NMR $^{\ominus}$C(CO$_2$Me)$_2$
a	*p*-NO$_2$	−48.32	65.4
b	*m*-NO$_2$	−43.17	65.4
c	*o*-NO$_2$	−41.73	65.2
d	*p*-MeO	−45.95	55.7
e	*p*-Ph	−44.93	64.9
f	*p*-Cl	−44.25	65.1

Figure 13. ^{13}C and ^{19}F chemical shift of selenonium ylides **19a–f**.

The application of IR and UV-VIS spectroscopies also has a standard character for the structural determination of selenonium ylides, which provides information on the incorporation of basic functional groups (carbonyl and aromatic rings) in a given structure. Thus, the carbonyl groups of selenonium ylide **11** gave a broad IR absorption at 1520 cm^{-1}. This value is strongly shifted to lower values from the standard value observed for the carbonyl group due to the delocalization resulting from the presence of the carbonyl groups [27]. Thus, the IR spectra of the cyclic *exo*-ylides, (3,4-dihydro-1*H*-2-benzoselenin-2-io)methanides **18a–e** (Figure 12) exhibited strong IR absorptions, shifted ca. 100 cm^{-1} to a lower frequency than the typical absorption for the carbonyl and cyano groups. These shifts were explained by assuming that the ylidic carbanions are delocalized over the electron-withdrawing carbonyl and/or cyano groups [37]. From time to time, UV-VIS data is attached to the spectroscopic characteristics of a given selenonium ylide. The relevant data for several selenonium ylides, **9** [40], **12** [28], and **15a** [32], already mentioned in this review are shown in Figure 14.

Ylide	L(nm)/Solvent	e [log e]	Ref.
9	232/MeOH	[430]	[35]
		290 [3.94]	
		322 [3.98]	
12	339/MeCN	7300	[23]
15a	250.3/MeOH	2.89 × 104	[27]

Figure 14. UV data for selenonium ylides, **9**, **12**, and **15a**.

In a single publication devoted to the use of circular dichroism spectroscopy as a tool in the structural determination of chiral selenonium ylides, the CD spectra of diastereomerically pure selenonium ylide (+)-**15a** and diastereoisomerically enriched ylide (−)-**15b** were analyzed. This analysis showed that the Cotton effects at 266 and 251 nm are related to the absolute configuration around a stereogenic selenium in the ylide **15**. Thus, the *R* configuration in the selenonium ylide **15a** is related to a positive Cotton effect at 266 nm, and a negative Cotton effect at 251 nm, and consequently, the *S* configuration in the ylide **15b** is related to a negative Cotton effect at 266 nm, and a positive Cotton effect at 251 nm [32].

There is a single publication dedicated specifically to the use of mass spectrometry as a tool in the structural determination of selenonium ylides [41]. Among the ylides, for which fragmentation modes are discussed in this paper, there are compounds **9–11**, already mentioned in this manuscript. Moreover, the detailed analysis of the mass spectrum of the selenonium ylide **11** showed that the molecular ion at $m/z = 332$ has the greatest abundance, thus indicating its high stability. Other fragments were observed at $m/z = 234$, which corresponds to Ph_2Se^+, and at $m/z = 157$, which corresponds to $C_6H_6Se^+$. The loss of one methyl group, which gave the peak with $m/z = 317$, was also observed [27]. Very recently, HRMS spectra were reported for a series of selenonium ylides **19a–f** [38].

The various spectroscopic techniques, which were mentioned above, were applied to determine the structural features of selenabenzene derivatives, which formally can be considered as the specific group of selenonium ylides [41,42]. One such example is stable 1-cyano-2-methyl-2-selenanaphthalene, **20** [43]. It was found that the IR absorption of its cyano group observed at 2130 cm^{-1} as a broad very strong band was shifted to the lower frequency than normal by about 100 cm^{-1}. This was suggested as strong evidence that the selenanaphthalene **20** is stabilized by the contribution of the ketenimine resonance structure **20a** (Figure 15).

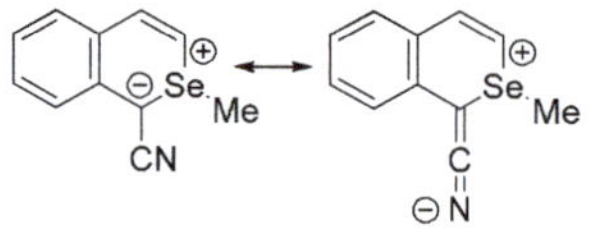

Figure 15. Stable selenabenzene **20**.

3. Synthesis

The major routes for the synthesis of selenonium ylides are as shown in Scheme 2.

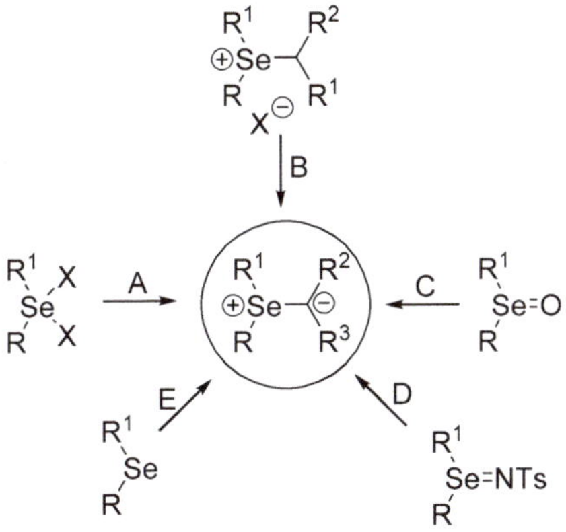

Scheme 2. Major synthetic routs to selenonium ylides; (A) Reaction of dihaloselenuranes with activated methylene compounds in the presence of bases, (B) deprotonation of selenonium salts with bases, (C) reaction of selenoxides with activated methylene compounds or electron-deficient alkynes, (D) reaction of selenonium (N-arylsulfon)imides with activated methylene compounds, and (E) reaction of selenides with aryliodonium zwitterions or diazocompounds.

3.1. Achiral and Racemic Compounds

The synthesis of the first stable selenonium ylide was reported by Lloyd and Singer in 1967 [21]. It was based on the reaction of a carbene generated by the thermal decomposition of diazotetraphenylcyclopentadiene with diphenylselenide (Scheme 3). After a simple workup, selenonium ylide **7** was obtained in a 93% yield as air stable yellow crystals.

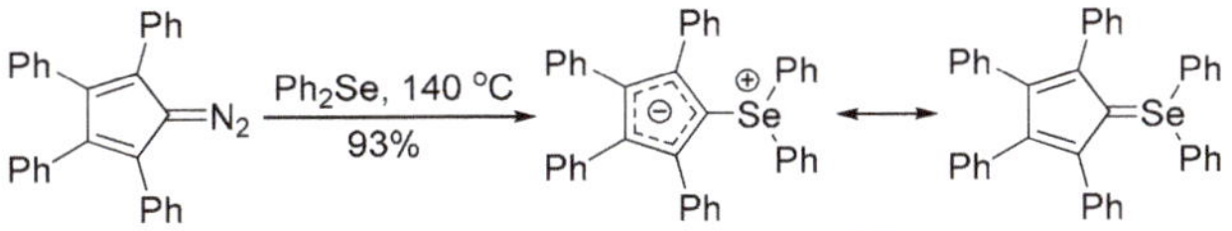

Scheme 3. Synthesis of the first stable selenonium ylide **7**.

The Cu(acac)$_2$-promoted reaction of diazodimedone (**21**) with bis(4-methoxyphenyl)selenide (**22**) was successfully applied in the synthesis of stable ylide **23** (Scheme 4) [44].

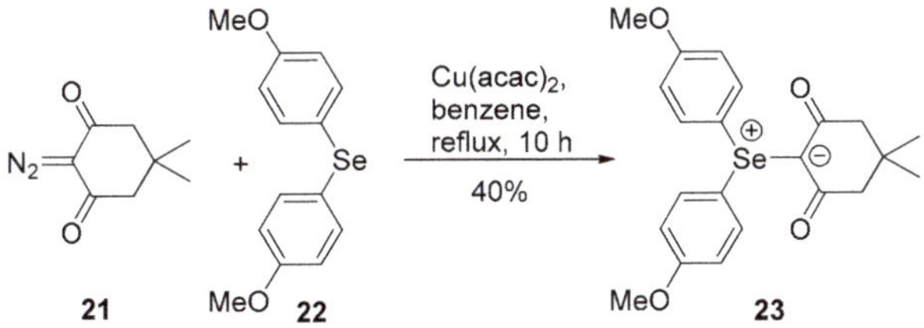

Scheme 4. Synthesis of ylide **23** via the reaction of diazocompound **21** with selenide **22**.

Recently, an efficient and robust carbenoid version of the so-called "diazo approach" to the synthesis of stable trifluoromethyl(aryl) selenonium ylides was developed by Ge and Shen [38]. They found that the treatment of trifluoromethyl(aryl)selenides with dimethyl diazomalonate in the presence of a catalytic amount of a rhodium salt (Rh$_2$(esp)$_2$ bis[rhodium($\alpha,\alpha,\alpha',\alpha'$-tetramethyl-1,3-benzenepropionic acid)]) for 1 h at 40 °C afforded air- and moisture-insensitive crystalline selenonium ylides **19a–f** in 45–91% yields (Scheme 5).

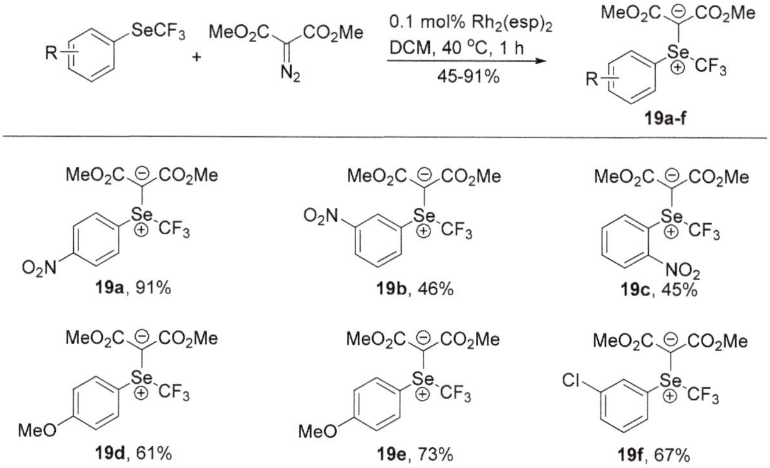

Scheme 5. Preparation of Se-trifluoromethyl-substituted selenonium ylides **19a–f**.

The displacement of an aryliodonium group from aryliodonium zwitterion **24** with diphenyl selenide was employed for the preparation of **25** [45]. After reflux for 1.5 h of a mixture of aryliodonium zwitterion **24** with diphenyl selenide in acetonitrile, stable selenonium ylide **25** was isolated in 24% (Scheme 6).

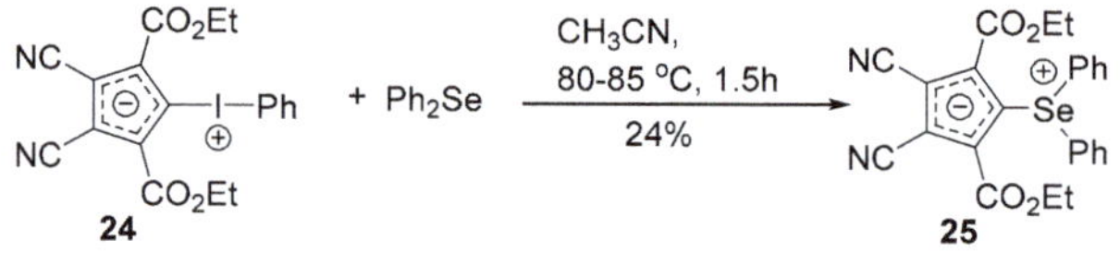

Scheme 6. Synthesis of selenonium ylide **25**.

Selenonium ylides stabilized by two electron-withdrawing substituents on the carbanionic center were generated by the reaction of the corresponding dihalogenoselenuranes and activated methylene compounds. For the first time, this approach was applied as early as in 1971 when 5-dimethylselanylidene-2.2-dimethyl-1,3-dioxane-4,6-dione (**26**) was prepared by the reaction of dibromodimethylselenurane with one equivalent of sodium salt of Meldrum acid in the presence of triethylamine (Scheme 7) [46].

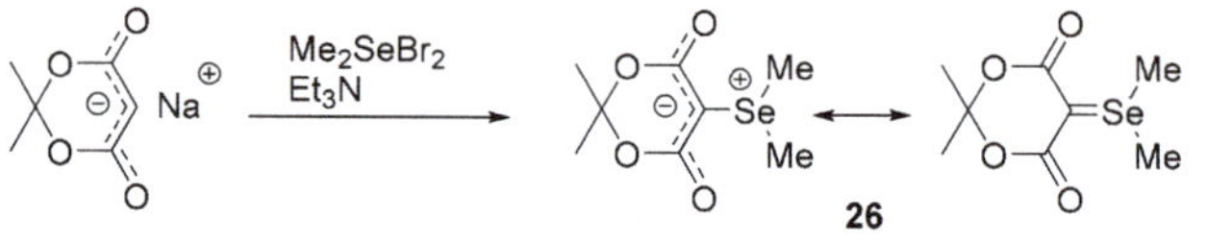

Scheme 7. Synthesis of 5-dimethylselanylidene-2.2-dimethyl-1,3-dioxane-4,6-dione (**26**).

Such an approach to the synthesis of selenonium ylides was also independently developed by Russian chemists for the preparation of diphenylselenonium dimedoneylide **10** [47]. Based on this strategy, this group and a number of others synthesized later on several stable acyclic and cyclic selenonium ylides **27** [22], **8–10, 28–38** [26,40], **11** [27], **39** [48], and **18a–e** [37] containing two electron acceptor groups, such as carbonyl, alkoxycarbonyl, or nitryl, attached to the ylide carbon atom (Scheme 8).

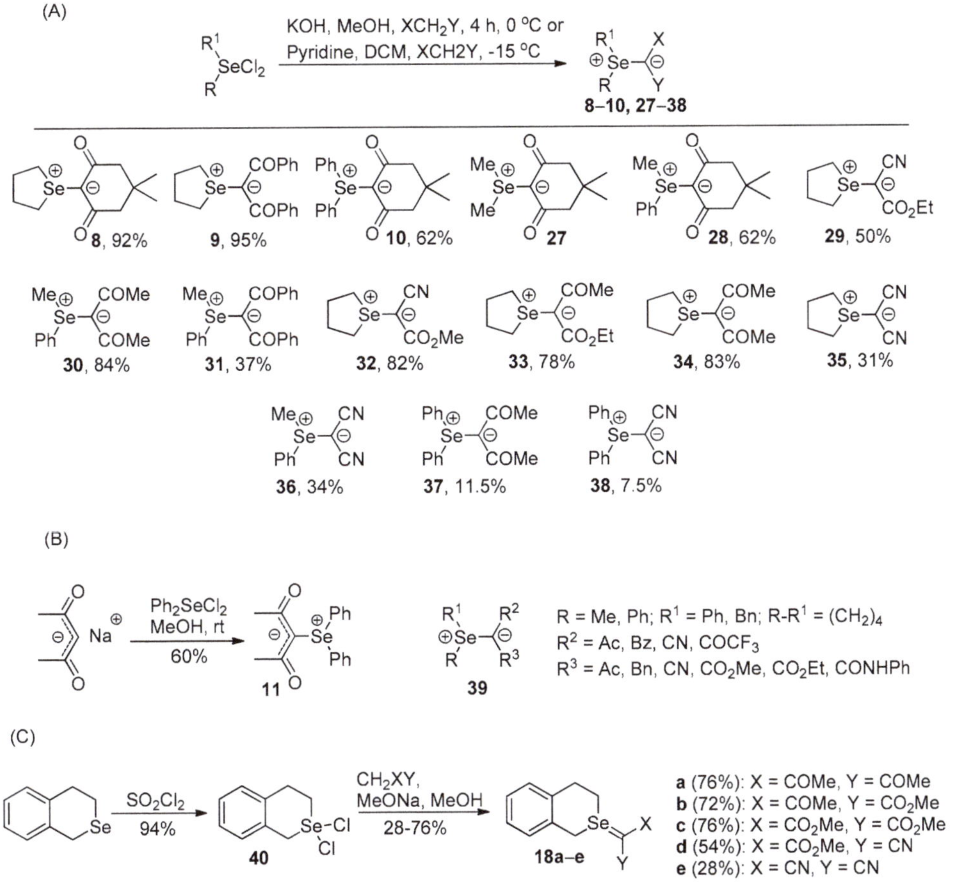

Scheme 8. Selenonium ylides synthesized from dihalogenoselenuranes and activated methylene compounds. (**A**) from dimethyl, methylphenyl, diphenyl and selenophene dihalogenoselenouranes; (**B**) from methylphenyl, diphenyl and selenophene dichloroselenouranes; (**C**) from cyclic dichloroselenouranes **40**.

Expanding the above strategy, Magdesieva and Kyandzhetsian worked out in 1973 a simple two-step protocol for the preparation of stable selenonium ylide salts [49,50]. It encompassed the treatment of stabilized phosphonium ylides **41** with dichloroselenurane **42**, affording double salts **43**, which in the presence of Al_2O_3 were converted into the white solid ylide salts **44** (Scheme 9).

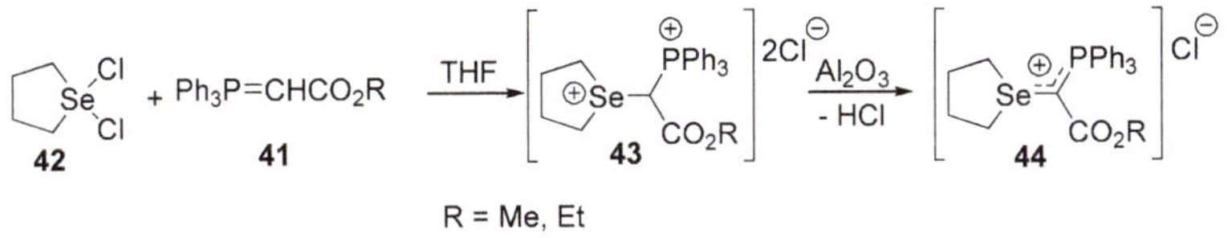

Scheme 9. Synthesis of selenonium ylide salts **44**.

Stable selenonium ylides have also been prepared by deprotonation of the corresponding selenonium salts. This approach was first applied by Lotz and Gosselck in the synthesis of acyclic ylide, stabilized by one benzoyl group, **46**, which was obtained from the corresponding selenonium bromide **45** upon treatment with sodium hydroxide (Scheme 10) [51].

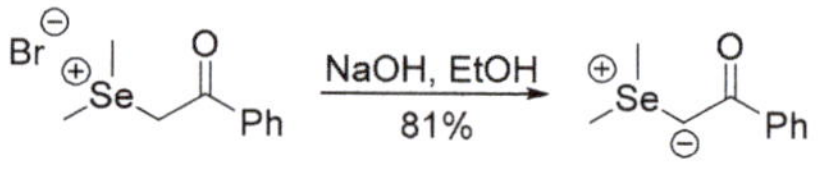

Scheme 10. Synthesis of ylide **46** via deprotonation of selenium salt **45**.

The same method was practiced for the preparation of a stable selenabenzene derivative with an electron-withdrawing group and the ylidic C-Se bond constituting a part of a cyclic conjugated six-electron system. In 1990, Hori and co-workers reported that methylation of 1-cyanoisoselenochromene (**47**) with methyl iodide and silver tetrafluoroborate followed by the reaction of diastereoisomeric 1-cyano-2-methylisoselenochromeniumte trafluoroborates (**48**) with triethylamine in ethanol gave in good yield l-cyano-2-methyl-2-selenanaphthalene **20** as orange needles (Scheme 11) [43].

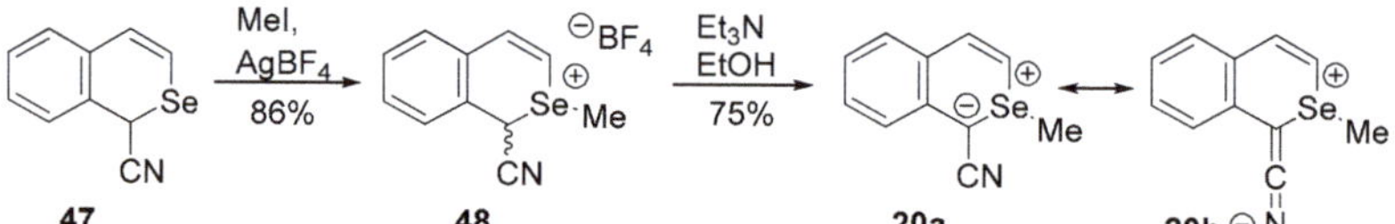

Scheme 11. Preparation of selenabenzene derivative **20**.

Another class of compounds that is widely used for the preparation of selenonium ylides are selenoxides. In 1975, Tamagaki and Sakaki reported a very simple and convenient procedure for the preparation of selenonium ylides involving the reaction of dialkyl or arylalkyl selenoxides with an equimolar amount of malononitrile or methyl cyanoacetate in chloroform at ambient temperature and with or without the addition of desiccating agents (Scheme 12) [52]. They found that the reaction of diphenyl selenoxide with malononitrile afforded a 53.4% yield of the reduction product, i.e., diphenyl selenide as the main product with a poor amount of ylide (**38**: 6.6%), whereas in that with methyl cyanoacetate, only the reduction product was detected. As it was reported a few years later, diphenyl and ditolyl selenoxides were effectively converted into the ylides **52** and **53** by refluxing with an equimolar amount of cyanoacetate or dimedone in CHCl$_3$, respectively (Scheme 13) [53].

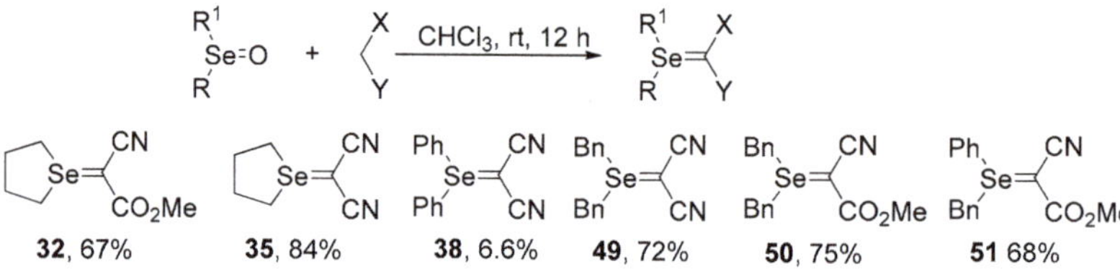

Scheme 12. Synthesis of selenonium ylides **32, 35, 38, 49–51** from dialkyl or arylalkyl selenoxides and activated methylene compounds.

In 1978, Shevetev and coworkers published an easy procedure for the preparation of selenonium ylides containing the nitro group attached directly to the ylide carbon atom [54]. Selenonium nitroylides were obtained in high yields (75–94%) by reacting equimolar amounts of aliphatic nitro compound with diphenylselenium oxide in the presence of acetic anhydride (Scheme 14). Selenonium nitroylides

12 and **54** are fairly stable in the crystalline form at room temperature, while **55** undergoes gradual decomposition (to the extent of 40% in 16 h at 20 °C). All compounds are stable as solutions in dimethyl sulfoxide (DMSO) and CH_3CN. Unlike the sulfonium analogs, the selenonium nitroylides are easily hydrolyzed by water to give diphenyl selenoxide and the corresponding nitroalkane.

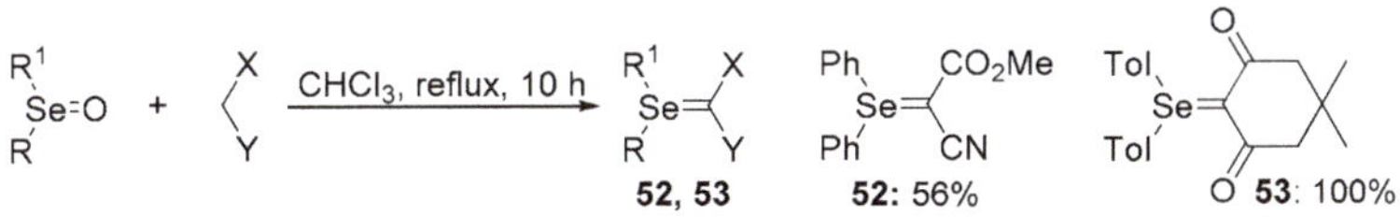

Scheme 13. Synthesis of selenonium ylides **52** and **53** from diaryl selenoxides.

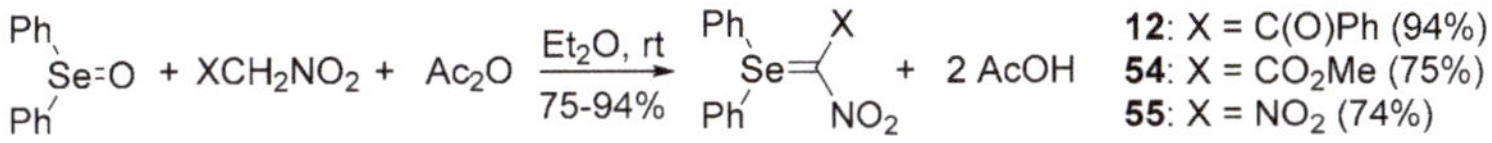

Scheme 14. Synthesis of selenonium nitroylides **12** and **54,55** from diphenyl selenoxide.

Condensation of stable selenoxides with activated methylene compounds promoted by the addition of dicyclohexylcarbodiimide (DCC) was employed by Magdesieva and coworkers for the preparation of selenonium ylides **56a–c** with a trifluoroacetyl group attached to the ylidic carbon atom (Scheme 15) [55].

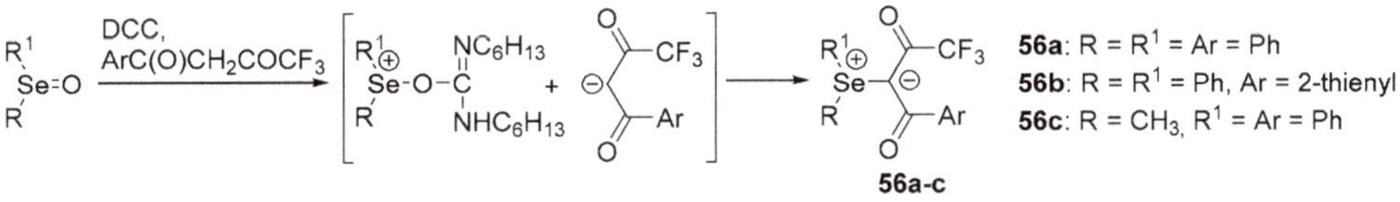

Scheme 15. DCC-promoted synthesis of ylides **56** from selenoxides.

Beside active methylene compounds, electron-deficient alkynes also react with selenoxides to give selenonium ylides. Usually, these reactions proceed smoothly even at ambient temperature and lead to the selenonium ylides in good yields. Based on this method, several stable selenonium ylides **57**, **58** [56,57], **59** [58], **13** [29], and **60a–i** [59] were prepared (Scheme 16).

As it was demonstrated by Tamagaki and Sasaki, selenonium ylides can also be easily prepared from selenonium sulfonimides [52]. Thus, treatment of selenonium N-p-toluenesulfonimides with activated methylene compounds afforded the corresponding stable selenonium ylides even at room temperature (Scheme 17).

This method was successfully applied in the synthesis of stable cyclic selenonium *exo*-ylides **18**, which were obtained in a two-step process from 3,4-dihydro-1H-2-benzoselenin (**63**) (Scheme 18) [37]. In the first step, selenide **63** was reacted with chloramine T trihydrate to give N-p-tolueneselenimide **64**, which in the next step was treated with five equivalents of activated methylene compounds, such as acetylacetone, methyl acetoacetate, dimethyl malonate, methyl cyanoacetate, and malononitrile, to give selenonium ylides **18a–e**, respectively.

3.2. Optically Active Selenonium Ylides

The first optically active diasteoisomerically pure selenonium ylide was reported by Kamigata and co-workers in 1991 [32,60]. According to the developed protocol, the esterification reaction of p-methylselenobenzoic acid (**65**) with l-menthol followed by the oxidation of ester **66** with t-butyl hypochlorite afforded selenoxide **67** in 69%, which upon treatment with dimedone gave a diastereomeric mixture of selenonium ylides **15a,b** in a quantitative yield (Scheme 19). Diastereoisomerically pure ylide (+)-**15a** was isolated as stable crystals by fractional recrystallization of the diastereomeric mixture

15a,b from hexane-diethyl ether. Diastereoisomer (−)-**15b**, obtained from a mother liquid, had only 27% diastereomeric purity.

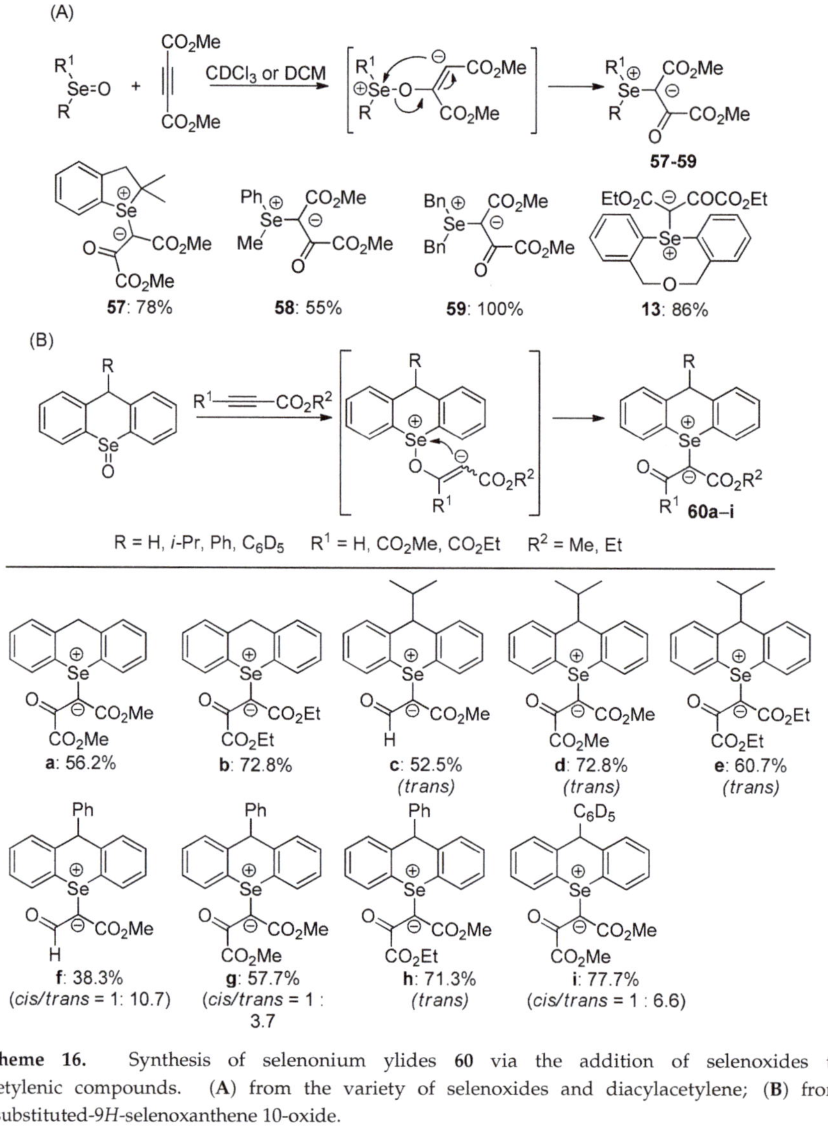

Scheme 16. Synthesis of selenonium ylides **60** via the addition of selenoxides to acetylenic compounds. (**A**) from the variety of selenoxides and diacylacetylene; (**B**) from 9-substituted-9H-selenoxanthene 10-oxide.

A few years later, another Japanese group reported the synthesis of a series of diastereoisomerically pure selenonium ylides **17** by using the 2-*exo*-hydroxy-10-bornyl group as a chiral auxiliary [34]. They found that the reaction of optically active (R_{Se})-selenoxide **68** and nucleophilic substitution reaction of (R_{Se})-chloroselenurane **69** with active methylene compounds proceeded with retention of the configuration, affording diastereoisomerically and enantiomerically pure selenonium ylides **17a–e** in high yields (Scheme 20).

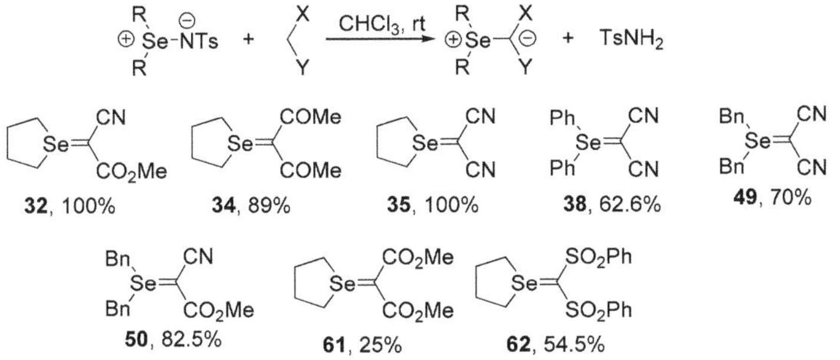

Scheme 17. Synthesis of selenonium ylides **32**, **34**, **35**, **38**, **49**, **50** and **61**, **62** from selenonium N-p-toluenesulfonimides.

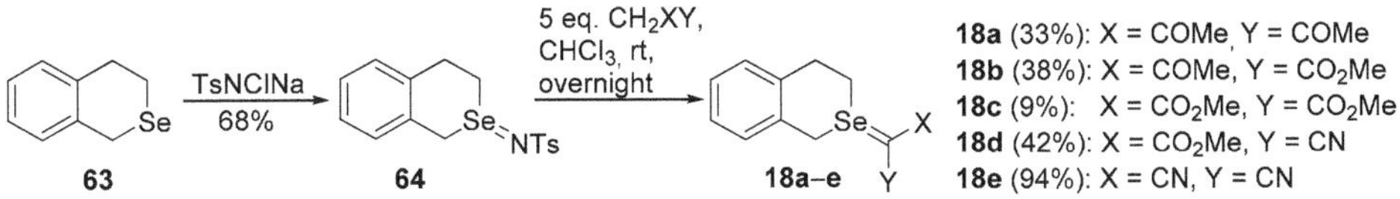

Scheme 18. Preparation of selenonium ylides **18** from selenonium N-p-toluenesulfonimide **64**.

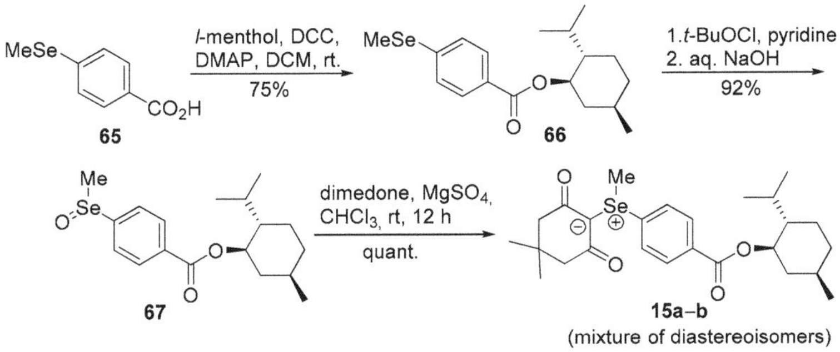

Scheme 19. Synthesis of optically active diastereoisomeric selenonium ylides **15a,b**.

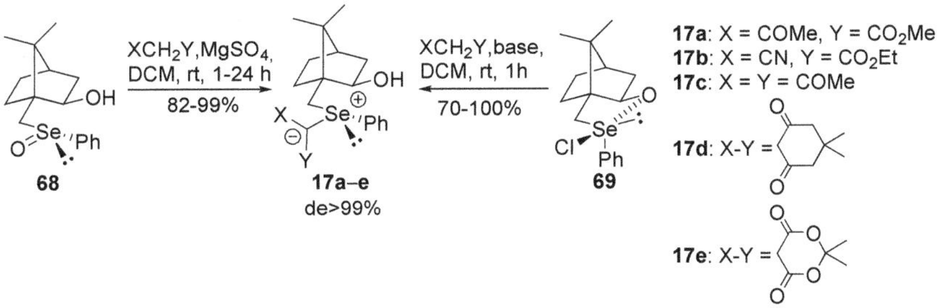

Scheme 20. Reaction of optically active selenoxide **68** and chloroselenurane **69** with activated methylene compounds.

4. Synthetic Applications

Selenium-containing compounds are highly valuable reagents and catalysts with widespread application in the organic chemistry (i.e., synthesis of complex natural products, pharmaceutical ingredients, new materials, and as a tool for the introduction of new functional groups). Due to the specific chemical reactivity, it could be expected that selenonium ylides should serve as useful synthetic reagents. Until now, their synthetic applicability, mainly to induce several types of C–C bond formation reactions, is still limited. In this part of the review, we comprehensively discuss such applications to the cyclopropanation, epoxidation reactions, synthesis of α,β-unsaturated ketones, and sigmatropic rearrangements.

4.1. Cyclopropanation Reactions

In 1973, Lotz and Gossleck described the use of selenonium ylides in the preparation of cyclopropanes [51]. The ylide **46** obtained from the appropriate selenonium bromide reacted with benzalacetophenone, giving *cis*-phenyl-dibenzoil-cyclopropane **70a** as the main product (Scheme 21).

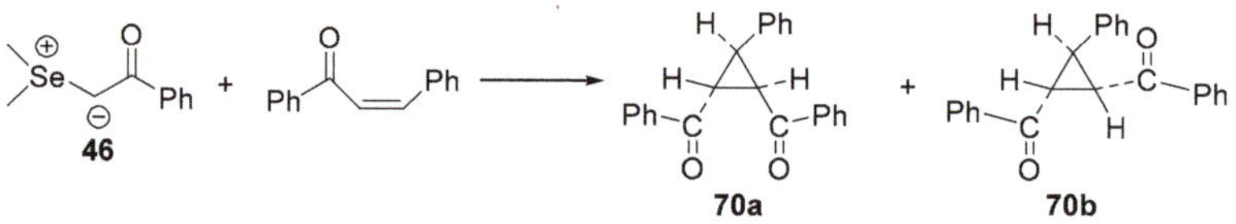

Scheme 21. Synthesis of cyclopropanes **70a,b**.

The reaction carried out with the isolated ylide **46** and benzalacetophenone afforded the *trans* isomer **70b**. Moreover, the use of a slight excess of sodium hydroxide solution and benzalacetophenone led to the mixture of *cis-trans* cyclopropanes. The termal and photolytic decomposition of selenonium ylide **46** afforded *trans*-tribenzoilcyclopropane **71** formed by the reaction sequence shown in Scheme 22. The decomposition of benzoildiazomethane **72** led to the carbene **73**, which dimerizes and forms dibenzoiloethylene **74**. In the presence of dimethyl selenide, which acts as a carbene catcher, the formed ylide **46** reacts with the activated double bond of **74** to form cyclopropane **71**.

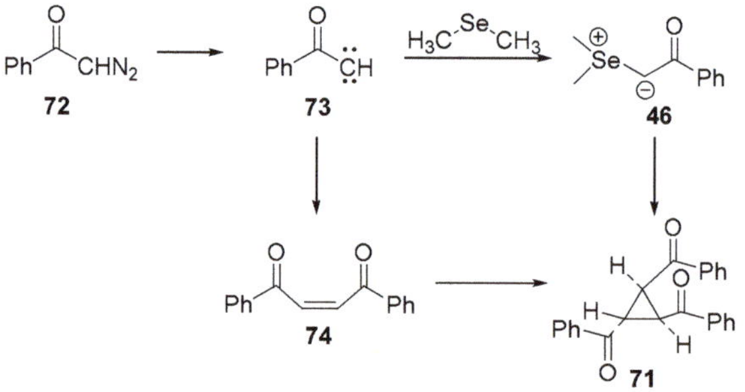

Scheme 22. The formation of *trans*-tribenzoilcyclopropane **71**.

The first application of the optically active selenonium ylides in asymmetric cyclopropanation was reported by Huang's group [61]. At first, they conducted the reactions of *exo*- and *endo*-camphor selenonium ylides **75a,b** and **76** with various α,β-unsaturated carbonyl compound **77a–l** (Scheme 23). For both *exo*-selenonium ylides **75a** and **75b**, the corresponding *cis*-(1R,2R,3R)-trisubstituted cyclopropanes **78** were obtained in good to excellent yields, high diastereoselectivities, and good to excellent enantioselectivities (Table 1).

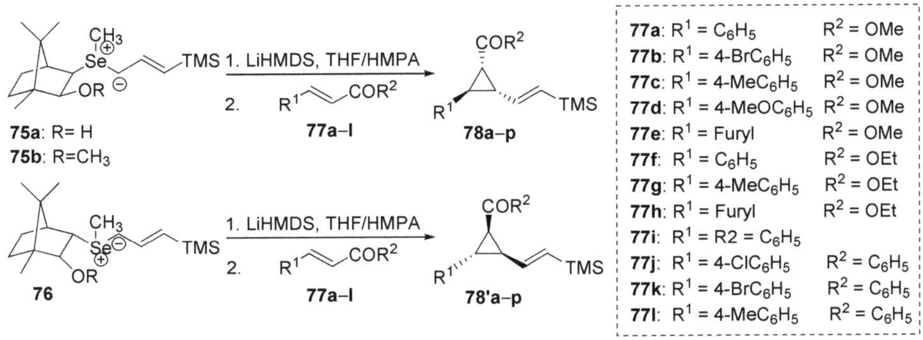

Scheme 23. Synthesis of *cis*-trisubstituted cyclopropanes **78** and **78** from *exo*- and *endo*-camphor selenonium ylides **75a,b** and **76**.

Table 1. Synthesis of *cis*-(1*R*,2*R*,3*R*)-trisubstituted cyclopropanes **78** from *exo*-camphor-derived selenonium ylides **75a,b**. [a]

Entry	Ylide 75	77	Product, (Yield, %) [b]	*cis/trans* [c]	*ee* [%] [d]
1	75a	77a	78a, (92)	>99:1	91
2	75a	77b	78b, (91)	>99:1	>99
3	75a	77c	78c, (87)	98:2	92
4	75a	77d	78d, (70)	90:10	>99
5	75a	77e	78e, (86)	>99:1	95
6	75a	77f	78f, (93)	>99:1	93
7	75a	77g	78g, (86)	90:10	>99
8	75a	77h	78h, (83)	95:5	93
9	75a	77i	78i, (90)	97:3	91
10	75a	77j	78j, (85)	92:8	92
11	75a	77k	78k, (92)	>99:1	>99
12	75a	77l	78l, (81)	95:5	95
13	75b	77a	78m, (90)	98:2	87
14	75b	77c	78n, (84)	97:3	81
15	75b	77f	78o, (91)	>99:1	90
16	75b	77i	78p, (80)	90:10	81

[a] The reaction was performed with the ratio of salt/base/**75** 1:2:1 at −78 °C for 3–5 h. [b] Isolated yields. [c] Determined by ^{1}H-NMR or GC. [d] Determined by chiral HPLC using Chiracel OD-H or AD-H column.

Similarly, for the reaction carried out with *endo*-selenonium ylide **76**, the asymmetric cyclopropanation reaction led to the *cis*-(1*S*,2*S*,3*S*)-trisubstituted cyclopropanes **78'** in good yield, with excellent diastereoselectivities and enantioselectivities (Table 2).

Table 2. Synthesis of *cis*-(1*S*,2*S*,3*S*)-trisubstituted cyclopropanes **78'** from *endo*-camphor selenonium ylide **76**. [a]

Entry	77	Product (Yield, %) [b]	*cis/trans* [c]	*ee* [%] [d]
1	77a	78'a, (90)	95:5	>99
2	77b	78'b, (88)	>99:1	95
3	77c	78'c, (83)	98:2	>99
4	77e	78'e, (84)	>99:1	85
5	77g	78'g, (82)	90:10	97
6	77h	78'h, (81)	98:2	70
7	77i	78'i, (90)	97:3	94
8	77l	78'l, (81)	95:5	>99

[a] The reaction was performed with the ratio of salt/base/**76** 1:2:1 at −78 °C for 3–5 h. [b] Isolated yields. [c] Determined by ^{1}H-NMR or GC. [d] Determined by chiral HPLC using Chiracel OD-H or AD-H column.

In the same paper, the asymmetric cyclopropanation via C_2-symmetric selenonium ylide **79** was described (Scheme 24). The corresponding *trans*-(1R,2R,3S)-cyclopropanes **80** were obtained in good yield, high diastereoselecitvities (d.r. 95:5 > 99:1), and excellent enantioselectivities (up to 99% *ee*) (Table 3).

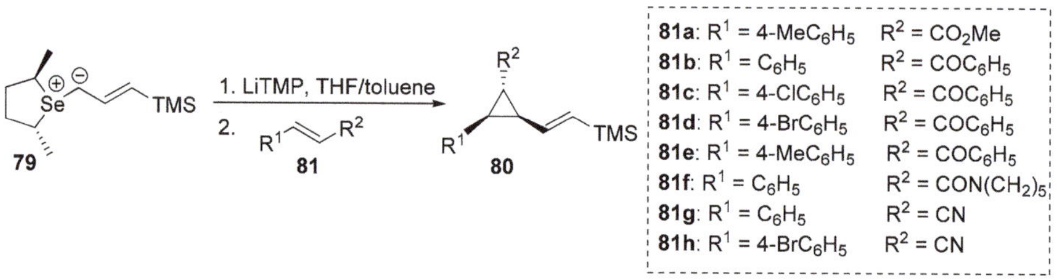

81a: R^1 = 4-MeC$_6$H$_5$ R^2 = CO$_2$Me
81b: R^1 = C$_6$H$_5$ R^2 = COC$_6$H$_5$
81c: R^1 = 4-ClC$_6$H$_5$ R^2 = COC$_6$H$_5$
81d: R^1 = 4-BrC$_6$H$_5$ R^2 = COC$_6$H$_5$
81e: R^1 = 4-MeC$_6$H$_5$ R^2 = COC$_6$H$_5$
81f: R^1 = C$_6$H$_5$ R^2 = CON(CH$_2$)$_5$
81g: R^1 = C$_6$H$_5$ R^2 = CN
81h: R^1 = 4-BrC$_6$H$_5$ R^2 = CN

Scheme 24. Synthesis of *trans*-(1R,2R,3S)-trisubstituted cyclopropanes **80** from selenonium ylide **79**.

Table 3. Stereoselective synthesis of *trans*-(1R,2R,3S)-trisubstituted cyclopropanes **80**. [a]

Entry	81	Product, (Yield, %) [b]	cis/trans [c]	ee [%] [d]
1	81a	80a, (93)	98:2	81
2	81b	80b, (92)	97:3	97
3	81c	80c, (89)	98:2	99
4	81d	80d, (91)	>99:1	98
5	81e	80e, (90)	95:5	98
6	81f	80f, (80)	>99:1	51
7	81g	80g, (82)	96:4	85
8	81h	80h, (83)	96:4	81

[a] The reaction was performed with the ratio of salt/base/**79** 2.5:3:1 at −78 °C for 4–5h. [b] Isolated yields. [c] Determined by ^{1}H-NMR or GC. [d] Determined by chiral HPLC using Chiracel OD-H or AD-H column.

In 2014, Midura and coworkers reported the asymmetric cyclopropanation of vinyl phosphonates using optically active selenonium ylides derived from (−)-menthol and (+)-limonene [62]. The asymmetric cyclopropanation of vinyl phosphonates **82** and **83** with benzyl terpenyl selenonium salts **84–86** occurred in moderate to good yields (20–54%), while the diastereoselectivity was observed only in the case of vinyl phosphonate **83**. Analysis of the enantiomers showed that their ratio depends on the chiral substituent bonded to the selenonium salts used in the reaction. Reaction of vinyl phosphinates **83** with menthol-derived selenonium salts **84** and **86** led to a cyclopropanation product with enantioselectivity of approximately 27% (Table 4, entry 1 and 4). The application of isoselenocineole-derived selenonium salt **85** led to enantioselectivities in the range of 88–92% (Table 4, entry 2).

The authors also performed the cyclopropanation reaction using the corresponding selenonium salt **89**, which contain the ethyl acetate substituent. The reactions afforded the *trans*- and *cis*-cyclopropanes **90** and **91** in good yield (75–86%), with moderate diastereoselectivity and excellent enantioselectivity (up to 99:1) (Table 5).

Table 4. Cyclopropanation reaction with selenonium salt containing a benzyl terpenyl substituent.

Entry	Salt	Michael Acceptor	Reaction Condition	trans/cis	Ratio of trans Diastereomers l/h	Ratio of cis Diastereomers l/h
1	84	82	K_2CO_3, CH_2Cl_2	47.0:53.0 [a]	43.5/56.5	40.3/59.7
2	85	82	DBU, acetone	56.0:44.0 [a]	5.9/94.1	9.4/90.6
3	86	83	K_2CO_3, CH_2Cl_2	80.0:20.0 [a]	—[b]	—[b]
4	86	83	DBU, MeCN	76.2:23.8 [a]	63.3/36.7	78.5/21.5

l—Lower R_f in HPLC; h—Higher R_f in HPLC. [a] The ratio of diastereomers determined by NMR. [b] Inseparable impurities disturbed the precise determination of the enantiomeric ratio.

Table 5. Cyclopropanation reaction with selenonium salt containing the ethyl acetate substituent.

Entry	Salt	Michael Acceptor	Reaction Condition	trans/cis	Ratio of cis Diastereomers l/h	Ratio of trans Diastereomers l/h
1	89	82	DBU, MeCN	65.0:35.0 [a]	98.0/2.0 [a]	99.0/1.0
2	89	83	DBU, MeCN	72.5:27.5 [a]	1.6/98.4	2.5/97.5

l—Lower R_f in HPLC; h—Higher R_f in HPLC. [a] The ratio of diastereomers determined by NMR.

4.2. Epoxidation Reactions

In 1974, Krief and his group reported the first example of the reaction of selenium ylides with carbonyl compounds, which provides epoxides [63]. Selenonium ylides **93a–c** generated in situ from selenium salts **92a–c** using potassium *tert*-butoxide as a base were found to react with aldehydes or ketones to form the corresponding epoxides **94–102** in good to high yields (50–90%) (Scheme 25, Table 6).

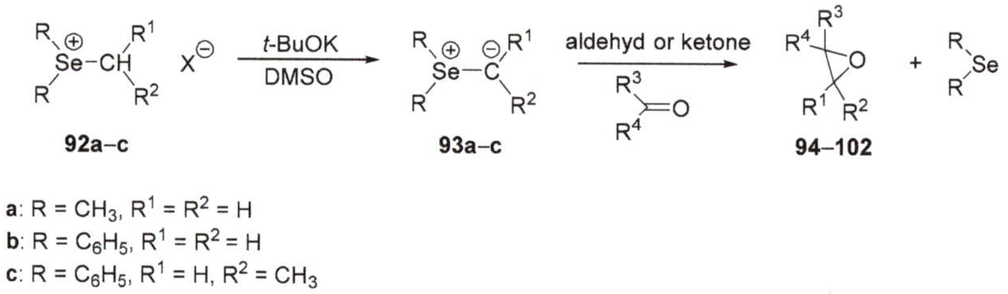

a: R = CH$_3$, R^1 = R^2 = H
b: R = C$_6$H$_5$, R^1 = R^2 = H
c: R = C$_6$H$_5$, R^1 = H, R^2 = CH$_3$

Scheme 25. Synthesis of epoxides **94–102** from selenonium salts **92a–c**.

Table 6. Reaction of selenonium salts **92a–c** with various aldehydes and ketones.

Entry	Selenonium Salt	Aldehyde or Ketone		Epoxides 94–102 (Yield, %)
		R^3	R^4	
1	92a	C$_6$H$_5$	H	**94**, (90)
2	92a	*p*-CH$_3$-OC$_6$H$_{14}$	H	**95**, (75)
3	92a	*p*-CN-C$_6$H$_{14}$	H	**96**, (54)
4	92a	mesityl	H	**97**, (79)
5	92a	C$_6$H$_5$CH=CH	H	**98**, (71)
6	92a	C$_6$H$_5$CH=CH	C$_6$H$_5$	**99**, (50)
7	92b	C$_6$H$_5$	H	**100**, (90)
8	92a	C$_6$H$_5$	C$_6$H$_5$	**101**, (90)
9	92c	C$_6$H$_5$	H	**102**, (69)

It is worth noting that in the reaction of selenonium salts with enolizable carbonyl compounds (i.e., heptanal, cyclohexanone, methyl ethyl ketone, and acetophenone), the corresponding epoxides were not formed. Such a result is caused by the formation of an acetophenone anion, which is subsequently methylated by the selenonium salt. The generation of the selenonium ylides prior to the addition of acetophenone allowed the avoidance of the methylation reaction.

Morihara's group reported the generation of the selenonium ylides by electrochemical reduction of the cyclic five-membered selenonium salts **103a–g** carried out in the presence or without benzaldehyde (Schemes 26 and 27) [64].

When electrochemical reduction of selenonium salts **103a–g** was carried out in the presence of acetophenone, the main reaction was epoxidation (products **104–108**); only in two cases, a product of a radical coupling (**109–110**) was formed. In most cases, moderate to good yields were observed (Table 7).

For electrochemical reduction carried out in the absence of benzaldehyde, the reaction course depends on the *R* substituent in the selenonium salt (Scheme 27). When the reactions were conducted on selenonium salts bearing a benzyl or allyl substituent, the products of the [2,3]-sigmatropic rearrangement (**111–114**) or radical coupling (**109–110**) were formed. In the case of a selenonium salt bearing a carbonyl group, formation of carbene led to olefins **115** or cyclopropanes **116** as products (Table 8).

In 2001, Metzner and coworkers reported the first application of an optically active selenonium ylide in the asymmetric epoxidation reaction [65]. The appropriate enantioenriched selenonium ylide was generated by the addition of benzyl bromide to C_2-symmetric (2R,5R)-2,5-dimethylselenolane **117** in the presence of NaOH. Its reaction with a variety of aldehydes **118–125** led to the corresponding epoxides. Thus, the reaction of aldehydes **118–120** with the stoichiometric amount of selenide **117** afforded the corresponding epoxides **126–128** in the yield from 71% to 97% and with excellent enantiomeric excesses (92–93%) (Scheme 28).

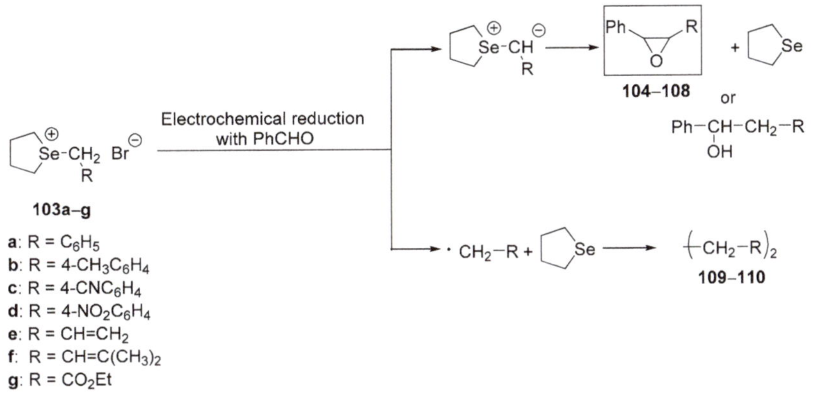

Scheme 26. Electrochemical reduction of substituted methyltetrahydroselenonium bromide **103a–g** in the presence of benzaldehyde.

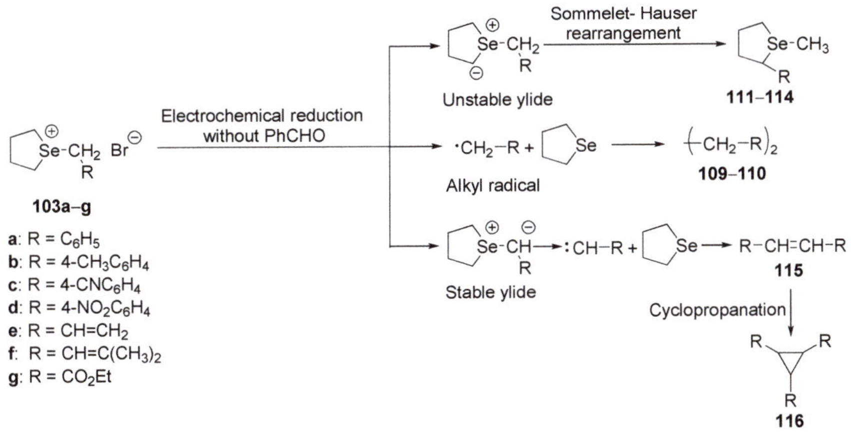

Scheme 27. Electrochemical reduction of selenonium salts **103a–g** without benzaldehyde.

Table 7. Electrochemical reduction of substituted methyltetrahydroselenonium bromide **103a–g** in the presence of benzaldehyde.

Entry	Selenonium Salt	Reaction	Product (Yield, %)
1	103a	Epoxidation	104 (79)
2	103b	Epoxidation	105 (63)
3	103c	Radical coupling	109 (68)
4	103d	Radical coupling	110 (72)
5	103e	Epoxidation	106 (69)
6	103f	Epoxidation	107 (30)
7	103g	Epoxidation	108 (32)

Table 8. Electrochemical reduction of selenonium salts **103a–g** without benzaldehyde.

Entry	Selenonium Salt	Reaction	Product (Yield, %)
1	103a	Sigmatropic rearrangement	111 (31)
2	103b	Sigmatropic rearrangement	112 (38)
3	103c	Radical coupling	109 (73)
4	103d	Radical coupling	110 (94)
5	103e	Sigmatropic rearrangement	113 (50)
6	103f	Sigmatropic rearrangement	114 (70)
7	103g	Carbene formation	115 (36), 116 (21)

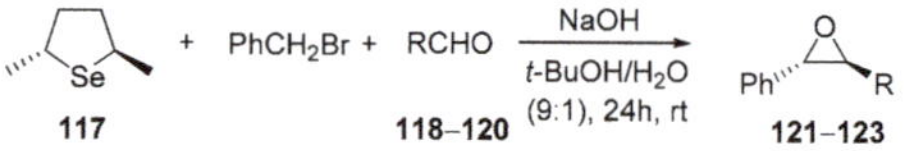

$$\text{117} + \text{PhCH}_2\text{Br} + \text{RCHO} \xrightarrow[\text{(9:1), 24h, rt}]{\text{NaOH, } t\text{-BuOH/H}_2\text{O}} \text{121–123}$$

118–120

		Yield [%]	%ee
118: R = C$_6$H$_5$	121: R = C$_6$H$_5$	71	92
119: R = 4-CH$_3$C$_6$H$_4$	122: R = 4-CH$_3$C$_6$H$_4$	86	93
120: R = 2-Naphthyl	123: R = 2-Naphthyl	97	92

Scheme 28. Asymmetric epoxidation of aldehydes by the reaction with selenonium ylides generated in situ from selenolane **117**.

In turn, the use of a catalytic amount of selenolane **117** (20% mol) in reaction with aldehydes **118–125** at ambient temperature led to the corresponding epoxides in good to excellent yields (65–97%). For more reactive heteroaromatic aldehydes (**124** and **125**), the reaction time was optimized to 4 h. In most cases, enantiomeric excesses were in the range 91–94%, except for aldehydes **121** and **122**, which bear electron-withdrawing groups (Scheme 29).

Four years later, Metzner's group also proved that (2R,5R)-2,5-dimethylselenolane (**117**) is an efficient catalyst for the benzylidenation of aromatic aldehydes [66]. The authors noted that as compared to the sulfur analogues, the selennium-based system leads to enhanced reactivity and higher asymmetric induction, with the same absolute configuration. The reaction of selenolane **117** with benzaldehyde **118** led to the epoxide **126**, which was formed, surprisingly, with a lack of diastereoselectivity and with an enantiomeric excess higher than 90%. The authors explained [67,68] that the formation of equal amounts of *trans* and *cis* diastereomers is caused by a reversible betaine formation, leading to the *cis* epoxide, which is formed from the betaine *syn* conformer (Scheme 30).

Watanabe and Kataoka described the use of ketodiphenylselenonium ylides generated from the corresponding alkynylselenonium salt for the synthesis of oxiranylketones [69]. The reaction of alkynylselenonium salt **134a–c** with various aromatic aldehydes in the presence of LiOH, silver triflate, and triethylamine gave oxiranylketones **135a–j** just as a *trans*-isomer in moderate to good yields (40–92%) (Scheme 31, Table 9).

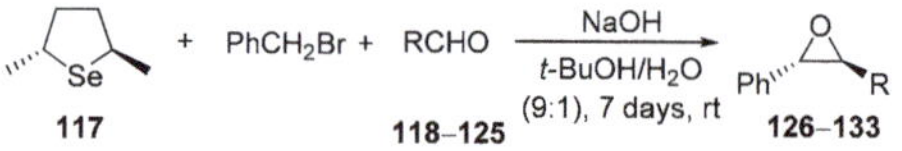

$$\text{117} + \text{PhCH}_2\text{Br} + \text{RCHO} \xrightarrow[\text{(9:1), 7 days, rt}]{\text{NaOH, } t\text{-BuOH/H}_2\text{O}} \text{126–133}$$

118–125

		Yield [%]	%ee
118: R = C$_6$H$_5$	126: R = C$_6$H$_5$	91	91
119: R = 4-CH$_3$C$_6$H$_4$	127: R = 4-CH$_3$C$_6$H$_4$	97	92
120: R = 2-Naphthyl	128: R = 2-Naphthyl	97	92
121: R = 4-ClC$_6$H$_4$	129: R = 4-ClC$_6$H$_4$	97	76
122: R = 4-CF$_3$C$_6$H$_4$	130: R = 4-CF$_3$C$_6$H$_4$	76	83
123: R = (E)-Cinnamyl	131: R = (E)-Cinnamyl	66	94
124: R = 2-Furyl	132: R = 2-Furyl	65	92
125: R = 2-Thiophenecarboxyl	133: R = 2-Thiophenecarboxyl	86	94

Scheme 29. Catalytic asymmetric epoxidation of aldehydes in the presence of a catalytic amount of selenolane **117**.

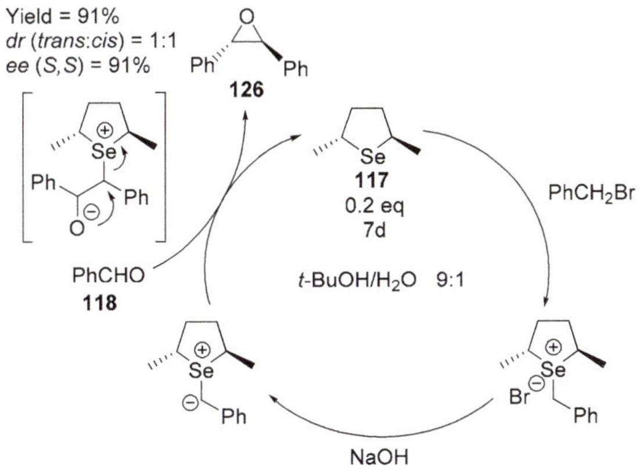

Scheme 30. Mechanism of formation epoxides in the reaction of the selenolane **117**/benzylbromide system with aldehydes.

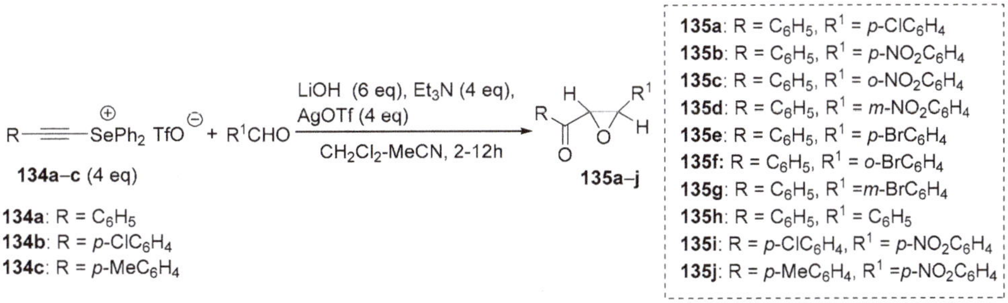

Scheme 31. Reaction of ketoselenonium salts **134a–c** with aromatic aldehydes.

Table 9. Reaction time and yields of oxiranylketones **135a–j** obtained in the reaction of ketoselenonium ylides **134a–c** with aromatic aldehydes.

Entry	134	Aldehyde R^{1}CHO	Time (h)	Product (Yield, %)
1	134a	R^1 = p-ClC$_6$H$_4$	12	135a (78)
2	134a	R^1 = p-NO$_2$C$_6$H$_4$	3.5	135b (84)
3	134a	R^1 = o-NO$_2$C$_6$H$_4$	1.5	135c (71)
4	134a	R^1 = m-NO$_2$C$_6$H$_4$	2	135d (58)
5	134a	R^1 = p-BrC$_6$H$_4$	9	135e (55)
6	134a	R^1 = o-BrC$_6$H$_4$	2	135f (92)
7	134a	R^1 = m-BrC$_6$H$_4$	5	135g (90)
8	134a	R^1 = Ph	6.5	135h (40)
9	134b	R^1 = p-NO$_2$C$_6$H$_4$	3	135i (89)
10	134c	R^1 = p-NO$_2$C$_6$H$_4$	3	135j (71)

In the case of aliphatic aldehydes, the desired oxiranylketones **136a–e** were formed in moderate yields (18–54%) under the same reaction conditions (Scheme 32, Table 10).

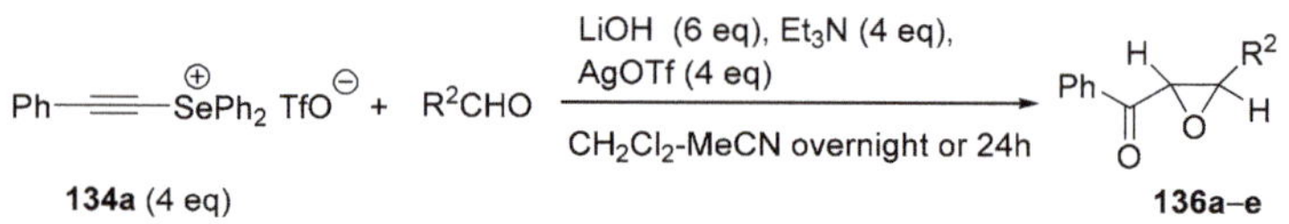

Scheme 32. Reactions of ketoselenonium ylide **134a** with aliphatic aldehydes.

Table 10. Reaction time and yields of oxiranylketones **136a–e** obtained from ketoselenonium ylide **134a** and aliphatic aldehydes.

Entry	Aldehyde R^2CHO	Time	Product (Yield, %)
1	$R^2 = CH_3CH_2$	overnight	137a (18)
2	$R^2 = CH_3(CH_2)_2$	24 h	137b (34)
3	$R^2 = Ph(CH_2)_2$	overnight	137c (54)
4	$R^2 = (CH_3)_2CH$	overnight	137d (37)
5	$R^2 = (CH_3)CHCH_2$	24 h	137e (63)

In turn, the reaction of alkynylselenonium salt **134a** with aromatic aldehydes in the presence of sodium *p*-toluenesulfonamide instead of LiOH led to the corresponding benzoyl aziridine derivatives **137a–d** in moderate yields (Scheme 33, Table 11). The comparison of the coupling constants values with literature data indicates that these isomers have the *cis* geometry (J_{HH} the methine protons on the aziridine ring is 7–8 Hz) [70].

Scheme 34 shows the plausible mechanism for the reactions of alkynylselenonium salt **134a** with aldehydes and the hydroxyl ion in the presence of a silver salt and triethylamine (Scheme 34). In the first step, the triple bond of the selenonium salt is activated by silver cation, and the hydroxyl ion attacks the β-carbon atom to form the vinyl ylide **138**. In the presence of Et$_3$N, the ylide **138** is transformed into the ketodiphenylselenonium ylide **139**, which reacts with an aldehyde to form appropriate oxiranylketones (route A). In turn, diphenyl selenoxide is formed by the attack of hydroxyl ion on a selenonium cation without activation of a triple bond by a silver ion (route B) [71,72].

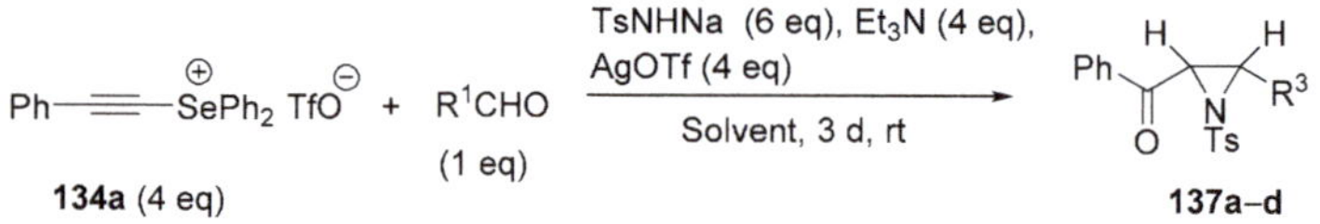

Scheme 33. Reactions of alkynylselenonium salt **134a** with aromatic aldehydes and TsNHNa.

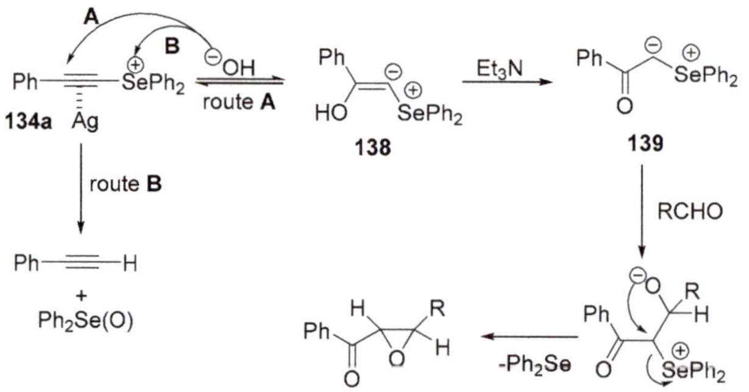

Scheme 34. Plausible mechanism of the reactions of alkynylselenonium salt **134a** with an aldehyde and hydroxide ion in the presence of silver cation and Et$_3$N.

Table 11. Aziridines **137a–d** obtained in the reaction of alkynylselenonium salt **134a** with aromatic aldehydes and TsNHNa.

Entry	Aldehyde	Solvent	Product (Yield, %)
1	R^1 = p-ClC$_6$H$_4$	CH$_2$Cl$_2$-MeCN	**137a** (44)
2	R^1 = p-NO$_2$C$_6$H$_4$	MeCN	**137b** (44)
3	R^1 = o-BrC$_6$H$_4$	MeCN	**137c** (48)
4	R^1 = o-MeOC$_6$H$_4$	CH$_2$Cl$_2$-MeCN	**137d** (30)

4.3. Synthesis of α,β-Unsaturated Ketones

Watanabe and Kataokan also reported the first application of vinylselenonium ylide, generated in situ from (Z)-vinylselenonium salts **140a** in the presence of sodium or potassium hydride as a base, in the synthesis of α,β-unsaturated ketones [73]. When the reactions of selenonium salt **140a** were carried out with sodium hydride as a base, the best results were obtained for the reaction with p-nitrobenzaldehyde, and the corresponding p-nitrophenyl styryl ketone **141a** was obtained in 65%. The reaction with p-chlorobenzaldehyde led to ketone **141b** only in an 11% yield. The use of 2 equiv. of sodium hydride instead of 1.3 equiv. increased the yield of the product to 58% (Scheme 35). In turn, the reactions with benzaldehyde or p-tolualdehyde afforded complex mixtures, including unreacted aldehydes, while the desired α,β-unsaturated ketones were not isolated.

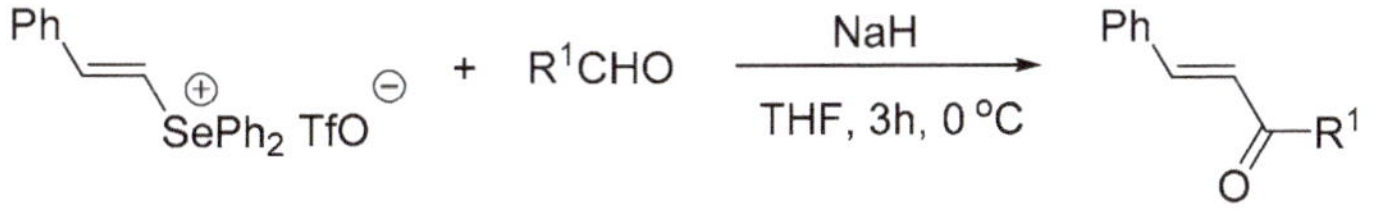

Scheme 35. Synthesis of α,β-unsaturated ketones **141a,b** from a vinylselenonium salt.

The formation of the vinylselenonium ylides in this reaction was confirmed by the experiment carried out on vinylselenonium salt **140b** with 1 equiv. of sodium hydride in tetrahydrofurane (THF) at 0 °C for 3 h without the aldehyde, followed by treatment with D$_2$O. The obtained mixture of **140b** and **140b'** while treated with sodium hydride in the presence of p-nitrobenzaldehyde under the same conditions as for the reaction of **140a** gave the compound **141c** in a 49% yield. In turn, the reaction of vinylselenonium salt **140b** with deuterated benzaldehyde led to the compound **141d** in a 14% yield (Scheme 36). In both cases, the obtained ketones did not contain a deuterium atom.

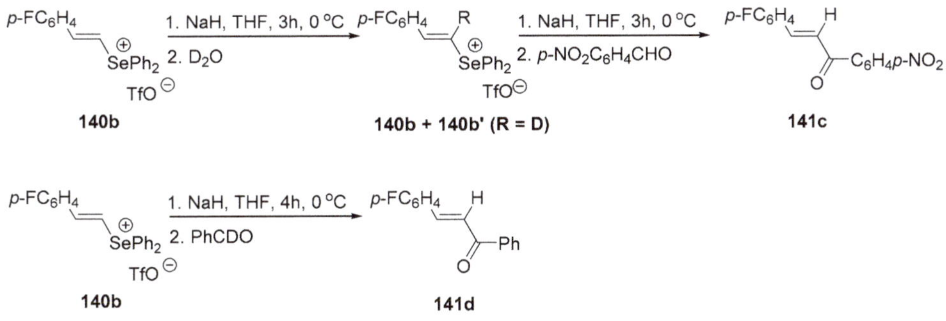

Scheme 36. Reaction of vinylselenonium salt **140b** with D$_2$O and PhCDO. Confirmation of the selenonium ylide formation.

When the reactions of vinylselenonium salt **140a** with aromatic aldehydes were carried out in the presence of potassium hydride as a base, the desired α,β-unsaturated ketones **141a,b** and **141e–g** were obtained in higher yields than in the case of the reactions carried out with sodium hydride (Table 12). Better yields were obtained when aldehydes with an electron-withdrawing group were used in the reaction instead of those with an electron-donating group.

Table 12. Reactions of vinylselenonium salt **140a** with aldehydes in the presence of KH. [a].

Entry	RCHO	Reaction Conditions	Product (yield, %)
1	p-NO$_2$C$_6$H$_4$CHO	KH, THF, 0 °C, 0.5 h	**141a** (94)
2	p-ClC$_6$H$_4$CHO	KH, THF, 0 °C, 0.5 h	**141b** (77)
3	p-BrC$_6$H$_4$CHO	KH, THF, 0 °C, 0.5 h	**141e** (76)
4	PhCHO	KH, THF, −10 °C, overnight	**141f** (43)
5	PhCHO	KH, THF-DMSO,[b] −30 °C, 2 h	**141f** (60)
6	p-MeC$_6$H$_4$CHO	KH, THF-DMSO,[b] −30 °C, 3.5 h	**141g** (49)

[a] **141a**: RCHO : KH = 2 : 1.3. [b] THF : DMSO = 13 : 1.

The plausible mechanism for the reactions of vinylselenonium salts with aldehydes is shown in Scheme 37. The reaction of vinylselenonium salt **140** with a base led to the formation of vinylselenonium ylide **142**, which in the next step reacted with an aldehyde and gave betaine **143**. Deprotonation of betaine **143** and β-elimination of diphenylselenide led to the adduct **144**, which isomerized to the corresponding α,β-unsaturated ketone **141**, probably via a hydride transfer.

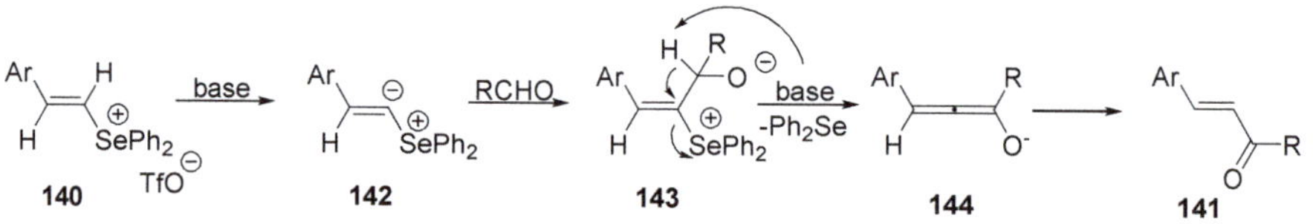

Scheme 37. The plausible mechanism of the reactions of vinylselenonium salts with aldehydes.

4.4. Sigmatropic Rearrangements

The reactions of dibenzylselenonium dicyanomethylide **145** and dibenzylselenonium cyanomethoxycarbonylmethylide **146** with triphenylphosphine were examined by Tamagaka and coworkers [74]. They found that the reaction of dibenzylselenonium dicyanomethylide **145** carried out at room temperature led to the mixture of products: Triphenylphosphine selenide **147** (87%), 2-benzyl-2-cyano-3-phenylpropanenitrile **148** (53%) and a small amount of dibenzyl diselenide (11%). The treatment of dibenzylselenonium cyanomethoxycarbonylmethylide **146** with triphenylphosphine afforded methyl 2-benzyl-2-cyano-3-phenylpropanoate **149**, triphenylphosphine selenide **147**, and dibenzyl diselenide in 29%, 49%, and 28% yields, respectively. In both cases, products obtained in the reactions were formed via the deselenization reaction and no dibenzyl selenide was observed (Scheme 38).

On the contrary, the reaction of dibenzylselenonium N-tosylimide **150** with triphenylphosphine at room temperature led to the formation of dibenzyl selenide (81%) as the main product, triphenyl N-tosylphosphimine **152** (54%), and only a trace of triphenylphosphine selenide (6%) (Scheme 39). The isolation of the phosphine selenide indicates that the selenonium imide **150** also undergoes deselenization but as a result of a minor process. In turn, the reaction of dibenzyl selenoxide with triphenylphosphine was found to be much more facile and led quantitatively to dibenzyl selenide and triphenylphosphine oxide **153**. No deselenization products were observed. Therefore, the reactivity order for the reduction into dibenzyl selenide is selenoxide > selenonium imide > selenonium ylide.

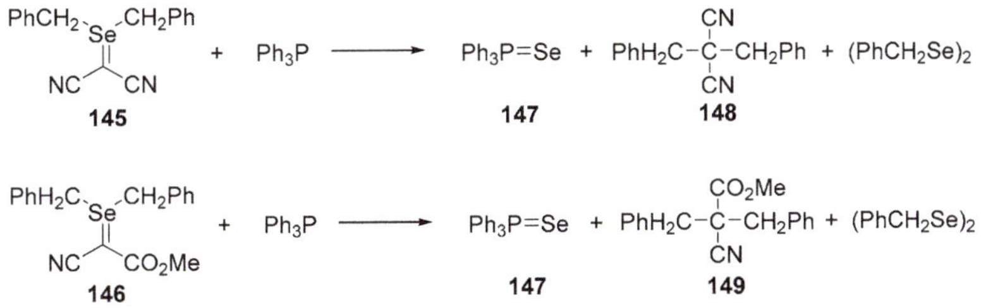

Scheme 38. Reaction of dibenzylselenonium dicyanomethylide **145** and dibenzylselenonium cyanomethoxycarbonylmethylide **146** with triphenylphosphine.

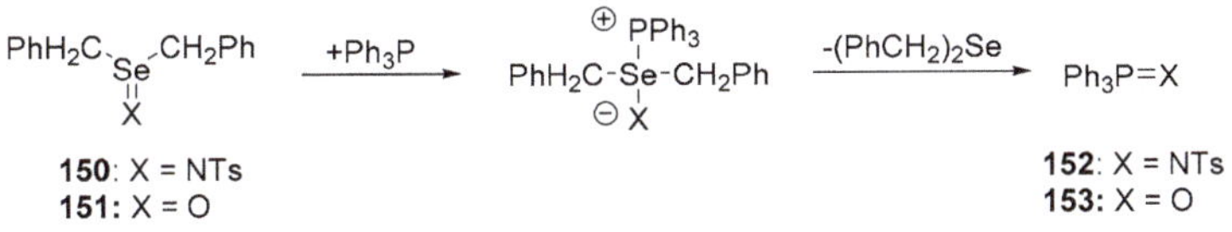

Scheme 39. The reaction of dibenzylselenonium *N*-tosylimide **150** with triphenylphosphine.

It was found that the addition of acetic acid or water to the reaction system changes the product distribution and reaction modes. The reaction of compounds **145** and **146** under these conditions gave dibenzyl diselenides as the main product. Meanwhile, the corresponding selenonium imide **150** and selenoxide **151** afforded dibenzyl selenide.

Reich and Cohen reported that the seleno-substituted ketone enolates can undergo an alkylation at the heteroatom [75]. Treatment of the appropriate enolate of α-(phenylseleno)acetophenone **154a** with prenyl iodide or bromide led to the alkylation product **155a** and unexpected product **156a** (Scheme 40).

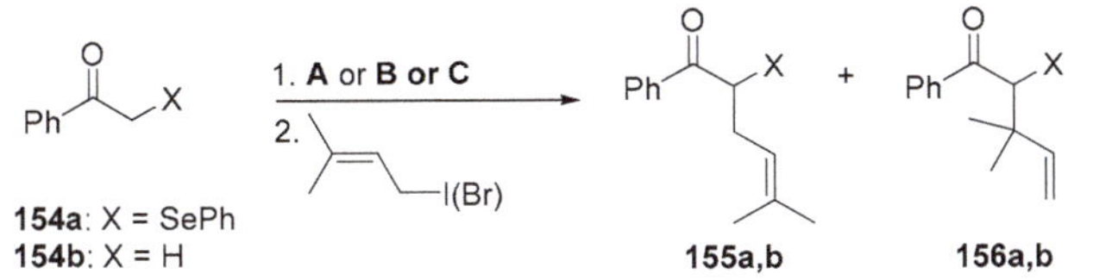

	155	:	**156**	(Yield, %)
154a: A: LDA, THF, 0 °C	47	:	53	(60)
154a: B: LDA, THF, HMPA, −78–25 °C	61	:	39	(66)
154b: **C**: LDA, THF, 0 °C	>99	:	1	(43)

Scheme 40. Reaction of α-(phenylseleno)acetophenone **154a** with prenyl iodide or bromide.

The formation of compound **156a** may result from two reaction pathways. The first one is the *O*-alkylation of enolate to give **157**, followed by the [3,3]-sigmatropic rearrangement, while the second one assumes alkylation at the selenium atom to form the ylide **158** and the subsequent [2,3]-sigmatropic rearrangement (Figure 16).

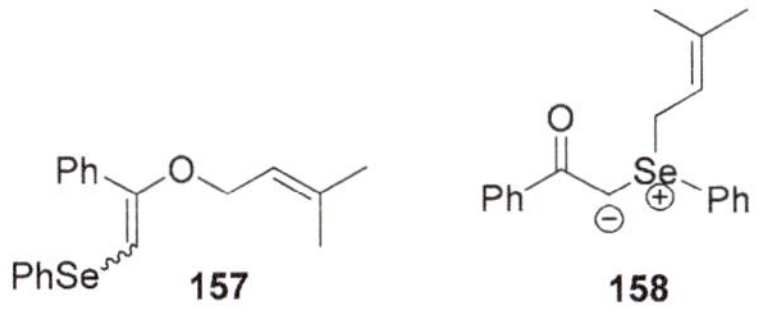

Figure 16. Enolate **157** and ylide **158**.

To confirm the ylide mechanism, the alkylation of α-allylselenoacetophenone **159** was performed. One of the reaction products was C-allyl product **160**, which must be formed by the [2,3]-sigmatropic rearrangement of the intermediate **161** capable of allyl migration [76] (Scheme 41).

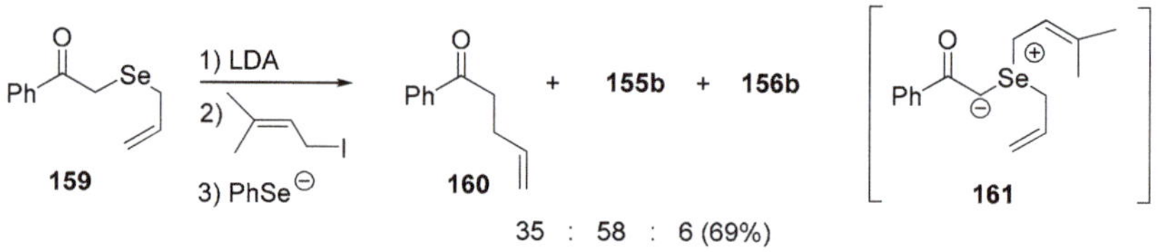

Scheme 41. Alkylation of α-allylselenoacetophenone (**159**).

Krief's group reported the [2,3]-sigmatropic rearrangement of allylic selenonium ylides and the application of the rearrangement to the synthesis of functionalized alkylidene cyclopropanes [77]. The alkylation reaction (method A, B, or C) of the corresponding 1-seleno-l-vinyl cyclopropanes **162a–c** led to the selenonium salts, which in the reaction with *t*-BuOK afforded appropriate selenonium ylide as an intermediate, which subsequently rearranged to alkylidenecyclopropanes **164a–c** (Scheme 42, Table 13).

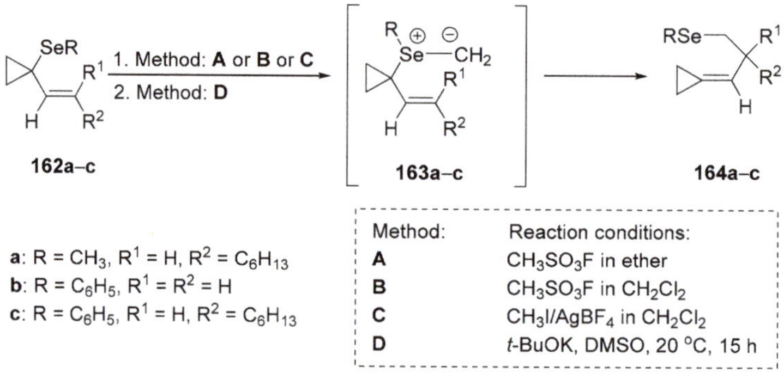

Scheme 42. Synthesis of alkylidenecyclopropanes **164a–c**.

It was found that the homoallyl selenides **164a** and **165** are good precursors of dienes. The alkylation reaction of the selenium atom (method A) followed by treatment with *t*-BuOK/DMSO (method D) led to the dienes **167** and **169** by an elimination reaction in the regioselective way (Scheme 43).

Table 13. Reaction conditions and the yields of alkylidenecyclopropanes **164a–c**.

Entry	Method	Product 164 (Yield, %)
162a	A then D	164a (85)
162a	C (MeI) then D	164a (53)
162b	C (MeI) then D	164b (60)
162b	C (MeI) then D	164b (56)
162c	B then D	164c (67)
162c	A then D	164c (85)

Braverman and coworkers reported a base-catalyzed [2,3]-sigmatropic rearrangement of bis-γ-substituted propargylic selenonium salts [78]. The reaction of ethyl bis-γ-cyclohexenylpropargyl selenium tetrafluoroborate **170a,b** with 1,8-diazabicyklo(5.4.0)undek-7-en (DBU) led to the appropriate selenonium ylide, which underwent a spontaneous [2,3]-sigmatropic rearrangement and gave the selenonium derivatives **171a,b**. The obtained compounds underwent a subsequent [1,3] shift to the appropriate dienynes **172a,b** (Scheme 44).

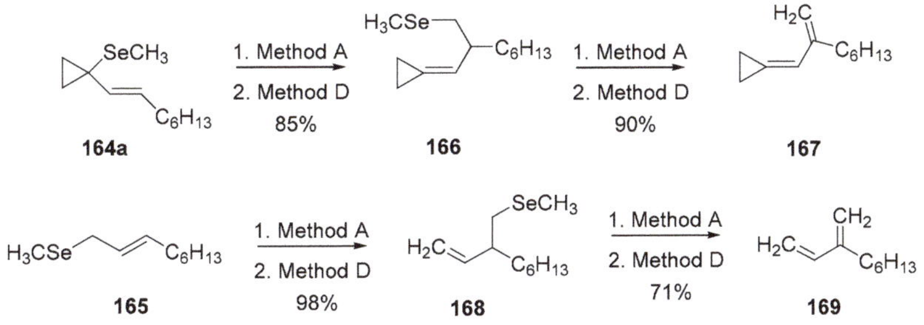

Scheme 43. Synthesis of dienes **167** and **169**.

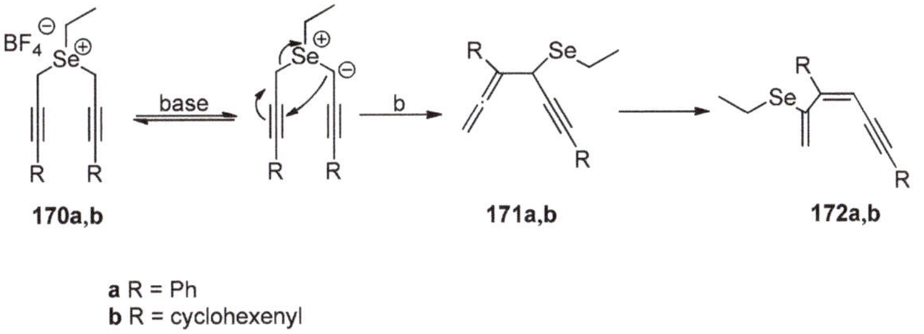

a R = Ph
b R = cyclohexenyl

Scheme 44. Base-catalyzed [2,3]-sigmatropic rearrangement of bis-γ-substituted bridged propargylic systems.

Similarly, the selenonium salt **173** in the presence of CH_3ONa undergoes [2,3]-sigmatropic rearrangements leading to the corresponding selenides **175** and **176**. Using weaker bases like 1,4-diazabicyclo[2.2.2]octane (DABCO) leads to mixtures of S_N2 products (Scheme 45). This result indicates the relatively high sensitivity of selenonium salts to nucleophilic displacement with respect to the corresponding sulfonium salts, which may be explained by the relatively higher polarizability of the selenium atom as well as the weaker Se-C bond [37].

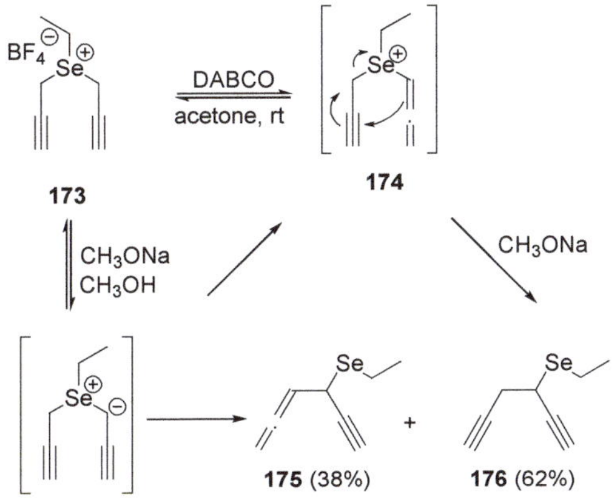

Scheme 45. Rearrangements of unsubstituted bridged propargylic systems **173**.

Uemura and coworkers described the first example of enantioselective addition of the carbenoid derived from ethyl diazoacetate to chalcogen atoms of aryl cinnamyl chalcogenides, which proceed via a [2,3]-sigmatropic rearrangement of the chalcogen ylide [79]. The reaction of (*E*)-cinnamyl aryl selenides **176a–c** with ethyl diazoacetate in the presence of a catalytic amount of copper or rhodium catalyst led to the mixture of diastereomeric ethyl 2-arylchalcogeno-3-phenylpent-4-enoates **177a–c**. When the reaction was carried out on (*E*)-cinnamyl phenyl selenide **176a** with a copper (I) salt and bisoxazoline, the desired products were obtained with an enantioselectivity up to 34%. It was found that the introduction of an electron-withdrawing group (*o*-nitro or *o*-trifluoromethyl) into the phenylselenium moiety improved the enantioselectivity of the corresponding products, while the introduction of an electron-donating group (i.e., *o*-methoxy, ferrocenylselenium) inhibited the reaction completely. Analogously, the reactions of (*E*)-cinnamyl phenyl selenide **176a** with the Doyle catalyst [Rh$_2$(5*S*-MEPY)$_4$ (1 mol%)] were carried out. At 40 °C, the reaction proceeded smoothly with slightly better but still low enantioselectivity (up to 41% *ee*) in comparison to that obtained in the reaction with a copper catalyst (Scheme 46, Table 14).

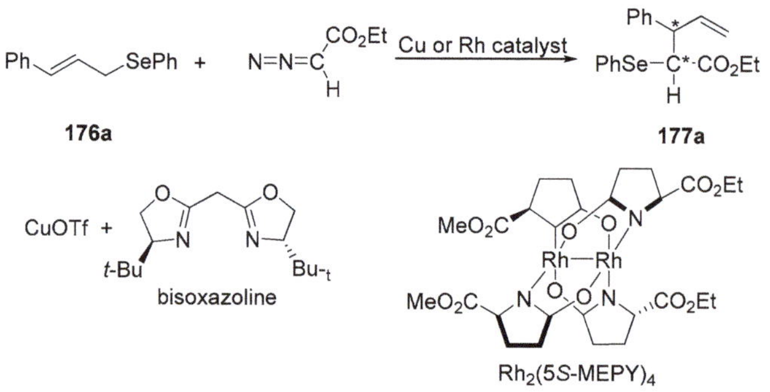

Scheme 46. Reaction of (*E*)-cinnamyl phenyl selenides **176** with ethyl diazoacetate in the presence of a catalytic amount of copper or rhodium catalyst.

Table 14. Reaction conditions for Scheme 46: Cu: CuOTf (5 mol%) + bisoxazoline (5 mol%); ii, cat. Rh: Rh$_2$(5*S*-MEPY)$_4$ (1 mol%). Tf = SO$_2$CF$_3$.

Entry	176	Reaction Conditions [a]	Yield (%)	dr of 177 [b] (*ee*, %)
1	**176a** (Ar = C$_6$H$_5$)	Cu, CHCl$_3$, 0 °C, 24 h	71	66:34 (22, 32)
2	**176b** (Ar = *o*-NO$_2$C$_6$H$_4$)	Cu, CHCl$_3$, 0 °C, 24 h	55	53:47 (13, 34)
3	**176c** (Ar = *o*-CCF$_3$C$_6$H$_4$)	Cu, CHCl$_3$, 0 °C, 24 h	35	69:31 (8, 30)
4	**176a**	Rh, CH$_2$Cl$_2$, 40 °C, 20 h	65	58:42 (25, 41)
5	**176a**	Rh, CH$_2$Cl$_2$, 15 °C, 20 h	10	-

[a] Cu: CuOTf (5 mol%) + bisoxazoline (5 mol%); Rh: Rh$_2$(5*S*-MEPY)$_4$ (1 mol%); [b] Determined by ^{1}H-NMR.

The reaction of (2-*tert*-butylseleno)propenenitrile **178a** with an excess of dimethylethynedicarboxylate provided dimethyl 5-cyano-4,5-dihydroselenophene-2,3-dicarboxylate (**179**) in a 78% yield [80]. In turn, the reaction carried out with 2-(ethylseleno)-, 2-(methylseleno)- and 2-(phenylseleno)propenenitrile **178b–d** and dimethylethynedicarboxylate led to polysubstituted butadienes **180b–d** in 63%, 34%, and 46% yields, respectively (Scheme 47).

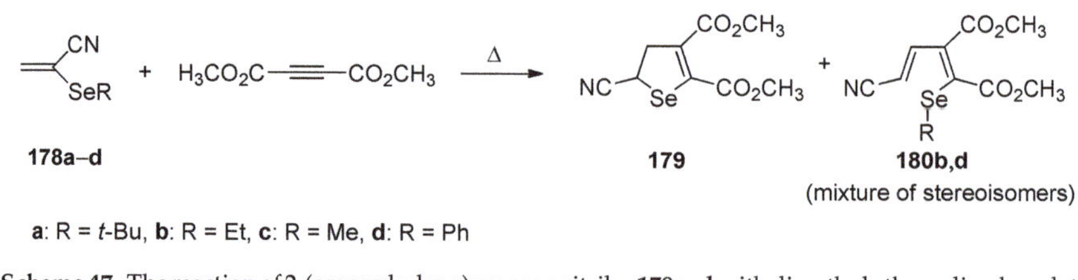

a: R = *t*-Bu, **b**: R = Et, **c**: R = Me, **d**: R = Ph

Scheme 47. The reaction of 2-(organylseleno)propenenitriles **178a–d** with dimethyl ethynedicarboxylate.

Two different reaction pathways leading to compound **179** and/or **180b–d** were postulated. In both cases, the intermediate selenonium ylides **181a–d** formed in the reaction of **178a–d** and dimethylethynedicarboxylate are involved. When the R group on Se in substrate **178a–d** is an alkyl unit, alkene can be eliminated (isobutene from **178a**, ethene from **178b**). In the case of **178a**, elimination of isobutene appears very facile and compound **179** is formed as the only product. On the other hand, elimination of ethene from **178b** is retarded by ring opening to **180b**, via intermediate **182b**, which results in the formation of a mixture of products. In turn, for derivatives **178c,d**, no olefin can be eliminated and thus the ring opening occurred and led to **180c,d** (Scheme 48).

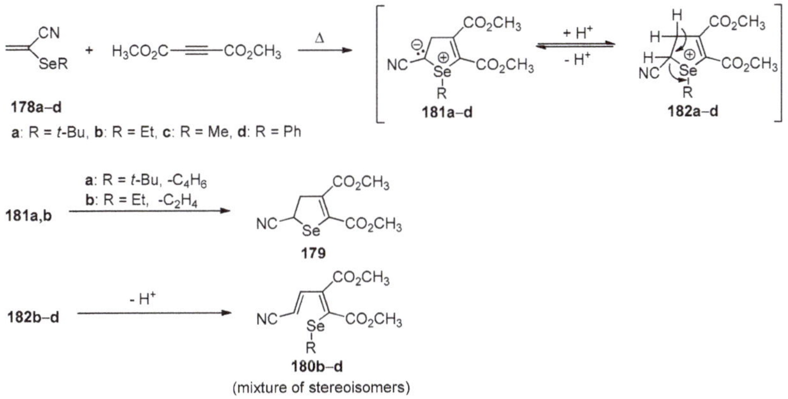

Scheme 48. Reaction pathways for the formation of 2,3-dihydroselenophenes or polysubstituted butadienes from selenonium ylides.

Shen and coworkers described the application of trifluoromethyl-substituted selenonium ylide **19a** as an electrophilic reagent in the reactions with various nucleophiles, including β-ketoesters and silyl enol ethers, aryl/heteroaryl boronic acids, electron-rich heteroarenes, and sulfonates [38]. The reactions of various β-ketoesters derived from indanone, tetralone, or 1-benzosuberone with **19a** in the presence of DBU led to the corresponding trifluoromethylated compound **183a–k** in high yields (79–99%). The reactions of non-phenyl fused or open-chain β-ketoesters were much slower and the formation of the desired products were not observed (Scheme 49).

The reaction of trifluoromethyl-substituted selenium ylide **19a** with various silyl enolethers in the presence of 10 mol% CuSCN afforded the α-trifluoromethyl ketones **184a–k** in high yields (Scheme 50). The obtained results showed that **19a** is a good electrophilic trifluoromethylating reagent not only for β-ketoesters but also for silyl enol ethers.

Compound **19a** was also tested in the reaction with various arylboronic acids in the presence of a copper catalyst. The highest yields of **185a–r** were obtained when the reactions were carried out with the use of 1.2 equiv. of CuCl and 0.8 equiv. of Cs_2CO_3 in DMF at room temperature (Scheme 51). It is worth noting that trifluoromethylated heteroarenes are important structural units in many agrochemicals and they can be used in the preparation of drugs.

The application of reagent **19a** as a precursor of the trifluoromethyl radical was also studied. The obtained results showed that under the irradiation of blue LED light, reagent **19a** reacted with electron-rich indole or pyrrole derivatives in the presence of 1.5 equiv. of DABCO to give the *m*-trifluoromethylated indoles or *o*-trifluoromethylated pyrroles **186a–q** in high yields (Scheme 52). Similar reactions with the corresponding electron-rich arenes were less successful. It was found that the addition of DABCO played a key role in promoting the reaction since the absence of DABCO significantly decreased the yield to 40%.

Additionally, it was found that the trifluoromethyl radical could be generated in the presence of sodium benzenesulfinate instead of an amine. Under the irradiation with visible light of **19a**, the complex collapsed to generate the trifluoromethyl radical, which reacts with the sulfinate radical cation to form the trifluoromethylated sulfone derivatives. Under these conditions, various benzenesulfinate derivatives were trifluoromethylated to give trifluoromethylated sulfones **187a–f** in excellent yields (Scheme 53).

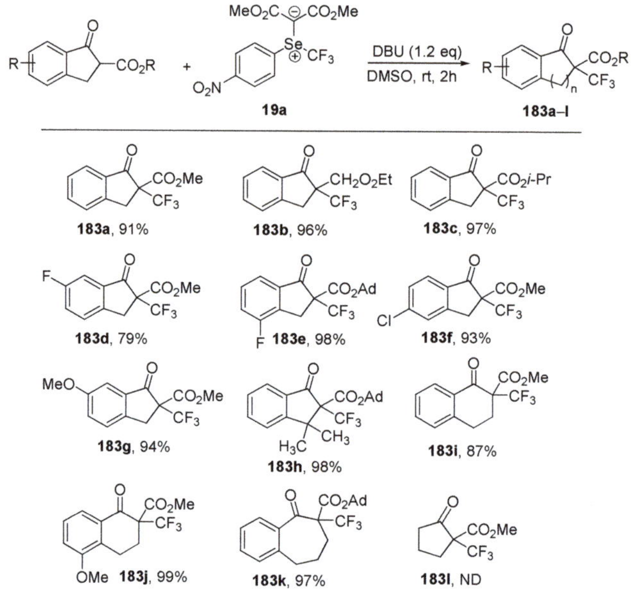

Scheme 49. Reaction of β-ketoesters with **19a**.

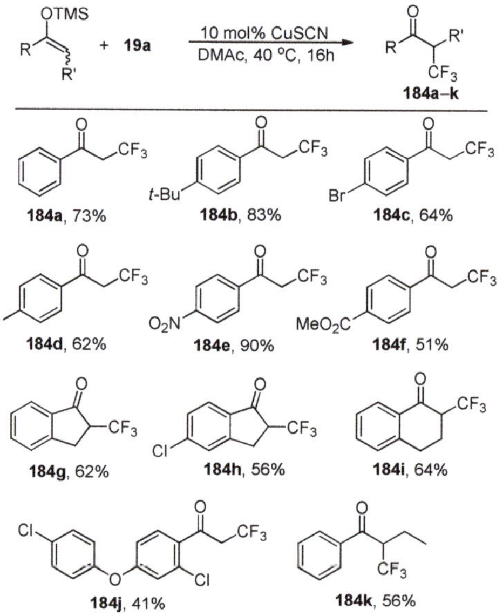

Scheme 50. Reaction of silyl enol ethers with **19a**.

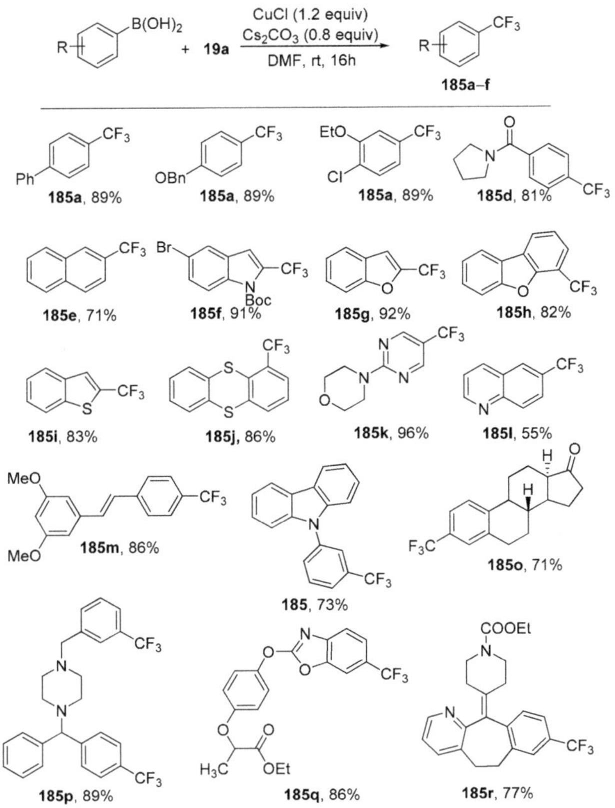

Scheme 51. The copper-mediated reactions of aryl/heteroaryl boronic acids with **19a**.

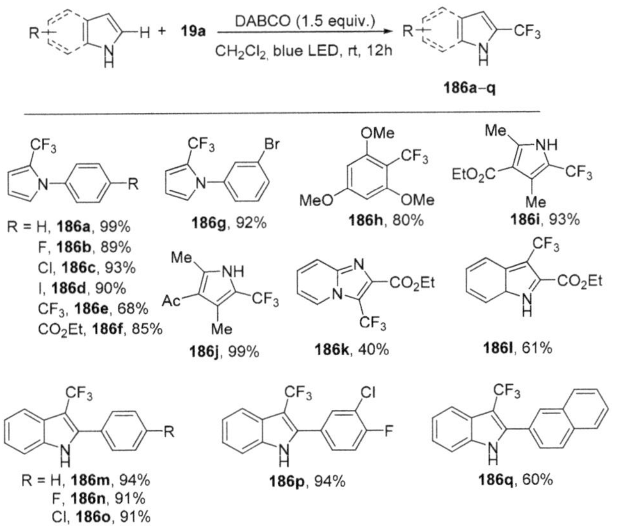

Scheme 52. Visible light-promoted trifluoromethylation of the arene C–H bond with **19a**.

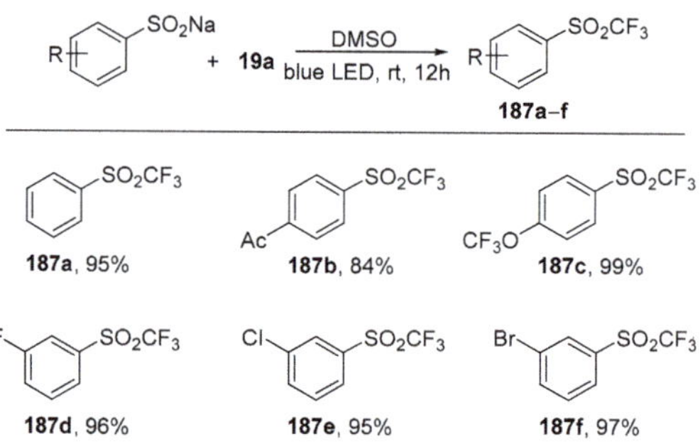

Scheme 53. Visible light-promoted trifluoromethylation of sulfinates with **19a**.

Another group discovered that the reaction of trifluoromethyl aryl selenonium ylides with aryl halides in the presence of copper salts provided diaryl selenides in good yields rather than the expected trifluoromethylated arenes [38].

Trifluoromethyl aryl selenonium ylides **19a–f** were suitable for the Cu-mediated arylselenylation of 4-iodo-1,1′-biphenyl (Scheme 54). A number of selenium ylides containing different substituents on the aromatic ring were tested. In most cases, the desired products were obtained in good to high yields (54–95%).

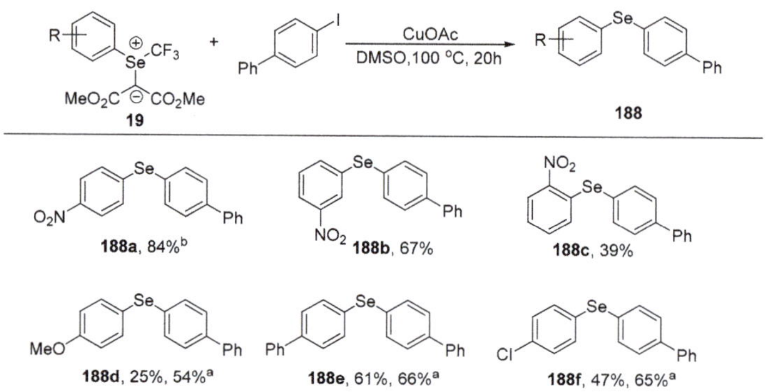

[a] 120 °C; [b] Diethyl 2-((4-nitrophenyl)(trifluoromethyl)-λ^4-selanylidene)malonate (**19b**) was used as a reagent instead of **19a**.

Scheme 54. Cu-mediated arylselenylation of phenyl iodide by different trifluoromethyl aryl selenonium ylides **19a–i**.

The reaction of dimethyl 2-((p-nitrophenyl)(trifluoromethyl)-λ^4-selanylidene)malonate **19a** with various aryl iodides or bromides bearing electron-donating groups, electron-withdrawing groups on the aryl rings led to the corresponding arylselenylated products **188a,b** and **j-ac** in good to high yields (Scheme 55). When the reaction was carried out with aryl chlorides, such as chlorobenzene and p-chlorobenzonitrile, no desired products were obtained.

On the basis of the experiments and previous reports [81,82], a plausible reaction mechanism for the copper-mediated arylselenylation of aryl halides with trifluoromethyl aryl selenonium ylides was proposed (Scheme 56). In the first step, the reduction of trifluoromethyl aryl selenonium ylide by copper via single electron transfer takes place and a radical intermediate (**I**) is formed. Next, the intermediate (**I**) rapidly decomposes to release a •CF$_3$ radical and form an anion intermediate (**II**). Then, α-elimination of an intermediate (**II**) leads to an Ar^{1}Se$^-$ anion, which combines with Cu(I) salt to generate the Ar^{1}SeCu complex (**III**) and release tetramethyl ethene-1,1,2,2-tetracarboxylate (path a). It is also possible that intermediate (**II**) undergoes protonation by traces of moisture in the solvent, which leads to dimethyl 2-(arylselanyl)malonate (**IV**) (path b). Reduction of compound **IV** by Cu afforded (phenylselanyl)copper (**III**) and/or diaryl diselenide (**V**). In the last step, Ar^{1}SeCu complex (**III**) reacts with aryl halides via oxidative addition to give a Cu(III) complex (**VI**), which undergoes reductive elimination to form diaryl selenide and regenerate Cu(I) species. It is worth noting that the •CF$_3$ radical can be reduced via single electron transfer to the $^-$CF$_3$ anion, which bonds to Cu(I) and forms CuCF$_3$. Coupling of CuCF$_3$ with aryl halides via oxidative addition and reductive elimination led to the trifluoromethylated product. Under standard reaction conditions, this pathway might be very slow and may not be the main process because only trace amounts of ArCF$_3$ were detected.

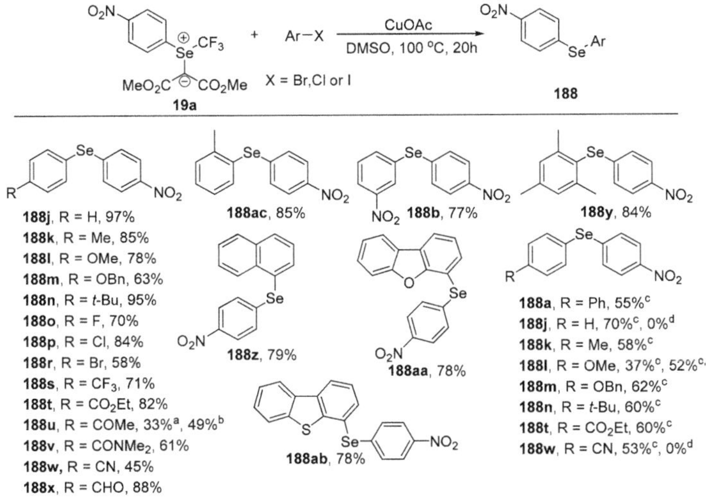

^{a} DMF was used instead of DMSO; ^{b} Cu (2 equiv.), DMF (2 mL), N$_2$, 100 °C, 3 h; ^{c} ArBr was used instead of ArI at 140 °C; ^{d} ArCl was used instead of ArI at 140 °C; ^{e} 48 h.

Scheme 55. Cu-mediated arylselenylation of aryl halides by ylides **19**.

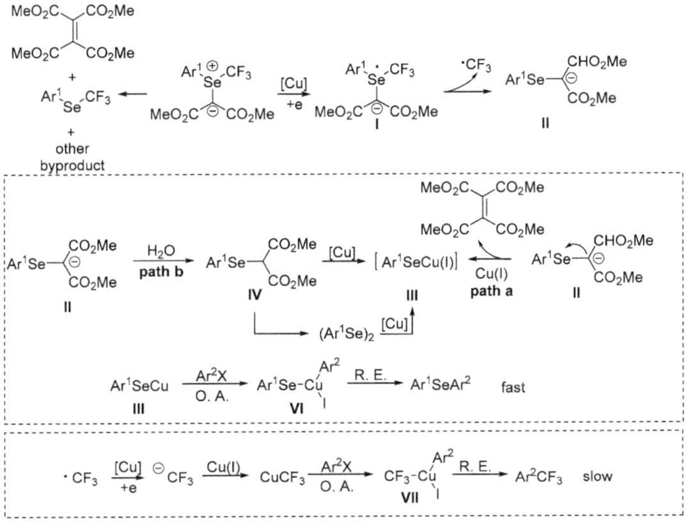

Scheme 56. A plausible mechanism for Cu-mediated arylselenylation of aryl halides with trifluoromethyl aryl selenonium ylides **19**.

Koengis and Jana recently reported the first study on rhodium-catalyzed generation and sigmatropic rearrangement of selenonium ylides and their synthetic applications. One of these applications allows access to important 1,1-disubstituted butadienes (Scheme 57) [83].

The most general application based on the generation of ylides in the reactions of allyl selenide **189** with different diazoesters **190** led to the desired homoallylic selenides **191** in excellent yields (Scheme 58). It was found that the type of substituent in the aromatic ring had little influence on the reaction yield, as various electron-donating groups as well as halides were compatible with the reaction. Additionally, other allylic selenides with a broad range of functional groups, such as nitro, cyano, and trifluoromethyl substituents, were investigated (Scheme 58). In this case, the seleno-Doyle–Kirmse reaction led to homoallylic selenides in good to high yields [83]. Thiophene and pyridine heterocycles were also compatible under these reaction conditions, and no poisoning of the rhodium catalyst occurred. The corresponding heterocycle-functionalized homoallylic selenides the rearrangement product in good yield but with only low diastereoselectivity, which is comparable to the diastereoselectivity range for the classic Doyle–Kirmse reactions [84–86].

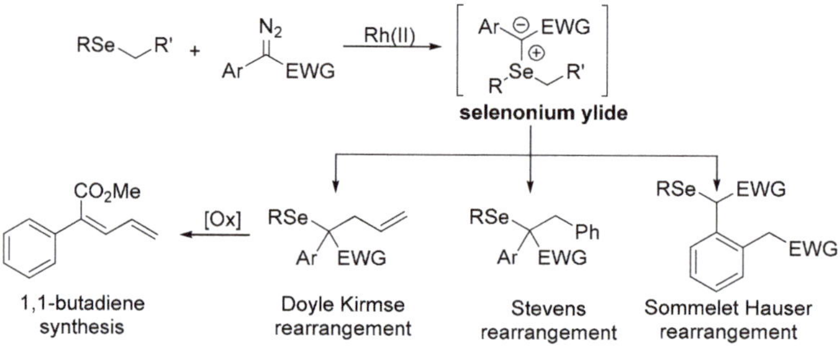

Scheme 57. Rhodium-catalyzed generation and sigmatropic rearrangement of selenonium ylides and their synthetic applications.

Under optimized conditions, the reaction of propargyl selenides **192** with α-aryldiazoacetates **193** afforded the desired allenyl selenides **194a–l** in excellent yields (Scheme 59).

The use of ethyl 2-(phenylselanyl)acetate **195a** led to the α-seleno-substituted esters **196a**, as products of Sommelet–Hauser or [2,3]-sigmatropic rearrangement. The reaction product corresponds to a formal o-C-H functionalization of the aromatic substituent of **190**. This transformation also took place for the cyano-substituted selenide **195b** and afforded the products o-C-H functionalization in good to high yields. In turn, *meta*-substituted diazoalkanes reacted in a highly regioselective manner to form the corresponding trisubstituted phenyl acetic acid ester **196i** in high yield (Scheme 60).

In the case of benzylic selenide **197**, the desired product of [1,2]-sigmatropic or Stevens rearrangement was obtained as a complex mixture. A change of the solvent used in the reaction to only water resulted in the rearrangement product **198a–f** in a good isolated yield. Similarly, the use of different donor–acceptor diazoesters smoothly led to the Stevens rearrangement product in a selective way (Scheme 61).

A one-pot protocol consisting of rhodium-catalyzed generation and rearrangement of selenonium ylides and a subsequent oxidation of the formed selenides in the synthesis of olefins is shown in Scheme 62. Thus, a two-step reaction of allyl selenide **189** with α-aryldiazoacetates **193** afforded Z-configured 1,1-disubstituted butadiene **199** in a 56% yield. A consecutive reaction protocol led to **199** in a similar yield (60%). The stereochemical outcome of this *syn* elimination was rationalized by the transition state in which the vinyl group and the phenyl ring have a *trans* conformation that results in the Z-configuration of the butadiene product (Scheme 62c). The stereochemistry of this reaction is complementary to that of the reaction of diazoalkanes with electrophilic palladium-allyl complexes [87]. A similar protocol was applied to the synthesis of trisubstituted olefin **200** as the product of the Stevens rearrangement of the generated ylide. The reaction led to the mixture of diastereoisomers in a 1:1 ratio (Scheme 62b), which is a result of the similar steric hindrance in both transition states (Scheme 62c).

In 2019, Anbarasan and coworkers described the rhodium-catalyzed rearrangement of selenonium ylides and their use in the synthesis of substituted vinylogous carbonates [88]. The reaction of various α-selenoesters **201** with diazocompound **202** in the presence of 2 %mol of $Rh_2(OAc)_4$ led to the desired products **203a–e** in a good yield (62–72%) (Scheme 63). Only in the case of ethyl α-phenylselenopropionate, the desired product **203f** was not observed, most probably due to the steric effect.

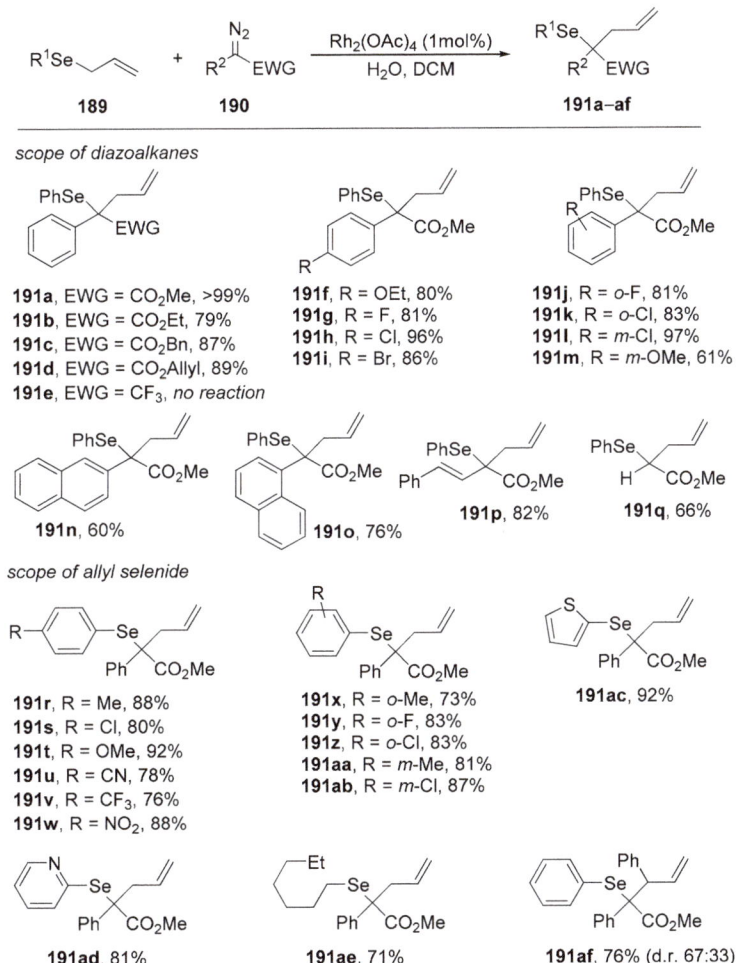

Scheme 58. [2,3]-Sigmatropic rearrangement of selenium ylides generated in situ by a rhodium catalysed reaction of selenides **189** with diazocompounds **190**.

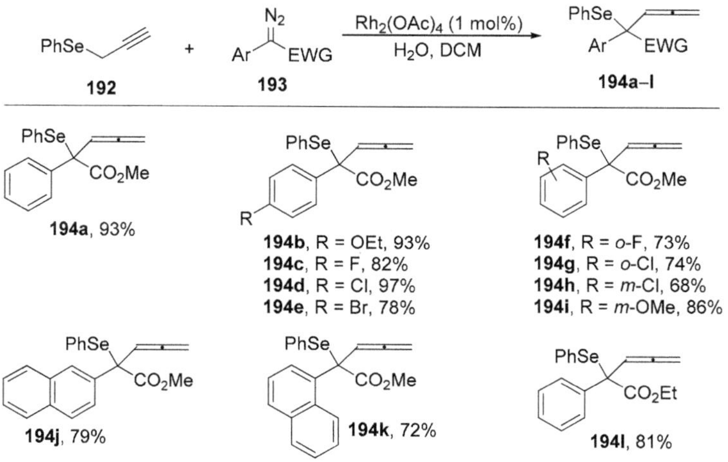

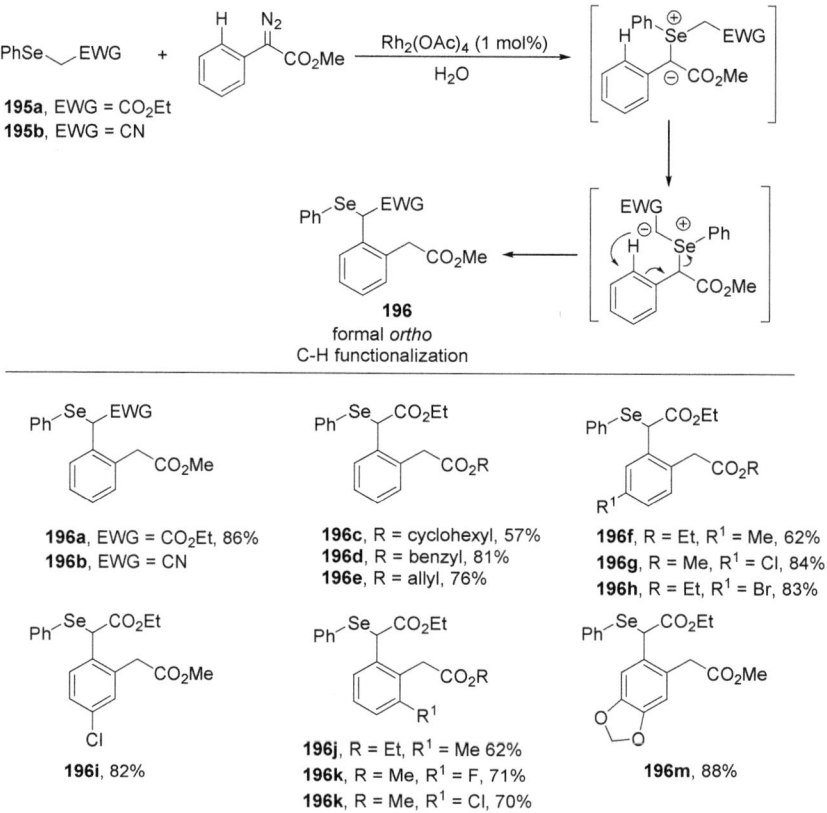

Scheme 59. [2,3]-Sigmatropic rearrangement of selenonium ylides generated in situ by a rhodium-catalyzed reaction of selenides **192** with diazocompounds **193**.

Scheme 60. The Sommelet–Hauser rearrangement of selenonium ylides generated in situ by a rhodium-catalyzed reaction of selenides **195** with α-phenyldiazoacetate.

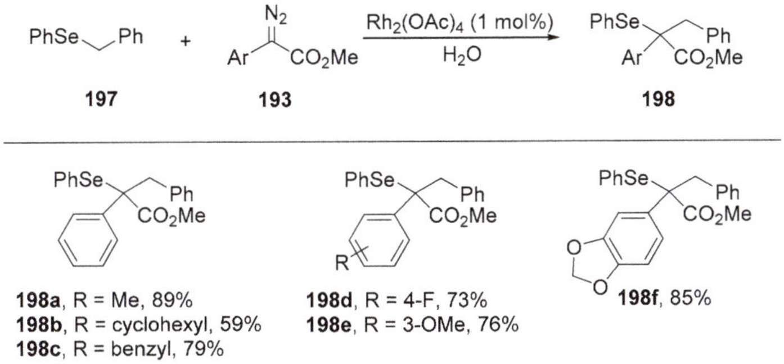

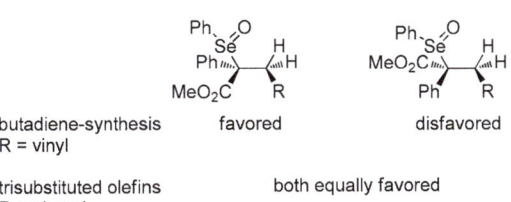

Scheme 61. Rhodium-catalyzed reaction of benzyl phenyl selenide **197** with α-aryldiazoacetates **197**.

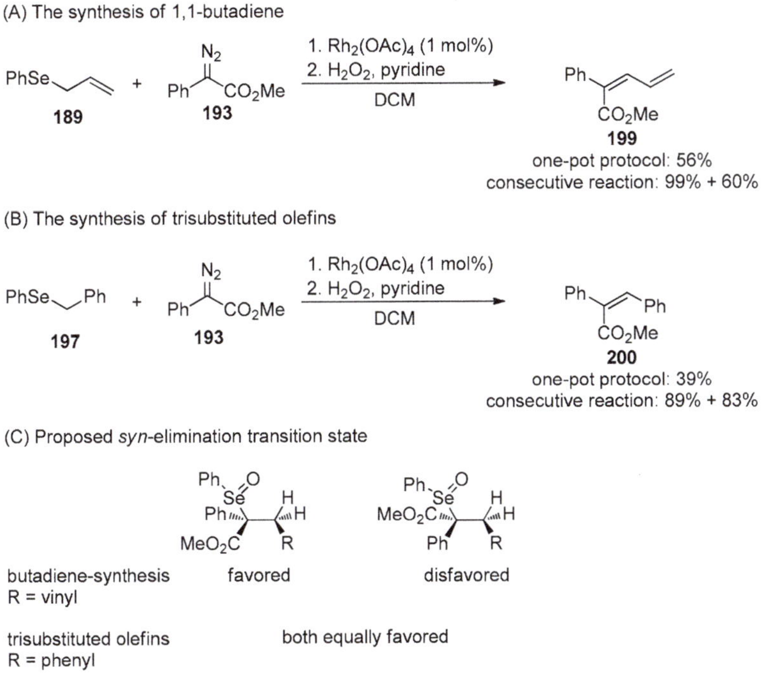

(A) The synthesis of 1,1-butadiene

(B) The synthesis of trisubstituted olefins

(C) Proposed *syn*-elimination transition state

butadiene-synthesis   favored   disfavored
R = vinyl

trisubstituted olefins   both equally favored
R = phenyl

Scheme 62. Applications of the in situ-generated selenonium ylides in the synthesis of olefins; (**A**) the synthesis of 1,1-butadiene; (**B**) the synthesis of trisubstituted olefins; (**C**) proposed *syn*-elimination state.

Hori and coworkers reported the reactions of α-selenanaphthalene stabilized by the cyano group, i.e., l-cyano-2-methyl-2-selenanaphthalene (**20a**) [43]. Its reaction with dimethyl acetylenedicarboxylate (DMAD) in benzene at room temperature gave benzocycloheptene derivative **204** in a 61% yield, whereas the same reaction in sulfolane led to the mixture of naphthalene derivatives **205** (37%) and **204**. Furthermore, the reaction was carried out in acetonitrile produced **204** (17%) and bisbenzocycloheptenyl derivative **206** (56%). Scheme 64 shows a plausible mechanism for the formation of the benzocycloheptene **204** and the naphthalene **205**.

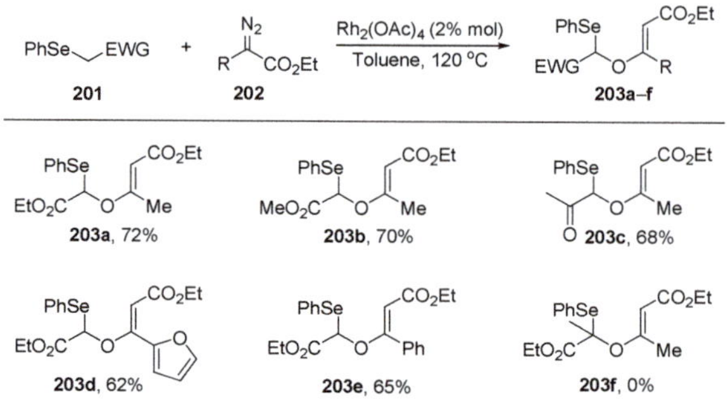

Scheme 63. Rhodium-catalyzed arrangement of selenonium ylides.

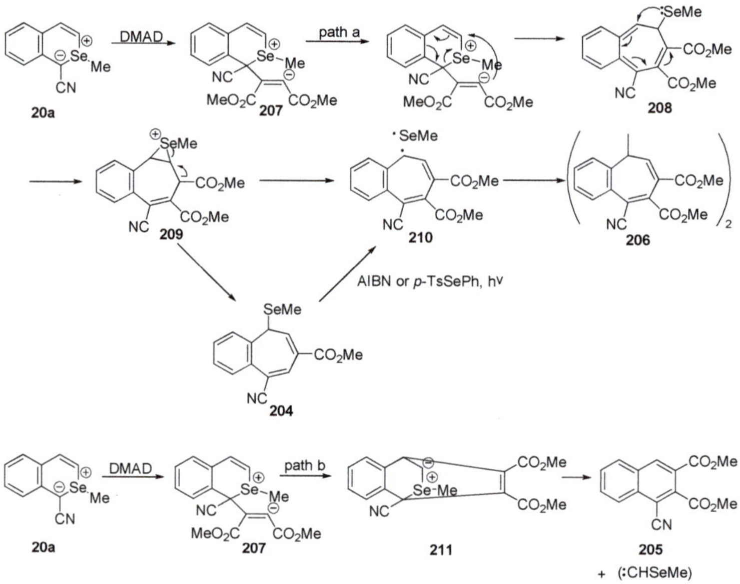

Scheme 64. The plausible mechanism for the formation of benzocycloheptene **204** and naphthalene **205**.

In contrast to the reaction with DMAD, reaction of **20a** with methyl propiolate afforded a mixture of adduct **212**, rearranged product **213**, and demethylated product **214** (Scheme 65).

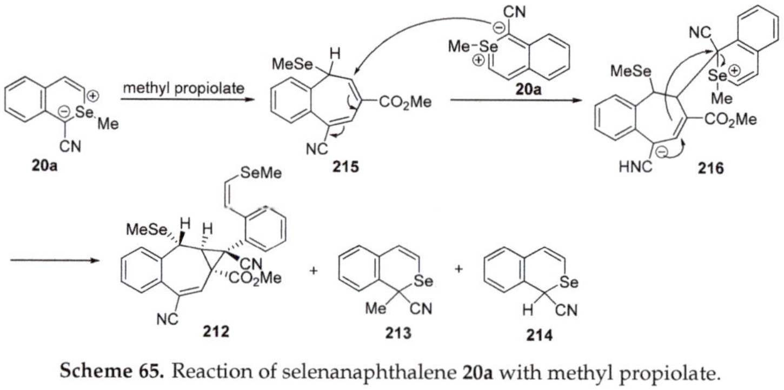

Scheme 65. Reaction of selenanaphthalene **20a** with methyl propiolate.

Moreover, the reactions of selenanaphthalene **20a** with olefins were examined (Table 15). The obtained results showed that the reaction of **20a** did not occur with styrene, dimethyl fumarate, and vinyl sulfones. However, when the reaction was conducted with vinyl sulfones, such as *trans*-styryl tolyl sulfone and 3-(*p*-tosyl)sulfolene, the yield of the 1,2-rearranged product **213** was reasonable.

Table 15. Reactions of selenanaphthalene **20a** with electron-deficient olefins.

Entry	Olefins (equiv.)	Solvent	Products (yield, %)
1	(*E*)-styryl *p*-tolyl sulfone (1.7)	MeCN	**213** (61)
2	(*E*)-styryl *p*-tolyl sulfone (1.7)	C_6H_6	**213** (59)
3	(*E*)-styryl *p*-tolyl sulfone (0.1)	C_6H_6	**213** (18), **214** (14)
4	3-(*p*-tosyl)sulfone (1.7)	MeCN	**213** (66), **214** (6)
5	styrene (1.7)	C_6H_6	**213** (17), **214** (9),
6	acrylonitrile (1.1)	MeCN	**214** (trace), **217** (29), **218** (53)
7	methyl acrylate (1.1)	MeCN	**213** (13), **219** (18), **220** (33)
8	methyl vinyl ketone (1.1)	MeCN	**213** (3), **221** (37), **222** (55)

Scheme 66 shows the reaction of selenanaphthalene **20a** with monosubstituted olefins. The reaction with acrylonitrile afforded *r*-1,*t*-2-dicyano-l-[2-(*cis*-2-methylselenovinyl)-phenyl] cyclopropane (**217**) and the *r*-1,*c*-2-dicyano isomer (**218**) in 29% and 53% yields, respectively. Methyl acrylate and methyl vinyl ketone reacted similarly with **7** to afford *cis-trans* mixtures of the cyclopropane derivatives **219**, **220**, **221**, and **222**, respectively.

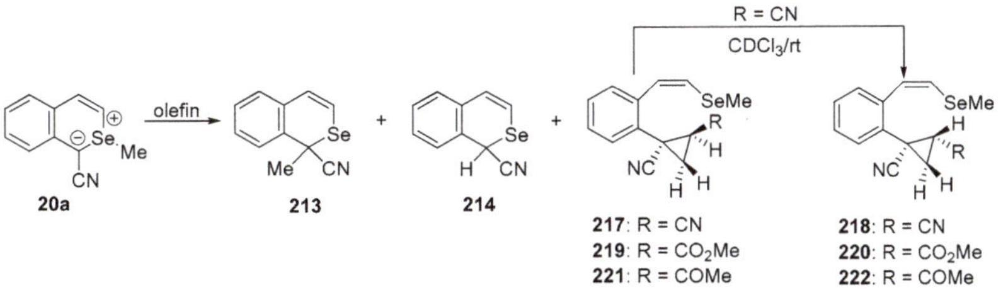

Scheme 66. Reaction of selenanaphthalene **20a** with olefins.

5. Conclusions and Perspectives

Synthetic approaches to the preparation of achiral and chiral selenonium ylides (including a few optically active ones) and the problem of their structural features, synthesis, reactivity, and application in organic synthesis were described in this manuscript. The purpose of this mini review was to provide the available information on all topics mentioned above in order to stimulate additional research in this field. The rationale for this research topic is the structural similarity between selenonium ylides and sulfonium ylides, which play a very important role as new synthetic reagents, biologically active compounds, and new functional materials [4–8]. Therefore, it is reasonable to expect that achiral and optically active selenonium ylides should be just as useful as sufonium ylides when they have sufficiently high chemical and optical stability. It is reasonable to expect that further research will allow the preparation of model compounds containing, for example, more sterically demanding substituents, which in turn enable the preparation of optically active selenonium ylides with an optical stability comparable to sulfonium ylides. First of all, it is worth checking their preparation by asymmetric synthesis. Moreover, access to a wider group of selenonium ylides, achiral and optically active, should open the way to the isolation of the corresponding oxoselenonium ylides, which, to our best knowledge, have not been reported in the chemical literature so far.

Author Contributions: The contribution of all authors in the preparation of the manuscript is equivalent. Conceptualization, J.D., A.R., R.Ż.; writing—original draft preparation, J.D., A.R., R.Ż.; writing—review and editing, J.D., A.R., R.Ż.; funding acquisition, J.D. All authors have read and agreed to the published version of the manuscript.

Funding: The writing of this manuscript was financially supported by the National Science Center, grant number UMO-2014/15/B/ST5/05329 (for JD).

Acknowledgments: We would thank Petro Onyko (Institute of Organic Chemistry, Ukrainian National Academy of Sciences, Kiev) for his help in getting copies of the selected Russian journals and Piotr Kiełbasiński for reading the final draft of this manuscript.

Conflicts of Interest: The authors declare no conflict of interest. The funders had no role in the writing of the manuscript.

References

1. Perkins, C.W.; Martin, J.C.; Arduengo, A.J.; Lau, W.; Alergia, A.; Kochi, K.J. An electrically neutral ε-sulfuranyl radical from hemolysis of a peresterwith neighboring sulfenyl sulfur: 9-S-3 species. *J. Am. Chem. Soc.* **1980**, *102*, 7753–7759. [CrossRef]
2. Hayes, R.A.; Martin, J.C. *Organic Sulfur Chemistry: Theoretical and Experimental Advances*; Bernardi, F., Csizmadia, J.G., Mangini, A., Eds.; Elsevier: Amsterdam, The Netherlands, 1985; Chapter 8; pp. 408–458.
3. Musher, J.I. The chemistry of hypervalent molecules. *Angew. Chem. Int. Ed. Engl.* **1969**, *8*, 54–68. [CrossRef]
4. Trost, B.M.; Melvin, L.S. *Sulfur Ylides, Emerging Synthetic Intermediates*; Academic Press: New York, NY, USA, 1975; Volume 2, pp. 13–156.
5. Lu, L.-Q.; Chen, J.-R.; Xiao, W.-J.N. Development of Cascade Reactions for the Concise Construction of Diverse Heterocyclic Architectures. *Acc. Chem. Res.* **2012**, *45*, 1278–1294. [CrossRef] [PubMed]
6. Neuhaus, J.D.; Oost, R.; Merad, J.; Maulide, N. Sulfur-based ylides in transition-metal-catalysed processes. *Top. Curr. Chem.* **2018**, *376*, 15. [CrossRef] [PubMed]
7. Mondal, N.; Chen, S.; Kerrigan, N.J. Recent Developments in Vinylsulfonium and Vinylsulfoxonium Salt Chemistry. *Molecules* **2018**, *23*, 738. [CrossRef] [PubMed]
8. Gessner, V.H. *Modern Ylide Chemistry: Applicationsin Ligand Design, Organic and Catalytic Transformations*; Springer: Berlin/Heidelberg, Germany, 2018; Volume 177.
9. Lloyd, D. Ylides of group V and VI elements. *Chem. Scr.* **1975**, *8*, 14–19.
10. Johnsons, A.W. Ylides of sulfur, selenium and tellurium, and related structures. In *Organic Compound of Sulphur, Selenium and Tellurium*; The Chemical Society: London, UK, 1973; Volume 2, pp. 288–340.
11. Johnsons, A.W. Ylides of sulfur, selenium and tellurium, and related structures. In *Organic Compound of Sulphur, Selenium and Tellurium*; The Chemical Society: London, UK, 1975; Volume 3, pp. 322–338. [CrossRef]
12. Block, E.; Haake, M. Ylides of sulfur, selenium and tellurium, and related structures. In *Organic Compound of Sulphur, Selenium and Tellurium*; The Chemical Society: London, UK, 1977; Volume 4, pp. 78–123.
13. Haake, M. Ylides of sulfur, selenium and tellurium, and related structures. *Org. Compd. Sulphur Selenium Tellurium* **1979**, *5*, 100–117.
14. Block, E.; Clive, D.L.; Furukawa, N.; Oae, S. Ylides of sulfur, selenium and tellurium and related structures. *Org. Compd. Sulphur Selenium Tellurium* **1981**, *6*, 79–147.
15. Krief, A. Synthesis of selenium and tellurium ylides and carbanions: Application to organic synthesis. In *PATAI'S Chemistry of Functional Groups*; Patai, S., Ed.; John Wiley & Sons, Ltd.: Chichester, UK, 1987; pp. 675–764.
16. Comasseto, J.V.; Piovan, L.; Wendler, E.P. Synthesis of selenium and tellurium ylides and carbanions. Application to organic synthesis. In *PATAI'S Chemistry of Functional Groups. Organic Selenium and Tellurium*; Rappoport, Z., Ed.; John Wiley & Sons, Ltd.: Chichester, UK, 2014; pp. 1–78.
17. Shimizu, T.; Kamigata, N. Isolation and stereochemistry of optically active tricoordinated selenium and tellurium compounds. *Rev. Heteroat. Chem.* **1998**, *18*, 11–35.
18. Nishubabayashi, Y.; Uemura, S. Selenoxide elimination and [2,3]-sigmatropic rearrangement. In *Organoselenium Chemistry: Syntsesis and Reactions*; Wirth, T., Ed.; Wiley-VCH: Weinheim, Germany, 2012.
19. Sadekov, I.O.; MInikin, V.I.; Semenov, V.V.; Shevelev, S.A. Twice stabilized chalcogenonium ylides. *Uspekhi Khimi.* **1981**, *50*, 813–859.
20. Hughes, E.D.; Kuriyan, K.I. Influence of poles and polar linkings on the course pursued by elimination reactions. Part XXIII. Stable Derivatives of the tercovalent-carbon compound of Ingold and Jessop. *J. Chem. Soc.* **1935**, 1609–1611. [CrossRef]
21. Lloyd, D.; Singer, M.I.C. A Selenonium Ylid. *Chem. Commun.* **1967**, 390. [CrossRef]

22. Saatsazov, V.V.; Kyandzhetsian, R.A.; Kuznetsov, S.I.; Madgesieva, N.N.; Khotsyanova, T.C. Interaction of dichlorides of organic selenides with carbalkoxymethylene triphenylphosphoranes. *Dakl. Akad. Nauk. SSSR* **1972**, *206*, 1130–1132.
23. Hope, H. The crystal structure of trimethylselenonium iodide, $(CH_3)_3SeI$. *Acta Crystallogr.* **1966**, *20*, 610–613. [CrossRef]
24. Hope, H.; Knobler, C.; McCullough, J.D. The crystal and molecular structure of dibenzoselenophene, $C_{12}H_8Se$. *Acta Crystallogr.* **1970**, *26*, 628–640. [CrossRef]
25. Beer, R.J.S.; Hatton, J.R.; Llaguno, E.C.; Paul, I.C. The Structure of a [1,2,5] oxaselenazolo [2,3-*b*] [1,2,5] oxaselenazole-7-Se^{IV} by X-Ray Crystallography and Nuclear Magnetic Resonance Spectroscopy. *J. Chem. Soc. D* **1971**, 594–595. [CrossRef]
26. Saatsazov, V.V.; Kyandzhetsian, R.A.; Kuznetsov, S.I.; Madgesieva, N.N.; Khotsyanova, T.C. X-ray diffraction of some selenium ylides. *Izv. Akad. Nauk SSSR Ser. Khim.* **1973**, *22*, 671–672.
27. Wei, K.-T.H.; Paul, I.C.; Chang, M.-M.Y.; Musher, J.I. Preparation and structural features of a selenium ylide, diacetylmethylenediphenylselenurane. *J. Am. Chem. Soc.* **1974**, *96*, 4099–4102. [CrossRef]
28. Shevelev, S.A.; Semenov, V.V.; Fainzilber, A.A. Synthesis of nitroylides and their conversions. *Izv. Akad. Nauk SSSR Ser. Khim.* **1978**, *27*, 1091–1098.
29. Fujihara, H.; Nakahodo, T.; Furukawa, N. Synthesis of 5*H*,7*H*-dibenzo [*b*,*g*] [1,5] selenoxocine from a selenonium salt of 5*H*,7*H*-dibenzo [*b*,*g*] [1,5] diselenocine and first X-ray evidence for the transannular oxygen-selenium interaction. *Tetrahedron Lett.* **1995**, *36*, 6275–6278. [CrossRef]
30. Comasseto, J.V.; Piovan, L.; Wendler, E.P. Synthesis of selenium and tellurium ylides and carbanions: Application to organic synthesis. In *PATAI'S Chemistry of Functional Groups*; Rappoport, Z., Ed.; John Wiley & Sons, Ltd.: Chichester, UK, 2013; pp. 657–734.
31. Paulmier, C. *Selenium Reagents and Intermediates in Organic Synthesis*; Organic Chemistry Series; Baldwin, J.E., Pergamon, J.E., Eds.; Pergamon Press: Oxford/Chichester, UK, 1986; Volume 4.
32. Kamigata, N.; Nakamura, Y.; Kikuchi, K.; Ikemoto, I.; Shimizu, T.; Matsuyama, H. Synthesis and stereochemistry of an optically active selenonium ylide. X-Ray molecular structure of (+)$_{Se}$-{4'-[(-)-menthyloxycarbonyl]phenyl} (methyl) selenonium 4,4-dimethyl-2,6-dioxocyclohexylide. *J. Chem. Soc. Perkin Trans. 1* **1992**, *13*, 1721–1728. [CrossRef]
33. Shimizu, T.; Kamigata, N. Synthesis and Stereochemistry of Optically Active Organic Selenium and Tellurium Compounds. *Yuki Gosei Kagaku Kyokaishi* **1997**, *55*, 35–43. [CrossRef]
34. Takahashi, T.; Kurose, N.; Kawanami, S.; Nojiri, A.; Arai, Y.; Koizumi, T.; Shiro, M. Nucleophilic substitution reaction of optically purechlorosulfurane with active methylene compounds: Formation of optically pure selenonium ylides. *Chem. Lett.* **1995**, *24*, 379–381. [CrossRef]
35. Kushnarev, D.F.; Kalabin, G.A.; Kyandzhetsian, R.A.; Magdesieva, N.N. NMR Spectroscopy of seleno- and telluroorganic compounds. X. ^{77}Se Chemical shifts of selenonium ylides. *J. Org. Chem. USSR (English Translation)* **1982**, *4*, 103–107, *Zhu. Org. Khim.* **1982**, *18*, 119–124.
36. Nozaki, H.; Tunemoto, D.; Morita, Z.; Nakamura, K.; Watanabe, K.; Takaku, M.; Kondo, K. Preparative and structural studies on certain sulphur-ylides. *Tetrahedron* **1967**, *23*, 4279–4290. [CrossRef]
37. Hori, M.; Kataoka, T.; Shimizu, H.; Tsutsumi, K.; Hu, Y.-Z.; Nishigiri, M. Cyclic selenonium *exo*-ylides (3,4-dihydro-1*H*-2-benzoselenin-2-io) methanides; syntheses and reactions. *J. Chem. Soc. Perkin Trans. 1* **1990**, 39–45. [CrossRef]
38. Ge, H.; Shen, Q. Trifluoromethyl-substituted selenium ylide: A broadly applicable electrophilic trifluoromethylating reagent. *Org. Chem. Front.* **2019**, *6*, 2205–2209. [CrossRef]
39. Wu, S.; Shi, J.; Zhang, C.-P. Cu-Mediated Arylselenylation of Aryl Halides with Trifluoromethyl Aryl Selenonium Ylides. *Org. Biomol. Chem.* **2019**, *17*, 7468–7473. [CrossRef] [PubMed]
40. Magdesieva, N.N.; Kandgetc, R.A.; Ibragimo, A.A. Synthesis of stable selenonium ylides. *J. Organomet. Chem.* **1972**, *42*, 399–404. [CrossRef]
41. Stackhouse, J.; Senklerb, G.H., Jr.; Maryanoff, B.E.; Mislow, K. Synthesis and characterization of a selenabenzene. *J. Am. Chem. Soc.* **1974**, *96*, 7835–7836. [CrossRef]
42. Honda, E.; Kataoka, T. Chemistry of selenabenzenes and related compounds. *Curr. Org. Chem.* **2004**, *8*, 813–825. [CrossRef]
43. Hori, M.; Kataoka, T.; Shimizu, H.; Tsutsumi, K.; Yoshimatsu, M. Synthesis and reactions of a sTable 2-selenanaphthalene, 1-cyano-2-mehtyl-2-selenanaphthalene. *J. Org. Chem.* **1990**, *55*, 2458–2463. [CrossRef]

44. Yamamoto, Y. Ylide-Metal Complexes. XI. The Preparation and Properties of VIA Group Metal (Te) Complexes of Alkylidenetriphenylphosphoranes and the Corresponding Selenium Compounds. *Bull. Chem. Soc. Jpn.* **1986**, *59*, 3053–3056. [CrossRef]
45. Friedrich, K.; Amann, W.; Fritz, H. Cyclopentadienid-Synthesen mit Iodonium-Yliden: Cyclopentadienide mit Schwefel, Selen, Phosphor und Arsen als Oniumzentrum. *Chem. Ber.* **1979**, *112*, 1267–1271. [CrossRef]
46. Ernstbrunner, E.; Lloyd, D. 5-(Dimethylselenanylidene)-2,2-dimethyl-1,3-dioxane-4,6-dione, a new stable selenonium ylide. *Liebigs Ann. Chem.* **1971**, *753*, 196–198. [CrossRef]
47. Magdesieva, N.N.; Kandgetcyan, R.A. Diphenylselenonium dimedoneylide. *Zh. Org. Khim.* **1971**, *7*, 2228–2229.
48. Zefirov, N.S. Stable selenium ylides. *Chem. Scr.* **1975**, *8*, 20–22.
49. Magdesieva, N.N.; Kyandzhetsian, R.A. Stable selenonium ylides. Reaction of selenolane dichloride with Carbethoxymethylenetriphenylphosphorane. *Zh. Org. Khim.* **1973**, *9*, 1755–1756.
50. Magdesieva, N.N.; Kyandzhetsian, R.A. Reaction of dichlorides of organic selenides with carbalkoxymethylenetriphenylphosphoranes. *Zh. Obshch. Khim.* **1974**, *44*, 1708–1711.
51. Lotz, W.W.; Gosselck, J. Synthesis and reactions of dimethylphenacylselenonium ylide. *Tetrahedron* **1973**, *29*, 917–919. [CrossRef]
52. Tamagaki, S.; Sakaki, K. A convenient synthesis of selenonium ylides. *Chem. Lett.* **1975**, 503–506. [CrossRef]
53. Tamagaki, S.; Akatsuka, R.; Kozuka, S. A convenient synthesis of telluronium ylides. *Bull. Chem. Soc. Jpn.* **1980**, *53*, 817–818. [CrossRef]
54. Shevelev, S.A.; Semenov, V.V.; Fainzilberg, A.A. Nitroylides. 4. Synthesis of selenonium nitroylides and their conversions. *Russ. Chem. Bull.* **1978**, *51*, 945–951. [CrossRef]
55. Magdesieva, N.N.; Kyandzhetsian, R.A.; Astafurov, V.M. Reaction of organic derivatives of selenium (IV) with benzoyl- and thenoyltrifluoroacetone. *Zh. Org. Khim.* **1975**, *11*, 508–511.
56. Reich, H.J.; Trend, J.E. Organoselenium Chemistry. Intra- and Intermolecular Trapping of Selenenic Acids Formed by Selenoxide Elimination. Formation of a Selenium Ylide. *J. Org. Chem.* **1976**, *41*, 2503–2504. [CrossRef]
57. Reich, H.J.; Wollowitz, S.; Trend, J.E.; Chow, F.; Wendelborn, D.F. Syn Elimination of Alkyl Selenoxides. Side Reactions Involving Selenenic Acids. Structural and Solvent Effects on Rates. *J. Org. Chem.* **1978**, *43*, 1697–1705. [CrossRef]
58. Tamagaki, S.; Akatsuka, R.; Kozuka, S. Additions of dibenzyl selenoxides and selenonium ylides to electron-deficient ethylene and acetylene. *Bull. Chem. Soc. Jpn.* **1977**, *50*, 1641–1642. [CrossRef]
59. Kataoka, T.; Tomimatsu, K.; Shimizu, H.; Hori, M. Stable selenoxanthenium ylides: Synthesis and new reductive cyclization of selenoxanthen-10-io (alkoxalyl alkoxycarbonyl) methanides and their related compounds. *Tetrahedron Lett.* **1983**, *24*, 75–78. [CrossRef]
60. Kamigata, N.; Nakamura, Y.; Matsuyama, H.; Shimizu, T. Synthesis of optically active selenonium ylide. *Chem. Lett.* **1991**, *20*, 249–250. [CrossRef]
61. Wang, H.-Y.; Yang, F.; Li, X.-L.; Yan, X.-M.; Huang, Z.-Z. First Example of Highly Stereoselective Synthesis of 1,2,3-Trisubstituted Cyclopropanes via Chiral Selenonium Ylides. *Chem. Eur. J.* **2009**, *15*, 3784–3789. [CrossRef]
62. Midura, W.H.; Ścianowski, J.; Banach, A.; Zając, A. Asymmetric synthesis of cyclopropyl phosphonates using chiral terpenyl sulfonium and selenonium ylides. *Tetrahedron Asymmetry* **2014**, *25*, 1488–1493. [CrossRef]
63. Dumont, W.; Bayet, P.; Krief, A. Synthesis and Reactions of Unstabilized—Selenonio Alkylides. *Angew. Chem. Int. Ed. Engl.* **1974**, *13*, 274–275. [CrossRef]
64. Morihara, K.; Matsunaga, H.; Kou, K.; Niyomura, O.; Ando, F.; Koketsu, J. Generation of Selenonium Ylides from Selenonium Salts by Electrochemical Reduction and their Reactions. *Electrochemistry* **2009**, *77*, 801–807. [CrossRef]
65. Takada, H.; Metzner, P.; Philouze, C. First chiral selenium ylides used for asymmetric conversion of aldehydes into epoxides. *Chem. Commun.* **2001**, 2350–2351. [CrossRef]
66. Briere, J.-F.; Takada, H.; Metzner, P. Chalcogen chiral ylides for the catalytic asymmetric epoxidation of aldehydes: From sulfur to selenium and tellurium. *Phosphorus Sulfur Silicon* **2005**, *180*, 965–968. [CrossRef]
67. Aggarwal, V.K.; Richardson, J. The complexity of catalysis: Origins of enantio- and diastereocontrol in sulfur ylide mediated epoxidation reactions. *Chem. Commun.* **2003**, 2644–2651. [CrossRef]

68. Aggarwal, V.K.; Charmant, J.P.H.; Ciampi, C.; Hornby, J.M.; O'Brien, C.J.; Hynd, G.; Parsons, R. Additions of stabilised and semi-stabilised sulfur ylides to tosyl protected imines: Are they under kinetic or thermodynamic control? *J. Chem. Soc. Perkin Trans. 1* **2001**, *23*, 3159–3166. [CrossRef]
69. Watanabe, S.; Asaka, S.; Kataoka, T. Michael-type addition of hydroxide to alkynylselenonium salt: Practical use as a ketoselenonium ylide precursor. *Tetrahedron Lett.* **2004**, *45*, 7459–7463. [CrossRef]
70. Matano, Y.; Yoshimune, M.; Suzuki, H. 3-Substituted 2-acyl-1-sulfonylaziridines from the reaction of triphenylbismuthonium 2-oxoalkylides and N-sulfonylaldimines. reversal of the *cis/trans*-isomer ratios depending on base and additive. *J. Org. Chem.* **1995**, *60*, 4663–4665. [CrossRef]
71. Detty, M.R. Oxidation of selenides and tellurides with positive halogenating species. *J. Org. Chem.* **1980**, *45*, 274–279. [CrossRef]
72. Harirchian, B.; Magnus, P.D. Preparation of dithio-, thioseleno-, thiosilyl-, and thiostannyl-keten acetals. *J. Chem. Soc. Chem. Commun.* **1977**, 522–523. [CrossRef]
73. Watanabe, S.; Kusumoto, T.; Yoshida, C.H.; Kataoka, T. The first example of enantioselective carbenoid addition to organochalcogen atoms: Application to [2,3] sigmatropic rearrangement of allylic chalcogen ylides. *J. Chem. Soc. Chem. Comunn.* **2001**, 839–840. [CrossRef]
74. Tamagaka, S.; Hatanaka, I.; Tamura, K. The reactions of dibenzylselenonium ylide, imide, and selenoxide with trtphenylphosphine. *Chem. Lett.* **1976**, *5*, 81–84. [CrossRef]
75. Reich, H.J.; Cohen, M.L. Selenium Stabilized Carbanions. Ylide Formation during Alkylation of Selenium and Sulfur Substituted Enolates. *J. Am. Chem. Soc.* **1979**, *101*, 1307–1308. [CrossRef]
76. Baldwin, J.E.; Tzodikov, N.R. Substituent rearrangement and elimination during noncatalyzed Fischer indole synthesis. *J. Org. Chem.* **1977**, *42*, 1878–1883. [CrossRef]
77. Halazy, S.; Krief, A. Synthetic routes to cyclopropylidenecarbinols and to cyclopropylidienes. *Tetrahedron Lett.* **1981**, *22*, 2135–2138. [CrossRef]
78. Braverman, S.; Zafrani, Y.; Rahimipourb, S. Base catalyzed [2,3] sigmatropic rearrangements of propargylic sulfonium and selenonium salts. *Tetrahedron Lett.* **2001**, *42*, 2911–2914. [CrossRef]
79. Nishibayashi, Y.; Ohe, K.; Uemura, S. The First Example of Enantioselective Carbenoid Addition to Organochalcogen Atoms: Application to [2,3] Sigmatropic Rearrangement of Allylic Chalcogen Ylides. *J. Chem. Soc. Chem. Commun.* **1995**, 1245–1246. [CrossRef]
80. Dopp, D.; Sturm, T. Reactions of 2-(organylseleno) propenenitriles with dimethyl ethynedicarboxylate. *Liebigs Ann. Recueil.* **1997**, *1997*, 541–546. [CrossRef]
81. Wang, S.M.; Han, J.-B.; Zhang, C.-P.; Qin, H.-L.; Xiao, J.-C. An overview of reductive trifluoromethylation reactions using electrophilic '+CF$_3$' reagents. *Tetrahedron* **2015**, *71*, 7949–7976. [CrossRef]
82. Zhang, C.-P.; Wang, Z.-L.; Chen, Q.-Y.; Zhang, C.-T.; Gu, Y.-C.; Xiao, J.-C. Copper-mediated trifluoromethylation of heteroaromatic compounds by trifluoromethyl sulfonium salts. *Angew. Chem. Int. Ed.* **2011**, *50*, 1896–1900. [CrossRef] [PubMed]
83. Jana, S.; Koenigs, R.M. Rhodium-Catalyzed Carbene Transfer Reactions for Sigmatropic Rearrangement Reactions of Selenium Ylides. *Org. Lett.* **2019**, *21*, 3653–3657. [CrossRef] [PubMed]
84. Zhang, Z.; Sheng, Z.; Yu, W.; Wu, G.; Zhang, R.; Chu, W.-D.; Zhang, Y.; Wang, J. Catalytic asymmetric trifluoromethylthiolation via enantioselective [2,3]-sigmatropic rearrangement of sulfonium ylides. *Nat. Chem.* **2017**, *9*, 970–976. [CrossRef]
85. Zhang, X.; Qu, Z.; Ma, Z.; Shi, W.; Jin, X.; Wang, J. Catalytic asymmetric [2,3]-sigmatropic rearrangement of sulfur ylides generated from copper (I) carbenoids and allyl sulfides. *J. Org. Chem.* **2002**, *67*, 5621–5625. [CrossRef]
86. Liang, Y.; Zhou, H.; Yu, Z.-X. Why Is Copper (I) Complex More Competent Than Dirhodium (II) Complex in Catalytic Asymmetric O-H Insertion Reactions? A Computational Study of the Metal Carbenoid O-H Insertion into Water. *J. Am. Chem. Soc.* **2009**, *131*, 17783–17785. [CrossRef]
87. Chen, S.; Wang, J. Palladium-catalyzed reaction of allyl halides with α-diazocarbonyl compounds. *Chem. Commun.* **2008**, 4198–4200. [CrossRef]
88. Reddy, A.C.S.; Anbarasan, P. Rhodium-Catalyzed Rearrangement of S/Se-Ylides for the Synthesis of Substituted Vinylogous Carbonates. *Org. Lett.* **2019**, *21*, 9965–9969. [CrossRef]

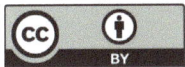

© 2020 by the authors. Licensee MDPI, Basel, Switzerland. This article is an open access article distributed under the terms and conditions of the Creative Commons Attribution (CC BY) license (http://creativecommons.org/licenses/by/4.0/).

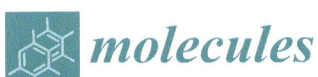

Article

Synthesis and Characterization of Ion Pairs between Alkaline Metal Ions and Anionic Anti-Aromatic and Aromatic Hydrocarbons with π-Conjugated Central Seven- and Eight-Membered Rings

Jan Bloch [1], Stefan Kradolfer [1], Thomas L. Gianetti [2], Detlev Ostendorf [1], Subal Dey [1], Victor Mougel [1] and Hansjörg Grützmacher [1,*]

[1] Department of Chemistry and Applied Biosciences, ETH Zürich, 8093 Zürich, Switzerland; bloch@inorg.chem.ethz.ch (J.B.); krastefa@inorg.chem.ethz.ch (S.K.); detos@gmx.de (D.O.); deys@ethz.ch (S.D.); mougel@inorg.chem.ethz.ch (V.M.)
[2] Department of Chemistry & Biochemistry, 1306 E. University Blvd., Tucson, AZ 85719, USA; tgianetti@email.arizona.edu
* Correspondence: hgruetzmacher@ethz.ch

Academic Editor: Yves Canac
Received: 21 September 2020; Accepted: 4 October 2020; Published: 15 October 2020

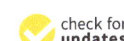

Abstract: The synthesis, isolation and full characterization of ion pairs between alkaline metal ions (Li^+, Na^+, K^+) and mono-anions and dianions obtained from 5H-dibenzo[a,d]cycloheptenyl ($C_{15}H_{11}$ = trop) is reported. According to Nuclear Magnetic Resonance (NMR) spectroscopy, single crystal X-ray analysis and Density Functional Theory (DFT) calculations, the trop$^-$ and trop$^{2-\bullet}$ anions show anti-aromatic properties which are dependent on the counter cation M^+ and solvent molecules serving as co-ligands. For comparison, the disodium and dipotassium salt of the dianion of dibenzo[a,e]cyclooctatetraene ($C_{16}H_{12}$ = dbcot) were prepared, which show classical aromatic character. A d^8-Rh(I) complex of trop$^-$ was prepared and the structure shows a distortion of the $C_{15}H_{11}$ ligand into a conjugated 10π-benzo pentadienide unit—to which the Rh(I) center is coordinated—and an aromatic 6π electron benzo group which is non-coordinated. Electron transfer reactions between neutral and anionic trop and dbcot species show that the anti-aromatic compounds obtained from trop are significantly stronger reductants.

Keywords: aromaticity; ion pairs; alkali metals; tropylidenyl ions; cyclooctatetraene ions; rhodium; electron paramagnetic resonance (EPR) spectroscopy; density functional theory (DFT); electrochemistry

1. Introduction

Transition metal complexes with 5H-dibenzo[a,d]cyclohepten-5-yl units (trivial name tropylidenyl = trop, see Scheme 1, right) as ligands are well established in the literature [1–4]. Their special properties give rise to complexes with extraordinary catalytic activities. For example, bis(trop)amine as ligand in d^8-Rh(I) complex **A** (Scheme 1, top) provokes an unusual butterfly-type structure for tetracoordinated sixteen electron configured transition metal complexes and can act as a cooperating ligand [5]. Both factors contribute to the high activities in the hydrogenation of ketone derivatives [6,7] or the dehydrogenative coupling of alcohols [8,9] under very mild reaction conditions. In another example, complexes of type **B** with the redox and chemically non-innocent cooperative diazadiene ligand trop$_2$dad (dad = diazadiene) [10] show an unprecedented high efficiency in dehydrogenation reactions of methanol or formaldehyde [10–12]. The olefinic double bond in the trop moiety acts as an electronically flexible ligand [13] and allows to stabilize low-valent metal centers [10].

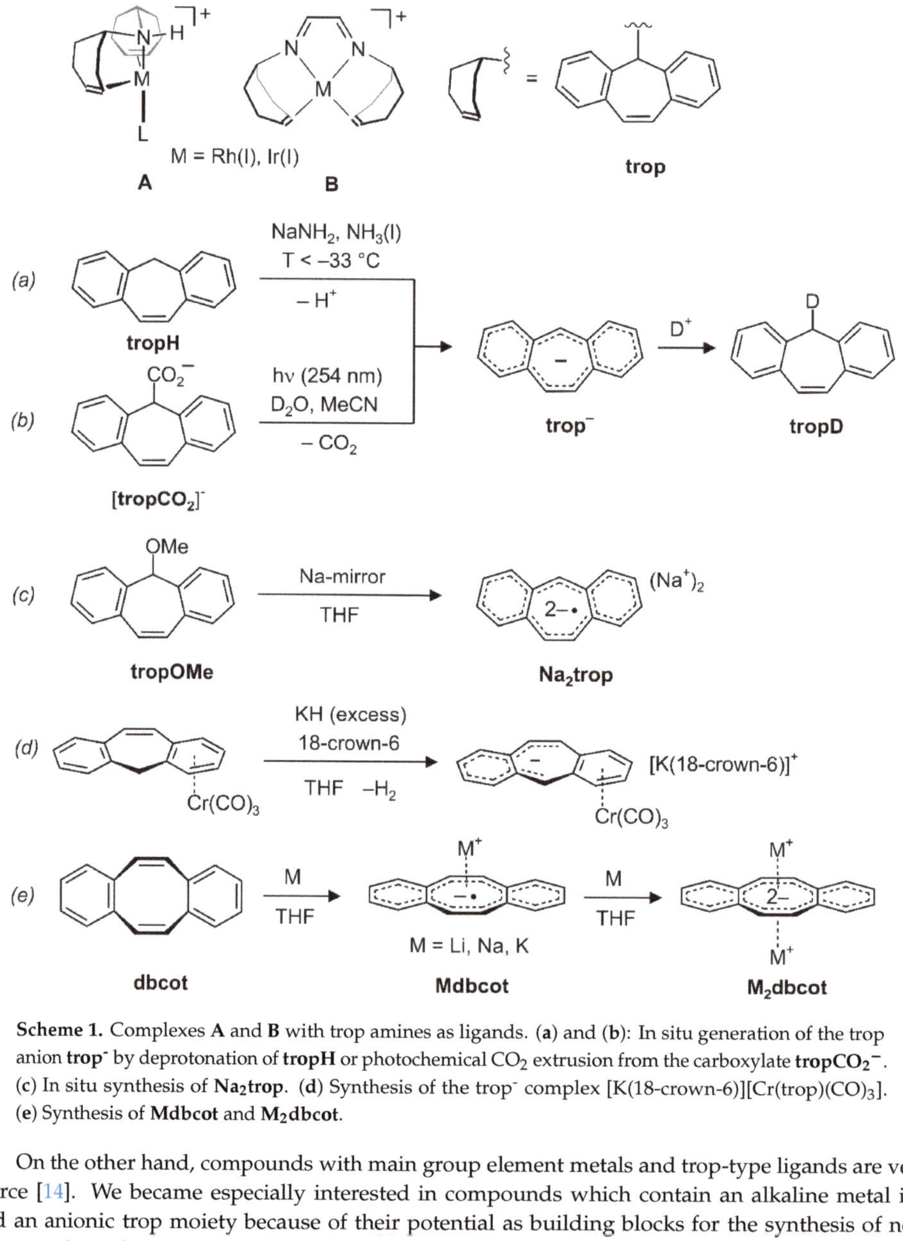

Scheme 1. Complexes **A** and **B** with trop amines as ligands. (**a**) and (**b**): In situ generation of the trop anion **trop**$^-$ by deprotonation of **tropH** or photochemical CO_2 extrusion from the carboxylate **tropCO$_2^-$**. (**c**) In situ synthesis of **Na$_2$trop**. (**d**) Synthesis of the trop$^-$ complex [K(18-crown-6)][Cr(trop)(CO)$_3$]. (**e**) Synthesis of **Mdbcot** and **M$_2$dbcot**.

On the other hand, compounds with main group element metals and trop-type ligands are very scarce [14]. We became especially interested in compounds which contain an alkaline metal ion and an anionic trop moiety because of their potential as building blocks for the synthesis of new trop-type ligands. Furthermore, these species, (M+)$_n$[trop]$^{n-}$, may form various forms of ion pairs with fascinating properties, and related species with reduced arenes as anions are interesting to explore on their own [15–17].

To the best of our knowledge, salts containing anionic 5H-dibenzo[a,d]cycloheptenides, [trop]$^{n-}$ (n = 1, 2) have never been isolated. Based on the 4n-Hückel-rule, the trop anion, $C_{15}H_{11}^-$, with its central 8π electron system flanked by two annulated benzo groups (giving a 16π electron system in total), should show anti-aromatic character. Indeed, when the trop anion is generated in situ in liquid ammonia by deprotonation of the neutral hydrocarbon suberene (**tropH**) ((a) in Scheme 1) [18], strongly shielded signals are observed in the ^{1}H NMR spectrum, as expected for an anti-aromatic compound [19]. Wan et al. suggested that the photodecarboxylation of the trop carboxylate anion **tropCO$_2^-$** [20,21] and the photochemical hydrogen–deuterium exchange of **tropH** [22,23] both proceed via the trop anion, **trop$^-$**, as intermediate ((b) in Scheme 1). This anion was also generated by deprotonation of suberene with n-butyllithium and characterized in situ by Ultraviolet/Visible (UV/Vis) spectroscopy [22,23]. In addition, the reduction of trop methoxide with elemental sodium was reported to give the trop dianion radical, $C_{15}H_{11}^{2-\bullet}$ ((c) in Scheme 1), which was characterized in situ by Electron Paramagnetic Resonance (EPR) spectroscopy [24].

The only compound we are aware of in which **trop$^-$** acts as a ligand to a transition metal was reported by Venzo et al., which showed that in complex **C**, the paratropic character of the trop anion significantly decreases upon coordination to a tricarbonylchromium group [25]. Based on ^{1}H and ^{13}C NMR spectroscopy, the authors suggested that the anti-aromatic 16π-electron structure is split into a 6π-electron system located on one of the benzo groups which coordinates to the Cr(CO)$_3$ fragment and an uncoordinated 10π-electron system, as shown in (d) in Scheme 1 [25,26].

Cyclooctatetraene, C_8H_8 (cot), is a textbook example in which the anti-aromatic character of a hypothetical planar molecule with an 8π-electron system leads to a severe structural distortion into a tub conformation. The same is true for its tub-shaped benzoannulated derivative dibenzo[a,e]cyclooctatetraene, **dbcot**, with alternating single and double bonds ($\overline{\Delta C=C}$ = 0.1170(10) Å) [27]. Reduction of **dbcot** with alkaline metals Li, Na and K ((e) in Scheme 1), proceeds stepwise to first give **Mdbcot** containing the dbcot$^{-\bullet}$ anion radical and then to M$_2$dbcot with the dbcot dianion (*vide infra*) [28,29]. The EPR spectra of **Mdbcot** suggest that there are contacts between the cations M$^+$ (M = Li, Na, K) and dbcot$^{-\bullet}$ [28,30]. Only the structure of the ion triple [Li(tmeda)]$_2$[dbcot] (tmeda = tetramethylethylenediamine) was determined. In this ion triple, the dianion adopts a planar structure with nearly equal C-C bond lengths in the central ring (the average bond length variation amounts to $\overline{\Delta C=C}$ = 0.024(2) Å). The Li(tmeda)$^+$ units are η^8-bound above and below the center of the dianion [31]. The ^{1}H NMR spectrum of the dianion shows that the proton resonances are significantly de-shielded. For example, the olefinic resonances in the central C8 ring are shifted from 6.72 ppm in dbcot [32] to 7.08 ppm in **Li$_2$dbcot** [28]. In combination with the structural data, the dbcot^{2-} dianion is therefore considered to be aromatic [19].

Herein, we report a new simple and clean synthesis of Mtrop and M$_2$trop which allows the isolation of various close and separated ion pairs which contain the trop mono- and di-anion. For comparison, the disodium and dipotassium salts of dbcot^{2-} were also prepared and structurally characterized. Their anti-aromatic or aromatic character is assessed experimentally based on structural and magnetic criteria. DFT-calculations on simplified model compounds, specifically calculation of the Nuclear Independent Chemical Shifts (NICS), were performed in order to bolster the conclusions derived from the experimental data.

2. Results

In order to obtain the trop anion trop$^-$ in pure form, the silylated trop derivatives **1a** (R = H) [3] or **1b** (R = Me) (**2**) were prepared by reacting tropCl [33] with an excess of Li and quenching the trop$^-$ as appearing intermediate with HMe$_2$SiCl or Me$_3$SiCl ((a) in Scheme 2). Both 1a and 1b can be easily purified and obtained in pure form as crystalline solids [3]. The trop silanes were subsequently treated with various alkali metal *tert*-butoxides to give the ion pairs **Litrop**, **Natrop** and **Ktrop** respectively, with trop$^-$ as the anion, as pure crystalline solids in moderate to good yields ((a) in Scheme 2).

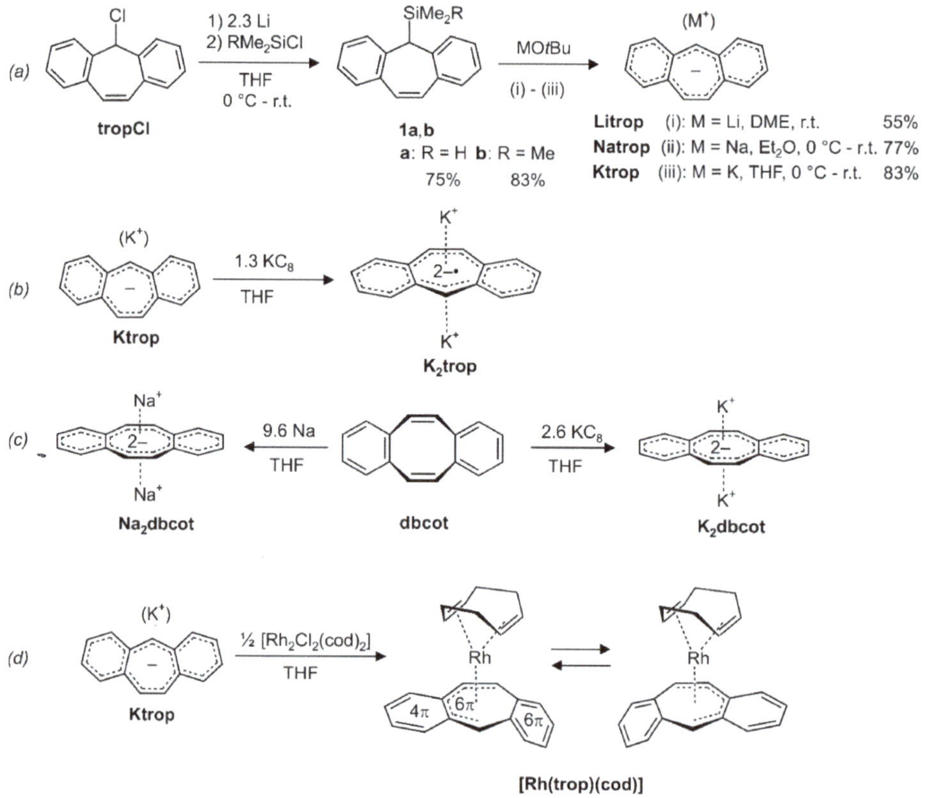

Scheme 2. (a) Synthesis of the silylated tropylidenes 1a, b and the trop⁻ containing ion pairs Mtrop (M = Li, Na, K). (b) Synthesis of trop$^{2-\bullet}$ dianion radical containing ion triple K$_2$trop by reduction of Ktrop. (c) Synthesis of the dbcot^{2-} dianion containing ion triples M$_2$dbcot (M = Na, K) by reduction of dbcot. (d) Synthesis of the organometallic d^8-Rh(I) complex [Rh(trop)(cod)]. r.t. = room temperature; DME: 1,2-dimethoxyethane; Et$_2$O: diethyl ether; THF: tetrahydrofuran.

Compound **Ktrop** can be further reduced with potassium graphite to give the ion triple **K$_2$trop**, which, apart from two K$^+$ ions, contains the trop dianion radical trop$^{2-\bullet}$ ((b) in Scheme 2). **K$_2$trop** was isolated as a dark green, micro-crystalline solid. We failed to prepare and isolate the dilithium and the disodium analogue so far. The synthesis of the disodium and the dipotassium derivatives of the dbcot^{2-} dianion, **Na$_2$dbcot** or **K$_2$dbcot**, is achieved in a straightforward manner by simply exposing dibenzo[a,e]cyclooctatetraene (dbcot) to elementary sodium or potassium graphite in anhydrous tetrahydrofuran ((c) in Scheme 2) as was likewise reported for the preparation of **Li$_2$dbcot** [28,31].

The trop anion can be used as a ligand in transition metal complexes, and reaction with half an equivalent of [Rh$_2$Cl$_2$(cod)$_2$] gives **[Rh(trop)(cod)]** as a dark red crystalline compound in moderate isolated yield (63%) ((d) in Scheme 2). In this complex, the d^8-valence electron configured Rh(I) center is exclusively coordinated to hydrocarbon ligands and represents to the best of our knowledge the first fully characterized mononuclear Rh(I) heptatrienide species. Only very few related compounds such as bimetallic Rh complexes [34,35], a Rh(I) azulene complex [36] and a Rh(III) cycloheptatrienide complex have been reported [37]. In contrast, the reaction with the dianion radical containing salt **K$_2$trop** did not yield any identifiable compound, likely due to the strongly reducing properties of the trop$^{2-\bullet}$ (vide infra).

2.1. Characterization by NMR, EPR and X-ray Diffraction Methods

All diamagnetic compounds were fully characterized by NMR spectroscopy. The paramagnetic compound **K₂trop** was analyzed by EPR spectroscopy. Single crystals of **Litrop, Natrop, Ktrop, K₂trop, Na₂dbcot, K₂dbcot** and **[Rh(trop)(cod)]** were grown and investigated with X-ray diffraction methods in order to determine the structures experimentally. In addition, the structures of compounds **Mtrop** (M = Li − K) and **[Rh(trop)(cod)]** and their degree of anti-aromatic or aromatic character was evaluated by calculating the Nuclear Independent Chemical Shifts (NICSs) (DFT, PBE [38,39] and 6-311+G (df, pd) [39] in a continuum solvation model (THF) [40,41]).

All compounds containing the trop⁻ anion show strongly shielded signals for all protons in the ^{1}H NMR spectra. In the dimer of the trop radical [23], namely $C_{15}H_{11} - C_{15}H_{11} = trop_2$ [42] (entry 1, Table 1), which has an electronic structure reminiscent of the conjugated hydrocarbon *cis*-stilbene, the olefinic protons $^1H_{ol}$ and the benzylic proton $^1H_{bz}$ attached to the central seven-membered ring are observed in the normal range at δ = 7.06 ppm and δ = 4.73 ppm. In the ion pairs, **Mtrop**, these resonances are significantly shifted to lower frequencies to δ ($^1H_{ol}$) < 2.6 ppm and δ ($^1H_{bz}$) < 0.56 ppm (M = Li, Na, K, entries 2–4, Table 1). Also, the protons of the annulated benzo groups are strongly shifted to lower frequencies by about 3 ppm.

Table 1. Characteristic properties of the trop anions, the dbcot dianions and the reference compounds trop₂ and dbcot. Abbreviations: δ ^{1}H and δ ^{13}C: ^{1}H and ^{13}C NMR chemical shifts (ppm) respectively, bz: benzylic, ol: olefinic, $^1J_{HC}$: coupling constant (Hz)) between the benzylic proton and carbon atom.

	δ $^1H_{ol}$	δ $^{13}C_{ol}$	δ $^1H_{bz}$	δ $^{13}C_{bz}$	$^1J_{HC}$
trop₂	6.90	131.43	4.90	52.18	
Litrop	2.64	139.03	0.50	83.67	139.8
Natrop	2.60	138.79	0.56	81.56	142.9
Ktrop	2.00	139.26	0.06	89.44	144.5
[Rh(trop)(cod)]	5.16	97.52	2.88	55.84	144.6
dbcot [32]	6.72	126.76			
Li₂dbcot [28]	7.08				
Na₂dbcot	7.17	93.37			
K₂dbcot	7.17	95.78			

The experimental structures of the contact ions pairs **Li^{thf}trop, Li^{dme}trop, Na^{dme}trop, K^{thf}trop** and **K^{18c6}trop** were determined with X-ray diffraction methods using a suitable single crystal of every compound and are depicted in Figure 1. Selected bond distances and angles are listed in Tables 2 and 3. The most remarkable feature is the bending of the central seven-membered ring in the trop⁻ moiety expressed by the fold angles Θ_1 and Θ_2 (Table 3). These angles vary strongly with the nature of the counter cation but also with the nature of the solvent molecules acting as co-ligands to M⁺. In **Li^{thf}trop**, the [Li(thf)₃]⁺ cation binds predominantly to C1 [Li-C1 2.279(3) Å] which provokes a rather strong bending (Θ_1 = 24.2°; Θ_2 = 14.1°), about half of the one observed in the hydrocarbon trop₂ (Θ_1 = 49.4°; Θ_2 = 22.5°). Encapsulation of Li⁺ by three dimethoxyethane (dme) solvent molecules leads to [Li (dme)₃]⁺[trop⁻] (**Li^{dme}trop**), in which no close contact between cation and anion occurs (shortest Li–C contact = 6.79 Å) and the trop⁻ anion adopts an almost flat structure (Θ_1 = 6°; Θ_2 = 3°). Likewise, in the structure of **Natrop**, which contains [Na(dme)₃]⁺, the contact between cation and anion is long (the distance between Na⁺ and the centroid (cnt) of the central C₇ ring is 5.25 Å) and the trop⁻ anion is flat (Θ_1 = 6.5°; Θ_2 = 4.7°).

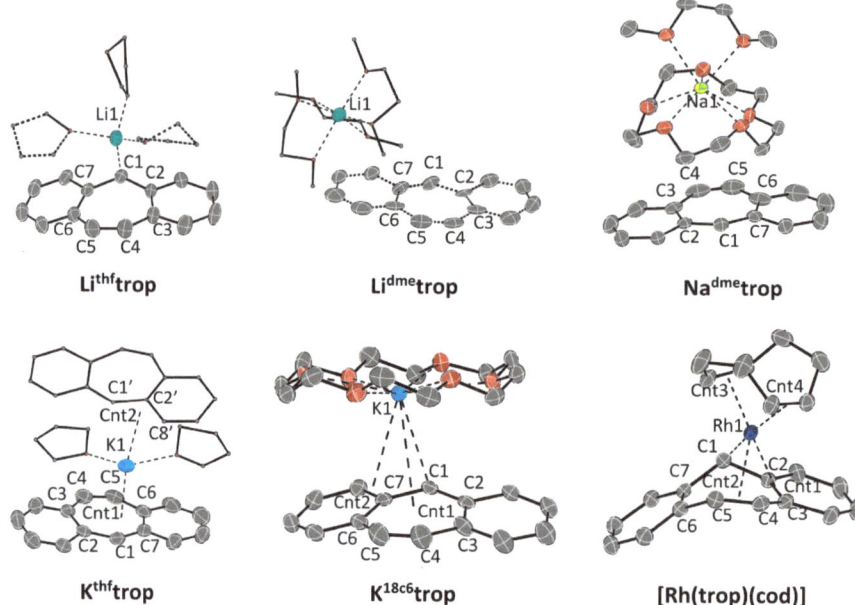

Figure 1. ORTEP plots **Li^{thf}trop**, **Li^{dme}trop**, **Na^{dme}trop**, **K^{thf}trop**, **K^{18c6}trop** and **[Rh(trop)(cod)]** at 50% ellipsoid probability (hydrogen atoms are omitted for clarity). **Li^{dme}trop**: only one of the two distorted trop moieties is shown. **[Rh(trop)(cod)]**: A co-crystallized toluene-molecule is omitted for clarity. Selected Rh-C bond distances [Å]: Rh1–C1 2.0912(16), Rh1–C2 2.3427(16), Rh1–C3 2.3995(16), Rh1–C4 2.2396(17), Rh1–C5 2.4044(18). Further selected structural parameters of all compounds are given in Tables 2 and 3.

Table 2. Selected bond lengths (Å) for the trop anions (Figure 1). Abbreviation: Cnt: centroid.

	Li^{thf}trop	Li^{dme}trop [a]	Na^{dme}trop	K^{thf}trop	K^{18c6}trop	[Rh(trop)(cod)]
C1–C2	1.440(2)	1.430(15)	1.420(16)	1.4265(19)	1.428(3)	1.429(3)	1.470(2)
C2–C3	1.423(2)	1.422(14)	1.435(17)	1.4342(19)	1.433(2)	1.430(3)	1.435(2)
C3–C4	1.468(2)	1.40(2)	1.54(2)	1.455(3)	1.463(3)	1.461(3)	1.458(3)
C4–C5	1.338(3)	1.325(14)	1.324(14)	1.308(3)	1.332(3)	1.339(3)	1.380(3)
C5–C6	1.464(3)	1.47(3)	1.46(3)	1.414(3)	1.467(3)	1.464(3)	1.482(3)
C6–C7	1.423(2)	1.422(16)	1.412(17)	1.419(2)	1.430(3)	1.434(3)	1.398(2)
C7–C1	1.434(2)	1.422(13)	1.414(15)	1.419(2)	1.425(3)	1.431(3)	1.492(2)
C1–M1	2.279(3)	6.788(17)	7.91(2)	5.3528(15)	3.0977(17) [b]	3.0213(18)	2.0912(16)
C4–M1	3.715(4)	7.63(2)	7.50(2)	5.4943(17)	3.4072(19)	4.937(3)	2.2397(17)
C5–M1	3.783(3)	8.35(2)	6.64(2)	5.5599(19)	3.346(2)	4.694(2)	2.4044(18)
M1–Cnt1		7.282(17)	7.34(2)	5.2530(15)	2.8223(4) [c]	3.8117(18)	2.2600(16)
M1–Cnt2					2.9708(4) [d]	3.303(2)	2.2186(18)
M1–Cnt3							1.9682(19)
M1–Cnt4							2.1139(19)

[a] The asymmetric unit contains two distorted trop moieties: a and b. [b] Distance to benzylic C of neighboring trop anion: C1'–K1: 3.0171(17) (see **K^{thf}trop** in Figure 1 for clarification). [c] Centroid of C1, C2, C5, C6, C7. [d] Allylic centroid of C1', C2' and C8'.

The most planar structure for a trop⁻ anion is observed in **K^thf trop** ($\Theta_1 = 1.7°$; $\Theta_2 = 2.4°$), which is best described as a close ion pair with a rather short distance between K1 and the centroid cnt1 of the C_7 ring of 2.82 Å. The K^+ is coordinated to the C_7 ring in a slightly asymmetric manner as indicated by the unequal K-C1 (3.098 Å) and K-C4/C5 distances (3.407 Å; 3.346 Å). Furthermore, the potassium ion has an additional contact at about 2.97 Å to another trop⁻ unit, such that $K^+ \cdots$ trop⁻ $\cdots K^+ \cdots$ trop⁻ chains are formed in the solid state. Remarkably, in **K^{18c6}trop**, the trop⁻ anion shows larger fold angles ($\Theta_1 = 12.4°$; $\Theta_2 = 12.3°$). In this ion pair, K^+ is rather asymmetrically bound and the distance to the centroid of to the central C_7 ring is large (3.812 Å). Instead, K^+ binds closer to the allylic fragment C1, C7, C15 (K1-cnt2 3.303 Å) with a rather short contact to the benzylic carbon center C1 (3.02 Å) and longer ones to C7 (3.263 Å) and C15 (3.490 Å). It is highly speculative to which extent these features of the solid-state structures are retained in solution. But, the coupling constants $^1J_{HC}$ of the benzylic carbon nucleus, $^{13}C_{bz}$, to the benzylic proton, $^1H_{bz}$, can be empirically correlated to the s-orbital character in the C_{bz}–H bond. In a bent trop anion, the C_{bz}–H bond will be closer to a sp³ configuration (25% s, smaller $^1J_{HC}$) that in a flat structure, where the C_{bz}–H is closer to a sp² configuration (33% s, larger $^1J_{HC}$). Indeed, $^1J_{HC}$ obtained in deuterated tetrahydrofuran, [D₈]THF, as solvent (Table 1) is larger for the potassium salt than in the bent lithium salts, indicating that the solid-state structures are retained to a certain degree in solution.

At this point, it is interesting to compare these main group metal complexes of trop⁻ with a "classical" organometallic complex such as **[Rh(trop)(cod)]**. In contrast to **Mtrop**, which shows strongly shielded ^1H NMR resonances for all protons, the signals for the ^1H nuclei at the benzo groups in **[Rh(trop)(cod)]** are in the same region (δ ^1H: 6.82–7.01 ppm) as in the reference compound **trop₂** (δ ^1H: 6.58–7.25 ppm). Also, the chemical shifts of the benzo ^{13}C nuclei are in the normal range for arenes in between δ = 127 and 137 ppm. Only the olefinic and benzylic ^1H and ^{13}C NMR signals (δ^1H_{ol}, δ^1H_{bz}, $\delta^{13}C_{ol}$, $\delta^{13}C_{bz}$) are significantly shifted to lower frequencies, indicating an interaction with the metal center, c.f. δ ($^{13}C_{ol}$) = 97.6 ppm, δ ($^{13}C_{bz}$) = 56.5 ppm in **[Rh(trop)(cod)]** vs. δ ($^{13}C_{ol}$) ~139 ppm and δ ($^{13}C_{bz}$) = 81.6–89.4 ppm in **Mtrop**, see Table 1). In solution, **[Rh(trop)(cod)]** is seemingly C_{2v}-symmetric which is not in agreement with the structure in solid state but can be explained by a dynamic phenomenon (*vide infra*). Complex **[Rh(trop)(cod)]** crystallizes as racemic mixture in the space group P2₁/c. The structure of one of the enantiomers is depicted in Figure 1 and is very different from the **Mtrop** compounds. The Rh(I)(cod) fragment binds to C1, C2, C3, C4 and C5 at distances between 2.09 to 2.40 Å (see legend to Figure 1) of the central seven-membered ring in a way which is also observed in other metal [43,44] and specifically, Rh(I) pentadienide complexes [43,44]. This pentadienide-type interaction donates 6π electrons to the Rh(I)(cod) fragment which thereby reaches an 18-electron configuration. Metal-to-ligand electron back donation leads to a slight elongation of all involved C–C bonds by about 0.03 Å with respect to the distances in the trop anion in the **Mtrop** contact pairs (M = Li, Na, K). The most notable structural feature is the strongly bent conformation of the trop⁻ unit: the intersection angle between the non-coordinated benzo group and the benzopentadienide unit is $\theta_3 = 49.9(1)°$ (cf. Figure 1). The η^5 coordination mode and non-symmetric structure observed in the solid state is in contrast with the apparent C_{2v} symmetry of the complex in solution. We therefore assume that in solution, **[Rh(trop)(cod)]** underlies a dynamic phenomenon by which the rhodium center rapidly exchanges between the two possible η^5 binding sites of the central seven-membered ring, as shown in Scheme 2d. This process must have a very low activation barrier because even at low temperatures, this process is not frozen out on the NMR time scale. This coordination mode is in stark contrast to the one of the only other dibenzo[a,d]cycloheptenide metal complex **C** (Scheme 1d) [25,26]. Here, NMR data indicate that the Cr(0)(CO)₃ fragment binds in a η^6 fashion to one of the annulated benzo groups of the trop moiety which leads to C_1 symmetric structure. The ^{13}C chemical shifts of this coordinated benzo group are characteristically shifted to lower frequencies [$\delta(^{13}C)$ = 70–100 ppm]. That is, in this case, the anti-aromatic π-electron system of trop⁻ is localized in a different way from the one in **[Rh(trop)(cod)]**, namely into a 6π-electron system at a terminal arene bound to the metal and an uncoordinated 10π-electron system.

The structures of the ion triples **K₂trop**, **Na₂dbcot** and **K₂dbcot** with the trop$^{2-\bullet}$ dianion radical or the dbcot^{2-} dianion respectively, are shown in Figure 2. Selected bond lengths and angles are listed in Tables 3 and 4.

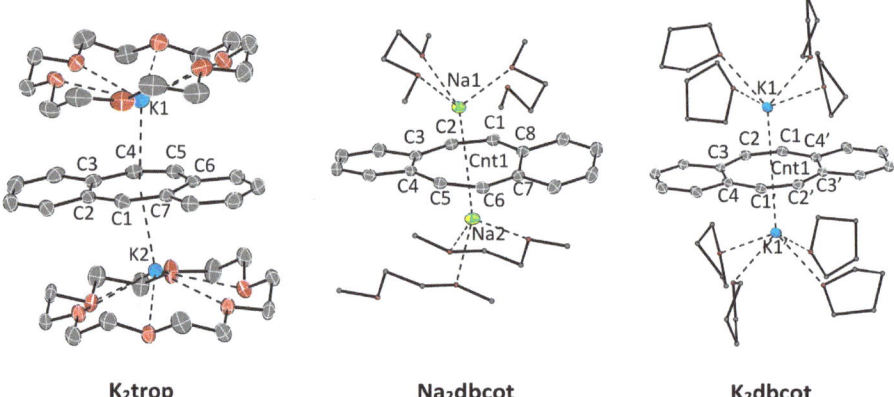

Figure 2. ORTEP plots of dianions at 50% ellipsoid probability (hydrogen atoms are omitted for clarity). **K₂trop**: A co-crystallized DME-molecule is omitted for clarity. **Na₂dbot**, **K₂dbot**: The second chemically identical but crystallographically unique compound in the asymmetric unit is omitted for clarity. Selected bond lengths (Å) and angles (°) are shown in Tables 3 and 4.

Table 3. Data from solid-state structures (Figure 1, Figure 2, and Figure 4). For comparison, **trop₂**, **trop⁺**, and **Li₂dbcot** are listed as well. Abbreviations: $\overline{C=C}$: average bond length in the central ring (Å), $\overline{\Delta C=C}$: average bond length difference in the central ring (Å), θ_1 and θ_2: dihedral angles in the trop scaffold (°), φ_1 and φ_2: dihedral angles in the **dbcot** scaffold (°), **K^{18c6}trop**: Ktrop with 18-crown-6.

Compound	Central Ring		Trop Angles		Dbcot Angles	
	$\overline{C=C}$	$\overline{\Delta C=C}$	θ_1	θ_2	φ_1	φ_2
trop₂ [42]	1.4451(7)	0.0802(10)	49.37(12)	22.46(9)		
trop⁺ [45],[a]	1.4134(11)	0.0283(15)	1.6(2)	3.44(14)		
Li^{thf}trop	1.4271(9)	0.0537(12)	24.16(19)	14.13(14)		
Li^{dme}trop	1.421(10)	0.060(14)	6(4)	2.9(25)		
Natrop	1.4108(9)	0.0420(13)	6.49(19)	4.66(12)		
K^{thf}trop	1.4253(11)	0.0491(15)	1.7(2)	2.37(14)		
K^{18c6}trop	1.4269(11)	0.0449(16)	12.4(3)	12.35(17)		
K₂trop	1.4346(10)	0.0337(14)	1.3(2)	2.30(13)		
[Rh(trop)(cod)]	1.4450(9)	0.0626(13)	55.49(18)	32.29(13)		
Li₂dbcot [31]	1.421(2)	0.024(2)			0 [b,c]	
Na₂dbcot	1.4281(5)	0.0234(7)			5.38(3)	4.88(3)
K₂dbcot	1.4279(7)	0.0263(10)			1.40(12) [b]	

[a] The counter ion is tetrakis(3,5-bis(trifluoromethyl)phenyl)borate. [b] The respective point group leads to pairwise identical dihedral angles. [c] The localization of dbcot on a crystallographic mirror plane leads to the perfect planarity [31].

Table 4. Selected bond lengths (Å) for ion pairs containing the trop^{2-} and dbcot^{2-} dianions (Figure 2). Abbreviation: Cnt: centroid.

	K$_2$trop	Na$_2$dbcot	K$_2$dbcot [a,b]	
C1–C2	1.426(3)	1.4121(15)	1.409(2)	1.409(2)
C2–C3	1.463(2)	1.4254(14)	1.426(2)	1.418(2)
C3–C4	1.434(3)	1.4555(14)	1.460(2)	1.463(2)
C4–C5	1.385(3)	1.4223(14)		
C5–C6	1.440(3)	1.4094(15)		
C6–C7	1.466(2)	1.4209(14)		
C7–C8		1.4596(14)		
C4–C1			1.420(2)	1.418(2)
C7–C1	1.428(2)			
C8–C1		1.4199(14)		
C1–M1	3.2455(18)	2.6792(11)	3.0482(15)	3.0905(14)
C2–M1		2.7258(11)	3.0093(15)	3.0728(14)
C4–M1	3.2607(18)			
C5–M1	3.1092(17)	2.6971(11)		
C6–M1		2.8896(11)		
C1–M2	3.0902(17)	2.7507(11)		
C2–M2		2.6557(11)		
C4–M2	3.3042(18)			
C5–M2	3.1789(18)	2.9216(11)		
C6–M2		2.7689(11)		
M1–Cnt1	2.7876(18)	2.0924(11)	2.4669(15)	2.5385(14)
M2–Cnt1	2.7495(17)	2.1348(11)		
K1-Cnt1-K2	166.507(12)	174.05(4)	180.00(5)	180.00(4)

[a] Two chemically identical, but crystallographically unique compounds are in the asymmetric unit. [b] The space group P2$_1$/n leads to pairwise identical C–C bond lengths.

As expected, the reduction of **Ktrop** to the radical dianion **K$_2$trop** leads to an overall elongation of all bonds within the central seven-membered ring (see increased average bond length $\overline{C=C}$ in Table 3). The average bond length difference ($\overline{\Delta C=C}$ in Table 3) becomes smaller and the C3–C4, C4–C5 and C5–C6 bond lengths' alternation is slightly diminished. The plots and structural data for **Na$_2$dbcot** and **K$_2$dbcot** are given in Figure 2 and Table 4 and are very similar to the ones reported for **Li$_2$dbcot** (Scheme 1 and Table 3) [31]. The dbcot^{2-} dianions in **K$_2$dbcot** and **Li$_2$dbcot** adopt a rather flat conformation while the one in **Na$_2$dbcot** shows a slightly twisted conformation likely because of crystal packing forces (see dihedral angles φ_1 and φ_2 in Table 3). All C–C bond lengths are longer than 1.4 Å and there is very little bond length variation (see $\overline{\Delta C=C}$ in Table 3).

The paramagnetic compound **K$_2$trop** was further characterized by EPR spectroscopy. In tetrahydrofuran (THF) as solvent, the EPR spectrum of **K$_2$trop** shows a rather complex hyperfine coupling pattern (Figure 3, line a) which can be simplified by the addition of two equivalents of 18-crown-6. This indicates that complexation of K$^+$ by 18-crown-6 significantly elongates the distances between the cation and dianion radical, which leads to much smaller and hence non-detectable ^{39}K-hyperfine splittings. Indirect proof comes from a comparison of the structures **K$_2$trop**, where one 18-crown-6 binds to every K$^+$ ion, and **K$_2$dbcot**, where each K$^+$ ion is coordinated by four THF molecules. In the former the K$^+$-Cnt distance is 2.79 Å while in the latter a shorter distance of 2.47 Å is observed (Cnt = centroid of the central ring). The less complex spectrum (Figure 3, line b) was used to simulate the hyperfine pattern (Figure 3, line c). The experimentally determined and calculated hyperfine coupling constants (HFCs) indicate delocalization of the unpaired electron over the whole dianion (see spin density plot in Figure 3). These data and the corresponding g-factor of 2.0064 are in fairly good agreement with the ones of the reported sodium analogue **Na₂trop** [24] more than 50 years ago (g = 2.0027 and HFCs shown in Figure 3).

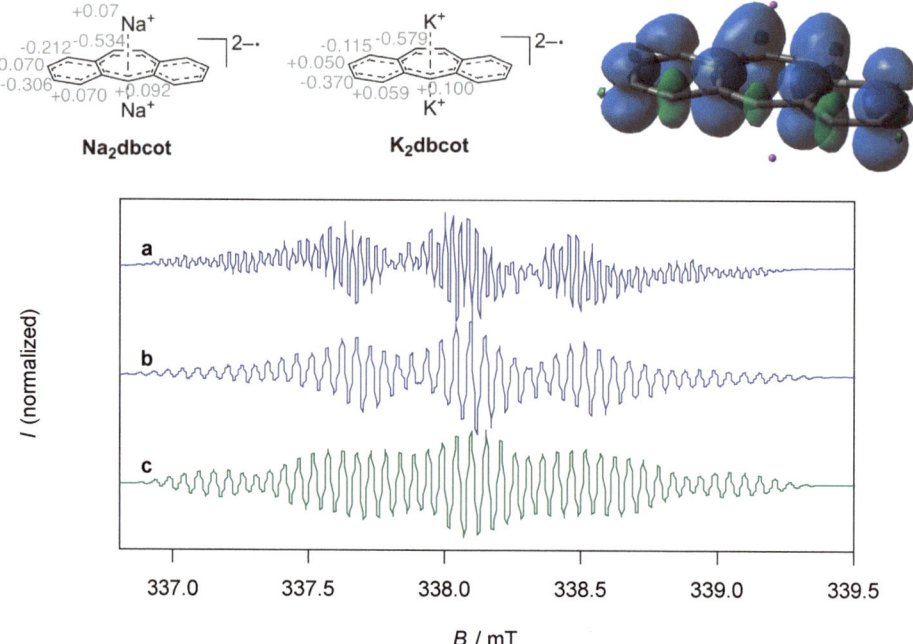

Figure 3. Top left: Reported hyperfine splittings (mT) of **Na₂trop**. Top middle: Calculated hyperfine coupling constants (HFCs) (mT) from the simulated spectrum of **K₂trop**. Top right: Spin density plot of **K₂trop** (isovalue = 0.0009, positive spin densities in blue and negative spin densities in green). DFT calculation: PBE [38] 6-311+G(df, pd) [39] in a continuum solvation model (THF). Bottom (**a**): EPR spectrum of **K₂trop** (0.5 mM) in THF, g = 2.0064. (**b**): EPR spectrum of **K₂trop** (0.5 mM) and 18-crown-6 (2 equivalents) in THF, g = 2.0067. (**c**): Simulated spectrum of **b**.

The ^{1}H NMR spectra of the contact ion pairs **M₂dbcot** (M = Na, K) show, in comparison to neutral dbcot, which is best described as a cyclic conjugated polyolefin, a diatopic ring current which leads to significantly de-shielded olefinic resonances, ^{1}H$_{ol}$ > 7 ppm (Table 1).

2.2. Evaluation of Anti-Aromaticity and Aromaticity by Calculation of NICS Values

Table 5 lists the calculated nuclear independent chemical shifts in the center of the rings, NICS(0), and 1 Å above and below the central plane of these, NICS(1) (DFT, PBE [38] 6-311+G(df, pd) [39]). The data for both six-membered rings A and C and the central seven-membered ring B is given. For comparison, also the data for the tropylium cation **trop⁺** are listed. As expected for an aromatic molecule with a 14 π-electron configuration, the NICSs data are strongly negative for all rings in **trop⁺**. On the other end of the scale, cyclobutadiene (CBD) is listed for comparison which is considered to be an archetypical anti-aromatic molecule with a 4-electron system and shows positive NICS values ((NICS(0) = 27.49, NICS(1) = 18.03). The values are largely exceeded by the NICS values of the central ring B in the flat and counter cation-free trop anion **trop⁻** which amount to 45.00 and 34.54. Even the flanking rings A and C in **trop⁻** reach positive values in the range of CBD. For simplicity, the NICS data were calculated for simplified model compounds of the contact ion pairs **Mtrop^m** (M = Li, Na, K; m indicates neglecting coordinated solvent molecules at M$^+$) and **K$_2$trop^m**, where the solvent molecules bound to M$^+$ were not considered. Nevertheless, the calculated π–π* transitions of the calculated UV/Vis spectra correspond well to the recorded UV/Vis spectra (Supplementary Figures S1–S4)—going from Li to K, the observed bathochromic shift is for example well reproduced by the model compounds. In addition, the overall structural agreement between these model compounds and the experimentally determined structures given in Table 3 is very good (e.g., the calculated distances C5-M are listed in Supplementary Table S1) and specifically, the decrease of the bent angles in the order **Litrop^m** > **Natrop^m** > **Ktrop^m** is well reproduced. The NICS values of the contact ion pairs are very sensitive to the bending of the central seven-membered ring. The stronger the ring B is bent, as in **Litrop^m** (θ_1 = 26.2°, θ_2 = 13.5°), the smaller the NICS values are and the less pronounced the anti-aromatic character. On the contrary, when the bending becomes small such as in **Ktrop^m**, the NICS values reach the ones of flat **trop$^-$**. While it may be debated whether CBD is an anti-aromatic compound because of its rectangular distortion [46], **Ktrop^m** can be truly considered as an anti-aromatic species which in the form of **K^{thf}trop** can be isolated as a substance. This claim is further bolstered by the fact that the averaged experimental C=C bond distances listed in Table 3 do not differ much between **trop$^+$** and **K^{thf}trop** and the C=C bond length variation $\Delta C=C$ is modest (0.028 Å in **trop$^+$**, vs. 0.049 Å in **K^{thf}trop**), indicating only small structural distortions. This is in contrast to CBD, where this variation is significant (C-C 1.576 Å, C=C 1.332 Å, $\overline{\Delta C = C}$ = 0.244 Å) [46].

Table 5. Calculated isotropic NICS(0) and NICS(1) values for **trop$^+$**, **trop$^-$**, model compounds **Mtrop^m** (M = Li, Na, K) and **K$_2$trop^m**, [Rh(trop)(cod)] and cyclobutadiene (CBD). The model compounds do not contain solvent molecules attached to the alkali cations. Computational details: PBE [38] 6-311+G(df, pd) [39] in a continuum solvation model (THF). Abbreviations: θ_1 and θ_2: dihedral angles of the optimized structures (°), CBD: 1,3-cyclobutadiene.

		A	B	C	θ_1	θ_2
trop$^+$	NICS(0)	−8.87	−4.71	−8.87	0.00	0.00
	NICS(1)	−11.76	−7.56	−11.76		
trop$^-$	NICS(0)	21.05	45.00	21.02	0.01	0.01
	NICS(1)	15.12	34.54	15.10		
Litrop^m	NICS(0)	6.41	25.23	6.66	26.19	13.54
	NICS(1) [a]	3.85	18.82	3.89		
	NICS(1) [b]	0.95	17.36	1.67		
Natrop^m	NICS(0)	10.23	30.78	10.23	19.99	11.00
	NICS(1) [a]	7.00	23.32	7.00		
	NICS(1) [b]	4.40	22.04	4.41		
Ktrop^m	NICS(0)	17.02	42.39	17.02	7.41	1.77
	NICS(1) [a]	12.03	32.38	12.02		
	NICS(1) [b]	11.18	32.86	11.18		

Table 5. Cont.

		A	B	C	θ_1	θ_2
[Rh(trop)(cod)]	NICS(0)	−6.04	−4.33	−5.79	58.20	34.54
	NICS(1) [a]	−7.41	−1.38	−7.90		
	NICS(1) [b]	−8.47	−26.89	−8.53		
K2trop[m]	NICS(0)	4.77	12.87	4.77	0.02	0.02
	NICS(1)	1.93	8.78	1.93		
CBD	NICS(0)		27.49			
	NICS(1)		18.03			

[a] NICS(1) opposite to the metal center. [b] NICS(1) on the same side as the metal center. CBD = cyclobutadiene, C_4H_4.

As already stated above, the trop⁻ anion as a ligand in a transition metal complex behaves very differently. The NICS data of the annulated benzo rings A and C in **[Rh(trop)(cod)]** are negative and indicate modest magnetic aromatic character.

The NICS data for the ion triple containing paramagnetic dianion radical trop$^{2-\bullet}$ are much smaller than for the mono-anions and indicate diminished anti-aromatic character in accord with conclusions derived from a comparison of the experimental structural data (the C=C bond lengths variation is slightly diminished in the less anti-aromatic dianion radical, see Table 3).

For completeness, the NICS(0) and NICS(1) data for the free dianion **dbcot^{2-}** and the model compounds **M$_2$dbcot[m]** (M = Li, Na, K) are listed in Table 6. As expected, all rings A, B, and C show negative NICS values indicating aromatic character. Note that the structural parameters and the UV/Vis spectra of the ion triples are accurately reproduced by DFT-calculations (Supplementary Figures S5–S7).

Table 6. Calculated isotropic NICS(0) and NICS(1) values (ppm) for dianionic dbcot compounds. Computational details: PBE [38] 6-311+G(df, pd) [39] in a continuum solvation model (THF). Abbreviations: φ_1 and φ_2: dihedral angles of the optimized structures (°).

		A	B	C	φ_1	φ_2
dbcot^{2-}	NICS(0)	−6.60	−17.20	−6.60	0.07	0.07
	NICS(1)	−7.39	−15.13	−7.39		
Li$_2$dbcot[m]	NICS(0)	−4.42	−15.27	−6.76	3.73	2.50
	NICS(1)	−6.51	−13.49	−8.45		
	NICS(1)	−5.31	−15.04	−7.77		
Na$_2$dbcot[m]	NICS(0)	−5.59	−14.57	−5.59	0.03	0.05
	NICS(1)	−7.06	−14.15	−7.06		
K$_2$dbcot[m]	NICS(0)	−5.41	−17.48	−5.42	0.03	0.04
	NICS(1)	−6.93	−16.96	−6.94		
Benzene	NICS(0)		−7.68			
	NICS(1)		−10.09			

2.3. Electrochemistry

The electrochemical properties of **trop₂**, **Ktrop** and **dbcot** were investigated to provide some understanding of the reactivity, especially with respect to mutual electron exchange processes. As previously reported, the cyclic voltammogram of **dbcot** shows two close lying reduction events at $E° = -2.24$ V and $E° = -2.33$ V vs. Fc/Fc$^+$, resulting from two consecutive one-electron transfer steps to give a planar dbcot^{2-} dianion (Fc = ferrocene, Fc$^+$ = ferrocenium) [28,29]. The dbcot$^{-\bullet}$ anion radical was detected by EPR at low temperatures but cannot be isolated. The formation of the trop$^{2-\bullet}$ dianion radical using **Ktrop** as starting material was investigated electrochemically and the cyclic voltammogram in a 0.1 M tetrabutylammonium hexafluorophosphate (TBAPF$_6$) solution in THF is presented in Figure 4. It shows two well-defined waves at −3.04 and −3.37 V vs. Fc/Fc$^+$. The redox process at −3.04 V is fully reversible, as indicated by the linear dependence of the anodic and cathodic peak heights as function of $v^{1/2}$ (Supplementary Figure S8). This reduction was determined to be a one-electron reduction and attributed to the reduction of trop$^-$ to the trop$^{2-\bullet}$ dianion radical. The second process at −3.37 V is irreversible and no anodic wave is recorded upon reversal of the potential scan, even at high scan rates (this could correspond to the formation of the trianion which was reported for [C$_7$H$_7$]$^{3-}$ [47]). The dependence of the cathodic peak current height of this process with $v^{1/2}$ is below the theoretical curve for a one electron Nernstian reaction (Supplementary Figure S9). In addition, the cathodic peak current decreases upon multiple cycling, while a new oxidation wave at −0.72 V appears, increasing upon multiple cycling (Supplementary Figure S10). This behavior is expected for a redox process coupled to a chemical reaction (EC mechanism) resulting in the deposition of the electrochemically generated species on the electrode. Indeed, a blue film formed after electrolysis on the electrode surface. The identity of that deposit could so far not be determined. The neutral hydrocarbon **trop₂** shows a comparable behavior. Two consecutive redox waves at −2.86 and −3.29 V vs. Fc/Fc$^+$ (Figure 4) are observed in its cyclic voltammogram. The first occurs at a significantly more anodic potential than for the potassium salt **Ktrop** ($\Delta E = 180$ mV). The redox process at −2.86 V is fully reversible whereas the second redox wave at −3.29 V is irreversible. Chronoamperometry and linear sweep voltammetry data indicate that the first reduction process at −2.86 V is a 1 e$^-$ reduction (see Supplementary for details, Figures S11–S12 and Table S2). In contrast to the reduction of trop$^-$, the variation of the cathodic peak current height of this process with $v^{1/2}$ follows the theoretical curve for a two-electron Nernstian reaction at low scan rates and a one-electron Nernstian reaction at high scan rates, suggesting an electron transfer-chemical reaction-electron transfer (ECE) mechanism (Supplementary Figure S9). The reversibility of the first reduction process at −2.86 V suggests therefore that the singly reduced radical trop₂$^{-\bullet}$ has a certain lifetime under electrochemical conditions. The ECE mechanism observed for the second reduction to the dianion trop₂$^{2-}$ suggests the cleavage of the C–C bond of trop₂$^{2-}$, forming two equivalents of the trop$^-$ mono-anion, which are further reduced at these potentials to give the dianion radical trop$^{2-\bullet}$. Hence, the electrochemical behavior of trop₂ can be summarized with the steps (1)–(4) indicated below:

$$\text{trop}_2 + 1e^- \rightarrow \text{trop}_2^{-\bullet} \tag{1}$$

$$\text{trop}_2^{-\bullet} + 1e^- \rightarrow \text{trop}_2^{2-} \tag{2}$$

$$\text{trop}_2^{2-} \rightarrow 2\ \text{trop}^- \tag{3}$$

$$2\ \text{trop}^- + 2\ e^- \rightarrow 2\ \text{trop}^{2-\bullet} \tag{4}$$

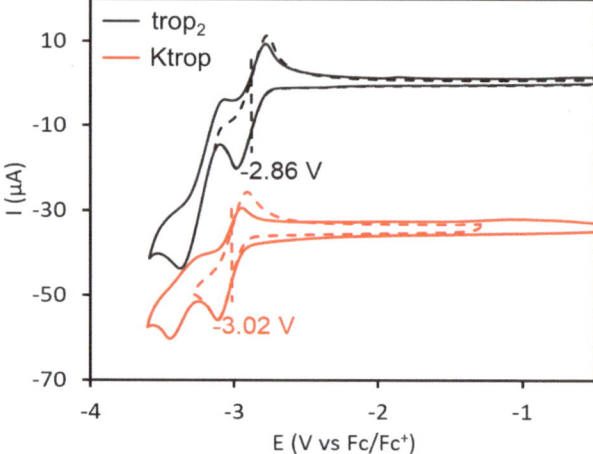

Figure 4. Cyclic voltammogram of **trop₂** (1 mM) in dry tetrahydrofuran at ambient temperature with scan rates ranging from 50 to 400 mV/s and referenced vs. Standard Calomel Electrode (SCE) [48]. [(nBu)$_4$N][PF$_6$] (100 mM) was used as a supporting electrolyte.

Interestingly, cyclic voltammetry studies of **trop₂** in the presence of 10 equivalents of KPF$_6$ showed anodically shifted redox waves, indicating that potassium ions contribute in stabilizing the trop anions and in facilitating the C–C bond cleavage of **trop₂** (Supplementary Figures S13–S14).

The electrochemical behavior of **trop₂** and **Ktrop** is reflected in the chemical reactivity of these species. First, the neutral hydrocarbon **trop₂** is cleanly converted with KC$_8$ under cleavage of the central C–C bond to give **Ktrop** (step (a) in Scheme 3). This reduction is reversible and addition of the ferrocenium salt FcPF$_6$ oxidizes **Ktrop** to reform **trop₂** (step (b) in Scheme 3). As already shown in Scheme 2, **Ktrop** is further reduced to **K₂trop** with potassium graphite (see (c) in Scheme 3). The anti-aromatic radical dianion salt **K₂trop** is a strong reductant (E° = –3.04 V). Addition of half an equivalent **trop₂** oxidizes **K₂trop** to give the mono-anion **Ktrop**, although heating to 60 °C is required ((d) in Scheme 3). Upon addition of half an equivalent of **dbcot** to **K₂trop**, the former is fully reduced to the aromatic dianion **K₂dbcot** ((e) in Scheme 3).

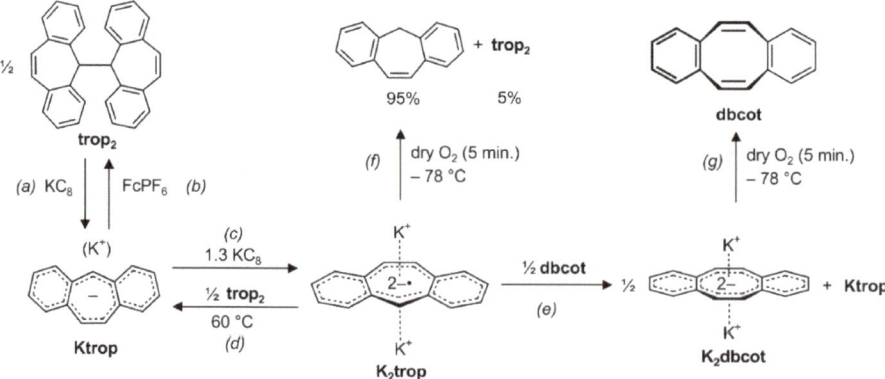

Scheme 3. Interconversions reactions between and within the trop and the dbcot scaffold. FePF$_6$: ferrocenium hexafluorophosphate.

When one equivalent of **dbcot** is used in the oxidation of the dianion radical **trop**$^{2-\bullet}$, a mixture of **K$_2$dbcot** (0.65 equivalents), aside 0.64 equiv. **Ktrop** and 0.16 equiv. of **trop$_2$** is obtained according to ^{1}H NMR spectroscopy. A featureless EPR signal (g = 2.00485) suggests that also K$^+$[dbcot$^{-\bullet}$] may be present [28,30,49]. Considering the stoichiometry of the reaction, we suspect that K$^+$[dbcot$^{-\bullet}$] (≈0.06 equiv.) is in a rapid equilibrium with the remaining neutral **dbcot** molecules (≈0.3 equiv.) which we could not detect by ^{1}H NMR spectroscopy. We also reacted two equivalents of the anti-aromatic mono-anionic ion pair **Ktrop** with **dbcot**. Also, in this reaction, a product mixture consisting of **K$_2$dbcot** (0.5 equiv.), unreacted **Ktrop** (0.9 equiv.) and **trop$_2$** (0.5 equiv.) is obtained. EPR spectroscopy indicates that, very likely, K$^+$[dbcot$^{-\bullet}$] (g = 2.00565) is formed in this reaction as well (Supplementary Scheme S1).

Finally, the oxidation of the dianion salts **K$_2$trop** and **K$_2$dbcot** with dry oxygen was investigated at low temperature. Remarkably, the oxidation of the paramagnetic **K$_2$trop** gives the hydrocarbon C$_{15}$H$_{12}$ (suberene = tropH) as a major product (95%) and not as expected **Ktrop** or **trop$_2$**, which is formed in only 5% yield ((f) in Scheme 3). On contrast, the reaction between oxygen and **K$_2$dbcot**, which contains the diamagnetic and aromatic dbcot^{2-} dianion, is very clean and gives the neutral hydrocarbon **dbcot** in almost quantitative yield ((g) in Scheme 3).

3. Materials and Methods

3.1. General Comments

All experiments were performed under an argon atmosphere using standard Schlenk and vacuum-line techniques or in a MBraun inert-atmosphere drybox (argon atmosphere). All reagents were used as received from commercial suppliers unless otherwise stated. The following compounds were synthesized according to literature procedure: KC$_8$ [50], dbcot [32] and [Rh$_2$Cl$_2$(cod)$_2$] [51]. THF, DME, diethyl ether, toluene and n-hexane were purified using an Innovative Technologies PureSolv system and stored over 4 Å molecular sieves. THF-d_8, C$_6$D$_6$ were distilled from sodium benzophenone ketyl. CDCl$_3$ was distilled from CaH$_2$. Solution NMR spectra were recorded on Bruker Avance 500, 400, 300, 250 and 200 MHz spectrometers. The chemical shifts (δ) are expressed in ppm relative to SiMe$_4$ for ^{1}H and ^{13}C respectively. Coupling constants (J) are given in Hertz (Hz) as absolute values. The multiplicity of the signals is indicated as s, d, t, q, or m for singlets, doublets, triplets, quartets, or multiplets. If the data allowed it, the assignment was based on the IUPAC recommendations for fused polycyclic hydrocarbons (Scheme 4) [52]. Further abbreviations were used in the assignment: br for broadened signals, Ar for aromatic signals, quart for quaternary ^{13}C signals.

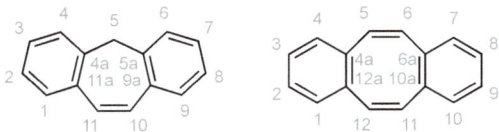

Scheme 4. The assignment in the NMR spectra are based on these numbering schemes.

EPR spectra were recorded by Dr. Reinhard Kissner on an X-band (9.50 GHz) Magnettech Miniscope 5000 EPR spectrometer with liquid nitrogen cooling. EPR spectra were simulated with Matlab R2016b, using EasySpin-5.2.11 package. UV/Vis spectra were recorded on a UV/Vis/NIR Lambda-19 spectrometer in a cell with a 2 mm path length. IR spectra were collected on a PerkinElmer Spectrum 2000 FT-IR-Raman spectrometer. Absorption bands are described as w, m or s for weak, medium or strong. Elemental analyses were performed by Peter Kälin in the Mikrolabor of the ETH Zürich. Melting points were determined with a Büchi melting-point apparatus and are not corrected. X-ray diffraction was performed at 100 K on an Oxford Xcalibur or Venture diffractometer with a CCD area detector and a molybdenum X-ray tube (0.71073 A). Using Olex^2 [53], the structure was solved by direct methods (SHELXS [54] or SHELXT [55]), followed by least-squares refinement against full matrix (versus F^2) with SHELXL [54]. All non-hydrogen atoms were refined anisotropically. The contribution of some hydrogen atoms, in their calculated positions, was included in the refinement using a riding model.

3.2. Synthesis

trop–Si(H)Me$_2$ (1a): 5-Chloro-5H-dibenzo[a,d]cycloheptene (10.02 g, 44.20 mmol, 1.0 equivalent) and elementary lithium (0.71 g, 102.31 mmol, 2.3 equivalents) were reacted in dry tetrahydrofuran (40 mL) at a.T. overnight. The resulting dark red liquid was added dropwise to a solution of chlorodimethylsilane (5.4 mL, 4.60 g, 48.63 mmol, 1.1 equivalents) in dry tetrahydrofuran (40 mL) over an ice bath. The resulting yellow liquid was allowed to warm to a.T. and stirred overnight. The turbid suspension was concentrated under reduced pressure and subsequently distilled in high vacuum (only one fraction was observed from 90 to 115 °C). The obtained yellow liquid was placed in the fridge to give a white, crystalline solid after three days, which was triturated with dry diethyl ether (10.0 mL) and dried in high vacuum (8.328 g, 33.26 mmol, yield: 75.3%).

^{1}H NMR (300 MHz, CDCl$_3$, jb071.1.4) δ 7.27–7.09 (m, 6H, H^{Ar}), 7.06 (dd, $^3J_{HH}$ = 7.4 Hz, $^4J_{HH}$ = 1.4 Hz, 2H, H-4,6), 6.74 (s, 2H, H-10,11), 4.18–4.07 (m, 1H, SiH), 3.49 (d, $^3J_{HH}$ = 4.1 Hz, 1H, H-5), −0.09 (d, $^3J_{HH}$ = 3.6 Hz, 6H, SiCH_3) ppm. ^{13}C NMR (75 MHz, CDCl$_3$, jb071.1.4) δ 140.83 (s, 2C, C^{quart}), 135.05 (s, 2C, C^{quart}), 132.59 (s, 2C, C-10,11), 129.59 (s, 2C, C^{Ar}), 129.13 (s, 2C, C-4,6), 128.96 (s 2C, C^{Ar}), 125.71(s, 2C, C^{Ar}), 47.60 (s, 1C, C-5), −3.71 (s, 2C, Si(CH$_3$)$_2$) ppm. ATR IR: λ^{-1}: 3015 (w, =C–H st), 2955 (w, –C–H st), 2143 (m, Si–H st), 868 (s), 796 (s), 726 (s), 446 (s) cm^{-1}. Elemental analysis: C (81.29%, calc.: 81.54%); H (7.37%, calc.: 7.24%).

trop–SiMe$_3$ (1b): 5-Chloro-5H-dibenzo[a,d]cycloheptene (4.32 g, 19.06 mmol, 1.0 equivalent) and elementary lithium (0.33 g, 47.55 mmol, 2.5 equivalents) were reacted in dry tetrahydrofuran (30 mL) at a.T. overnight. The resulting deep red liquid was added dropwise to a colorless solution of trimethylsilyl chloride (3.2 mL, 2.74 g, 25.21 mmol, 1.3 equivalents) in dry tetrahydrofuran (35 mL). The reaction mixture was allowed to warm to a.T. and stirred overnight. The solvent of the orange solution was removed under reduced pressure to give an orange solid. The crude product was purified by sublimation (up to 150°C, HV) to give a yellow, crystalline solid (4.20 g, 15.88 mmol, yield: 83.3%).

^{1}H NMR (300 MHz, C$_6$D$_6$, jb121.1.3) δ 7.08 (ddd, $^3J_{HH}$ = 7.5 Hz, $^3J_{HH}$ = 6.1 Hz, $^4J_{HH}$ = 2.7 Hz, 2H, H-3,7), 7.06–6.92 (m, 4H, H-1,2,8,9), 6.86 (d, $^3J_{HH}$ = 7.4 Hz, 2H, H-4,6), 6.48 (s, 2H, H-10,11), 3.41 (s, 1H, H-5), −0.06 (s, 9H, SiCH_3) ppm. ^{13}C NMR (75 MHz, C$_6$D$_6$, jb121.1.3) δ 140.91 (s, 2C, C-4a,5a), 135.49 (s, 2C, C-9a,11a), 132.86 (s, 2C, C-10,11), 129.95 (s, 2C, C-1,9), 129.73 (s, 2C, C-4,6), 129.07 (s, 2C, C-3,7), 125.71 (s, 2C, C-2,8), 50.24 (s, 1C, C-5), −0.39 (s, 3C, SiCH$_3$) ppm. Elemental analysis: C (81.70%, calc.: 81.76%); H (7.74%, calc.: 7.62%).

Litrop: Method A: Lithium sand (0.348 g, 50.20 mmol, 2.3 equivalents) was suspended in dry tetrahydrofuran (10 mL) and placed in a cooling bath (propan-2-ol and dry ice). 5-Chloro-5H-dibenzo[a,d]cyclo-heptene (5.00 g, 22.06 mmol, 1.0 equivalent) was dissolved in dry tetrahydrofuran (30 mL). The resulting light yellow solution was added dropwise (during 25 min) to the brown suspension. The reaction mixture was allowed to warm to a.T. and a color change to dark red was observed under heat development. After two hours, the dark red liquid was concentrated to approximately 25 mL and filtered over a plug of celite. The resulting red solution was layered with dry n-hexane (71 mL) and stored in the freezer (−23 °C, 6 days). A first crop of green, crystalline needles was obtained (0.479 g, 1.26 mmol, yield: 2.5%; according to ^{1}H NMR spectroscopy, the compound contained 2.5 equivalents of THF). The supernatant was layered with dry n-hexane (30 mL) and stored in the freezer (−23 °C, 1 day) and a second crop was obtained (7.448 g, 19.68 mmol,[1] yield: 94.0%, overall yield: 95.0%).

Method B: (5H-Dibenzo[a,d]cyclohepten-5-yl)-dimethyl-silane (**1a**, 0.159 g, 0.64 mmol, 1.0 equivalent) was dissolved in dry 1,2-dimethoxyethane (2.0 mL). The resulting slightly yellow solution was added to a white suspension of lithium *tert*-butoxide (0.051 g, 0.64 mmol, 1.0 equivalent) in dry 1,2-dimethoxyethane (2.0 mL) (in a solvent with lower polarity (such as diethyl ether or tetrahydrofuran), a significantly lower yield was obtained). A swift color change to dark red was observed and the reaction mixture was stirred at a.T. (3 h). The dark red liquid was filtered over glass filter paper and celite, layered with dry *n*-hexane (10.0 mL) and stored in the freezer (−30 °C, overnight). The light yellow supernatant was discarded and the obtained green crystals were washed with dry *n*-hexane (3 × 1 mL) and dried under a stream of argon (0.1170 g, 0.35 mmol, yield: 55.2%; according to ^{1}H NMR spectroscopy, the compound contained 1.5 equivalents of dme).

^{1}H NMR (300 MHz, C$_6$D$_6$/THF-d_8, jb070.1.6) δ 5.70 (td, $^3J_{HH}$ = 7.5 Hz, $^4J_{HH}$ = 1.6 Hz, 2H, *H-3,7*), 5.15 (td, $^3J_{HH}$ = 7.1 Hz, $^4J_{HH}$ = 1.3 Hz, 2H, *H-2,8*), 4.87 (dd, $^3J_{HH}$ = 7.1 Hz, $^4J_{HH}$ = 1.6 Hz, 2H, *H-1,9*), 4.59 (dd, $^3J_{HH}$ = 7.9 Hz, $^4J_{HH}$ = 1.3 Hz, 2H, *H-4,6*), 3.92 (s, 2H, *H-10,11*), 1.54 (s, 1H, *H-5*) ppm. ^{1}H NMR (400 MHz, THF-d_8, jb070.1.7) δ 4.80–4.73 (m, 2H, *H-3,7*), 4.12–4.05 (m, 2H, *H-2,8*), 3.73–3.66 (m, 2H, *H-1,9*), 3.48–3.42 (m, 2H, *H-4,6*), 2.64 (s, 2H, *H-10,11*), 0.50 (s, 1H, *H-5*) ppm. ^{13}C NMR (101 MHz, THF-d_8, jb070.1.7) δ 163.60 (s, 2C, *C-4a,5a*), 139.03 (s, 2C, *C-10,11*), 138.27 (s, 2C, *C-9a,11a*), 132.65 (s, 2C, *C-3,7*), 132.05 (s, 2C, *C-1,9*), 120.67 (s, 2C, *C-4,6*), 112.44 (s, 2C, *C-2,8*), 83.67 (s, 1C, *C-5*) ppm. UV/Vis (THF): λ$_{max}$ 233 (ε: 1276(321) m^{2}mol^{-1}), 287 (ε: 2984(340) m^{2}mol^{-1}), 443 (ε: 631(102) m^{2}mol^{-1}), 513 (shoulder, ε: 411(65) m^{2}mol^{-1}) nm. ATR IR: λ^{-1}: 2985 (w, –C–H st), 2926 (w, –C–H st), 1364 (s), 1068 (s), 912 (s), 724 (s), 436 (s) cm^{-1}. Elemental Analysis for Litrop(dme)$_{1.7}$: C (74.79%, calc.: 75.07%); H (7.78%, calc.: 7.95%). MP: 62 °C (decomp.).

Natrop: (5*H*-Dibenzo[*a,d*]cycloheptene-5-yl)-dimethyl-silane (**1a**, 2.005 g, 8.01 mmol, 1.0 equivalent) was dissolved in dry diethyl ether (30 mL). The resulting colorless solution was added to a white suspension of sodium *tert*-butoxide (0.769 g, 8.00 mmol, 1.0 equivalent) in dry diethyl ether (60 mL) over an ice bath. After 30 min, the reaction mixture was allowed to warm to a.T. and a dark red liquid was obtained. The solvent was removed under reduced pressure and dry 1,2-dimethoxyethane (30 mL) was added to the red residue. The liquid was filtered over a plug of celite, layered with dry *n*-hexane (80 mL) and stored in the freezer (−23 °C, 2 days). The light yellow supernatant was discarded and the obtained dark green crystals were washed with dry *n*-hexane (2 × 10 mL) and briefly dried in vacuo (1.931 g, 6.16 mmol, yield: 77.0%; according to ^{1}H NMR spectroscopy the compound contained 1.1 equivalents of dme).

^{1}H NMR (300 MHz, THF-d_8, jb075.3) δ 4.76 (ddd, $^3J_{HH}$ = 7.8 Hz, $^3J_{HH}$ = 7.1 Hz, $^4J_{HH}$ = 1.6 Hz, 2H, *H-3,7*), 4.08 (td, $^3J_{HH}$ = 7.1 Hz, $^4J_{HH}$ = 1.2 Hz, 2H, *H-2,8*), 3.68 (dd, $^3J_{HH}$ = 7.1 Hz, $^4J_{HH}$ = 1.6 Hz, 2H, *H-1,9*), 3.43 (d, $^3J_{HH}$ ≈ 6.9 Hz§, 2H, *H-4,6*), 2.60 (s, 2H, *H-10,11*), 0.56 (s, 1H, *H-5*) ppm. ^{1}H NMR (400 MHz, C$_6$D$_6$/THF-d_8, krastefa.50) δ 5.18 (td, $^3J_{HH}$ = 7.5 Hz, $^4J_{HH}$ = 1.6 Hz, 2H, *H-3,7*), 4.54 (td, $^3J_{HH}$ = 7.1 Hz, $^4J_{HH}$ = 1.3 Hz, 2H, *H-2,8*), 4.11 (dd, $^3J_{HH}$ = 7.1 Hz, $^4J_{HH}$ = 1.6 Hz, 2H, *H-1,9*), 3.93 (dd, $^3J_{HH}$ = 7.9 Hz, $^3J_{HH}$ = 1.4 Hz, 2H, *H-4,6*), 2.98 (s, 1H, *H-10,11*), 1.10 (s, 1H, *H-5*) ppm. ^{13}C NMR (101 MHz, C$_6$D$_6$/THF-d_8, krastefa.51) δ 161.95 (s, 2C, *C-4a,5a*), 138.79 (s, 2C, *C-10,11*), 136.39 (s, 2C, *C-9a,11a*), 133.16 (s, 2C, *C-3,7*), 132.57 (s, 2C, *C-1,9*), 120.12 (s, 2C, *C-4,6*), 113.22 (s, 2C, *C-2,8*), 81.56 (s, 1C, *C-5*) ppm. UV/Vis (THF): λ$_{max}$ 285 (ε: 3074(349) m^{2}mol^{-1}), 459 (ε: 803(158) m^{2}mol^{-1}) nm. ATR IR: λ^{-1}: 3039 (w, =C–H st), 3003 (w, =C–H st), 2978 (w, –C–H st), 2932 (w, –C–H st), 2913 (w, –C–H st), 2869 (w, –C–H st), 2823 (w, –C–H st), 1553 (s), 1443 (s), 1362 (s), 1118 (s), 1082 (s), 1028 (s), 734 (s) cm^{-1}. Elemental Analysis for Natrop(dme)$_{1.1}$: C (74.20%, calc.: 74.36%); H (6.92%, calc.: 7.08%). MP: 45 °C (decomp.).

§ The upper part of the multiplet lies underneath the signal of the solvent DME.

Ktrop: Method A: (5*H*-Dibenzo[*a,d*]cyclo-hepten-5-yl)-dimethyl-silane (**1a**, 1.500 g, 5.99 mmol, 1.0 equivalent) and potassium *tert*-butoxide (0.693 g, 6.18 mmol, 1.0 equivalent) were placed under argon. Dry tetrahydrofuran (20 mL) was added and a dark red liquid was obtained immediately. The reaction mixture was stirred at a.T. (10 hr) and filtered over a plug of celite. The dark red filtrate was layered with dry *n*-hexane (68 mL) and stored in the freezer (−23 °C, 4 days). A first crop of red crystals was isolated (0.624 g, 2.34 mmol, yield: 39.1%; according to ^{1}H NMR spectroscopy the compound contained 0.5 equivalent of THF). The supernatant was layered with dry *n*-hexane (60 mL), stored in the freezer (−23 °C, 3 days) and a second crop was obtained (0.461 g, 2.00 mmol, yield: 32.4%, overall yield: 71.5%).

Method B: (5H-Dibenzo[a,d]cycloheptene-5-yl)-trimethyl-silane (**1b**, 4.909 g, 18.57 mmol, 1.0 equivalent) and potassium *tert*-butoxide (2.085 g, 18.58 mmol, 1.0 equivalent) were placed under argon. Dry tetrahydrofuran (35 mL) was added over an ice bath. The yellow solution was allowed to warm to a.T. and a gradual color change to dark red was observed. The reaction mixture was stirred overnight. The solvent was removed under reduced pressure. The red residue was triturated with dry diethyl ether (2 × 20 mL) and then washed with dry diethyl ether (40 mL). The resulting red solid was briefly dried in vacuo (3.552 g, 15.42 mmol, yield: 83.1%). The red solid (0.271 g, 1.18 mmol) was recrystallized in dry tetrahydrofuran (5.0 mL), filtered over glass filter paper and celite, layered with dry *n*-hexane (10.0 mL) and stored in the freezer (−30 °C, 2.5 days). The long, crystalline needles were washed with dry *n*-hexane (4 × 1.5 mL) and dried under a stream of argon (0.171 g, 0.74 mmol, yield of recrystallization: 63%).

^{1}H NMR (300 MHz, THF-d_8, jb073.1.1EA) δ 4.47 (ddd, $^3J_{HH}$ = 7.9 Hz, $^3J_{HH}$ = 7.1 Hz, $^4J_{HH}$ = 1.6 Hz, 2H, *H-3,7*), 3.74 (td, $^3J_{HH}$ = 7.1 Hz, $^4J_{HH}$ = 1.2 Hz, 2H, *H-2,8*), 3.26 (dd, $^3J_{HH}$ = 7.1 Hz, $^4J_{HH}$ = 1.6 Hz, 2H, *H-1,9*), 2.97 (dd, $^3J_{HH}$ = 8.0 Hz, $^4J_{HH}$ = 1.3 Hz, 2H, *H-4,6*), 2.00 (s, 2H, H-10,11), 0.06 (s, 1H, H-5) ppm. ^{1}H NMR (400 MHz, THF-d_8, krastefa.11, T = 273 K) δ 4.40 (ddd, $^3J_{HH}$ = 8.2 Hz, $^3J_{HH}$ = 7.1 Hz, $^4J_{HH}$ = 1.6 Hz, 2H, *H-3,7*), 3.65 (td, $^3J_{HH}$ = 7.0 Hz, $^4J_{HH}$ = 1.3 Hz, 2H, *H-2,8*), 3.18 (dd, $^3J_{HH}$ = 7.1 Hz, $^4J_{HH}$ = 1.6 Hz, 2H, *H-1,9*), 2.89 (dd, $^3J_{HH}$ = 8.0 Hz, $^4J_{HH}$ = 1.3 Hz, 2H, *H-4,6*), 1.91 (s, 2H, H-11,10), −0.01 (s, 1H, *H-5*) ppm. ^{13}C NMR (101 MHz, THF-d_8, krastefa.12, T = 273 K) δ 162.96 (s, 2C, *C-4a,5a*), 139.26 (s, 2C, *C-10,11*), 138.42 (s, 2C, *C-9a,11a*), 133.95 (s, 2C, *C-3,7*), 132.89 (s, 2C, *C-1,9*), 120.17 (s, 2C, *C-4,6*), 111.87 (s, 2C, *C-2,8*), 89.44 (s, 1C, *C-5*) ppm. UV/Vis (THF): λ$_{max}$ 286 (ε: 3343(566) m^{2}mol^{-1}), 296 (shoulder, ε: 3086(595) m^{2}mol^{-1}), 478 (ε: 1025(277) m^{2}mol^{-1}) nm. ATR IR: λ^{-1}: 3006 (w, =C–H st), 2985 (w, –C–H st), 2939 (w, –C–H st), 2924 (w, –C–H st), 1366 (m), 1121 (s), 1039 (m), 914 (m), 797 (m), 740 (s), 436 (m) cm^{-1}. Elemental Analysis: C (78.25%, calc.: 78.21%); H (4.94%, calc.: 4.81%). MP: 240 °C (decomp.).

K$_2$trop: Ktrop (0.461 g, 2.00 mmol, 1.0 equivalent) was dissolved in dry tetrahydrofuran (5.0 mL). The resulting dark red solution was added to a golden suspension of potassium graphite (0.355 g, 2.62 mmol, 1.3 equivalents) in dry tetrahydrofuran (5.0 mL) and stirred at a.T. (3 days). The dark red suspension was filtered over a plug of celite and the dark red filter cake was washed with dry tetrahydrofuran (3.5 mL). The dark red filtrate was split into two portions and each was layered with dry *n*-hexane (6.0 mL) and stored in the freezer (−30 °C, 3 days). The dark red, microcrystalline solid of both fractions was washed with dry *n*-hexane (2 × 2 mL each) and briefly dried in vacuo (0.372 g, 0.77 mmol, yield: 38.3%). The supernatant of both fractions was concentrated under reduced pressure and the dark residue was recrystallized again from dry tetrahydrofuran (3.0 mL) and dry *n*-hexane (6.0 mL) at −30 °C to give a second crop of dark red, microcrystalline solid (0.060 g, 0.12 mmol, yield: 6.2%, overall yield: 44.5%).

UV/Vis (THF): λ$_{max}$ 286 (ε: 4098(190) m^{2}mol^{-1}), 297 (shoulder, ε: 3857(204) m^{2}mol^{-1}), 361 (ε: 1988(237) m^{2}mol^{-1}), 482 (ε: 1633(37) m^{2}mol^{-1}) nm. ATR IR: λ^{-1}: 3020 (w, =C–H st), 2970 (w, –C–H st), 2868 (w, –C–H st), 1324 (m), 1015 (m), 736 (m), 686 (m), 433 (m) cm^{-1}. Elemental Analysis for K$_2$trop(thf)(*n*-hexane)$_{0.2}$: C (67.95%, calc.: 67.62%); H (5.92%, calc.: 6.12%). MP: >250 °C.

Na$_2$dbcot: Dibenzo[a,e]cyclooctatetraene (0.507 g, 2.48 mmol, 1.0 equivalent) was dissolved in dry tetrahydrofuran (10 mL). The colorless solution was added to a Schlenk tube with a sodium mirror (0.55 g, 23.92 mmol, 9.6 equivalents). A swift color change to dark red was observed. The reaction mixture was stirred at a.T. (1 day). The solvent was removed under reduced pressure. The purple residue was suspended in dry tetrahydrofuran (7 mL) and filtered over a plug of celite to give a dark red filtrate (a) and a dark red filter cake (b). (a) The dark red filtrate was layered with dry *n*-hexane (10 mL) and stored at a.T. (7 days). The obtained dark crystals were washed with dry *n*-hexane (2 mL) and dried under a stream of argon (0.145 g, 0.34 mmol, yield: 13.6%). (b) The filter cake was extracted with dry 1,2-dimethoxyethane (6 mL). The dark red filtrate was layered with dry *n*-hexane (8 mL) and stored in the freezer (−30 °C, 6 days). The obtained dark crystals were washed with dry *n*-hexane (2 × 2 mL) and dried under a stream of argon (0.256 g, 0.45 mmol, yield: 18.3%, overall yield: 31.9%).

^{1}H NMR (300 MHz, THF-d_8, jb105.1.2) δ 7.87 (dd, $^3J_{HH}$ = 6.6 Hz, $^4J_{HH}$ = 3.3 Hz, 4H, H-1,4,7,10), 7.17 (s, 4H, H-5,6,11,12), 6.21 (dd, $^3J_{HH}$ = 6.6 Hz, $^4J_{HH}$ = 3.4 Hz, 4H, H-2,3,8,9) ppm. ^{13}C NMR (75 MHz, THF-d_8, jb105.1.2) δ 135.26 (s, 4C, C-1,4,7,10), 108.90 (s, 4C, C-2,3,8,9), 107.43 (s, 4C, C-4a,6a,10a,12a), 93.37 (s, 4C, C-5,6,11,12) ppm. UV/Vis (THF): λ$_{max}$ 238 (ε: 2523(2) m^{2}mol^{-1}), 261 (shoulder, ε: 1842(132) m^{2}mol^{-1}), 328 (ε: 5293(512) m^{2}mol^{-1}), 392 (ε: 853(87) m^{2}mol^{-1}), 514 (ε: 94(12) m^{2}mol^{-1}), 553 (ε: 106(13) m^{2}mol^{-1}), 597 (ε: 76(9) m^{2}mol^{-1}) nm.

K$_2$dbcot: Dibenzo[*a,e*]cyclooctatetraene (0.301 g, 1.47 mmol, 1.0 equivalent) was dissolved in dry tetrahydrofuran (12 mL). Potassium graphite (0.526 g, 3.89 mmol, 2.6 equivalents) was added. The resulting dark red suspension was allowed to stir at a.T. (1 day). The reaction mixture was filtered over a plug of celite. The filter cake was washed with dry tetrahydrofuran (3 mL). The filtrate was split into two portions and each layered with dry *n*-hexane (8 mL) and stored in the freezer (−30 °C, 3 days). The obtained dark green crystals were washed with dry *n*-hexane (2 × 1 mL) and briefly dried in vacuo (0.450 g, 1.15 mmol, yield: 78.3%). The supernatant was concentrated under reduced pressure and the black residue was recrystallized in the same manner to give a second crop (0.047 g, 0.12 mmol, yield: 8.2%, overall yield: 86.6%).

^{1}H NMR (300 MHz, THF-d_8, jb085.1.1) δ 7.87 (dd, $^3J_{HH}$ = 6.7 Hz, $^4J_{HH}$ = 3.5 Hz, 4H, H-1,4,7,10), 7.17 (s, 4H, H-5,6,11,12), 6.19 (dd, $^3J_{HH}$ = 6.7 Hz, $^4J_{HH}$ = 3.3 Hz, 4H, H-2,3,8,9) ppm. ^{13}C NMR (75 MHz, THF-d_8, jb085.1.1) δ 135.72 (s, 4C, C-1,4,7,10), 109.36 (s, 4C, C-4a,6a,10a,12a), 108.91 (s, 4C, C-2,3,8,9), 95.78 (s, 4C, C-5,6,11,12) ppm. UV/Vis (THF): λ$_{max}$ 235 (ε: 3997(184) m^{2}mol^{-1}), 261 (shoulder, ε: 1053(87) m^{2}mol^{-1}), 326 (ε: 1959(338) m^{2}mol^{-1}), 388 (ε: 334(53) m^{2}mol^{-1}), 502 (ε: 38(6) m^{2}mol^{-1}), 544 (ε: 42(7) m^{2}mol^{-1}), 587 (ε: 31(5) m^{2}mol^{-1}) nm. MP: >250 °C.

[Rh(trop)(cod)]: Cyclooctadiene rhodium(I) chloride dimer (0.050 g, 0.10 mmol, 1.0 equivalent) and **Ktrop** (0.047 g, 0.20 mmol, 2.0 equivalents) were stirred in dry toluene (6 mL) at a.T. (12 hr). The dark red liquid was filtered over a plug of celite, layered with dry *n*-hexane (6 mL) and stored in the freezer (−30 °C, 13 days). The obtained dark red crystals were washed with dry *n*-hexane (0.5 mL) and dried under a stream of argon (0.052 g, 0.13 mmol, yield: 63.0%).

^{1}H NMR (400 MHz, C$_6$D$_6$, jb083.8A) δ 7.01–6.88 (m, 6H, H^{Ar}), 6.85 (dd, $^3J_{HH}$ = 7.1 Hz, $^1J_{HH}$ = 1.7 Hz, 2H, H-4,6), 5.16 (d, $^2J_{RhH}$ = 1.2 Hz, 2H, H-10,11), 4.09 (s$_{br}$, 2H, CH^{COD}), 3.59 (s$_{br}$, 2H, CH^{COD}), 2.88 (s, 1H, H-5), 2.21 (s$_{br}$, 4H, CH_2^{COD}), 1.76 (s$_{br}$, 4H, CH_2^{COD}) ppm. ^{13}C NMR (101 MHz, C$_6$D$_6$, jb083.8A) δ 137.43 (s, 2C, C-4a,5a), 132.63 (s, 2C, C-9a,11a), 128.06 (s, 2C, C-1,9/3,7§), 126.86 (s, 2C, C-4,6), 126.66 (s, 2C, C-3,7/1,9), 126.13 (s, 2C, C-2,8), 97.52 (d, $^1J_{RhC}$ = 5.4 Hz, 2C, C-10,11), 91.23 (s, 2C, CH^{COD}), 70.69 (s, 2C, CH^{COD}), 55.84 (d, $^1J_{RhC}$ = 13.2 Hz, 1C, C-5), 35.22 (s, 2C, CH_2^{COD}), 29.91 (s, 2C, CH_2^{COD}) ppm.

§ The peak is buried under the signal for C$_6$D$_6$.

^{1}H NMR (500 MHz, THF-d_8, jb083.8.2A, −40 °C) δ 7.10–6.99 (m, 6H, H^{Ar}), 6.89–6.84 (m, 2H, H-4,6), 5.46 (s, 2H, H-10,11), 3.92 (m$_{br}$, 2H, CH^{COD}), 3.70 (m$_{br}$, 2H, CH^{COD}), 2.81 (s, 1H, H-5), 2.30 (m, 4H, CH_2^{COD}), 1.76 (m, 4H, CH_2^{COD}) ppm. ^{13}C NMR (126 MHz, THF-d_8, jb083.8.2A, −40 °C) δ 137.75 (s, 2C, C-4a,5a), 133.25 (s, 2C, C-9a,11a), 128.54 (s, 2C, C-1,9/3,7), 127.42 (s, 2C, C-3,7/1,9), 127.24 (s, 2C, C-4,6), 126.78 (s, 2C, C-2,8), 97.57 (d, $^1J_{RhC}$ = 5.0 Hz, 2C, C-10,11), 90.61 (d, $^1J_{RhC}$ = 6.9 Hz, 2C, CH^{COD}), 70.35 (d, $^1J_{RhC}$ = 15.6 Hz, 2C, CH^{COD}), 56.45 (d, $^1J_{RhC}$ = 13.0 Hz, 1C, C-5), 35.09 (s, 2C, CH_2^{COD}), 30.46 (s, 2C, CH_2^{COD}) ppm.

4. Conclusions

A desilylation reaction using silyl trop derivative which proceeds by addition of KO*t*Bu allowed the very clean synthesis of larger amounts of the salts of the trop anion, **trop**$^-$, which contain alkali metal counter cations M$^+$ = Li, Na, K. With these at hand, an in-depth study on the electronic configuration of these conjugated hydrocarbons exclusively composed from sp^2-valence electron hybridized carbon centers could be performed. As the Hückel counting rules imply, the 16π-electron configuration of **trop**$^-$ predicts this to be anti-aromatic. This is indeed the case as NMR data and as well as calculated NICS data clearly show. A number of contact ion pairs, **Mtrop**, could be structurally characterized by X-ray diffraction methods. In these, ethereal molecules complete the coordination sphere around the

M$^+$ cation. From tetrahydrofuran (THF), close ion pairs are obtained which show an intimate contact between cation and trop$^-$ anion. In these, the trop$^-$ anion is bent and its anti-aromaticity lowered. On the contrast, crystallization from solvents, which have a higher solvation energy for alkali cations, lead to separated ion pairs in which the trop$^-$ anion is flatter and consequently, more anti-aromatic. Moreover, Li$^+$ shows a higher tendency to form contact ion pairs than the larger potassium cation with a significantly reduced charge density. This culminates in the isolation of [K(thf)$_2$][trop]$_\infty$, which forms a one-dimensional coordination polymer in the solid state with long K$^+$ trop$^-$ distances. This compound contains a flat trop$^-$ anion which shows very little variation of the C=C bond lengths, strongly shielded NMR signals, strongly positive NICS values and as such, fulfils all formal criteria requested for an anti-aromatic compound. In this light, the ease of synthesis from trop silyl ethers and alcoholates is somewhat surprising, indicating that **Mtrop** salts are remarkably stable. The trop$^-$ monoanion can be further reduced to give salts **M$_2$trop** with a paramagnetic dianion radical, trop$^{2-\bullet}$, which was isolated and fully characterized as **K$_2$trop**. In this species, the anti-aromaticity is reduced compared to the mono-anion. In a reaction between a Rh(I) halide complex and trop$^-$, the complex **[Rh(trop)(cod)]** was prepared. Not unexpected, this pure organometallic 18 electron complex shows a very different structure in which the trop unit—especially its annulated benzo groups—is aromatized. This reaction also shows that trop anions may have potential as ligands for transition metal complexes and as a building block for main group element compounds. It remains to be seen in how far trop-type anions can be used as electron carriers related to the well-established use of arenes for that purpose [15].

Supplementary Materials: The following are available online: 1. DFT-Calculations; Table S1: Selected bond lengths [Å] for the calculated trop mono- and dianions; Table S2: Key parameters for the determination of the number of electrons; Figure S1: Bottom: Recorded (red) vs. calculated (blue) spectrum of **Litrop** in THF; Figure S2: Bottom: Recorded (red) vs. calculated (blue) spectrum of **Natrop** in THF; Figure S3: Bottom: Recorded (red) vs. calculated (blue) spectrum of **Ktrop** in THF; Figure S4: Stacked spectra of **Litrop**, **Natrop** and **Ktrop** in THF; Figure S5: Bottom: Recorded (red) vs. calculated (blue) spectrum of **K$_2$trop** in THF; Figure S6: Recorded (red) vs. calculated (blue) spectrum of **Na$_2$dbcot** in THF; Figure S7: Recorded (red) vs. calculated (blue) spectrum of **K$_2$dbcot** in THF; 2. Electrochemical data for **Ktrop** and **trop$_2$** on GC electrode; Figure S8: Scan rate dependence of the 1st reduction process for **Ktrop** and **trop$_2$** in 0.1 M TBAPF$_6$ solution in THF on glassy carbon electrode; Figure S10: Overlay of the I$_p$ currents vs. scan rate$^{1/2}$ plot of **Ktrop**$^{2-/3-}$ and **trop$_2$**$^{1-/2-}$ redox processes with theoretical 1e$^-$ and 2e$^-$ plot slopes; Figure S9: Overlay of the successive CV scans for 1 mM of **Ktrop** solution in THF (0.1 M TBAPF$_6$) at 100 mVs^{-1}; Figure S11: I vs. t$^{-1/2}$ plot of the chronoamperometry data obtained from a 10 mM **trop$_2$** solution at −3.07 V vs. Fc/Fc$^+$ and a 10 mM ferrocene solution at 0.23 V vs. Fc/Fc$^+$ in 0.1 M TBAPF$_6$ in THF; Figure S12: Overlay of linear sweep voltammograms of a 10 mM **trop$_2$** solution and a 10 mM ferrocene in a 0.1 M TBAPF$_6$ solution in THF obtained in stationary regime at a carbon microelectrode (5 mVs^{-1} scan rate); Figure S13: Overlay of the CVs recorded for **Ktrop**, **trop$_2$**, and **trop$_2$** in presence of 10 mM KPF$_6$; Figure S14: Overlay of the cyclic voltammograms at various scan rates with 1 mM **trop$_2$** in 0.1 M TBAPF$_6$ solution in THF on glassy carbon electrode; Scheme S1: Selected interconversion reactions between the **trop** and the **dbcot** scaffold.

Author Contributions: Conceptualization, H.G., T.L.G., and V.M.; investigation, J.B, S.K., D.O., S.D.; writing—original draft preparation, J.B. and H.G.; writing—review and editing, T.L.G., V.M., H.G.; supervision, H.G.; funding acquisition, H.G. All authors have read and agreed to the published version of the manuscript.

Funding: This research was funded by the Swiss National Science Foundation (SNF) through grant number 2-77199-18.

Conflicts of Interest: The authors declare no conflict of interest. The funders had no role in the design of the study; in the collection, analyses, or interpretation of data; in the writing of the manuscript, or in the decision to publish the results.

References

1. Thomaier, J.; Boulmaâz, S.; Schönberg, H.; Rüegger, H.; Currao, A.; Grützmacher, H.; Hillebrecht, H.; Pritzkow, H. Dibenzotropylidene Phosphanes (TROPPs): Synthesis and Coinage Metal Complexes. *New J. Chem.* **1998**, *22*, 947–958. [CrossRef]
2. Schönberg, H.; Boulmaâz, S.; Wörle, M.; Liesum, L.; Schweiger, A.; Grützmacher, H. A Monomeric d^9-Rhodium(0) Complex. *Angew. Chem. Int. Ed.* **1998**, *37*, 1423–1426. [CrossRef]
3. Ostendorf, D.; Landis, C.; Grützmacher, H. Trigonal Pyramids: Alternative Ground-State Structures for Sixteen-Electron Complexes. *Angew. Chem. Int. Ed.* **2006**, *45*, 5169–5173. [CrossRef] [PubMed]

4. Lichtenberg, C.; Viciu, L.; Adelhardt, M.; Sutter, J.; Meyer, K.; de Bruin, B.; Grützmacher, H. Low-Valent Iron(I) Amido Olefin Complexes as Promotors for Dehydrogenation Reactions. *Angew. Chem. Int. Ed.* **2015**, *54*, 5766–5771. [CrossRef]
5. Grützmacher, H. Cooperating Ligands in Catalysis. *Angew. Chem. Int. Ed.* **2008**, *47*, 1814–1818. [CrossRef]
6. Maire, P.; Büttner, T.; Breher, F.; Le Floch, P.; Grützmacher, H. Heterolytic Splitting of Hydrogen with Rhodium(I) Amides. *Angew. Chem. Int. Ed.* **2005**, *44*, 6318–6323. [CrossRef]
7. Zweifel, T.; Naubron, J.-V.; Büttner, T.; Ott, T.; Grützmacher, H. Ethanol as Hydrogen Donor: Highly Efficient Transfer Hydrogenations with Rhodium(I) Amides. *Angew. Chem. Int. Ed.* **2008**, *47*, 3245–3249. [CrossRef]
8. Zweifel, T.; Naubron, J.-V.; Grützmacher, H. Catalyzed Dehydrogenative Coupling of Primary Alcohols with Water, Methanol, or Amines. *Angew. Chem. Int. Ed.* **2009**, *48*, 559–563. [CrossRef]
9. Gianetti, T.L.; Annen, S.P.; Santiso-Quinones, G.; Reiher, M.; Driess, M.; Grützmacher, H. Nitrous Oxide as a Hydrogen Acceptor for the Dehydrogenative Coupling of Alcohols. *Angew. Chem. Int. Ed.* **2016**, *55*, 1854–1858. [CrossRef] [PubMed]
10. Rodríguez-Lugo, R.E.; Trincado, M.; Vogt, M.; Tewes, F.; Santiso-Quinones, G.; Grützmacher, H. A Homogeneous Transition Metal Complex for Clean Hydrogen Production From Methanol–Water Mixtures. *Nat. Chem.* **2013**, *5*, 342. [CrossRef]
11. Trincado, M.; Sinha, V.; Rodriguez-Lugo, R.E.; Pribanic, B.; de Bruin, B.; Grützmacher, H. Homogeneously Catalysed Conversion of Aqueous Formaldehyde to H_2 and Carbonate. *Nat. Commun.* **2017**, *8*, 14990. [CrossRef] [PubMed]
12. Sinha, V.; Pribanic, B.; de Bruin, B.; Trincado, M.; Grützmacher, H. Ligand- and Metal-Based Reactivity of a Neutral Ruthenium Diolefin Diazadiene Complex: The Innocent, the Guilty and the Suspicious. *Chem. Eur. J.* **2018**, *24*, 5513–5521. [CrossRef] [PubMed]
13. Defieber, C.; Grützmacher, H.; Carreira, E.M. Chiral Olefins as Steering Ligands in Asymmetric Catalysis. *Angew. Chem. Int. Ed.* **2008**, *47*, 4482–4502. [CrossRef] [PubMed]
14. Harder, S.; Martin, J.; Langer, J.; Wiesinger, M.; Elsen, H. Dibenzotropylidene Substituted Ligands for Early Main Group Metal-Alkene Bonding. *Eur. J. Inorg. Chem.* **2020**, *2020*, 2582–2595. [CrossRef]
15. Bock, H.; Ruppert, K.; Näther, C.; Havlas, Z.; Herrmann, H.-F.; Arad, C.; Göbel, I.; John, A.; Meuret, J.; Nick, S.; et al. Distorted Molecules: Perturbation Design, Preparation and Structures. *Angew. Chem. Int. Ed.* **1992**, *31*, 550–581. [CrossRef]
16. Bock, H.; Gharagozloo-Hubmann, K.; Sievert, M.; Prisner, T.; Havlas, Z. Single Crystals of an Ionic Anthracene Aggregate with a Triplet Ground State. *Nature* **2000**, *404*, 267–269. [CrossRef]
17. Müllen, K. Reduction and Oxidation of Annulenes. *Chem. Rev.* **1984**, *84*, 603–646. [CrossRef]
18. Vos, H.W.; Bakker, Y.W.; Maclean, C.; Velthorst, N.H. Paramagnetic Ring Currents in the Carbanion of 5*H*-dibenzo[*a,d*]cycloheptene and the Nitranion of 5*H*-dibenz[*b,f*]azepine. *Chem. Phys. Lett.* **1974**, *25*, 80–83. [CrossRef]
19. von Schleyer, P.R.; Jiao, H. What is Aromaticity? *Pure Appl. Chem.* **1996**, *68*, 209–218. [CrossRef]
20. McAuley, I.; Krogh, E.; Wan, P. Carbanion Intermediates in the Photodecarboxylation of Benzannelated Acetic Acids in Aqueous Solution. *J. Am. Chem. Soc.* **1988**, *110*, 600–602. [CrossRef]
21. Krogh, E.; Wan, P. Photodecarboxylation of Diarylacetic Acids in Aqueous Solution: Enhanced Photogeneration of Cyclically Conjugated Eight π Electron Carbanions. *J. Am. Chem. Soc.* **1992**, *114*, 705–712. [CrossRef]
22. Wan, P.; Krogh, E.; Chak, B. Enhanced Formation of 8π(4n) Conjugated Cyclic Carbanions in the Excited State: First Example of Photochemical C–H Bond Heterolysis in Photoexcited Suberene. *J. Am. Chem. Soc.* **1988**, *110*, 4073–4074. [CrossRef]
23. Budac, D.; Wan, P. Excited-State Carbon Acids. Facile Benzylic Carbon-Hydrogen Bond Heterolysis of Suberene on Photolysis in Aqueous Solution: A Photogenerated Cyclically Conjugated Eight π Electron Carbanion. *J. Org. Chem.* **1992**, *57*, 887–894. [CrossRef]
24. Bauld, N.L.; Brown, M.S. Dianion Radicals. II. Tropenide Systems. *J. Am. Chem. Soc.* **1967**, *89*, 5417–5421. [CrossRef]
25. Ceccon, A.; Gambaro, A.; Pizzato, L.; Romanin, A.; Venzo, A. Metal Stabilized Carbanions. Kinetic Acidity and ^1H NMR Spectrum of the π-(Tricarbonylchromium)-5*H*-dibenzo[*a,d*]cycloheptenyl Anion. *J. Chem. Soc. Chem. Commun.* **1982**, *16*, 907–908. [CrossRef]

26. Ceccon, A.; Gambaro, A.; Venzo, A. Metal-Stabilized Carbanions. *J. Organomet. Chem.* **1984**, *275*, 209–222. [CrossRef]
27. Irngartinger, H.; Reibel, W.R.K. Structures of Dibenzo[*a*,*e*]cyclooctatetraene and Tetrabenzo[*a*,*c*,*e*,*g*]cyclooctatetraene (*o*-Tetraphenylene). *Acta Cryst. B* **1981**, *37*, 1724–1728. [CrossRef]
28. Katz, T.J.; Yoshida, M.; Siew, L.C. The *sym*-Dibenzcyclooctatetraene Anion Radical and Dianion. *J. Am. Chem. Soc.* **1965**, *87*, 4516–4520. [CrossRef]
29. Kojima, H.; Bard, A.J.; Wong, H.N.C.; Sondheimer, F. Electrochemical Reduction of *sym*-Dibenzocyclooctatetraene, *sym*-Dibenzo-1,5-cyclooctadiene-3,7-diyne, and *sym*-Dibenzo-1,3,5-cyclooctatrien-7-yne. *J. Am. Chem. Soc.* **1976**, *98*, 5560–5565. [CrossRef]
30. Gerson, F.; Martin, W.B., Jr.; Plattner, G.; Sondheimer, F.; Wong, H.N.C. ESR. Spectra and Structures of Radical Anions in the Dibenzo[*a*,*e*]cyclooctene Series. *Helv. Chim. Acta* **1976**, *59*, 2038–2048. [CrossRef]
31. Sygula, A.; Fronczek, F.R.; Rabideau, P.W. The First Example of η^8 Coordination of Lithium Cations with a Cyclooctatetraene Dianion: Crystal Structure of Li_2(dibenzo[*a*,*e*]cyclooctatetraene)(TMEDA)$_2$. *J. Organomet. Chem.* **1996**, *526*, 389–391. [CrossRef]
32. Franck, G.; Brill, M.; Helmchen, G. Dibenzo[*a*,*e*]cyclooctene: Multi-gram Synthesis of a Bidentate Ligand. *Org. Synth.* **2012**, *89*, 55–65.
33. Berti, G. Communications - Dibenzo[*a*,*e*]tropylium and 5-Phenyldibenzo[*a*,*e*]tropylium Cations. *J. Org. Chem.* **1957**, *22*, 230. [CrossRef]
34. Ball, R.G.; Edelmann, F.; Kiel, G.Y.; Takats, J.; Drews, R. Cycloheptatrienyl-Bridged Heterobimetallic Complexes: Facile Phosphine Substitution Reactions of (μ-C_7H_7)Fe(CO)$_3$Rh(CO)$_2$. *Organometallics* **1986**, *5*, 829–839. [CrossRef]
35. Dickson, R.S.; Jenkins, S.M.; Skelton, B.W.; White, A.H. The Addition of Small Molecules to (η-C_5H_5)$_2$Rh$_2$(CO)(CF$_3$C$_2$CF$_3$)—IX. C–H Bond Activation in the Reactions with Dienes, Polyenes and Arenes; the Crystal and Molecular Structure of [(η-C_5H_5)$_2$Rh$_2${C(CF$_3$)=C(CF$_3$)H}]$_2$(C$_6$H$_4$). *Polyhedron* **1988**, *7*, 859–870. [CrossRef]
36. Oro, L.A.; Valderrama, M.; Cifuentes, P.; Foces-Foces, C.; Cano, F.H. Azulene as a Ligand in Cationic Rhodium and Iridium Complexes. Crystal Structure of [Rh(TFB)(az)]PF$_6$. *J. Organomet. Chem.* **1984**, *276*, 67–77. [CrossRef]
37. Kunkely, H.; Vogler, A. Ligand-to-Ligand Charge Transfer in [(η-C_5Me_5)Rh^{III}(η-C_7H_7)]$^{3+}$: Absorption and Emission. *Inorg. Chem. Commun.* **2004**, *7*, 650–653. [CrossRef]
38. Perdew, J.P.; Burke, K.; Ernzerhof, M. Generalized Gradient Approximation Made Simple. *Phys. Rev. Lett.* **1996**, *77*, 3865, Erratum in **1997**, *78*, 1396–1396. [CrossRef]
39. Krishnan, R.; Binkley, J.S.; Seeger, R.; Pople, J.A. Self-Consistent Molecular Orbital Methods. XX. A Basis Set for Correlated Wave Functions. *J. Chem. Phys.* **1980**, *72*, 650–654. [CrossRef]
40. von Schleyer, P.R.; Maerker, C.; Dransfeld, A.; Jiao, H.; van Eikema Hommes, N.J.R. Nucleus-Independent Chemical Shifts: A Simple and Efficient Aromaticity Probe. *J. Am. Chem. Soc.* **1996**, *118*, 6317–6318. [CrossRef]
41. Chen, Z.; Wannere, C.S.; Corminboeuf, C.; Puchta, R.; von Schleyer, P.R. Nucleus-Independent Chemical Shifts (NICS) as an Aromaticity Criterion. *Chem. Rev.* **2005**, *105*, 3842–3888. [CrossRef] [PubMed]
42. Lichtenberg, C.; Prokopchuk, D.E.; Adelhardt, M.; Viciu, L.; Meyer, K.; Grützmacher, H. Reactivity of an All-Ferrous Iron–Nitrogen Heterocubane under Reductive and Oxidative Conditions. *Chem. Eur. J.* **2015**, *21*, 15797–15805. [CrossRef] [PubMed]
43. Zhong, H.M.; Rawal, V.H. 1,3-Pentadiene. In *Encyclopedia of Reagents for Organic Synthesis*; John Wiley & Sons, Ltd.: New York, NY, USA, 2001.
44. Ernst, R.D. Structural and Reactivity Patterns in Transition-Metal-Pentadienyl Chemistry. *Chem. Rev.* **1988**, *88*, 1255–1291. [CrossRef]
45. Cordoneanu, A.; Drewitt, M.J.; Bavarian, N.; Baird, M.C. Synthesis and Characterization of Weakly Coordinating Anion Salts of a New, Stable Carbocationic Reagent, the Dibenzosuberenyl (Dibenzotropylium) ion. *New J. Chem.* **2008**, *32*, 1890–1898. [CrossRef]
46. Wu, J.I.C.; Mo, Y.; Evangelista, F.A.; von Ragué Schleyer, P. Is Cyclobutadiene really highly Destabilized by Antiaromaticity? *Chem. Commun.* **2012**, *48*, 8437–8439. [CrossRef]
47. Bahl, J.J.; Bates, R.B.; Beavers, W.A.; Launer, C.R. Cycloheptatrienyl and Heptatrienyl Trianions. *J. Am. Chem. Soc.* **1977**, *99*, 6126–6127. [CrossRef]

48. Connelly, N.G.; Geiger, W.E. Chemical Redox Agents for Organometallic Chemistry. *Chem. Rev.* **1996**, *96*, 877–910. [CrossRef]
49. Salcedo, R.; Sansores, L.E.; Fomina, L. Theoretical Study about the Radicals and Anions of [8]annulenes. *J. Mol. Struct.* **1997**, *397*, 159–166. [CrossRef]
50. Viculis, L.M.; Mack, J.J.; Mayer, O.M.; Hahn, H.T.; Kaner, R.B. Intercalation and Exfoliation Routes to Graphite Nanoplatelets. *J. Mater. Chem.* **2005**, *15*, 974–978. [CrossRef]
51. Giordano, G.; Crabtree, R.H.; Heintz, R.M.; Forster, D.; Morris, D.E. Di-µ-Chloro-Bis(η^4-1,5-Cyclooctadiene)-Dirhodium(I). In *Inorganic Syntheses*; Angelici, R.J., Ed.; John Wiley & Sons, Ltd.: New York NY, USA, 2007.
52. IUPAC. Section A -Hydrocarbons. In *Nomenclature of Organic Chemistry*; Pergamon Press: Oxford, UK, 1979.
53. Dolomanov, O.V.; Bourhis, L.J.; Gildea, R.J.; Howard, J.A.K.; Puschmann, H. OLEX2: A Complete Structure Solution, Refinement and Analysis Program. *J. Appl. Crystallogr.* **2009**, *42*, 339–341. [CrossRef]
54. Sheldrick, G. A Short History of SHELX. *Acta Cryst. A* **2008**, *64*, 112–122. [CrossRef] [PubMed]
55. Sheldrick, G. SHELXT-Integrated Space-Group and Crystal-Structure Determination. *Acta Cryst. A* **2015**, *71*, 3–8. [CrossRef] [PubMed]

Sample Availability: Samples of the compounds **tropCl**, **1a**, **1b**, and **dbcot** are available from the authors.

Publisher's Note: MDPI stays neutral with regard to jurisdictional claims in published maps and institutional affiliations.

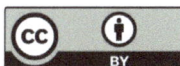

© 2020 by the authors. Licensee MDPI, Basel, Switzerland. This article is an open access article distributed under the terms and conditions of the Creative Commons Attribution (CC BY) license (http://creativecommons.org/licenses/by/4.0/).

MDPI
St. Alban-Anlage 66
4052 Basel
Switzerland
Tel. +41 61 683 77 34
Fax +41 61 302 89 18
www.mdpi.com

Molecules Editorial Office
E-mail: molecules@mdpi.com
www.mdpi.com/journal/molecules

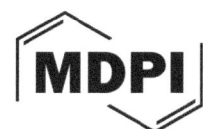

www.ingramcontent.com/pod-product-compliance
Lightning Source LLC
LaVergne TN
LVHW072319090526
838202LV00019B/2314